Neurocultural Health and Wellbeing

Aim of this devoted book Series in neurology is to highlight the relationship between neuroscience and culture. Nowadays, there is more evidence of how our brain is influenced by the various artistic and cultural disciplines, both in the form of entertainment as well as – and above all – through the emotions and gratification which lead to wellbeing. The emotional mechanisms, the different cultural manifestations provided, are due to the activation of a perceptual and cognitive range that constitute the basis of the social behaviors. All this makes us aware of the benefits the arts have on personal and collective health.

This concept was already known to philosophers in ancient times, who were convinced that inner balance was influenced by culture and in particular by music.

During the centuries, men understood that the *cultivation of the spirit*, or *humanitas*, had a certain role on behavior and from the beginning of modern experimental science, in the fifteenth, the spread of the notions of neuroanatomy allowed artists to get closer to the knowledge of the brain's mechanisms and reveal the emotional and empathic responses at the basis of creativity, and indeed of their own psychophysical wellbeing. A dialogue between the science of the mind and artistic disciplines was born. The results of this meeting made it possible to better define which mental processes are involved when we come into contact with the various humanistic disciplines, and how they can be applied, for instance, to the treatment of mental disorders and neuropsychiatric diseases.

The goal of this Series is both to prove the role of biological brain mechanisms and the influence of various artistic forms on clinical practice, especially in neuro-psychiatric disorders, as well as to trace different therapeutic and psycho-physical well-being applications based on scientific evidence from medical literature.

Volumes of the Series will be edited by experts under the supervision of an international editorial committee. Each book, focused on a specific discipline, will provide knowledge on relationship between the brain activity and different forms of language, communication, art. This close inter-relationship with specific focus on different forms of art will explain the effectiveness of this kind of approaches in neuro-psychiatric diseases.

This Series will allow to understand how the culture is one of the fundamental tools to improve general well-being, quality of life and motivation in neurological diseases.

This Series also find a correlation with SDG3 goal "ensuring healthy lives and promoting wellbeing for all at all ages" for the progress of the health and wellbeing considering that neurological diseases are on the rise worldwide including in the developing countries.

Alfredo Raglio
Editor

Music and Music Therapy Interventions in Clinical Practice

A Textbook for Music Therapy Professionals, Clinicians and Researchers

Springer

Editor
Alfredo Raglio
Music Therapy Research Laboratory
Istituti Clinici Scientifici Maugeri IRCCS
Pavia, Italy

ISSN 2731-4464 ISSN 2731-4472 (electronic)
Neurocultural Health and Wellbeing
ISBN 978-3-031-88577-8 ISBN 978-3-031-88578-5 (eBook)
https://doi.org/10.1007/978-3-031-88578-5

This Springer imprint is published by the registered company Springer Nature Switzerland AG
The registered company address is: Gewerbestrasse 11, 6330 Cham, Switzerland

Preface

This textbook was primarily conceived to establish an international reference point for individuals who are pursuing or plan to pursue an academic training in the field of music therapy.

After many years of clinical and research experience, I felt the desire to delineate the current state of the art in the discipline, using Evidence-Based Music Therapy as a guiding framework. This approach, which has shaped my professional experience, serves as the foundation for this work.

The volume begins with a redefined perspective on music therapy, introducing the main and most established music therapy approaches, both active and receptive, as well as more recent and innovative approaches.

Innovation itself is a core theme of this manual, with a focus on how technology and novel advancements could open new scenarios and expand the therapeutic potential of music. This innovative perspective remains rigorously grounded, with a primary goal: to make therapeutic interventions with music more effective and accessible.

Additionally, the textbook aims to raise awareness and encourage clinicians and institutions to adopt music as a valuable resource in prevention, therapy, and rehabilitation, adhering to the scientific rigor and ethical principles that all forms of care demand.

The structure of the textbook is organized as follows. The initial chapters (Chaps. 2, 3, and 4) establish the scientific foundations of the discipline. Subsequent chapters (Chaps. 5, 6, 7, 8, 9, and 10) detail main active and receptive approaches, followed by a chapter (Chap. 11) dedicated to outlining the framework of a music therapy intervention. The next section (Chaps. 12, 13, 14, 15, 16, 17, and 18) presents the most significant literature and evidence on the key areas of application. The concluding section focuses on research (Chaps. 19 and 20), offering a general overview (Chapter 18) and an innovative perspective on process analysis using objective tools such as neuroimaging techniques and motion detection systems (Chap. 20).

One of the goals of this work is to strengthen the dialogue between music and science, as well as between music and medicine. These relationships are reaching nowadays a significant turning point, driven by different aspects: on the one hand, the remarkable growth in music therapy research; on the other hand, the increasing need to develop nonpharmacological therapies grounded in a holistic evidence-based approach.

I would like to express my deep gratitude to the individual contributors who made this manual possible—colleagues and, in many cases, friends with whom I have shared part of my professional journey. Their expertise and willingness have been fundamental in the publication of this work.

I hope that the contents presented here will serve as an inspiration for music therapy professionals, clinicians, researchers, and anyone interested in approaching this field from a scientific perspective.

Pavia, Italy Alfredo Raglio

Contents

1 Introduction: What Can We Consider Music Therapy?

Alfredo Raglio

If we were to give a shared definition of music therapy even today, many years after this discipline sought its space among therapeutic rehabilitation interventions, we would encounter some difficulties. The term "music therapy" is indeed particularly complex because it includes the term "music" associated with the term "therapy." Already these words, individually, are challenging to define.

The international music therapy community has attempted to provide various definitions in highly inclusive ways, aiming to encompass a large portion of experiences related to the use of music in a clinical context (Fig. 1.1). The risk of many of these definitions is to consider any intervention involving music in a pathological context as therapeutic. The more inclusive the definitions are, the greater this risk becomes.

On the other hand, this aspect reflects a condition where music therapy remains rather heterogeneous and only partially codified as therapy. This heterogeneity involves training, content, and the recognition of the discipline, which vary significantly, even from a geographical perspective.

In any therapeutic context, the presence of reference models contributes to defining boundaries and formalizing the purposes and contents of different approaches, respecting often disparate perspectives. It is not about creating fractures or emphasizing differences but rather bringing clarity and awareness to a complex field. The process of defining a therapeutic discipline often takes decades and, above all, is in continuous evolution.

In the field of music therapy, the idea of approaches based on theoretical reference models materialized during the IX World Congress of Music Therapy in Washington (1999). There was an early attempt in this direction through the

A. Raglio (✉)
Music Therapy Research Laboratory, Istituti Clinici Scientifici Maugeri IRCCS, Pavia, Italy
e-mail: alfredo.raglio@icsmaugeri.it

A. Raglio (ed.), *Music and Music Therapy Interventions in Clinical Practice*, Neurocultural Health and Wellbeing,
https://doi.org/10.1007/978-3-031-88578-5_1

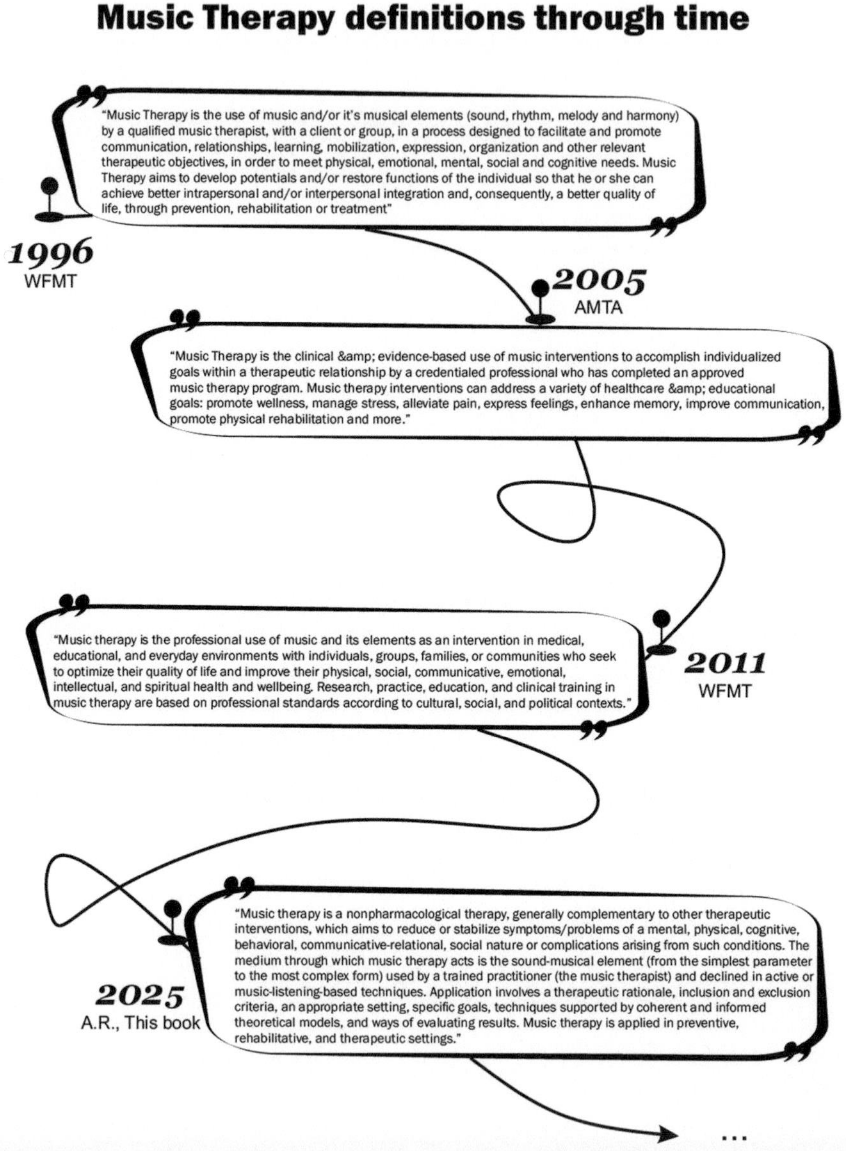

Fig. 1.1 From the 1996 World Federation of Music Therapy definition of music therapy to a possible current definition

definition of five models considered consolidated and widely spread: Nordoff-Robbins Music Therapy (Nordoff and Robbins 1977), Analytical Music Therapy (Priestley 1994), Guided Imagery and Music (Bonny 2002), Benenzon Music Therapy (Benenzon 1981), and Behavioral Music Therapy (Madsen et al. 1968).

The Neurologic Music Therapy (Thaut and Volker 2025) was later added to these models, as well as other forms of music therapy application, such as the psychodynamic approach in music therapy (De Backer and Sutton 2014), remaining strictly relational, or, for example, Community Music Therapy (Pavlicevic and Ansdell 2004) and Songwriting (Baker et al. 2008, 2009) if moving toward less traditional approaches.

In general, the central point of these approaches is that it is not always easy to convey applications that are consistent with these models and have produced verifiable results to theoretical reference models.

Among the more established models, we can certainly mention Nordoff-Robbins Music Therapy, Guided Imagery of Music, and later, Neurologic Music Therapy.

Once again, the risk is to confuse certain terms, for example, the "model" (the set of theories, applicable modes, and generalizable verification methods) with the "technique" (the practice through which a model is applied).

Furthermore, the solidity of a therapeutic intervention model, whatever it may be, is also based on concrete results attributable to the model itself and produced by scientifically credible studies. In this case, especially concerning some models, the literature highlights significant gaps.

Identifying approaches in which the theoretical perspective is clear and the subsequent practice is consistent is rather rare for music therapy. It is particularly difficult to define a specificity of the sonorous-music element in therapeutic action that gives music therapy a defining value. It is more common to adapt psychological or neuroscientific theories to the use of music. However, in this case, the model of therapeutic intervention appears less related to the musical mediator, that is, the proposed musical content.

After the 1999 World Congress in Washington, no other formal moments of in-depth exploration or reflection concerning possible music therapy approaches have followed. Frequently, the applied "models" have manifested as techniques implemented freely by professionals or researchers, with the inevitable risk of bypassing any reflection on the theoretical foundations of music therapy, often reducing the discipline to pragmatic approaches that are challenging to replicate.

In other cases, theoretical reflection has led to the use of terms describing psychological or neuroscientific approaches without any correspondence or coherence with the specific context of music therapy. The concept of possible music therapy models thus remains an ongoing part, especially when considering the "model" as a set of elements that consistently include a theoretical, applied, and verification component (Raglio and Oasi 2015).

Robb's invitation (Robb et al. 2011) for a precise definition of music therapy interventions is undoubtedly an important stimulus in this regard. Until the early 2000s, the vague definition of music therapy experiences led to considering any music-related intervention in care contexts as "music therapy."

Especially in the initial phases, the international music therapy community associated a relational component, essential for conferring therapeutic qualities on the intervention (Gold et al. 2009). Any form of music intervention disconnected from a relational process was considered distinct from music therapy, defining interventions lacking this component as "music medicine," an approach not contextualized within the scope of music therapy.

Certainly, the training of the music therapist influences the type of intervention, and the prevalence of the relational aspect has oriented many interventions in this direction. What this chapter (and more generally, this manual) aims to highlight is the possibility of attributing an intrinsically therapeutic value to the musical component of the intervention if appropriately oriented.

The therapeutic value of an intervention, in fact, stems from a series of factors not necessarily attributable to the relational component: (a) a specific training of the music therapist, (b) a therapeutic rationale from which specific techniques based on theoretical models supporting the intervention derive, (c) the presence of specific therapeutic-rehabilitative objectives, (d) an appropriate setting, and (e) the assessment of the intervention (Raglio and Oasi 2015).

In detail: (a) The training of a music therapist should encompass a set of knowledge and skills oriented specifically to the application domain but, in a general sense, should involve musical, psychological, clinical-rehabilitative, and, of course, music therapy-related aspects. What the music therapist should acquire is a design and application ability that responds appropriately to the needs of the patient/client using specific techniques. Ideally, a basic music therapy training should be conceived, in addition to tailored competencies in different application contexts. From this perspective, there is still considerable heterogeneity in academic training experiences that, depending on the realities, focus on "MUSIC therapy" interventions rather than "music THERAPY" interventions. Emphasis can be placed on the musical component or the therapeutic component. A similar distinction is reflected in the concept of "music as therapy" (emphasis on the therapeutic component inherent in the musical element) or the concept of "music in therapy" (emphasis on the therapeutic process in which music serves as a mediator in the healing process). These concepts were originally introduced by Kenneth Bruscia (Bruscia 2014). Probably, overcoming these positions is achieved through the integration of the concept of music and therapy into a logic where the approach becomes "MUSIC THERAPY," in a dimension where therapy and music merge and assume equal value; (b) it is of fundamental importance to define the therapeutic rationale of the intervention: every therapy requires theoretical and applicative assumptions that make the intervention plausible and appropriate. Once again, the term that defines this necessity is the word "therapy," which has scientific but also ethical implications. This emphasizes the difference between a musical intervention and a music therapy intervention. A patient/client must be aware of the peculiarities of the intervention and what the therapeutic project implies, which must be necessarily embraced and shared; (c) the concept of therapy implies the possibility of identifying specific therapeutic objectives, outlining intervention strategies aimed at their achievement. These objectives, in therapeutic logic, should ideally be achieved, at least in part, and maintained over time, ideally producing a relatively stable change; (d) the therapeutic process requires a setting, i.e., flexible conditions that make its implementation possible: a space, a time, a set of means, and rules that facilitate the implementation of therapy; (e) equally important is the assessment of results, through appropriate qualitative and quantitative tools that may vary depending on the context. A result, therefore, to be considered as such, must be tangible and not only subjectively perceived. The extent of the result must also be related to the severity of the problem addressed. It follows that in cases of complex or degenerative pathologies, the results may be of small magnitude and not necessarily enduring.

The presence of these points can therefore be helpful in determining which interventions with music potentially take on therapeutic value: the absence of one or more of these elements reduces the therapeutic scope of the intervention and places it, more likely, among the proposals that may provide indirect benefits even in the absence of a specific therapeutic intentionality.

I believe that reference to the aspects that define the intervention as therapeutic may result in overcoming the possible gap between the musical and therapeutic components.

It is a matter of drawing attention to how, in every area of application, a rationale can be found that emphasizes and declines the musical component in a curative logic.

The relational component, emphasized by the international music therapy community as a foundational element of the discipline, has defined music therapy models based on content derived from psychology. Importantly, the development of such models has not taken into account, except partially, the prevalent use in music therapy practice of the sonorous-music element and nonverbal communication. Psychological models, often used in verbal therapies, have simply been translated into music therapy.

On the contrary, I believe it is essential to trace music therapy back to therapeutic principles inherent in the nonverbal/sonorous-music mediator as the defining element of music therapy interventions. This helps to increase the therapeutic specificity of sound and to define music therapy as an intervention in which the sonorous-music element assumes a definite and fundamental role.

Many music therapy interventions or therapeutic effects of music are documented on the basis that they are mediated by the relationship between patient/client and music therapist (think of active or receptive approaches), or by music-induced pleasure (in music listening experiences) with consequent neurochemical repercussions. But, in these cases, a question arises: does the therapeutic effect come from the relationship or pleasure experienced, or from a specific role that music takes in the therapeutic approach?

In other words, do relationship-based interventions (e.g., psycho-educational approaches) or reward system-based interventions (e.g., doing something that produces pleasure) produce the same effect as music therapy? What is specific about the intervention based on the use of the sonorous-music element?

From this point of view, the effort should be aimed at identifying therapeutic models that use the sonorous-music element, at various levels, based on a psychophysiological rationale that gives scientific credibility and application rigor to the interventions.

Hence the need for congruence between theoretical references and the application part and the implementation of approaches supported by evidence-based practice.

The basic questions of tracing them back to this point of view are:

1. What population?
2. What goals?
3. What approach to music?
4. What therapeutic rationale?
5. What evidence?
6. What assessment tools?

The more a music therapist is able to relate adequately and answer these questions, the more we are in the presence of an intervention that can contextualize itself in the therapeutic field, regardless of whether it is based on the relational component or on other assumptions. From these considerations, a definition of music therapy can be derived that includes the therapeutic elements that are indispensable for the intervention to be therapeutically connoted:

Music therapy is a nonpharmacological therapy, generally complementary to other therapeutic interventions, which aims to reduce or stabilize symptoms/problems of a mental, physical, cognitive, behavioral, communicative-relational, social nature or complications arising from such conditions. The medium through which music therapy acts is the sound-musical element (from the simplest parameter to the most complex form) used by a trained practitioner (the music therapist) and declined in active or music-listening-based techniques. Application involves a therapeutic rationale, inclusion and exclusion criteria, an appropriate setting, specific goals, techniques supported by coherent and informed theoretical models, and ways of evaluating results. Music therapy is applied in preventive, rehabilitative, and therapeutic settings.

In this definition we find characterizing elements that try to contextualize therapeutic intervention with music by distinguishing it from generic musical interventions. People often confuse the positive effect of music that is generally produced by, for example, singing in a choir or making and listening to music together, with the specificity that the use of the voice or certain active and receptive techniques takes on in certain psychopathological conditions. In these cases, the voice, instrument, or listening are not used simply for singing, playing, or listening to music but are declined into specific techniques, motivated by a therapeutic rationale and specific goals that will be the subject of careful evaluations. This makes music potentially effective, thus something not exclusively aesthetic and pleasurable. The pleasure given by making or listening to music can certainly constitute a "plus" but not the "core" of music therapy. This is equivalent to saying that, for example, a patient suffering from a form of chronic pain will benefit from music (performed or listened to) not only in relation to the pleasure felt during the musical experience, but, more importantly, in relation to the fact that the action of a specific use of music may counteract the perception of pain and the level of stress produced by it. If this is done based on conscious and replicable choices implemented by the music therapist, we will be able to attribute therapeutic value to the intervention.

It is evident how this thinking takes the focus to a level of greater depth and defines what the training standard of the music therapist should be and what the specificity of his or her training should be. The shift is from an empirical-applicational to a scientific level. I believe that the future of music therapy, if this is the direction, involves a high level of specialization and the need to create guidelines for the different clinical settings to which music therapy can be directed.

While supporting the general idea of the value and positive action of music on human beings at all levels and stages of life, music therapy should be characterized as a discipline that studies why and how this happens. The music therapist should be able to hypothesize and shape a specific therapeutic project, distinguishing his or her intervention from a generic music intervention.

A topic of relevance is also the role that new technologies will play in defining new applications of music therapy. Some experiences of music therapy at a distance, thus technology-mediated, have already been activated in the pandemic period and have been maintained thereafter (Clements-Cortés et al. 2023; Cephas et al. 2022). These experiences documented the possibility of introducing new ways of intervention that might have seemed distant or impractical before this shocking event. The concept of settings and the content of interventions can thus be considered flexible and adaptable to therapeutic needs. This has been demonstrated by the extreme need to do so by opening new, even unexpected, therapeutic perspectives. In my opinion, it is not a matter of comparing traditional interventions with new application perspectives, but rather of implementing the best possible strategy to effectively achieve our goals.

Some examples.

Therapeutic Music Listening is a new receptive technique (Raglio 2023) (see also the Chapter devoted to it in this volume). This approach ensures that it can also be used at a distance, for example, through Telemedicine (Raglio 2020).

This setting, of course, on the one hand modifies the relational impact given by direct contact but, on the other hand, allows its implementation in any context and condition, with the possible presence of a web connection and a formal or informal caregiver.

It is therefore a matter of rethinking therapeutic interventions with music from a new perspective by introducing technological support wherever possible.

Another example of technological support again related to music listening is the use of algorithms for composing music thought for therapeutic purposes (Raglio and Vico 2017).

This, too, may seem completely unrelated to a music therapy intervention if we limit ourselves to considering the relational component and conventional musical material. However, the possibility of creating pieces that follow ad hoc compositional criteria to produce therapeutic effects helps us to think about musical material and its effectiveness regardless of the relational implications.

A piece of music conceived for therapeutic purposes through the aid of an algorithm can be modeled and varied, allowing us to relate its parameters and structural characteristics to its potential effects. The result given by using algorithmic music is directly related to the musical component by-passing the effects of the relationship and the cultural factor associated with conventional music listening. This makes easier to try to answer the following question: can music itself, based on specific characteristics, pursue targeted therapeutic goals?

It will be research that will give an answer to this challenging question, but some ongoing and partially completed studies have shown how algorithmic music can produce effects very similar to those of conventional music proposed for the same purposes (Raglio et al. 2021a).

The use of other technologies, e.g., Machine Learning techniques or Artificial Neural Networks (Raglio et al. 2020, 2021b, 2023b), will help us understand which populations are better suited for algorithmic music listening than for conventional music listening. This means, then, that with appropriate tools we can now be able to identify target populations in relation to specific music-therapeutic techniques. This echoes the idea that, as in any therapy, not all interventions can be equally effective in a specific therapeutic-rehabilitation context.

A final example of how the concept of music-based therapy can find various declinations is the use of "sonification" techniques in neurorehabilitation settings (Raglio et al. 2021c, 2023c).

Such techniques allow the sonorous representation of an event/behavior. In rehabilitation, these techniques can be used with the mediation of sensors that map the movements involved in rehabilitation training and associate them with musical patterns, defining a progression of sounds. This progression constitutes important audio-motor feedback for the patient. If the movements are performed correctly, the patient will perceive a regular and natural pattern of sound-music production. Conversely, if the movements are irregular, the sound-music production heard will also reflect that irregularity. This allows the patient to modulate/regulate and plan movements. Also, this approach can improve proprioception as well as potentially reduce the perception of fatigue and pain during rehabilitation.

The above examples are intended to draw attention to different ways of using sound and music in therapeutic-rehabilitation settings and, consequently, to what can be defined as music therapy, but also to the role of the music therapist in these new contexts.

These new interventions, if we consider the definition of music therapy given in this chapter, can be included within the scope of activities aimed at therapeutic-rehabilitative purposes.

This is possible because we are in the presence of approaches that have solid theoretical foundations, application protocols associated with specific techniques, and produce potential clinically verifiable outcomes. What changes in these interventions is the type of relationship that is developed between therapist and patient, the type of techniques and the consequent role of the music therapist who is sometimes involved in the preparatory and supervisory aspects of the interventions (as in the case of "sonification" and algorithmic music) and, beyond that, in a relationship with the patient/client that precedes and follows the sessions (as in the case of Therapeutic Music Listening).

The music therapist's role and skills remain irreplaceable and given by specific training that brings together clinical, psychological, musical, technological, and, of course, music therapy knowledge and skills.

It is evident how music therapy practice should go hand in hand with research to define, as anticipated, guidelines of the discipline concerning different areas of application.

Greater uniformity and standardization do not necessarily mean limiting and binding clinical practice to common rules, but rather normalizing it, making it more appropriate and effective.

This implies a process to focus on music therapy vocabulary (often heterogeneous and inconsistent), application protocols (often absent), and basic and advanced academic and professional training based on shared standards.

Scientific evidence should guide and support this process.

From what has emerged, it is therefore possible to consider a series of approaches characterized by a greater or lesser therapeutic-rehabilitative connotation. This connotation is attributable not so much to the relational factor but, rather, to the presence of all those aspects mentioned above and synthesized in Fig. 1.2: theoretical reference models that make the therapeutic rationale clear, specific intervention techniques used in a defined setting, specific therapeutic objectives defined (generally in a team context) by an appropriately trained professional, and the possibility of verifying the results.

These indicators allow for orientation in identifying music interventions in a clinical context as music therapeutic interventions. This effectively leads to overcoming and significantly expanding the spectrum of potentially therapeutic

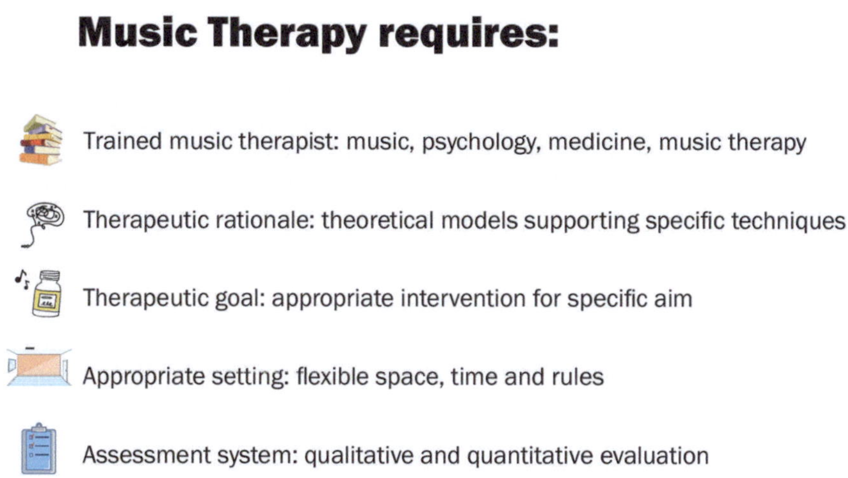

Fig. 1.2 Main therapeutic factors characterizing music therapy approaches

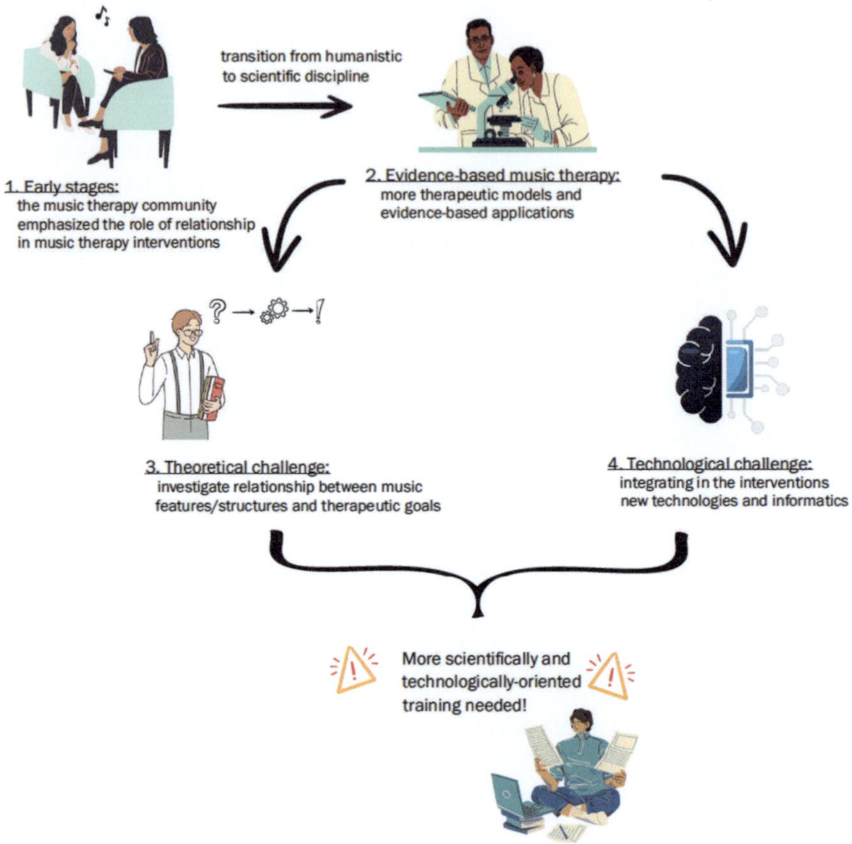

Fig. 1.3 Key points of the chapter

interventions by introducing a continuum on which we can place interventions based on the presence or absence of the mentioned factors.

The rigor in the classification of interventions is consistent with the fact that, as in any therapy, not all approaches used in clinical settings can be considered therapeutic. In the field of music therapy, this refers to the idea that only specific interventions can produce specific results but also underscores that the generic use of music does not have intrinsic therapeutic value.

Research can provide answers regarding the real effectiveness of each intervention in order to determine therapeutic appropriateness and the relevant applicative guidelines (Fig. 1.3).

References

Baker F, Wigram T, Stott D, et al. Therapeutic songwriting in music therapy. Part I: Who are the therapists, who are the clients, and why is songwriting used? Nord J Music Ther. 2008;17(2):105–23.

Baker F, Wigram T, Stott D, et al. Therapeutic songwriting in music therapy. Part II: Comparing the literature with practice across diverse clinical populations. Nord J Music Ther. 2009;18(1):32–56.

Benenzon RO. Music therapy manual. Springfield: Charles C Thomas Pub Ltd; 1981.

Bonny HL. Music & consciousness: the evolution of guided imagery and music. Gilsum: Barcelona Publishers; 2002.

Bruscia KE. Defining music therapy. 3rd ed. Barcelona Publishers; 2014.

Cephas AS, Sofield S, Millstein A. Embracing technological possibilities in the telehealth delivery of interactive music therapy. Nord J Music Ther. 2022;31(3):214–27.

Clements-Cortés A, Pranjić M, Knott D, et al. International music therapists' perceptions and experiences in telehealth music therapy provision. Int J Environ Res Public Health. 2023;20(8):5580.

De Backer J, Sutton J. The music in music therapy. Psychodynamic music therapy in Europe: clinical, theoretical and research approaches. London: Jessica Kingsley Publishers; 2014.

Gold C, Solli HP, Krüger V, Lie SA. Dose-response relationship in music therapy for people with serious mental disorders: systematic review and meta-analysis. Clin Psychol Rev. 2009;29(3):193–207.

Madsen CK, Cotter V, Madsen CH. A behavioural approach to music therapy. J Mus Ther. 1968;5:15–23.

Nordoff P, Robbins C. Creative music therapy. New York: John Day; 1977.

Pavlicevic M, Ansdell G. Community music therapy. London: Jessica Kingsley Publishers; 2004.

Priestley M. Essays on analytical music therapy. Gilsum: Barcelona Publishers; 1994.

Raglio A. Therapeutic music listening as telehealth intervention. Complement Ther Clin Pract. 2020;41:101245.

Raglio A. A novel music-based therapeutic approach: the therapeutic music listening. Front Hum Neurosci. 2023;17:1204593.

Raglio A, Oasi O. Music and health: what interventions for what results? Front Psychol. 2015;6:230.

Raglio A, Vico F. Music and technology: the curative algorithm. Front Psychol. 2017;8:2055.

Raglio A, Imbriani M, Imbriani C, et al. Machine learning techniques to predict the effectiveness of music therapy: a randomized controlled trial. Comput MethodsPrograms Biomed. 2020;185:105160.

Raglio A, Baiardi P, Vizzari G, et al. Algorithmic music for therapy: effectiveness and perspectives. Appl Sci. 2021a;11:8833.

Raglio A, Bellandi D, Manzoni L, et al. Communication improvement reduces BPSD: a music therapy study based on artificial neural networks. Neurol Sci. 2021b;42(5):2103–6.

Raglio A, Panigazzi M, Colombo R, et al. Hand rehabilitation with sonification techniques in the subacute stage of stroke. Sci Rep. 2021c;11(1):7237.

Raglio A, Grossi E, Manzoni L. Artificial neural networks for a semantic map of variables in a music listening-based study. Appl Sci. 2023b;13(21):11811.

Raglio A, De Maria B, Parati M, et al. Movement sonification techniques to improve balance in Parkinson's disease: a pilot randomized controlled trial. Brain Sci. 2023c;13(11):1586.

Robb SL, Burns DS, Carpenter JS. Reporting guidelines for music-based interventions. J Health Psychol. 2011;16(2):342–52.

Thaut M, Volker H. Handbook of neurologic music therapy (Second Edition). Oxford: Oxford University Press; 2025.

Part I

Psychological, Neuroscientific, and Biological Bases of Therapeutic Use of Music

The Contribution of Music Psychology to Music Therapy

2

Gianni Nuti

Key Points

- Music that transforms and moves from the body's biochemical and psychomotor reactions.
- Promoting flow experiences to foster forms of psychic integration.
- Thinking of music as a symbolic representation of vital and dynamic phenomena evolving in time and space.

2.1 Foreword

Every musical phenomenon—always complex, even when it is developed in the form of a dry monody or in a sequence of percussion instruments with a fixed pitch—is the synthetic manifestation of a living organism, which hides its expressiveness in a global complex of features and movements, styles and moods: in short, it is the polyphony of a unique and indivisible essence, which loses its meaning if it is dissected into individual strings, separated from the context. This approach prevents one from analysing the psychological effects of a melody stripped of the harmonic framework in which it is embedded, of a rhythmic model outside the antecedent and consequent temporal segmentations.

It has taken us several decades to free psychological studies applied to music from that basic misunderstanding that saw subjects exposed to completely unstructured sound stimulations—rhythmic patterns, melodic fragments, harmonic cadences, timbral mixtures, dynamic or agogic conductance—that were perhaps

G. Nuti (✉)
Aosta Valley University, Aosta, AO, Italy
e-mail: g.nuti@univda.it

A. Raglio (ed.), *Music and Music Therapy Interventions in Clinical Practice*, Neurocultural Health and Wellbeing,
https://doi.org/10.1007/978-3-031-88578-5_2

strongly connoted, but completely incomparable with the real object of investigation, i.e. a musical phenomenon that implies complexity, narrativity and expressive intentionality. The shattering of musical syntax into simple elements conceals the *raison d'être* of music itself. Admittedly, a psychological reading of the mechanisms implemented by a performer, a composer, a musician practicing improvisation allows one to refine learning strategies, prevent performance stress factors, non-functional muscular tensions, manage psychomotor commitment for ever greater time arcs with precision and efficiency, but it remains a self-referential study, oriented to refine the weapons of the discipline but not to recover its meaning.

Fortunately, in addition to this, psychology today:

- Studies the profound reasons why music—in the sense just defined—represents a primary need for human beings, helping to build their balance in whatever anthropic and natural context they are called upon to adapt.
- Analyses the reactions it provokes in living bodies in terms of transformations.
  - Psychophysiological and functional.
  - Behaviour and relational dynamics.
  - In the imaginative dimension that every mind nurtures, continually modifying lived reality, sometimes creating others, by abstraction.
- It provides, to those who use this vehicle of intersubjective relations for therapeutic and rehabilitative purposes, the keys to selecting the best possible strategies to increase the level of well-being of the individual and of entire social groups.

This contribution aims precisely to offer a more circumstantial interpretative slant with respect to the great quantity of scientific studies that have dealt with music in recent years, limiting itself to emphasising the transformative and evolutionary value that this practice represents for the individual and for the whole of humanity in its temporal dimension, offering it some opportunity to heal its wounds, to attenuate its fragilities. It is precisely of Time that we speak, since Bernstein (1954) spoke of music as a combination of mathematics and magic, of the organisation and qualification of temporal experience—"(…) Music exists in time, and it is time that must be cut, modelled and reshaped until, like a statue, it becomes a living form…"[1]—and at the same time an open gateway to an ineffable, immeasurable, in fact, metatemporal phenomenon. In the interaction between consciousness and this perception of the flowing of events that appear and disappear, undergo metamorphoses, contract and expand, unite or shatter, compact or fray, personal well-being and the relationship with people and nature around is at stake, but it also substantiates the sense of making and listening to music. We will therefore try to talk about the direct and indirect benefits fostered by listening to and making music, particularly for those with motor, cognitive, psychological, psychiatric, but also existential and social frailties, i.e. in their relationship with their neighbours and with their context of life.

We will do this starting from an assumption and a provocation.

[1] L. Bernstein, La gioia della Musica, Milano, Longanesi, 1982 p. 9 (trad. it Raffaele Mammalella, prima ed. statunitense, The Joy of Music 1954).

The assumption is that, if music is a human artifice born out of profound needs for communication and expression, it can only assume therapeutic functions to the extent that it affects the quality and complexity of the interaction between the person, his or her inner life and the world. Only if musical language does not exhaust its sense in itself, is not the object of constant and intensive dedication as opaque to its profound meanings, but is a vehicle for human promotion, does it acquire its meaning. Music is an elective instrument, the privileged theatre in which to meet the other: only if one understands that it is the relationship between people, between people and nature that generates emotional states, profiles of affectivity, the most authentic cognitions about one's own living and that of the Universe in motion can music be given its most appropriate role. This is why it must be conceived not as the voice of an exuberant ego, but as part of a polyphony that, thanks to imagination, knows how to construct an intermediate space derived from several vital presences stretched towards the desire to build a memorable event because it is shared, which does not water down the personal style of each individual but enhances it, thanks to the intertwined coexistence of different styles engaged to build a polychrome and unitary one. Communicating—a theme that is so emergent in this era—is therefore not exchanging messages by assuming now the role of transmitter, now that of receiver, but is tantamount to creating a 'third' phenomenon as the result of two or more people 'stepping out of themselves' to create a third essence, the result of a union, provisional and constantly evolving, a temporal structure, such as that evoked by Bernstein, symbolically analogous to a living form. We do not speak of 'states', therefore of immobile entities like still frames, nor of simple action-reaction dynamics between stimulus and individual response, but of *flows*, energies and phenomenal evolutions that symbolically represent restless motions towards encounter, recognition, symbiosis between living bodies forced by centripetal forces to separation, fragmentation, isolation. Every form of pathology, existential malaise, every experience of pain is connected with a limitation of one's field of action and sensitive experience, it is a denial of the desire for encounter and unity and an impediment to expression. This is where expressivity is understood as that permanent tension of the human being towards its emergence, unveiling, a sort of self-revelation or, as Hillman would say, the concretisation of one's own *daimon*: it is certainly made up of an articulated and multiform destiny, partly the result of destinations predefined by a genetic heritage, for another part more relevant by the road one has taken and has decided to travel, with all the changing landscape around it.

Instead, the provocation concerns the negation of the dichotomy between listening and music practice: contact with music is always active, it stimulates, among the many areas of the brain, the motor cortex in a similar way, whether or not it receives direct or implicit signals from the peripheral neurotransmitters. This is due to the fact that musical communication is based on a principle: it is the fruit of the distillation into symbolic codes of experiences of the body in movement and in contact with the anthropic and natural environment of proximity, the translation into feelings and emotional states is the prerogative of other cerebral areas always ready to activate when they perceive complexes of organised sounds and bearers of meaning whether the body actually moves or does so by isomorphic mirroring (Hjelmslev 1968).[2]

[2] Hjelmslev L. (1968), *I fondamenti della teoria del linguaggio*, tr. it. di G.C. Lepschy, Einaudi, Torino [19611] 1968, pp. 121–122.

2.2 The Body at the Centre

The first key-concept to start from for this brief excursus is the deep relationship between the sound-musical phenomenon and the body: aroused, evoked, represented, solicited in a transmodal manner, only apparently by hearing, in fact as part of a vibrational phenomenon involving the entire living organism, together with the forms and matter around it. Multisensoriality is implicated in a direct or indirect way: in addition to hearing, sight—if one listens to or produces music live, even with electronic instruments—proprioceptive and enteroceptive receptors are involved by virtue, precisely, of the contact with physical stimuli determined by air vibrations, but also by visceral and interosseous ones, especially if one plays an instrument or is in the womb in the prenatal phase. A close affinity, within the five best-known senses, is between hearing and touch, since, as Ed Yong (2023)[3] argues, both are mechanical senses, recorders of external movements by receiving biomechanical signals through cells that are pressed, bent, pulled away or rubbed: the cochlear or vestibular hair cells in the former case, the fingertips (or vibrissae in felines or rodents, the tip of the beak in birds, the Eimer's organs in moles), for example in the latter. The advantages of hearing are linked to the fact that, unlike touch, proximity is not necessary: encounters can take place from a distance, without contact surfaces but only the mediation of air or water; furthermore, unlike sight, hearing also works in the dark and travels at the speed of sound, which is much faster than the speed at which the molecules of smell propagate: this is the reason why many animals rely almost entirely on this channel of information.

Therefore, sound is an immersive experience—particularly performing in terms of exactness, speed and penetration capacity—that allows the acquisition of knowledge through the body in its entirety, which captures, assimilates and transforms in an embodied manner and is moved to act in the environmental context, continuously forging its own representation of reality. The human being can dedicate to the musical experience a level of centring and focusing so high as to desensitise the consciousness with respect to everything that runs outside that 'bubble', thanks to a total engagement in the assumed task of the perceptive, but also cognitive and metacognitive mechanisms: direct or indirect perception, emotional and affective movement, comprehension of the complex sound message that activates anticipatory, predictive processes contributing to co-constructing the collective experience, influencing the climate of the performance or interacting directly in the realisation of the musical event.

As in a psychological treatment, the interfering factors within a musical setting produce intermittencies in the therapeutic relationship: in the sound–music relationship these factors resist in the face of such an all-embracing involvement of body and mind of the people involved.

The reflexive activity follows the experience of contact with the sound-musical phenomenon by investigating the reasons why there was such an intense and

[3]Yong, E. (2023). *Un mondo immenso. Come i sensi degli animali rivelano il mondo nascosto intorno a noi*, Milano, La Nave di Teseo.

involving emotional impact. We have evidence of changes in the body's biochemical balances following exposure to a musical phenomenon.

With regard to neurotransmitters, hormones in particular, it must be said that the pleasure of listening to music increases levels of dopamine, a neurotransmitter associated with pleasure and reward. A study conducted by Salimpoor et al. (2011)[4] shows that when a subject listens to music that is pleasurable for him or her to the point of *chills*, this is associated with the release of *dopamine*. A sample of listeners was subjected to *diffusion tensor imaging* (DTI), a kind of magnetic resonance imaging that, by exploiting the *anisotropy* of certain anatomically homogeneous brain tissues, detects the movements of water molecules, making it possible to detect connections even on a three-dimensional scale. It emerges that in the mapped cases, the *auditory cortex* connects with the *anterior insular cortex*, which is involved in subjective emotional experiences, and the *medial prefrontal cortex*, which assesses risks, grasps the weight of dangers linked to the most intense emotional states. This cerebral stimulation recalls the possibility of training the mind, through contact with symbolic forms of life, to recognise and cope with stressful situations by training it to activate predictive reactions and handle real situations of emotional tension (Alexander and Brown 2011).[5] On the other hand, it should be emphasised that each person presents variables in the frequency and intensity of the neural interconnections between these areas, demonstrating the uniqueness of one's own way of experiencing an aesthetic experience and the different plasticity that each brain is capable of defining on the basis of its initial conformation, but above all of the type and quantity of meaningful experiences with which it has come into contact (Sachs et al. 2016).[6]

On the subject of stress, there have been studies in experimental settings that recorded a more rapid decrease in *cortisol* levels in those who listened to music after episodes of psychosocial stress than in those who were immersed in silence (Thoma et al. 2013),[7] but the results did not seem unambiguous. What is certain, however, is the reduction in levels of this hormone in premature infants when stimulated by the mother's voice and singing (Filippa et al. 2017).[8] It is yet another matter when it comes to activities in collective contexts: listening to music in the presence of peers produces a decrease in stress levels and an increase in the sense of belonging, of feelings of social cohesion, regardless of the degree of familiarity of the group members: thus, the social dimension of the musical experience favours the attenua-

[4] Salimpoor, V. N., Benovoy, M., Larcher, K., Dagher, A., & Zatorre, R. J. (2011). "Anatomically distinct dopamine release during anticipation and experience of peak emotion to music". *Nature Neuroscience*, 14(2), 257–262.

[5] Alexander, W. H., & Brown, J. W. (2011). "Medial prefrontal cortex as an action-outcome predictor". *Nature Neuroscience*, 14(10), 1338–1344.

[6] Sachs, M. E., Ellis, R. J., Schlaug, G., & Loui, P. (2016). "Brain connectivity reflects human aesthetic responses to music". *Social cognitive and affective neuroscience*, 11(6), 884–891.

[7] Thoma, M.V., La Marca, R., Brönnimann, R., Finkel, L., Ehlert, U., Nater, U.M., 2013. *The effect of music on the human stress response*. PLoS One 8, e70156.

[8] Filippa, M., Kuhn, P., & Westrup, B. (2017*), Early vocal contact and preterm infant brain development.* Cham, Switzerland: Springer International Publishing.

tion of negative and wearisome emotional states and the at least temporary removal of differences (Boer and Abubakar 2014).[9] A further indicator of the close commonality between musical practice and affectivity is the amount of oxytocin present in the blood under conditions of exposure to musical phenomena, in particular choral activities Kreutz et al. (2004)[10]: this peptide hormone produced by the hypothalamic nuclei and secreted in the neurohypophysis is present in all mammals because it stimulates uterine contractions, milk duct cells and has important supportive actions during labour and childbirth, also as a pain reducer. More generally, the substance decreases the activity of the sympathetic nervous system, which is deputed to promote propulsive actions—in cases of danger or flight in particular—in favour of an increase in the parasympathetic system, which produces states of calm. But even more emblematic is the similarity of the musical experience in terms of oxytocin value to the erotic experience of physical contact in intimacy, of sharing food, of affectively meaningful social unity (Algoe et al. 2017).[11]

To complete the picture of the changes elicited by music for a human being, let us emphasise a complementary field to the one addressed so far, namely that which measures the ability of music to modulate metabolic responses, thus helping to maintain homeostasis between the body's various functions such as heart rate, blood pressure, hunger and thirst stimuli, wake–sleep cycles, and energy balance. Research has established a role for music in regulating the hypothalamic–pituitary axis, the autonomic nervous system as a stimulant or relaxant (Trappe 2010)[12] and as a producer of mood-stabilising endorphins (Levitin 2011).[13] Recent findings have, finally, demonstrated a role of music in recovery in gastric and intestinal motility, in particular in the modulation of cancer-related gastrointestinal symptoms, and in increasing lipid metabolism and lactic acid clearance during exercise and recovery after exertion (Yamasaki et al. 2012)[14] as well as in increasing defences against antigens and increasing the activity of natural killer cells (Charnetski et al. 1998).[15]

[9] Boer, D., Abubakar, A., 2014. "Music listening in families and peer groups: benefits for young people's social cohesion and emotional well-being across four cultures". *Front. Psychol.* 5, 392.

[10] Kreutz, G., Bongard, S., Rohrmann, S., Hodapp, V., & Grebe, D. (2004). "Effects of choir singing or listening on secretory immunoglobulin A, cortisol, and emotional state". *Journal of behavioral medicine*, 27, 623–635.

[11] Algoe, S. B., Kurtz, L. E., & Grewen, K. (2017), "Oxytocin and Social Bonds: The Role of Oxytocin in Perceptions of Romantic Partners' Bonding Behavior", *Psychological Science*, 28(12), 1763–1772.

[12] Trappe, H. J. (2010). "The effects of music on the cardiovascular system and cardiovascular health". *Heart*, 96(23), 1868–1871.

[13] Levitin, D. J. (2011). *This is your brain on music: Understanding a human obsession*. Atlantic Books Ltd.

[14] Yamasaki, A., Booker, A., Kapur, V., Tilt, A., Niess, H., Lillemoe, K. D., … & Conrad, C. (2012). "The impact of music on metabolism". *Nutrition*, 28(11–12), 1075–1080.

[15] Charnetski, C. J., Brennan Jr., F. X., & Harrison, J. F. (1998). "Effect of music and auditory stimuli on secretory immunoglobulin A (IgA)". *Perceptual and Motor Skills*, 87(3_suppl), 1163–1170.

All these modifications in the biochemical and psychomotor set-up of the person are not, of course, in themselves, the exclusive consequence of an active or receptive exposure to music, but it is the co-presence, the reticular integration between most of the reactions described in the face of an immersive experience that makes the language of sounds one of the most complete endeavours to express—precisely express, to bring out—pooling the humanity of the human being. In fact, all creative, attentive, analysing, organising and constructive processing capacities, short- and long-term memorisation, psychomotor control and coordination (especially of fine mobility in the case of active practice), predictive anticipation (Lumaca et al. 2019),[16] problem solving, and affective-emotional symbolisation are engaged in a musical activity with consequent systemic and reticular cerebral dynamism. What is still to be consolidated is the demonstration of how long, in the medium to long term, these benefits last in regulatory, protective and balancing terms with respect to people's lives, what relationships exist between systematic and continuous sound–music practice and the evolution, growth and transformation of people, particularly those with inhibited communication channels, forms of social and relational fragility and/or with motor deficits: only a persistent, circumstantiated and measurable change on precise clinical objectives can make it legitimate to associate the term therapy with music, otherwise, we will speak of forms of relief, of temporary conditions of induced well-being (Pietschnig et al. 2010)[17] or, when related to the increase of specific technical skills and mastery of the discipline, of music education (Tóth-Bakos 2016).[18]

2.3 Not Fragments, But Flow Experiences

What was said at the beginning about the distortion of music research when it is analysed with autopsy techniques and administered in a mercurial manner, thus by isolated particles, is confirmation of the fact that contact with sounds manipulated by man only becomes an authentic experience to the extent that it is perceived as a fluid, articulated and complex phenomenon. Freud (1913) did not like music but only the plastic arts and sculpture in particular[19] precisely because the becoming of

[16] Lumaca, M., Trusbak Haumann, N., Brattico, E., Grube, M., & Vuust, P. (2019). "Weighting of neural prediction error by rhythmic complexity: A predictive coding account using mismatch negativity". *European Journal of Neuroscience*, 49(12), 1597–1609.

[17] Pietschnig, J., Voracek, M., & Formann, A. K. (2010). "Mozart effect–Shmozart effect: A meta-analysis". *Intelligence*, 38(3), 314–323.

[18] Tóth-Bakos, A. (2016). "Music education and music therapy". In *INTED2016 Proceedings* (pp. 1643–1652). IATED.

[19] Works of art make a strong impression on me, particularly literary works and plastic works, more rarely paintings. Thus I am led, on favourable occasions, to contemplate them at length in order to feel them in my own way, that is, to discover through what they produce an effect. When I cannot do so, as with music for example, I am almost unable to enjoy them. A rationalist or perhaps analytical disposition struggles within me against emotion when I cannot know why I am moved nor what it is that grips me. Freud S. (1913). *Il Mosè di Michelangelo*. O.S.F., p. 7

complex sound presences does not allow us to grasp their constituent elements and rationally describable meanings: his capacity for analysis and logical interpretation requires firm elements on which to rest gazes from several perspectives, while music, on the contrary, eludes. Proust (1913) says it well when, in describing a chamber concerto for violin and piano, he describes the bewitching surprise of a phrase or a harmony that arouses a «purely musical» impression, that is «inextensive, completely original, irreducible to any other order of impressions» and the graspability of meanings is eluded by the whirling succession of appearances and disappearances, overlaps and evolutions of the musical texture:

> Perhaps the notes we hear at that moment already tend, according to pitch and quantity, to cover before our eyes, surfaces of various sizes, to trace arabesques, to give us sensations of width, lightness, stability and whimsy. But the notes vanish before these sensations have sufficiently formed in us not to be submerged by those that already awaken the following or even simultaneous notes and this impression would continue to envelop us with its liquidity (…) the motifs that at times emerge from it (…) impossible to describe, impossible to recall (…). impossible to describe, to recall, to define, ineffable if memory, like a labourer working to build lasting foundations in the midst of the waves, fabricating for us facsimiles of those fleeting phrases, did not allow us to compare them to the following ones and differentiate them.[20]

It is memory, therefore, that allows the fixation of identification codes, of patterns of relationships useful for constructing over time recognition systems, profiles of motor activation, of relationships with space to which are associated emotional states, autobiographical memories, synaesthesias reconstructed according to plots that are always new, albeit full of familiar fragments. This short-term cognitive faculty processes between seven and nine items (notes, chords, patterns, engravings); however, through the use of chunking, i.e. organic groupings of microcells and the use of repetition, it is possible to store longer and more complex musical phrases. Long-term memory, on the other hand, stores information in the form of episodic sequences, linguistic symbols and codes and even unconscious motor conducts (Imberty et al. 1993)[21]: music permeates all these types of storage, colouring them with affective-emotional states, capable of becoming powerful triggers in the case of mnestic retrieval, particularly with people suffering from degenerative pathologies.

Let us analyse these assumptions starting from our point of observation: in active music therapy practices, it is evident that complexity does not refer to performative aspects—pieces that are difficult to perform—or compositional aspects—music written or improvised on the basis of sophisticated technical constructs, but as essential distillations of profound knowledge, gestures that are also elementary but

[20] Proust M. (1913), *Dalla parte di Swann*, trad. it Milano, Bur, 1985, pp. 304–306.

[21] Imberty M., Baroni M., Porzionato G. (1993), Memoria musicale e valori sociali. Metodi d'indagine e aspetti educativi, I Quaderni della SIEM, Milano, Ricordi.

multiple and interconnected. Such organisms are vectors of expressive power to the extent that they invoke multifaceted and authentic meanings, made up as much of personal studies and experiences as of an authentic desire to encounter the other through the mediation of music. An isolated sound, a pattern surrounded by silence may represent a signal, they may contain within themselves a meaning of recall, a warning, but they do not possess any coefficient of expressiveness: it is necessary to construct a narrative plot, a concatenation of correlated events that allow them to be identified as a system of evolving meanings, thus flows of sounds in motion, structures of time.

In this regard, the concept of flow experience (flow), coined by Mihály Csíkszentmihályi (1990),[22] is well-suited to the sound–music relationship: it indicates the immersive and permeating state achieved during the performance of an activity so involving that it makes one lose track of chronological time, favouring a high concentration to the point of excluding any interfering factor and allowing the enjoyment of intense pleasure. The connection of this concept with the practice of music has the following characteristics:

1. Listening to music or playing an instrument requires a high level of attention and concentration on the piece of music listened to or produced, which becomes a vehicle through which to experience symbolic body adventures without actually moving: floating, falling, rising, jumping, etc., according to a design of successions, deviations and anticipations, continuities and discontinuities that produce intrinsic temporal plots in which overlaps, intersections, co-presences, irregularities and recurrences are permissible (Keeler et al. 2015).[23]
2. When people are completely absorbed in music, they can experience a reduction in awareness of everything around them, thus entering an exclusive state in which they experience a suspension of existential time in order to enter a symbolic time nourished by an alternation between tension and relaxation, continuity and discontinuity, complexity and intelligibility according to a flow of pneumatic energy, adherent to the rhythms of the breath, attuned to their desires to listen or perform and at the same time inspiring them.
3. In both listening and active practice, a balance must be maintained between the skills possessed and the challenge thrown down by the musical experience, in order to address and appreciate a repertoire that presents analogies with what one already possesses and appreciates, but also more enigmatic elements, elusive and far removed from one's sensibilities yet inducing curiosity.
4. This balance between possibility and risk, the desired concentration, the mobilisation of the entire body towards a goal extended along a time string suspends the state of consciousness and envelops people in a metareal bubble: while deter-

[22] Czikszentmihalyi, M. (1990). *Flow: The psychology of optimal experience*, New York, Harper & Row.

[23] Keeler, J. R., Roth, E. A., Neuser, B. L., Spitsbergen, J. M., Waters, D. J. M., & Vianney, J. M. (2015). "The neurochemistry and social flow of singing: bonding and oxytocin", *Frontiers in human neuroscience*, 9, 158442.

mined by the most visceral contact with matter, it challenges its laws to the point of transcending them. This applies as much to those who are direct and concrete protagonists of the musical production as to those who witness it with transport and full participation.

5. An immersive experience such as music produces intrinsic gratification, pleasure and motivates the continuation of this practice throughout existence, perhaps in different ways and forms, even and especially in persons with various frailties (Hallam 2010).[24]

The flow is guaranteed by a focus on the sound gesture in terms of immediate and constant feedback with respect to what has just been played and prediction of what can be determined in the immediate future. In this regard, one is creative when one hypothesises or produces unpredictable deviations as well as reinforcing reiterations, but also when one demonstrates mastery in how and what to play, not so much for the precision of the gesture according to standard aesthetic canons, but for evolving expressive poignancy.

The practice of musical improvisation presents exemplary characteristics with respect to what has just been said, because it plays its game in the extemporaneity, in the full independence of the performer from predetermined and written forms, although it draws from a wealth of prior knowledge combined with innate aptitudes and faculties that it can employ in the "here and now" in the "presence in the moment" that is deemed useful to develop a coherent and effective expressive plan. Thus, the 'I' manifests itself in a temporal stretch separated from the chronological flow, from the inexorable timing of real life, and becomes the creator of a flow that keeps external and internal, distinct substances and independent rhythms, united. All this through a creative relationship of the person with matter—a sound object, a musical instrument—that is, with exogenous substances that come into contact for a reciprocal transformative and revelatory process.

But the human activity that synthetically projects vital experiences onto a system of symbols always involves, directly or indirectly, the participation of several people united around a shared intention. The psychologist Keith Sawyer, in his book Group Genius, first of all argues that even an idea matured in the mind of one man is always the end result of a long and articulated social process, decanted in individual memory but always born together with someone. This also applies to musical composition, interpretation or solo improvisation. Secondly, the author reads any experience of intersubjective creativity under the lens of the musician practising group improvisation. He emphasises how the collective flow is determined by total dedication to listening to each other, free from all planning and constructive predetermination, is invigorated by the open breath that great flexibility contains and inspired by a fascination with the unpredictable: none of the actors knows precisely what is going to happen. This status imposes on everyone, in their reciprocal attention, continuous adaptations to what the others create in order to build correspondences,

[24] Hallam, S. (2010). "The power of music: Its impact on the intellectual, social and personal development of children and young people". *International journal of music education*, 28(3), 269–289.

consonances, contrasts in a conscious and intentional way for a mysterious outcome: all are focused on the final outcome without knowing what it will be like, all are busy sculpting the same block of marble each with their own chisel to bring out of the material a face whose features they do not have in mind, whose definitive features they do not know. It is very much like the fate of all of us, busy living in the present with an ever-changing idea of self-according to what the environment around us inspires and with no idea of how our form will be completed before we close our eyes forever.

2.4 Every Change Is Collective, Every Healing Is a Social Fact

A musical phenomenon therefore shakes and is co-acted upon by the surrounding environment (Ongaro and Ward 2017),[25] expresses a will of the creator to expand and, at the same time, marks the limits of a relationship with the world, constricted within limited sensory envelopes, incapable of transcending towards broader understandings of which, we know, matter is made. This enactivist approach inaugurated by Varela, Thompson and Rosch (2017)[26] attributes to the environment a synergetic role with each subject in its embodied integrity and complexity, as an inspirer of sensorimotor behaviour and conduct: the actions performed by man are inspired by the characteristics of which the sensory elements with which we come into contact are composed, by the fragments of the world of which each of us is a part. Knowledge therefore takes place not only through cognitive processes, reasoning, logic and calculations, but by immersion, through the bodies that capture, move and undergo continuous transformations. The plasticity of the brain, which is particularly developed in experienced musicians and in all those who frequent musical practices for medium to long periods of time, is but a mirror of these more embodied metamorphoses. This new scientific awareness makes it possible to attribute to sound–musical communication a more relevant role than hitherto acknowledged, since they are vibratory complexes that induce reasoning only after an awareness of the significant impact recorded by the sensory–motor and affective-emotional dimensions that is effective in itself. Thanks to this, the frontier of possible learning also opens up for those who see their verbal communication channels inhibited or partially impaired: both the principle of educability for all and that of rehabilitation and the improvement of intersubjective relations and a sense of belonging to the world are thus applicable to all without distinction (Nuti 2019).[27]

The environment, according to our selective filters that pick up what the organism in its wholeness needs, is made up of parts of sensitive nature and people: the latter are close to us by similarity and involved by a mysterious, invisible and

---

[25] Ongaro, G., & Ward, D. (2017). "An enactive account of placebo effects". *Biology & Philosophy*, 32, 507–533.

[26] Varela, F. J., Thompson, E., & Rosch, E. (2017). *The embodied mind, revised edition: Cognitive science and human experience.* MIT press.

[27] Nuti G. (2019), *Pedagogia dell'Appartenenza*, Louvain La Neuve, Paris, L'Harmattan.

reciprocal attractive energy that does not exhaust its functions in defence against dangers, in the empowerment gained from hunting in groups or cultivating the land in collectives to ensure abundant food in every season of the year.

Even in times of collective crises, music exerts a thaumaturgic function: Nicola Massa (1549) prescribed that pestilential fever patients should sing for at least an hour a day, while Saint Charles Borromeo obliged plague-stricken citizens to gather in song by going out into the street or looking out of the window seven times a day to the sound of bells, intoning propitiatory litanies with an apotropaic function. It was also seen during the recent pandemic how entire populations suddenly compacted around musical rituals in the form of hymns sung from windows between apartment blocks or by attending singing performances by inspired soloists on the roofs of houses (Sarasso et al. 2021).[28]

We need to synchronise ourselves, to experience moments of social bonding in order to strengthen social ties by exorcising intimate fears and at the same time perceiving them as common factors among like-minded people, counteracting the emptiness of isolation and the terror of death. As Damasio (2000)[29] teaches us, cultivating emotional states, abandoning oneself to them and at the same time attempting to give them a form, to free them within a system of coordinated and shared actions, does not invalidate the human capacity to understand the world; on the contrary, it puts one in closer contact with the truth of things, albeit without revealing it. Art making, as James Hillman (2005)[30] reminds us, counteracts our dangerous tendency to adopt some kind of collective anaesthesia in order to survive: without it, we would become insensitive to the environment, dehumanising ourselves irreparably.

In collective contexts, music plays important roles and, as the anthropologist Alan Merriam (2000)[31] has aptly documented, it punctuates the times of communities at every latitude. We are interested in highlighting some of these contexts that are useful in giving value to the relationship between psychology and music for therapy:

- The *rituality* associated with transitions between life stages, aimed at celebrating crucial events in families and individuals;
- *dance* as an indispensable moment of energetic concentration, of exchange between bodies, of symbolisation of intercourse;
- *play* as a form of escape from the prison of functions, from the stranglehold of daily needs for protection, nourishment, hygiene, which have obligatory rules in order to engineer their own, shared with peers, with no aim other than the plea-

[28] Sarasso, P., Ronga, I., Neppi-Modona, M., & Sacco, K. (2021). "The role of musical aesthetic emotions in social adaptation to the Covid-19 pandemic". *Frontiers in Psychology*, 12, 611639.

[29] Damasio, A. (2000). *Emozione e coscienza*, Milano, Adelphi.

[30] Hillman, J., Donfrancesco, F., & Donfrancesco, P. (2005). *Politica della bellezza*. Milano, Moretti & Vitali.

[31] Merriam, A. P., Carpitella, D., & Di Piazza, E. (2000). *Antropologia della musica*. Palermo, Sellerio.

sure of measuring oneself in a challenge, aiming at a goal, challenging an adversary or just oneself;

In all these formulas of coexistence, a search for *beauty* is implicitly pursued, understood as a combination of proportions and entropy, of recognisable geometries and hidden volumes, of known forms and unknown features. The ways and forms of these actions are deposited in a body of beliefs, *cultural values* and *models of coexistence* on which a strong collective identity is founded, one that is compatible with and not a substitute for the individual. Each individual embodies similar needs within him or herself even when his or her relationships with the world are limited: someone has to recognise them and give them a satisfactory response.

2.5 Reflections on Music Therapy

What has been described so far serves to underline some points of attention that music therapy, in its various declinations and application modalities and currents of thought should, in our opinion, consider.

First and foremost, the body, which should be taken into account for the totality of its communicative potential: even if we are talking about people with severe cognitive and psychomotor limitations, the forms with which they organise their movements and/or vocalisations possible in terms of speed, curvature, intonation, timbre and frequency, are evidence of a specific style, of a personal existential cross-section and not just the tangible vital residue from the outside of a prisoner and annihilated existence: from this it is necessary to start in order to grasp the open communication channel and enlarge its capacity, the amount of information and to probe its extensibility beyond what at that moment seems the only possible scenario. The therapist's observation must be profound during the treatment and the inter-subjective relationship, so that he/she is able to grasp all the nuances of change taking place, emerging from the measurable neuropsychophysiological indicators even in the face of a stereotypical picture or in any case resistant to any modification, at least at a first glance.

It should be added that the relationship between musical production and listening and bodily expression, even structured ones such as dance, is a research front that has yet to be explored in neuro-psychological terms, except for some recent initial in-depth studies that pave the way towards identifying the causes that lead to the limitation of rhythmic movements in some individuals (Theofanopoulou 2023),[32] but in art-therapies it produces clear evidence from which hard science researchers could take useful cues.

The *experience of flow* represents an effective image of the sound–musical relationship as it unfolds in the suspended time in which, within any therapeutic setting, the experience needs to take substance: it is centred on a precise objective of

[32] Theofanopoulou, C. (2023). "A journey from speech to dance through the field of oxytocin". *Comprehensive Psychoneuroendocrinology*, 100193.

reciprocal liberation of the respective expressive space through the dynamic and mutable construction of a third place, not only shared, but co-created and nurtured, the progressive opening of forms, techniques, instruments and strategies through which to communicate vital states and their emotional implications, to kindle and strengthen profiles of affectivity and thus of bonds. In the specific case, for example, of having to strengthen the verbalisation abilities in a person with articulation and syntactic construction difficulties, it may be effective to enhance what is profoundly musical, that is, the involvement of the body in psychomotor actions that are coherent in terms of profile, intensity and form organised according to logics of relative solidarity, not too hierarchised and sculpted, but fluidised by the interweaving of complexities so vital as to involve the person as a whole because they are irregular, unpredictable and therefore mobilising, capable of activating emulation processes without too many logical–rationalistic superstructures and desires for absolute control. In short, one can learn by embodied cognition if one immerses oneself in an experiential flow in which one forgets one's own difficulties, letting oneself be carried away by a force that drags one towards overcoming the obstacle without fear.

It goes without saying that sound–musical improvisation, moreover freed from idiomatic or genre affiliations (jazz or western baroque), is the most natural way to entertain a non-verbal inter-subjective relationship because, with its *aesthetics of the unexpected* (Siron 2005),[33] it allows one to play the dialectic by constructing a predictable frame of reference by proposing or indulging in conventional musical constructs, but at the same time seeking surprise, the unexpected revealer of new horizons to explore and consolidate together. It is a process analogous to that which is created in an interpersonal relationship when it starts from some common, even superficial assumptions, but then develops through reciprocal discoveries that influence each other through emulation and rethinking, periodically coming closer to comfort each other and moving apart to breathe.

Certainly the creation of flow experiences favours the refinement of attentional capacities, of self-control of one's own motricity, concentrating it on functional aspects and attenuating or eliminating interfering and energetically wasteful ones; but the fluidity of the sound–music relationship in a music-therapeutic context is a terrain to be conquered: It often starts from psychically shattered clinical pictures, from memories full of black chasms, from interminable silences or glossolalia repeated a thousand and one times without apparent evolution, and must arrive at structured and metamorphic products. In particular, silences must become spaces of waiting, stretched like violin strings because they are filled with the will to understand, with a look of care and research at the same time, even when, especially at the beginning of a therapeutic pathway, they can be almost interminably long.

The social and relational dimension of musical practice, even when the relationships are dual, symbolically reflects forms of belonging to collectives, aggregations of people with their dynamics and rituals. This dimension can also find spaces of inclusion in group musical contexts in which people with different abilities,

[33] Siron, J. (2005). "L'improvvisazione nel jazz e nelle musiche contemporanee. L'imperfetto del momento attuale". J. J. Nattiez (a cura di), *Enciclopedia della musica*, 5, 737–756.

expertise and personal and technical instrumental histories cooperate, provided that therapeutic goals are focused on the basis of appropriate preliminary anamnesis, processes are monitored and outcomes are assessed in a punctual, circumstantial and expert manner.

With regard to the relationship between regularity and irregularity, between synchrony and syncopation, music therapy must interrogate itself in search of the most appropriate key, from case to case, to deal with the sound–music relationship starting from an investigation of the prevalences expressed by the person or the group being cared for in order to identify with respect to these fundamental dualisms for the organisation of a precise temporal style, the starting point to hypothesise a falling one, so that both opposites are contemplated in the search for a personalised balance, because every human relationship is made of their mixture and alternation, but each one has a measure of this unique co-presence. Let us start with some evidence: it has been discovered that the urge to dance is linked to a succession of beats over time. The so-called groove experience, however, is not made up of exactness, but of microscopic inaccuracies and obvious accent diffractions. The co-presence of isochronous tactus and syncopated elements allows, on the one hand, to adhere to a reassuring trend and, on the other hand, to enjoy an occasional, surprising unpredictability: to mark the co-presence of different elements, it is noted that it is two different brain areas—the primary auditory cortex and the dorsal auditory pathway, i.e. the area connecting the auditory cortex to the movement cortex—that follow the rhythm of the melody and the basic tactus respectively. Finally, the pleasure and desire to move the body in time is connected to the dialectic between predictive abilities and the actual continuation of the musical construct when the occasional elements present recurrences and periodic repetitions that lead one to predict what will happen next (Zalta et al. 2024).[34]

If being together on music demands certainty and surprises in order to maintain a relational interest, the heart of the exchange is rooted in the representation of emotional states. Already Darwin, in his essay *The Origin of Man* (1882),[35] argued that language and music derived from a musical protolanguage useful to strengthen defence against dangers and enemies, to encourage mating and to express emotional states. Today, studies on the effects of amusia (Thompson et al. 2012)[36] in the recognition of emotional states described by the intonational variables with which verbal sentences are pronounced show how the musicality of human action—that is, the rhythms, the curvatures of voice and colour, the temporal segmentation of one's gestures as well as of words and songs—is the strongest and most penetrating form of expression of emotional states, always mixed, ambivalent, never univocal

---

[34] Zalta, A., Large, E. W., Schön, D., & Morillon, B. (2024). "Neural dynamics of predictive timing and motor engagement in music listening". *Science Advances*, 10(10), eadi2525.

[35] Darwin, C. (1882). *L'origine dell'uomo e la scelta in rapporto col sesso*. Unione tipografico-editrice.

[36] Thompson, W. F., Marin, M. M., & Stewart, L. (2012). "Reduced sensitivity to emotional prosody in congenital amusia rekindles the musical protolanguage hypothesis". *Proceedings of the National Academy of Sciences*, 109(46), 19027–19032.

between people who meet around the same event experienced in a similar, but not identical way: the ground of communion is constituted by these matrices of trans-modal expressivity—thus alluding without rekindling them to multiple sensory experiences and united by coherent morphologies—which develop in pathways of polysemic narrativity, thus, as J. J. Nattiez (2011),[37] never descriptive but evocative and infinitely interpretable.

The role of music therapy, from a psychological perspective, should be to exploit the expressive charge of each intentionally proposed sound sequence to activate and develop a gradually more variegated and complex intersubjective relationship, arranged along articulated and extended narrative flows: this would be the mirror of a progressive psychic integration and, at the same time, the manifestation of a beneficial interpersonal recognition. However, it should also go down this road in collective contexts in which a more open practice of social inclusion is reconciled with the definition of personalised therapeutic goals, addressing each situation of discomfort in a broad context, which benefits, symbiotically, from the transformative process of each and every one.

References

Alexander WH, Brown JW. Medial prefrontal cortex as an action-outcome predictor. Nat Neurosci. 2011;14(10):1338–44.

Algoe SB, Kurtz LE, Grewen K. Oxytocin and social bonds: the role of oxytocin in perceptions of romantic partners' bonding behavior. Psychol Sci. 2017;28(12):1763–72.

Bernstein L. La gioia della Musica. Milano: Longanesi; 1982. p. 9. (trad. it Raffaele Mammalella, prima ed. statunitense, The Joy of Music 1954)

Boer D, Abubakar A. Music listening in families and peer groups: benefits for young people's social cohesion and emotional well-being across four cultures. Front Psychol. 2014;5:392.

Charnetski CJ, Brennan FX Jr, Harrison JF. Effect of music and auditory stimuli on secretory immunoglobulin A (IgA). Percept Mot Skills. 1998;87(3_suppl):1163–70.

Czikszentmihalyi M. Flow: the psychology of optimal experience. New York: Harper & Row; 1990.

Damasio A. Emozione e coscienza. Milano: Adelphi; 2000.

Darwin C. L'origine dell'uomo e la scelta in rapporto col sesso. Unione tipografico-editrice; 1882.

Filippa M, Kuhn P, Westrup B. Early vocal contact and preterm infant brain development. Cham: Springer; 2017.

Freud S. Il Mosè di Michelangelo. OSF. 1913:7.

Hallam S. The power of music: its impact on the intellectual, social and personal development of children and young people. Int J Music Educ. 2010;28(3):269–89.

Hillman J, Donfrancesco F, Donfrancesco P. Politica della bellezza. Milano: Moretti & Vitali; 2005.

Hjelmslev L. I fondamenti della teoria del linguaggio, tr. it. di G.C. Lepschy, Einaudi, Torino [19611]; 1968. p. 121–2.

Imberty M, Baroni M, Porzionato G. Memoria musicale e valori sociali. Metodi d'indagine e aspetti educativi, I Quaderni della SIEM. Milano: Ricordi; 1993.

Keeler JR, Roth EA, Neuser BL, Spitsbergen JM, Waters DJM, Vianney JM. The neurochemistry and social flow of singing: bonding and oxytocin. Front Hum Neurosci. 2015;9:158442.

[37] Nattiez, J. J. (2011). "La Narrativisation de la musique. La musique: récit ou proto-récit?". *Cahiers de Narratologie. Analyse et théorie narratives*, (21).

Kreutz G, Bongard S, Rohrmann S, Hodapp V, Grebe D. Effects of choir singing or listening on secretory immunoglobulin A, cortisol, and emotional state. J Behav Med. 2004;27:623–35.
Levitin DJ. This is your brain on music: understanding a human obsession. Atlantic Books Ltd; 2011.
Lumaca M, Trusbak Haumann N, Brattico E, Grube M, Vuust P. Weighting of neural prediction error by rhythmic complexity: a predictive coding account using mismatch negativity. Eur J Neurosci. 2019;49(12):1597–609.
Merriam AP, Carpitella D, Di Piazza E. Antropologia della musica. Palermo: Sellerio; 2000.
Nattiez JJ. La Narrativisation de la musique. La musique: récit ou proto-récit? Cahiers de Narratologie. Analyse et théorie narratives. 2011;21
Nuti G. Pedagogia dell'Appartenenza. Louvain La Neuve/Paris: L'Harmattan; 2019.
Ongaro G, Ward D. An enactive account of placebo effects. Biol Philos. 2017;32:507–33.
Pietschnig J, Voracek M, Formann AK. Mozart effect–Shmozart effect: a meta-analysis. Intelligence. 2010;38(3):314–23.
Proust M. Dalla parte di Swann, trad. it Milano. Bur. 1913;1985:304–6.
Sachs ME, Ellis RJ, Schlaug G, Loui P. Brain connectivity reflects human aesthetic responses to music. Soc Cogn Affect Neurosci. 2016;11(6):884–91.
Salimpoor VN, Benovoy M, Larcher K, Dagher A, Zatorre RJ. Anatomically distinct dopamine release during anticipation and experience of peak emotion to music. Nat Neurosci. 2011;14(2):257–62.
Sarasso P, Ronga I, Neppi-Modona M, Sacco K. The role of musical aesthetic emotions in social adaptation to the Covid-19 pandemic. Front Psychol. 2021;12:611639.
Siron J. L'improvvisazione nel jazz e nelle musiche contemporanee. L'imperfetto del momento attuale. J. J. Nattiez (a cura di). Enciclopedia della musica. 2005;5:737–56.
Theofanopoulou C. A journey from speech to dance through the field of oxytocin. Comp Psychoneuroendocrinol. 2023:100193.
Thoma MV, La Marca R, Brönnimann R, Finkel L, Ehlert U, Nater UM. The effect of music on the human stress response. PLoS One. 2013;8:e70156.
Thompson WF, Marin MM, Stewart L. Reduced sensitivity to emotional prosody in congenital amusia rekindles the musical protolanguage hypothesis. Proc Natl Acad Sci. 2012;109(46):19027–32.
Tóth-Bakos A. Music education and music therapy. In: INTED2016 proceedings. IATED; 2016. p. 1643–52.
Trappe HJ. The effects of music on the cardiovascular system and cardiovascular health. Heart. 2010;96(23):1868–71.
Varela FJ, Thompson E, Rosch E. The embodied mind. Revised edition: Cognitive science and human experience. MIT Press; 2017.
Yamasaki A, Booker A, Kapur V, Tilt A, Niess H, Lillemoe KD, Conrad C. The impact of music on metabolism. Nutrition. 2012;28(11–12):1075–80.
Yong E. Un mondo immenso. Come i sensi degli animali rivelano il mondo nascosto intorno a noi. Milano: La Nave di Teseo; 2023.
Zalta A, Large EW, Schön D, Morillon B. Neural dynamics of predictive timing and motor engagement in music listening. Sci Adv. 2024;10(10):eadi2525.

Music Under the Lens of Neuroscience

3

Eleonora Fullone, Giorgio Lazzari, Carlotta Lega, and Laura Ferreri

Key Points

- Since the 1940s, the development and implementation of new brain investigation techniques have significantly stimulated research in the field of the neuroscience of music.
- Music is a highly complex stimulus that involves multiple cognitive and neural mechanisms, making it an ideal lens for studying brain function.
- Engaging in musical activities stimulates several brain regions involved in various functions, including language, movement, memory, attention, and emotions.
- Musical training generates neuroplasticity in the brain and enables transfer effects on other cognitive functions.
- Because it activates the whole brain, music represents a useful tool for neurostimulation and rehabilitation in clinical domains, such as language, motor, and memory disorders.

E. Fullone
Department of Brain and Behavioral Sciences, University of Pavia, Pavia, Italy

School for Advanced Studies – IUSS, Pavia, Italy
e-mail: eleonora.fullone01@universitadipavia.it

G. Lazzari · C. Lega · L. Ferreri (✉)
Department of Brain and Behavioral Sciences, University of Pavia, Pavia, Italy
e-mail: giorgio.lazzari01@universitadipavia.it; carlotta.lega@unipv.it; laura.ferreri@unipv.it

A. Raglio (ed.), *Music and Music Therapy Interventions in Clinical Practice*, Neurocultural Health and Wellbeing,
https://doi.org/10.1007/978-3-031-88578-5_3

3.1 Introduction

Music is a universal aspect of human life, with musical behaviors present in every culture and throughout all historical periods. This ubiquity has made music a subject of interest across numerous fields of study, from the earliest theoretical work on music, the Harmonika Stoicheia by Greek Aristoxenou (Aristoxenus and Macran 1902), to various modern scientific approaches. Although music is generally associated with the arts, it was considered a consistent part of scientific knowledge—alongside mathematics, geometry, and astronomy—until the second half of the eighteenth century. Moreover, the universality of music has sparked various theories about its evolutionary origins. While the nonadaptationist perspectives suggest that music is pleasant but evolutionarily nonessential (see, e.g., Pinker 1999), adaptationist theories consider musical behavior naturally shaped by evolutionary processes. For example, Darwin (1871), later supported by Miller (1999), speculated that music evolved as a protolanguage for mate choice and sexual selection. Other theories emphasize music's role in facilitating group cohesion (Savage et al. 2021) or helping infant emotional regulation (for an overview of music evolution, see Hallam et al. 2012).

In the field of psychology and neuroscience, pioneering publications from the 1940s to the 1960s led to a significant increase in research in the 2000s (Thaut and Donald 2018). This burst of publications is largely due to the development and implementation of new brain investigation techniques in the latter half of the twentieth century. Electroencephalography (EEG) and magnetoencephalography (MEG) provide direct measures of electrical and magnetic activity, respectively, offering insights into neural temporal dynamics. One of the first music studies dates back to 1947 (Shaw and Hill 1947) and used EEG to investigate the neural correlates of musicogenic epilepsy. Given their good temporal resolution, EEG and MEG have been used over the decades to explore several aspects of auditory cognition and its temporal dynamics. For example, many studies have investigated musical syntax (e.g., Maess et al. 2001; Sammler et al. 2013), neural entrainment to rhythms (Nozaradan et al. 2011), and interbrain synchrony in joint musical activity (Babiloni et al. 2012). Neuroimaging measures such as positron emission tomography (PET) and functional magnetic resonance imaging (fMRI) also offer important insights into the interplay between the brain and music, thanks to their high spatial resolution. In one of the first PET studies, Roland et al. (1981) demonstrated focal activations of the cerebral cortex (specifically, the right temporal and parietal lobe, and right posterior inferior frontal area) associated with the discrimination of nonverbal auditory stimuli. Over the following years, these techniques facilitated the study of neural correlates of a wide variety of musical experiences, ranging from music perception (Janata 2015) and production (Zatorre et al. 2007) to memory (Jäncke 2008) and emotions (Blood and Zatorre 2001).

Moreover, other techniques such as diffusion tensor imaging (DTI) and voxel-based morphometry (VBM) provide information about brain changes due to musical training (see also Sect. 3.3). For example, greater cortical thickness has been observed in musicians (compared to nonmusicians), particularly in the superior temporal cortex (Foster and Zatorre 2010; Karpati et al. 2017), dorsolateral frontal (Bermudez et al. 2009), and motor regions (Elbert et al. 1995; Gaser and Schlaug 2003). In addition, pianists exhibit greater brain plasticity adaptations, including both decreases and increases in gray matter, which result from their system's optimization guided by early musical training (Vaquero et al. 2016). Music listening also influences brain function and structure, as evidenced by changes observed when listening to enjoyable or favorite music (Wilkins et al. 2014) and white matter variations related to individual differences in music reward sensitivity (Martínez-Molina et al. 2019).

In the field of brain stimulation research, techniques such as transcranial magnetic stimulation (TMS) and transcranial direct current stimulation (tDCS) have been employed to establish cause–effect relationships between music cognitive processes and brain activations. More specifically, studies have investigated the underpinning mechanisms of musical emotions (Stupacher et al. 2013; Mansouri et al. 2017; Mas-Herrero et al. 2021), fine auditory processing (Lega et al. 2016b), motor prediction during music listening (Stephan et al. 2018; Gordon et al. 2018), and music-driven memory processes (Chow et al. 2021). Finally, promising techniques like functional near-infrared spectroscopy (fNIRS) are emerging in the study of music cognition. fNIRS offers advantages over traditional methods by allowing researchers to study music processes in more ecological settings, overcoming the technical limitations of other neuroimaging tools (Curzel et al. 2024).

Research in the neuroscience of music over the last few decades has shown that playing or listening to music involves nearly all human cognitive functions, which can be explored through different neuroimaging and neurostimulation techniques. Studies have shown that musical activities involve several brain regions associated with other cognitive and behavioral processes, such as speech, movement, memory, attention, and the reward system (Zatorre 2005). In this context, understanding the neuroscientific foundations of music cognition appears pivotal for using music as "a mediating language in the therapy process" (Thaut and Hoemberg 2014). In this vein, this chapter aims to present a general overview of neuroscientific research on music, offering scientific evidence for its applicability in various cognitive domains. To this aim, we will delve into music perception and motor processes, its connection with language, emotional and rewarding aspects, its intrinsic link with memory components, as well as its role in social cognition. Furthermore, we will focus on the role of musical expertise in modulating brain processes. Finally, based on this evidence, we will discuss how such neuroscientific insights can be applied in music-based interventions.

3.2 Music and Cognitive Processing

3.2.1 Perception

Music is a highly complex stimulus that evolves over time and engages several cognitive and neural mechanisms. Its components of rhythm, melody, and harmony are processed by distinct yet overlapping neural networks, contributing to the unique cognitive and emotional experiences that music can evoke.

When listening to music, acoustic information is converted into neural signals within the cochlea and then gradually processed in the auditory brainstem, decoding several properties of external stimuli such as pitch, timbre, intensity, and periodicity of sounds (Koelsch 2011). For example, an fMRI study found that pitch height (i.e., the sound frequency used to segregate sound sources) and pitch chroma (i.e., a circular dimension of pitch used for tracking information from a particular sound source) are processed differently in the brain. Height changes are represented posterior to the primary auditory cortex, while chroma changes are represented anterior to the primary auditory cortex (Warren et al. 2003). Moreover, in the case of melodies, it has been shown that pitch recognition involves a ventral stream connecting primary auditory areas to the inferior frontal gyrus (Vuust et al. 2022). In pitch perception research, several studies have also focused on the so-called amusia, a neurogenetic disorder with impairment of pitch processing that results in deficits in music production and perception. Amusia individuals struggle to understand when someone, including themselves, sings off-key, to recognize familiar tunes without lyrics, to detect incorrect or out-of-tune notes, and to memorize even short melodies (Tillmann et al. 2015). This inability of amusic individuals to access acquired musical pitch knowledge is attributed to neural transmission abnormalities between the auditory cortex and the inferior frontal gyrus in the right cerebral hemisphere (Peretz 2016).

Beyond pitch and melody perception, neuroscience research investigating harmony has also yielded several important findings that deepen our understanding of how the brain processes music. Harmony, defined as the combinatorial arrangement of chords within musical sequences characterized by local and nonlocal dependencies (Swain 1995; see also Bianco et al. 2016), adheres to harmonic principles that govern musical structure and are usually considered part of a musical "syntax" (see e.g., Bharucha 1983; Rohrmeier and Koelsch 2012). In this vein, EEG and MEG studies on harmony showed that violating hierarchical harmonic rules in a sequence of chords elicits the so-called early right anterior negativity brain potential (ERAN, Koelsch et al. 2001; Maess et al. 2001), localized by fMRI investigations in the inferior frontal gyrus (Tillmann et al. 2003; Koelsch et al. 2005a). Altogether, these studies confirmed the existence of a musical syntax or grammar intimately related to listeners' perceptual and predictive abilities (as further developed in Sect. 3.2.3).

Rhythm is also a crucial musical component and one of the most extensively studied musical features. Rhythmic behavior encompasses several processes, from beat extraction to the temporal coordination of movements in response to it. These processes rely on the listener's ability to synchronize internal oscillations with the perceived beat of the auditory signal, known as neural entrainment (Large 2008). Neural entrainment involves the activation of the brain's auditory and motor regions (e.g., the cerebellum, the supplementary motor area, and the premotor cortex) during rhythm perception (for a review, see Levitin et al. 2018; Cannon and Patel 2021), with neural responses reflecting the hierarchical metric nature of musical rhythm (Nozaradan et al. 2011). Several brain areas have been found to be implicated in rhythm perception besides motor-related regions (Zatorre and Salimpoor 2013). For instance, the basal ganglia are activated in both beat finding (Grahn and Rowe 2013) and continuation tasks (Kung et al. 2013). In addition, the cerebellum is involved in the elaboration of absolute timing, which involves a metrical representation of defined temporal intervals (Spencer and Ivry 2013). However, all these brain regions do not play as soloists but rather as part of an ensemble. Accordingly, studies have revealed brain connectivity between auditory and premotor areas (Chen et al. 2006), as well as between the basal ganglia and supplementary motor, premotor, and auditory cortical areas when processing beat-based rhythms compared to non-beat-based rhythms (Grahn and Rowe 2009; Toiviainen et al. 2020).

Taken together, these findings underscore that listening to music not only engages our auditory system but also deeply involves motor processes, even in the absence of overt movement. Importantly, this highlights the interconnectedness between perception and action in the context of musical experience, as further developed in the next section.

3.2.2 Movement

The connection between music and movement is evident in every musical experience. Consider, for example, the urge to tap your foot to a beat or the intricate finger movements of a pianist. Neuroscientific studies have shown that both active synchronization with music and passive listening to music activate brain regions involved in planning and executing movements, such as the premotor cortex and supplementary motor area (Grahn and Brett 2007; Chen et al. 2008a; Bengtsson et al. 2009; Grahn 2009, p. 200; Grahn and Rowe 2013; Proksch et al. 2020). This occurs because the brain's auditory and motor systems are closely interconnected, forming a network that supports both the perception and production of musical and rhythmic patterns. Specifically, the dorsal auditory–motor network integrates auditory and motor information (Hickok and Poeppel 2004; Chen et al. 2008a; Rauschecker 2011; Lega et al. 2016a) and creates fine temporal predictions (Patel and Iversen 2014; Ross et al. 2016, 2018a, b; Cannon and Patel 2021), thus supporting both rhythm perception (Chen et al. 2008a; Siman-Tov et al. 2022) and sensorimotor synchronization (Chen et al. 2008b; Giovannelli et al. 2014). Furthermore, learning to play an instrument involves the integration of sensory and motor information, as well as fine motor skills. During musical training, the interaction between auditory and motor systems is particularly intriguing: each action taken while playing an instrument produces sound, which in turn influences the next action, creating a continuous loop of sensory feedback (Zatorre et al. 2007). Musicians engage the premotor and auditory cortex when either listening to music without performing or performing music silently, suggesting that these regions are crucial in linking sound with action (Bangert et al. 2006; Baumann et al. 2007; Brown et al. 2015). Years of musical training likely solidify this sound–action association by establishing strong connections between the sounds produced and the movements needed to create them (Elsner and Hommel 2001; Chen et al. 2008a; see also Sect. 3.3 on musical expertise). Importantly, studies have demonstrated that this co-activation of auditory and motor regions arises even after a few days of musical practice (Lahav et al. 2007; Chen et al. 2012; Wollman et al. 2018).

Music's ability to engage motor regions highlights the deep connection between our auditory and movement systems, with potential applications in motor rehabilitation. For instance, the action-related processes in music perception underscore its potential, particularly in rehabilitation for motor disorders like Parkinson's disease (as further developed in Sect. 3.4).

3.2.3 Language

The connection between music and language has long been recognized. Darwin's theory suggests that music evolved as a form of protolanguage (Darwin 1871; see also introductory Sect. 3.1). Neuroscience research has revealed anatomical overlaps and functional connections between music and language. Several brain areas, including the primary and secondary auditory regions, the supramarginal gyrus, and Broca's area, are engaged in both activities (for reviews, see Besson and Schön 2001; Slevc and Okada 2015). Moreover, white matter traits, such as the arcuate fasciculus, exhibit increased connectivity in both musicians and bilinguals (Vaquero et al. 2020). An example of their neuroanatomical and functional overlap lies in studies investigating syntactic processing (Patel 2003), and showing the elicitation of the same event-related potential components (such as the so-called P600) in detecting musical and linguistic incongruities (Patel et al. 1998; Maess et al. 2001; Koelsch et al. 2004). The semantics of music and language have also been extensively explored, with studies revealing shared neural correlates at both regional and network levels (e.g., Koelsch et al. 2004; Koelsch 2012; Yu et al. 2017). In the same vein, some studies have explored changes in the detection of musical and language irregularities from neurophysiological and behavioral perspectives. For instance, Koelsch et al. (2005b) showed that left anterior negativity, typically elicited by syntactically incorrect words, was reduced when these words were presented simultaneously with syntactically irregular musical chords but not with linguistic–semantic incongruences. In another study, an enhanced garden–path effect (an initial incorrect interpretation by the reader due to syntactic ambiguities) was found when structurally unexpected words were presented with harmonically unexpected chords, compared to critical words violating semantic expectancy and critical chords violating timbral expectancy (Slevc et al. 2009). However, it is worth mentioning that other data indicate certain regions within the anterior superior temporal gyrus and temporal lobes respond more strongly to music than speech. In addition, studies have shown that music and language activate different neural populations within overlapping regions (for a review, see Peretz et al. 2015).

All this evidence has prompted new research questions about the possible advantages of the joint activities of music and language. For example, Schön et al. (2008) demonstrated that learning a new language might benefit from the musical properties of song compared to speech alone. The ability to form mental representations of statistical structures based on predictions and expectations, through the perception of relationships between sounds, could explain the transfer effect of music on language processing (Schön et al. 2008; see also Sect. 3.3). Moreover, this prediction mechanism, rooted in the anticipation of various musical features, is crucial not only for musical perception, action, and language processing but also for emotional responses to music.

3.2.4 Emotions and Reward

Music is an exceptionally powerful emotional stimulus. Humans primarily engage with music to regulate their emotions and improve their mood (Juslin and Västfjäll 2008). Emotions commonly studied in relation to music include joy and sadness, as well as more nuanced emotions such as nostalgia, surprise, tension, wonder, power, and transcendence, all of which can be strongly and efficiently elicited by musical experiences. From a cognitive perspective, emotions result from the interplay between several components such as appraisal, physiological responses, emotional expressions, and action tendencies (Mauss et al. 2005).

According to the circumplex model of emotions (Russell 1980; Juslin and Sloboda 2001), the broad spectrum of emotions evoked by music can be represented on two main dimensions: valence (ranging from very negative to very positive) and arousal (ranging from very relaxed to very excited). For instance, joy and power are defined by high valence and arousal, sadness by low levels of both dimensions, nostalgia and transcendence by high valence and low arousal, and fear by low valence and high arousal. Music allows listeners to navigate efficiently within this emotional space by modulating different features, with mode and tempo (among others, such as timbre and cadences) playing pivotal roles. At a neural level, musical changes in these two components are associated with neural activity in specific brain regions involved in emotions. At the subcortical level, these regions involve: (I) limbic and paralimbic structures such as the amygdala, involved in processing all stimuli with a universal socio-affective message; (II) the dopaminergic mesolimbic reward system with the nucleus accumbens, activated in response to pleasurable music; (III) the hippocampal formation, functionally connected with the hypothalamus, involved in both positive and negative as well as in social attachments-related emotions; (IV) the insula, with its role in autonomic regulation and interoceptive representation of music-evoked bodily emotional reactions. At the cortical level, we can observe: (I) the rostral cingulate zone, acting as a hub for interoceptive awareness, internal selection of movements, and regulation of autonomic functions; (II) the orbitofrontal cortex, which controls emotional behavior and is activated by expectancy violations; (III) the pre-supplementary motor area, implicated in motor preparation and programming when there is an urge to move with the music (for a review, see Koelsch 2014).

Studies on neurochemical and psychophysiological reactions to music emotions have provided new insights into the mechanisms underlying the elicitation of highly intense emotions, such as chills (Mas-Herrero et al. 2023). Intense pleasure elicited by music is not only subjectively reported but also objectively measured through physiological responses such as skin conductance (Mas-Herrero et al. 2023) and changes in heart and respiration rates (Salimpoor et al. 2011). These responses are strongly associated with changes in the autonomic nervous system and the reward pathway. For example, Salimpoor et al. (2011) found, through an fMRI–PET study, that music-related intense pleasure leads to dopamine release in the striatal system, with an anatomical pathway dissociation between the anticipation of the reward (in the caudate) and peak pleasure itself (in the nucleus accumbens). The causal role of dopamine in music reward responses was further confirmed by TMS (Mas-Herrero et al. 2017, 2021) and pharmacological (Ferreri et al. 2019) interventions, which can up- and downregulate music reward responses by stimulating or inhibiting the dopaminergic reward system, respectively.

Interestingly, while the experience of pleasure in music is universal across cultures, there are individual differences in the degree to which it is experienced. In the general population, individuals can be divided into musical hedonics, hyperhedonics, and anhedonics, with the latter being unable to experience pleasure in response to music specifically (Mas-Herrero et al. 2013). At the brain level, differences in structural connectivity between the perceptual and subcortical brain regions predict individual differences in sensitivity to music reward (the so-called musical hedonia). Indeed, less connectivity between the auditory cortex and nucleus accumbens is observed in musical anhedonics compared to musical hedonics and hyperhedonics (Martínez-Molina et al. 2016, 2019).

3.2.5 Memory

Music is an integral part of daily life for many, and most of us can remember some music excerpts, their lyrics, or even some associated personal events. Consequently, cognitive and neuroscientific research has increasingly focused on the mnemonic aspects of music. Two distinct systems of music memory have been explored: semantic and episodic. This distinction, first pointed out by Tulving (1972), separates memories of events tied to specific times and places (episodic) from memories of factual knowledge (semantic). In the realm of music, semantic memory involves recognizing familiar songs or melodies, while episodic memory entails recalling musical excerpts along with the spatiotemporal context in which they were encoded. Through a PET study, Platel et al. (2003) showed a functional distinction in music memory systems. Episodic memory was found to activate bilaterally the middle and superior frontal gyri and precuneus, while semantic memory involved activation in the medial and orbital frontal cortex (bilaterally), the left angular gyrus, and the left anterior part of the middle temporal gyri (see also Watanabe et al. 2008). Further investigations have revealed that musical and verbal semantic memory share a network (i.e., left temporal and prefrontal), but with topographical specificities (i.e., an anterior activation for memory of musical material, and a posterior activation for verbal one; Groussard et al. 2010).

Autobiographical memory, which includes memories related to personal history, is particularly intriguing in the context of music. It comprises both a semantic (self-representation) and an episodic component (recollection of spatiotemporally located personal events). Music is intricately intertwined with autobiographical memories, often serving as a potent cue for recalling significant moments from one's past (Jakubowski and Ghosh 2021). When individuals listen to melodies associated with specific events, they frequently vividly recall those times. This phenomenon likely arises because music evokes strong emotions linked to personal experiences, forging a lasting association between a particular song and the memory of that event

(Janata et al. 2007; Centomo et al. 2023). At a neural level, music-driven autobiographical memory has been associated with the activation of the medial prefrontal cortex with lateral prefrontal and posterior cortices (Janata 2009).

Collectively, this evidence suggests that musical memory encompasses not only memory for musical elements such as pitch (Vines et al. 2006; Graves et al. 2019) and rhythm contour (Schmuckler and Moranis 2023), but also extends to nonmusical associated information. Music has been shown to prime the semantic language memory system, influencing the processing of specific abstract and concrete words (Koelsch et al. 2004). Moreover, musicians tend to outperform nonmusicians in verbal long-term memory (e.g., Jakobson et al. 2008) and verbal working memory (e.g., Franklin et al. 2008) (see Sect. 3.3). Interestingly, musical pleasure, by stimulating the reward system, has been demonstrated to enhance episodic memory for music (Ferreri and Rodriguez-Fornells 2017; Ferreri et al. 2021) and associated verbal stimuli (Cardona et al. 2020), suggesting that music, through its emotional component, modulates higher cognitive functions such as memory (Jäncke 2008).

3.2.6 Social Cognition

The inclination toward music is widespread among humans. As previously discussed, music can evoke emotions that profoundly influence our emotional regulation, making it a commonly chosen coping strategy during crises. Even during challenging times, such as the COVID-19 lockdowns, people found solace in music, singing, and playing instruments from their balconies to confront the crisis and alleviate isolation (Granot et al. 2021; Ferreri et al. 2021; Mas-Herrero et al. 2023). Accordingly, music-related activities—both playing an instrument and listening to music—have been demonstrated to promote social connections (e.g., Tarr et al. 2014). In this vein, Savage et al. (2021) have proposed that the primary evolutionary function of music is to promote social bonding through musical interactions. More specifically, through active engagement in music and its emotional power, humans can form, strengthen, and sustain relationships, fostering cooperation within a group and contributing to members' and groups' self-identity. Researchers studying music from a developmental perspective have highlighted that infants possess an innate ability to process pitch and rhythmic structures, enabling their early engagement with both music and caregivers (Trainor and Hannon 2013; Nguyen et al. 2023). A significant form of early musical interaction in early development is the so-called infant-directed singing (e.g., lullabies), a typical parents' behavior that can be observed cross-culturally. This practice not only strengthens bonding between caregivers and infants but also enhances emotional co-regulation and supports social interactions (Lense et al. 2022). Musical communication in infancy has been shown to strengthen parent–infant bonding and enhances attachment (Vlismas et al. 2013). As children grow, preferred music plays a role in establishing social group membership and selecting friends (Soley and Spelke 2016; Cirelli et al. 2018). This trend continues into adulthood when rhythmic synchronization fosters prosocial behavior and feelings of connectedness, such as among dancers in the same group (Savage et al. 2021; Curzel et al. 2024). At a neural level, several mechanisms, including sensory-motor coupling (Harry et al. 2023), reward processes (Savage et al. 2021) (see Sects. 3.2.2 and 3.2.4), and the endogenous opioid system and oxytocin release (Chanda and Levitin 2013) are implicated in music-related prosociality. Thus, from infancy through adulthood, music continues to play a pivotal role in forming and maintaining social bonds, fostering a sense of belonging within communities, and enabling groups of individuals to synchronize their moods, emotions, actions, and perspectives.

3.3 The Case of Musical Expertise

Playing a musical instrument is a multifaceted activity that engages several cognitive, emotional, and motor functions, which likely stimulate diverse neural processes over years of training. Specifically, the intense engagement of motor, perceptual, and visual systems along with multimodal integration processes required during musical practice has been shown to shape musicians' brains through neuroplasticity mechanisms (Schlaug 2015). In particular, learning to play a musical instrument is associated with distinct changes in both white and gray matter architecture (Olszewska et al. 2021). Regarding white matter, differences between musicians and nonmusicians have been observed in regions linked to fine motor control and sensory processing. For instance, musically trained subjects (as compared to nontrained) have been found to exhibit a higher volume and enhanced microstructure of the arcuate fasciculus, a crucial white-matter tract connecting temporal and frontal brain regions involved in sound perception and production (Halwani et al. 2011). Likewise, musicians have shown increased connectivity in the corpus callosum, a group of fibers connecting motor-related areas of the hemispheres (first evidenced by Schlaug et al. 1995). In addition, musical training strongly influences the organization of gray matter in multiple brain networks related to sensory processing and higher-order cognitive function. For instance, musicians have been found to present greater cortical thickness than nonmusicians, with peaks in superior temporal and dorsolateral frontal regions (Bermudez et al. 2009). Interestingly, in another study, pianists (compared to non-musicians) presented a pattern of both increase and decrease of gray matter associated with expertise. More specifically, they showed decreased gray matter volume in areas related to sensorimotor control, auditory processing, and score reading (i.e., in the right supramarginal, right superior temporal, and right postcentral gyri), while increased gray matter volume in a network involved in the reinforcement of learning (i.e., in bilateral putamen with hippocampus and amygdala, right thalamus, bilateral lingual gyri and left superior temporal gyrus). Furthermore, these neuroplastic adaptations were also dependent on the age of musical training onset, as pianists with an early onset of piano playing showed smaller gray matter volume in the right putamen and better piano performance (Vaquero et al. 2016).

Altogether, these findings underscore the profound impact of musical training on brain structure. As a result, various cognitive processes influenced by music training have been observed to be enhanced in musicians (the so-called transfer effect). At a perceptual level, musicians (vs. nonmusicians) distinguished better among different melodies and had more precise predictive processing (Vuust et al. 2022). For instance, musicians demonstrated better performance at detecting unexpected rhythmic violations compared to nonmusicians. At the neural level, this improvement is reflected in a shorter latency of the event-related potential mismatch-negativity to violations (Vuust et al. 2009). Musicians also exhibited a stronger representation of metrical structures (Palmer and Krumhansl 1990) and better performance in processing both temporal and nontemporal rhythmic features. In this case, their fine temporal predictions might be enabled by their precise body control and the series of statistical regularities learned from practice and study (Novembre and Keller 2018).

Detection of incongruities and prediction mechanisms are present in both music and language (see also Sect. 3.2.3). Intriguingly, children and adults with music training (compared to non-music-trained subjects) showed higher sensitivity to violations of both linguistic and musical syntax (Fitzroy and Sanders 2013). In addition, musically trained adults demonstrated better semantic processing, but not phonological processing, than individuals without training (Yu et al. 2017), while expert musicians exhibited superior pitch processing in both music and language compared to nonmusicians (Schön et al. 2004). As both music and language are based on statistical learning mechanisms (see also Sect. 3.2.3), the transfer effect of music on language might be explained by musicians' better ability to form mental representations of statistical structure based on predictions and expectations (Schön et al. 2008). Another explanation of this effect is provided by the OPERA hypothesis (Patel 2011). According to this hypothesis, the transfer effect occurs due to the Overlapping of subcortical and cortical networks in acoustic features of both music and speech, the higher Precision of processing in these networks in music (being more demanding than speech), the elicitation of Emotions in response to music due also to the frequent Repetition requested by musical activities, and their association with focused Attention.

Besides language, a positive transfer effect has also been identified in memory processes, with musicians performing better than nonmusicians in retrieving tonal stimuli but also in recalling verbal and, in some cases, visuospatial stimuli during working and long-term verbal memory tasks (e.g., Franklin et al. 2008; see Talamini et al. 2017 for a meta-analysis). In addition, musicians benefit from their expertise in nonmusical visuospatial (Sluming et al. 2007; Patston et al. 2007) and attentional skills (Talamini et al. 2017; Criscuolo et al. 2019).

Although the transfer effect of musical expertise on nonmusical cognitive skills constitutes a highly debated topic in literature (see Sala and Gobet 2020; Bigand and Tillmann 2022; Schellenberg and Lima 2024), converging evidence points to music-driven neuroplastic changes, also reflected in improved behavior. In light of the neural and cognitive advantages of music training, and considering the earlier discussion about the engagement of several cognitive processes during musical experiences, a natural next step would be to explore if and how music interventions could effectively serve as a neurocognitive stimulation tool in both clinical and educational settings.

3.4 Neuroscience-Based Music Interventions

All the neuroscientific evidence presented so far forms an ideal foundation for music-applied research in clinical settings. Indeed, music activities engage the whole brain through various cognitive and neural operations, many of which are commonly employed in our daily lives for nonmusical activities. This has led to the growing idea that music can constitute a reliable and efficient cognitive stimulation tool.

The main findings highlighted in this chapter align with a model proposed by Koelsch (2009; borrowed from the "heuristic working factor model for music therapy" by Hillecke et al. 2005). This model attempts to identify specific factors modulating the effects of music therapy. According to Koelsch (2009), the perceptual factor, related to music's ability to shape the decoding of acoustic features, also involved in the language domain, might explain the efficacy of a musical intervention in language impairments. Thanks to the attentiveness factor, music might distract attention from negative stimuli and experiences, thus enhancing positive emotions also in case of anxiety or attention disorder. The emotional factor, related to the previously discussed musical power, might constitute an important resource for affective disorders, while the cognitive factor would explain music-driven stimulation on higher cognitive functions, such as memory and language. The interconnection and overlap between cognition and action related to music activities, constituting the behavioral factor, may enable beneficial effects in both directions, as it is for example observed in Parkinsonian patients. Finally, social engagement during music listening or playing (i.e., the interpersonal factor) makes it a communication tool promoting social cohesion and others' understanding. In line with this model and drawing from the previously discussed processes, we now provide some examples of how music can be efficiently used to stimulate, and in some cases rehabilitate cognitive functions. When focusing on music-driven sensorimotor integration processes, one of the most promising neuroscience-based music application concerns stroke patients affected by motor impairments. Music-supported therapy (MST) has been developed to aid motor recovery, employing techniques such as hitting drum pads (whether pitch-tuned or not), playing melodies on the piano, and coordinating limb movements with rhythm through rhythmic auditory stimulation (RAS; Chen 2018). In a seminal single-case study, Rojo et al. (2011) implemented MST using a midi piano and an electronic drum set emitting piano sounds to target fine and gross motor movements of the paretic upper extremity in a chronic stroke patient. Using an fMRI–TMS design study, they observed an improvement in motor quality and changes in motor cortical excitability, thus highlighting how the auditory–motor coupling leverages music's temporal regularities to enhance movement coordination and planning. In addition, the real-time manipulation of rhythmic patterns can provide feedback to adjust accuracy and quality of movements (Chen 2018). This beneficial effect could also be helpful in Parkinson's disease, where patients often experience gait issues characterized by slowness, temporal variability, and freezing, especially in sequential and rhythmic movements (Thaut et al. 2019). Accordingly, RAS training, which synchronizes gait movements to predictable time cues, has been shown to improve key gait kinematics in Parkinson's patients (Thaut et al. 2019) with long-lasting effects (Benoit et al. 2014).

We previously considered the intrinsic link between music and language. Among the music-based applications in this domain, dyslexia is one of the most investigated. Dyslexia is a learning disability affecting spelling and print decoding abilities in the absence of other comorbidities, resulting in a core phonological deficit related to a deficit in temporal processing (Goswami 2011). Hornickel and Kraus (2013) claimed that poor readers have an impaired representation of the fine structure of speech sound necessary for articulation. Importantly, children with musical training have shown enhanced verbal intelligence compared to nonmusically trained children, with better detection of pitch changes in speech, higher reading abilities, and a better ability to segment a new language (Moreno et al. 2011). Thus, researchers have provided proof of the positive effect of musical training on dyslexics' reading skills and phonological awareness, attributing improvements to enhanced rhythmical and metrical abilities (Flaugnacco et al. 2014, 2015). Music interventions have also been implemented with aphasic patients and have been shown to enhance functional communication, repetition, and naming abilities (Racette 2006; Liu et al. 2022). In this context, the singing-based melodic intonation therapy (MIT), widely utilized for aphasia, apraxia of speech, and articulation disorders, offers potential benefits through several mechanisms. The significant results observed with MIT in patients can be attributed to the neural overlaps in music and language representations, the neuroplastic reorganization of language function, the activation of an auditory–vocal pathway to improve articulatory motor function, and the modulation of positive emotions through music listening (Merrett et al. 2014).

The emotional engagement facilitated by music makes it an excellent tool for modulating moods in cases of depressive and anxiety symptoms. Music interventions, when combined with standard treatments, have been shown to offer short-term benefits for people with depression compared to standard treatment alone (for a review, see Aalbers et al. 2017). Similarly, Särkämö and colleagues (2008) observed that stroke patients participating in music interventions during rehabilitation exhibited better recovery in verbal memory and focused attention, along with reduced feelings of depression and confusion, compared to those undergoing an audiobook intervention. Accordingly, music interventions have been further shown as particularly beneficial for Alzheimer patients, who can also benefit from musical interventions (for a review, see Matziorinis and Koelsch 2022), particularly concerning memory and emotional processes. Alzheimer's disease (AD), a progressive neurodegenerative disorder widely prevalent among elderly individuals, is characterized by impairments in several cognitive domains (e.g., memory, visuospatial ability, executive function, language, and speech production), as well as by behavioral and psychological symptoms of dementia, such as depression, anxiety, apathy, and difficulties in emotional control. Despite difficulties in recalling autobiographically salient information, AD patients often retain the ability to recognize familiar melodies and to sing with music even without song recognition (Cuddy et al. 2015). Therefore, memory for music remains relatively spared in these patients. Jacobsen et al. (2015) found that brain regions (i.e., pre-supplementary motor area and caudal anterior cingulate cortex) involved in musical memory and music-evoked emotions are the last to degenerate in this disease. Moreover, music-evoked emotions activate the anterior hippocampal formation, a brain region also involved in memory functions that are impaired in AD (Koelsch 2020). Furthermore and crucially, music interventions with these patients have been shown to reduce stress levels and alleviate anxiety and depression significantly (De La Rubia Ortí et al. 2018), improving also mood and quality of life compared, for example, to other recreational activities such as cooking classes (Samson et al. 2009).

All in all, the scientific evidence reviewed so far suggests that, by tapping into several cognitive processes, music interventions might constitute a useful neuro-stimulation and rehabilitation tool in several clinical domains.

3.5 Conclusions

This chapter aimed to explore music through the lens of neuroscience. A neuroscientific approach, elucidating how music influences the brain and behavior, can help music therapists better understand their practice and develop new techniques to achieve practical, functional, and enduring outcomes that extend beyond general well-being.

Throughout the different sections, we showed how much music research has benefited from new advanced research technologies (e.g., brain imaging, and brain wave recordings) along with the possibility to individualize neurological, biological, and physiological processes activated during musical experiences. Indeed, the involvement of music-related brain processes in other non-musical domains—such as movement, language, emotions, and memory—with the subsequent promotion of interaction between these networks can explain the intriguing results obtained with music therapy approaches and can guide future research. Moreover, the ability of music learning to change the brain through neuroplastic mechanisms makes it a perfect tool for clinical interventions based on music activities and training. Finally, another advantage of music in this context is its noninvasive and feasible nature compared to other equivalent pharmaceutical therapies (e.g., Huang and Huang 2023). All these benefits justify the encouraging enthusiasm of this interdisciplinary research field.

Altogether, the reviewed studies suggest that the psychological and musicological complexity of music makes it an ideal instrument for understanding how the brain works and for gaining insights into our understanding of the environment–brain interplay (Zatorre 2005). Human life is universally pervaded by music. It finds its place as much in the environment and social contexts as in the brain world of each individual, in a continuous exchange that allows music to be experienced on several levels. The neuroscientific and psychological perspective tries to explore these mechanisms, thus disclosing the opportunity to apply the benefits of music in clinical and educational fields and improving human well-being in both pathological and nonpathological contexts.

References

Aalbers S, Fusar-Poli L, Freeman RE, et al. Music therapy for depression. Cochrane Database Syst Rev. 2017;2017:CD004517. https://doi.org/10.1002/14651858.CD004517.pub3.

Aristoxenus, Macran HS. The harmonics of Aristonexus. Oxford: At the Clarendon Press; 1902.

Babiloni C, Buffo P, Vecchio F, et al. Brains "in concert": frontal oscillatory alpha rhythms and empathy in professional musicians. NeuroImage. 2012;60:105–16. https://doi.org/10.1016/j.neuroimage.2011.12.008.

Bangert M, Peschel T, Schlaug G, et al. Shared networks for auditory and motor processing in professional pianists: evidence from fMRI conjunction. NeuroImage. 2006;30:917–26. https://doi.org/10.1016/j.neuroimage.2005.10.044.

Baumann S, Koeneke S, Schmidt CF, et al. A network for audio–motor coordination in skilled pianists and non-musicians. Brain Res. 2007;1161:65–78. https://doi.org/10.1016/j.brainres.2007.05.045.

Bengtsson SL, Ullén F, Henrik Ehrsson H, et al. Listening to rhythms activates motor and premotor cortices. Cortex. 2009;45:62–71. https://doi.org/10.1016/j.cortex.2008.07.002.

Benoit C-E, Dalla Bella S, Farrugia N, et al. Musically cued gait-training improves both perceptual and motor timing in Parkinson's disease. Front Hum Neurosci. 2014;8 https://doi.org/10.3389/fnhum.2014.00494.

Bermudez P, Lerch JP, Evans AC, Zatorre RJ. Neuroanatomical correlates of musicianship as revealed by cortical thickness and voxel-based morphometry. Cereb Cortex. 2009;19:1583–96. https://doi.org/10.1093/cercor/bhn196.

Besson M, Schön D. Comparison between language and music. Ann N Y Acad Sci. 2001;930:232–58. https://doi.org/10.1111/j.1749-6632.2001.tb05736.x.

Bharucha J. The representation of harmonic structure in music: hierarchies of stability as a function of context. Cognition. 1983;13:63–102. https://doi.org/10.1016/0010-0277(83)90003-3.

Bianco R, Novembre G, Keller PE, et al. Neural networks for harmonic structure in music perception and action. NeuroImage. 2016;142:454–64. https://doi.org/10.1016/j.neuroimage.2016.08.025.

Bigand E, Tillmann B. Near and far transfer: is music special? Mem Cogn. 2022;50:339–47. https://doi.org/10.3758/s13421-021-01226-6.

Blood AJ, Zatorre RJ. Intensely pleasurable responses to music correlate with activity in brain regions implicated in reward and emotion. Proc Natl Acad Sci USA. 2001;98:11818–23. https://doi.org/10.1073/pnas.191355898.

Brown RM, Zatorre RJ, Penhune VB. Expert music performance: cognitive, neural, and developmental bases. In: Progress in brain research. Elsevier; 2015. p. 57–86.

Cannon JJ, Patel AD. How beat perception co-opts motor neurophysiology. Trends Cogn Sci. 2021;25:137–50. https://doi.org/10.1016/j.tics.2020.11.002.

Cardona G, Rodriguez-Fornells A, Nye H, et al. The impact of musical pleasure and musical hedonia on verbal episodic memory. Sci Rep. 2020;10:16113. https://doi.org/10.1038/s41598-020-72772-3.

Centomo F, Wyttenbach IM, Bencivenni A, Raglio A. Music and autobiographical memory: a new experimental protocol. Psychogeriatrics. 2023;23:547–9. https://doi.org/10.1111/psyg.12947.

Chanda ML, Levitin DJ. The neurochemistry of music. Trends Cogn Sci. 2013;17:179–93. https://doi.org/10.1016/j.tics.2013.02.007.

Chen JL. Music-supported therapy for stroke motor recovery: theoretical and practical considerations. Ann N Y Acad Sci. 2018;1423:57–65. https://doi.org/10.1111/nyas.13726.

Chen JL, Zatorre RJ, Penhune VB. Interactions between auditory and dorsal premotor cortex during synchronization to musical rhythms. NeuroImage. 2006;32:1771–81. https://doi.org/10.1016/j.neuroimage.2006.04.207.

Chen JL, Penhune VB, Zatorre RJ. Listening to musical rhythms recruits motor regions of the brain. Cereb Cortex. 2008a;18:2844–54. https://doi.org/10.1093/cercor/bhn042.

Chen JL, Penhune VB, Zatorre RJ. Moving on time: brain network for auditory-motor synchronization is modulated by rhythm complexity and musical training. J Cogn Neurosci. 2008b;20:226–39. https://doi.org/10.1162/jocn.2008.20018.

Chen JL, Rae C, Watkins KE. Learning to play a melody: an fMRI study examining the formation of auditory-motor associations. NeuroImage. 2012;59:1200–8. https://doi.org/10.1016/j.neuroimage.2011.08.012.

Chow R, Noly-Gandon A, Moussard A, et al. Effects of transcranial direct current stimulation combined with listening to preferred music on memory in older adults. Sci Rep. 2021;11:12638. https://doi.org/10.1038/s41598-021-91977-8.

Cirelli LK, Trehub SE, Trainor LJ. Rhythm and melody as social signals for infants. Ann N Y Acad Sci. 2018;1423:66–72. https://doi.org/10.1111/nyas.13580.

Criscuolo A, Bonetti L, Särkämö T, et al. On the association between musical training, intelligence and executive functions in adulthood. Front Psychol. 2019;10:1704. https://doi.org/10.3389/fpsyg.2019.01704.

Cuddy LL, Sikka R, Vanstone A. Preservation of musical memory and engagement in healthy aging and Alzheimer's disease. Ann N Y Acad Sci. 2015;1337:223–31. https://doi.org/10.1111/nyas.12617.

Curzel F, Osiurak F, Trân E, et al. Enhancing musical pleasure through shared musical experience. iScience. 2024;27:109964. https://doi.org/10.1016/j.isci.2024.109964.

Darwin C. The descent of man. D. Appleton and Company; 1871.

De La Rubia Ortí JE, García-Pardo MP, Iranzo CC, et al. Does music therapy improve anxiety and depression in Alzheimer's patients? J Altern Complement Med. 2018;24:33–6. https://doi.org/10.1089/acm.2016.0346.

Elbert T, Pantev C, Wienbruch C, et al. Increased cortical representation of the fingers of the left hand in string players. Science. 1995;270:305–7. https://doi.org/10.1126/science.270.5234.305.

Elsner B, Hommel B. Effect anticipation and action control. J Exp Psychol Hum Percept Perform. 2001;27:229–40. https://doi.org/10.1037/0096-1523.27.1.229.

Ferreri L, Rodriguez-Fornells A. Music-related reward responses predict episodic memory performance. Exp Brain Res. 2017;235:3721–31. https://doi.org/10.1007/s00221-017-5095-0.

Ferreri L, Mas-Herrero E, Zatorre RJ, et al. Dopamine modulates the reward experiences elicited by music. Proc Natl Acad Sci USA. 2019;116:3793–8. https://doi.org/10.1073/pnas.1811878116.

Ferreri L, Mas-Herrero E, Cardona G, et al. Dopamine modulations of reward-driven music memory consolidation. Ann N Y Acad Sci. 2021;1502:85–98. https://doi.org/10.1111/nyas.14656.

Fitzroy AB, Sanders LD. Musical expertise modulates early processing of syntactic violations in language. Front Psychol. 2013;3 https://doi.org/10.3389/fpsyg.2012.00603.

Flaugnacco E, Lopez L, Terribili C, et al. Rhythm perception and production predict reading abilities in developmental dyslexia. Front Hum Neurosci. 2014;8 https://doi.org/10.3389/fnhum.2014.00392.

Flaugnacco E, Lopez L, Terribili C, et al. Music training increases phonological awareness and reading skills in developmental dyslexia: a randomized control trial. PLoS One. 2015;10:e0138715. https://doi.org/10.1371/journal.pone.0138715.

Foster NEV, Zatorre RJ. A role for the intraparietal sulcus in transforming musical pitch information. Cereb Cortex. 2010;20:1350–9. https://doi.org/10.1093/cercor/bhp199.

Franklin MS, Sledge Moore K, Yip C-Y, et al. The effects of musical training on verbal memory. Psychol Music. 2008;36:353–65. https://doi.org/10.1177/0305735607086044.

Gaser C, Schlaug G. Brain structures differ between musicians and non-musicians. J Neurosci. 2003;23:9240–5. https://doi.org/10.1523/JNEUROSCI.23-27-09240.2003.

Giovannelli F, Innocenti I, Rossi S, et al. Role of the dorsal premotor cortex in rhythmic auditory-motor entrainment: a perturbational approach by rTMS. Cereb Cortex. 2014;24:1009–16. https://doi.org/10.1093/cercor/bhs386.

Gordon CL, Iacoboni M, Balasubramaniam R. Multimodal music perception engages motor prediction: a TMS study. Front Neurosci. 2018;12:736. https://doi.org/10.3389/fnins.2018.00736.

Goswami U. A temporal sampling framework for developmental dyslexia. Trends Cogn Sci. 2011;15:3–10. https://doi.org/10.1016/j.tics.2010.10.001.

Grahn JA. The role of the basal ganglia in beat perception: neuroimaging and neuropsychological investigations. Ann N Y Acad Sci. 2009;1169:35–45. https://doi.org/10.1111/j.1749-6632.2009.04553.x.

Grahn JA, Brett M. Rhythm and beat perception in motor areas of the brain. J Cogn Neurosci. 2007;19:893–906. https://doi.org/10.1162/jocn.2007.19.5.893.

Grahn JA, Rowe JB. Feeling the beat: premotor and striatal interactions in musicians and non-musicians during beat perception. J Neurosci. 2009;29:7540–8. https://doi.org/10.1523/JNEUROSCI.2018-08.2009.

Grahn JA, Rowe JB. Finding and feeling the musical beat: striatal dissociations between detection and prediction of regularity. Cereb Cortex. 2013;23:913–21. https://doi.org/10.1093/cercor/bhs083.

Granot R, Spitz DH, Cherki BR, et al. "Help! I need somebody": music as a global resource for obtaining wellbeing goals in times of crisis. Front Psychol. 2021;12:648013. https://doi.org/10.3389/fpsyg.2021.648013.

Graves JE, Pralus A, Fornoni L, et al. Short- and long-term memory for pitch and non-pitch contours: insights from congenital amusia. Brain Cogn. 2019;136:103614. https://doi.org/10.1016/j.bandc.2019.103614.

Groussard M, Viader F, Hubert V, et al. Musical and verbal semantic memory: two distinct neural networks? NeuroImage. 2010;49:2764–73. https://doi.org/10.1016/j.neuroimage.2009.10.039.

Hallam S, Cross I, Thaut M, editors. Oxford handbook of music psychology. Oxford University Press; 2012.

Halwani GF, Loui P, Rüber T, Schlaug G. Effects of practice and experience on the arcuate fasciculus: comparing singers, instrumentalists, and non-musicians. Front Psychol. 2011;2 https://doi.org/10.3389/fpsyg.2011.00156.

Harry BB, Margulies DS, Falkiewicz M, Keller PE. Brain networks for temporal adaptation, anticipation, and sensory-motor integration in rhythmic human behavior. Neuropsychologia. 2023;183:108524. https://doi.org/10.1016/j.neuropsychologia.2023.108524.

Hickok G, Poeppel D. Dorsal and ventral streams: a framework for understanding aspects of the functional anatomy of language. Cognition. 2004;92:67–99. https://doi.org/10.1016/j.cognition.2003.10.011.

Hillecke T, Nickel A, Bolay HV. Scientific perspectives on music therapy. Ann N Y Acad Sci. 2005;1060:271–82. https://doi.org/10.1196/annals.1360.020.

Hornickel J, Kraus N. Unstable representation of sound: a biological marker of dyslexia. J Neurosci. 2013;33:3500–4. https://doi.org/10.1523/JNEUROSCI.4205-12.2013.

Huang E, Huang J. Music therapy: a noninvasive treatment to reduce anxiety and pain of colorectal cancer patients – a systemic literature review. Medicina. 2023;59:482. https://doi.org/10.3390/medicina59030482.

Jacobsen J-H, Stelzer J, Fritz TH, et al. Why musical memory can be preserved in advanced Alzheimer's disease. Brain. 2015;138:2438–50. https://doi.org/10.1093/brain/awv135.

Jakobson LS, Lewycky ST, Kilgour AR, Stoesz BM. Memory for verbal and visual material in highly trained musicians. Music Percept. 2008;26:41–55. https://doi.org/10.1525/mp.2008.26.1.41.

Jakubowski K, Ghosh A. Music-evoked autobiographical memories in everyday life. Psychol Music. 2021;49:649–66. https://doi.org/10.1177/0305735619888803.

Janata P. The neural architecture of music-evoked autobiographical memories. Cereb Cortex. 2009;19:2579–94. https://doi.org/10.1093/cercor/bhp008.

Janata P. Neural basis of music perception. In: Handbook of clinical neurology. Elsevier; 2015. p. 187–205.
Janata P, Tomic ST, Rakowski SK. Characterisation of music-evoked autobiographical memories. Memory. 2007;15:845–60. https://doi.org/10.1080/09658210701734593.
Jäncke L. Music, memory and emotion. J Biol. 2008;7:21. https://doi.org/10.1186/jbiol82.
Juslin PN, Sloboda JA, editors. Music and emotion: theory and research. Oxford/New York: Oxford University Press; 2001.
Juslin PN, Västfjäll D. Emotional responses to music: the need to consider underlying mechanisms. Behav Brain Sci. 2008;31:559–75. https://doi.org/10.1017/S0140525X08005293.
Karpati FJ, Giacosa C, Foster NEV, et al. Dance and music share gray matter structural correlates. Brain Res. 2017;1657:62–73. https://doi.org/10.1016/j.brainres.2016.11.029.
Koelsch S. A neuroscientific perspective on music therapy. Ann N Y Acad Sci. 2009;1169:374–84. https://doi.org/10.1111/j.1749-6632.2009.04592.x.
Koelsch S. Toward a neural basis of music perception – a review and updated model. Front Psychol. 2011;2 https://doi.org/10.3389/fpsyg.2011.00110.
Koelsch S. Brain and music. Wiley Blackwell; 2012.
Koelsch S. Brain correlates of music-evoked emotions. Nat Rev Neurosci. 2014;15:170–80. https://doi.org/10.1038/nrn3666.
Koelsch S. A coordinate-based meta-analysis of music-evoked emotions. NeuroImage. 2020;223:117350. https://doi.org/10.1016/j.neuroimage.2020.117350.
Koelsch S, Gunter TC, Schröger E, et al. Differentiating ERAN and MMN: an ERP study. Neuroreport. 2001;12:1385–9. https://doi.org/10.1097/00001756-200105250-00019.
Koelsch S, Kasper E, Sammler D, et al. Music, language and meaning: brain signatures of semantic processing. Nat Neurosci. 2004;7:302–7. https://doi.org/10.1038/nn1197.
Koelsch S, Fritz T, Schulze K, et al. Adults and children processing music: an fMRI study. NeuroImage. 2005a;25:1068–76. https://doi.org/10.1016/j.neuroimage.2004.12.050.
Koelsch S, Gunter TC, Wittfoth M, Sammler D. Interaction between syntax processing in language and in music: an ERP study. J Cogn Neurosci. 2005b;17:1565–77. https://doi.org/10.1162/089892905774597290.
Kung S-J, Chen JL, Zatorre RJ, Penhune VB. Interacting cortical and basal ganglia networks underlying finding and tapping to the musical beat. J Cogn Neurosci. 2013;25:401–20. https://doi.org/10.1162/jocn_a_00325.
Lahav A, Saltzman E, Schlaug G. Action representation of sound: Audiomotor recognition network while listening to newly acquired actions. J Neurosci. 2007;27:308–14. https://doi.org/10.1523/JNEUROSCI.4822-06.2007.
Large EW. Resonating to musical rhythm: theory and experiment. In: Grondin S, editor. The psychology of time. Cambridge: Emerald; 2008. p. 189–231.
Lega C, Stephan MA, Zatorre RJ, Penhune V. Testing the role of dorsal premotor cortex in auditory-motor association learning using Transcranical Magnetic Stimulation (TMS). PLoS One. 2016a;11:e0163380. https://doi.org/10.1371/journal.pone.0163380.
Lega C, Vecchi T, D'Angelo E, Cattaneo Z. A TMS investigation on the role of the cerebellum in pitch and timbre discrimination. Cerebellum Ataxias. 2016b;3:6. https://doi.org/10.1186/s40673-016-0044-4.
Lense MD, Shultz S, Astésano C, Jones W. Music of infant-directed singing entrains infants' social visual behavior. Proc Natl Acad Sci USA. 2022;119:e2116967119. https://doi.org/10.1073/pnas.2116967119.
Levitin DJ, Grahn JA, London J. The psychology of music: rhythm and movement. Annu Rev Psychol. 2018;69:51–75. https://doi.org/10.1146/annurev-psych-122216-011740.
Liu Q, Li W, Yin Y, et al. The effect of music therapy on language recovery in patients with aphasia after stroke: a systematic review and meta-analysis. Neurol Sci. 2022;43:863–72. https://doi.org/10.1007/s10072-021-05743-9.
Maess B, Koelsch S, Gunter TC, Friederici AD. Musical syntax is processed in Broca's area: an MEG study. Nat Neurosci. 2001;4:540–5. https://doi.org/10.1038/87502.

Mansouri FA, Acevedo N, Illipparampil R, et al. Interactive effects of music and prefrontal cortex stimulation in modulating response inhibition. Sci Rep. 2017;7:18096. https://doi.org/10.1038/s41598-017-18119-x.

Martínez-Molina N, Mas-Herrero E, Rodríguez-Fornells A, et al. Neural correlates of specific musical anhedonia. Proc Natl Acad Sci USA. 2016;113:E7337. https://doi.org/10.1073/pnas.1611211113.

Martínez-Molina N, Mas-Herrero E, Rodríguez-Fornells A, et al. White matter microstructure reflects individual differences in music reward sensitivity. J Neurosci. 2019;39:5018–27. https://doi.org/10.1523/JNEUROSCI.2020-18.2019.

Mas-Herrero E, Marco-Pallares J, Lorenzo-Seva U, et al. Individual differences in music reward experiences. Music Percept. 2013;31:118–38. https://doi.org/10.1525/mp.2013.31.2.118.

Mas-Herrero E, Dagher A, Zatorre RJ. Modulating musical reward sensitivity up and down with transcranial magnetic stimulation. Nat Hum Behav. 2017;2:27–32. https://doi.org/10.1038/s41562-017-0241-z.

Mas-Herrero E, Dagher A, Farrés-Franch M, Zatorre RJ. Unraveling the temporal dynamics of reward signals in music-induced pleasure with TMS. J Neurosci. 2021;41:3889–99. https://doi.org/10.1523/JNEUROSCI.0727-20.2020.

Mas-Herrero E, Ferreri L, Cardona G, et al. The role of opioid transmission in music-induced pleasure. Ann N Y Acad Sci. 2023;1520:105–14. https://doi.org/10.1111/nyas.14946.

Matziorinis AM, Koelsch S. The promise of music therapy for Alzheimer's disease: a review. Ann N Y Acad Sci. 2022;1516:11–7. https://doi.org/10.1111/nyas.14864.

Mauss IB, Levenson RW, McCarter L, et al. The tie that binds? Coherence among emotion experience, behavior, and physiology. Emotion. 2005;5:175–90. https://doi.org/10.1037/1528-3542.5.2.175.

Merrett DL, Peretz I, Wilson SJ. Neurobiological, cognitive, and emotional mechanisms in melodic intonation therapy. Front Hum Neurosci. 2014;8 https://doi.org/10.3389/fnhum.2014.00401.

Miller G. Evolution of human music through sexual selection. In: Wallin NL, Merker B, Brown S, editors. The origins of music. The MIT Press; 1999. p. 329–60.

Moreno S, Bialystok E, Barac R, et al. Short-term music training enhances verbal intelligence and executive function. Psychol Sci. 2011;22:1425–33. https://doi.org/10.1177/0956797611416999.

Nguyen T, Flaten E, Trainor LJ, Novembre G. Early social communication through music: state of the art and future perspectives. Dev Cogn Neurosci. 2023;63:101279. https://doi.org/10.1016/j.dcn.2023.101279.

Novembre G, Keller PE. Music and action. In: Bader R, editor. Springer handbook of systematic musicology. Berlin/Heidelberg: Springer; 2018. p. 523–37.

Nozaradan S, Peretz I, Missal M, Mouraux A. Tagging the neuronal entrainment to beat and meter. J Neurosci. 2011;31:10234–40. https://doi.org/10.1523/JNEUROSCI.0411-11.2011.

Olszewska AM, Gaca M, Herman AM, et al. How musical training shapes the adult brain: predispositions and neuroplasticity. Front Neurosci. 2021;15:630829. https://doi.org/10.3389/fnins.2021.630829.

Palmer C, Krumhansl CL. Mental representations for musical meter. J Exp Psychol Hum Percept Perform. 1990;16:728–41. https://doi.org/10.1037/0096-1523.16.4.728.

Patel AD. Language, music, syntax and the brain. Nat Neurosci. 2003;6:674–81. https://doi.org/10.1038/nn1082.

Patel AD. Why would musical training benefit the neural encoding of speech? The OPERA hypothesis. Front Psychol. 2011;2 https://doi.org/10.3389/fpsyg.2011.00142.

Patel AD, Iversen JR. The evolutionary neuroscience of musical beat perception: the Action Simulation for Auditory Prediction (ASAP) hypothesis. Front Syst Neurosci. 2014;8 https://doi.org/10.3389/fnsys.2014.00057.

Patel AD, Gibson E, Ratner J, et al. Processing syntactic relations in language and music: an event-related potential study. J Cogn Neurosci. 1998;10:717–33. https://doi.org/10.1162/089892998563121.

Patston LLM, Hogg SL, Tippett LJ. Attention in musicians is more bilateral than in non-musicians. Laterality: asymmetries of body. Brain Cogn. 2007;12:262–72. https://doi.org/10.1080/13576500701251981.

Peretz I. Neurobiology of congenital amusia. Trends Cogn Sci. 2016;20:857–67. https://doi.org/10.1016/j.tics.2016.09.002.

Peretz I, Vuvan D, Lagrois M-É, Armony JL. Neural overlap in processing music and speech. Philos Trans R Soc B. 2015;370:20140090. https://doi.org/10.1098/rstb.2014.0090.

Pinker S. How the mind works. Ann N Y Acad Sci. 1999;882:119–27. https://doi.org/10.1111/j.1749-6632.1999.tb08538.x.

Platel H, Baron J-C, Desgranges B, et al. Semantic and episodic memory of music are subserved by distinct neural networks. NeuroImage. 2003;20:244–56. https://doi.org/10.1016/S1053-8119(03)00287-8.

Proksch S, Comstock DC, Médé B, et al. Motor and predictive processes in auditory beat and rhythm perception. Front Hum Neurosci. 2020;14:578546. https://doi.org/10.3389/fnhum.2020.578546.

Racette A. Making non-fluent aphasics speak: sing along! Brain. 2006;129:2571–84. https://doi.org/10.1093/brain/awl250.

Rauschecker JP. An expanded role for the dorsal auditory pathway in sensorimotor control and integration. Hear Res. 2011;271:16–25. https://doi.org/10.1016/j.heares.2010.09.001.

Rohrmeier MA, Koelsch S. Predictive information processing in music cognition. A critical review. Int J Psychophysiol. 2012;83:164–75. https://doi.org/10.1016/j.ijpsycho.2011.12.010.

Rojo N, Amengual J, Juncadella M, et al. Music-supported therapy induces plasticity in the sensorimotor cortex in chronic stroke: a single-case study using multimodal imaging (fMRI-TMS). Brain Inj. 2011;25:787–93. https://doi.org/10.3109/02699052.2011.576305.

Roland PE, Skinhøj E, Lassen NA. Focal activations of human cerebral cortex during auditory discrimination. J Neurophysiol. 1981;45:1139–51. https://doi.org/10.1152/jn.1981.45.6.1139.

Ross JM, Iversen JR, Balasubramaniam R. Motor simulation theories of musical beat perception. Neurocase. 2016;22:558–65. https://doi.org/10.1080/13554794.2016.1242756.

Ross JM, Iversen J, Balasubramaniam R. Dorsal premotor contributions to auditory rhythm perception: causal transcranial magnetic stimulation studies of interval, tempo, and phase. 2018a.

Ross JM, Iversen JR, Balasubramaniam R. The role of posterior parietal cortex in beat-based timing perception: a continuous theta burst stimulation study. J Cogn Neurosci. 2018b;30:634–43. https://doi.org/10.1162/jocn_a_01237.

Russell JA. A circumplex model of affect. J Pers Soc Psychol. 1980;39:1161–78. https://doi.org/10.1037/h0077714.

Sala G, Gobet F. Cognitive and academic benefits of music training with children: a multilevel meta-analysis. Mem Cogn. 2020;48:1429–41. https://doi.org/10.3758/s13421-020-01060-2.

Salimpoor VN, Benovoy M, Larcher K, et al. Anatomically distinct dopamine release during anticipation and experience of peak emotion to music. Nat Neurosci. 2011;14:257–62. https://doi.org/10.1038/nn.2726.

Sammler D, Koelsch S, Ball T, et al. Co-localizing linguistic and musical syntax with intracranial EEG. NeuroImage. 2013;64:134–46. https://doi.org/10.1016/j.neuroimage.2012.09.035.

Samson S, Dellacherie D, Platel H. Emotional power of music in patients with memory disorders: clinical implications of cognitive neuroscience. Ann N Y Acad Sci. 2009;1169:245–55. https://doi.org/10.1111/j.1749-6632.2009.04555.x.

Sarkamo T, Tervaniemi M, Laitinen S, et al. Music listening enhances cognitive recovery and mood after middle cerebral artery stroke. Brain. 2008;131:866–76. https://doi.org/10.1093/brain/awn013.

Savage PE, Loui P, Tarr B, et al. Music as a coevolved system for social bonding. Behav Brain Sci. 2021;44:e59. https://doi.org/10.1017/S0140525X20000333.

Schellenberg EG, Lima CF. Music training and nonmusical abilities. Annu Rev Psychol. 2024;75:87–128. https://doi.org/10.1146/annurev-psych-032323-051354.

Schlaug G. Musicians and music making as a model for the study of brain plasticity. In: Progress in brain research. Elsevier; 2015. p. 37–55.

Schlaug G, Jäncke L, Huang Y, et al. Increased corpus callosum size in musicians. Neuropsychologia. 1995;33:1047–55. https://doi.org/10.1016/0028-3932(95)00045-5.

Schmuckler MA, Moranis R. Rhythm contour drives musical memory. Atten Percept Psychophys. 2023;85:2502–14. https://doi.org/10.3758/s13414-023-02700-w.

Schön D, Magne C, Besson M. The music of speech: music training facilitates pitch processing in both music and language. Psychophysiology. 2004;41:341–9. https://doi.org/10.1111/1469-8986.00172.x.

Schön D, Boyer M, Moreno S, et al. Songs as an aid for language acquisition. Cognition. 2008;106:975–83. https://doi.org/10.1016/j.cognition.2007.03.005.

Shaw D, Hill D. A case of musicogenic epilepsy. J Neurol Neurosurg Psychiatry. 1947;10:107–17. https://doi.org/10.1136/jnnp.10.3.107.

Siman-Tov T, Gordon CR, Avisdris N, et al. The rediscovered motor-related area 55b emerges as a core hub of music perception. Commun Biol. 2022;5:1104. https://doi.org/10.1038/s42003-022-04009-0.

Slevc LR, Okada BM. Processing structure in language and music: a case for shared reliance on cognitive control. Psychon Bull Rev. 2015;22:637–52. https://doi.org/10.3758/s13423-014-0712-4.

Slevc LR, Rosenberg JC, Patel AD. Making psycholinguistics musical: self-paced reading time evidence for shared processing of linguistic and musical syntax. Psychon Bull Rev. 2009;16:374–81. https://doi.org/10.3758/16.2.374.

Sluming V, Brooks J, Howard M, et al. Broca's area supports enhanced visuospatial cognition in orchestral musicians. J Neurosci. 2007;27:3799–806. https://doi.org/10.1523/JNEUROSCI.0147-07.2007.

Soley G, Spelke ES. Shared cultural knowledge: effects of music on young children's social preferences. Cognition. 2016;148:106–16. https://doi.org/10.1016/j.cognition.2015.09.017.

Spencer RMC, Ivry RB. Cerebellum and timing. In: Manto M, Schmahmann JD, Rossi F, et al., editors. Handbook of the cerebellum and cerebellar disorders. Dordrecht: Springer; 2013. p. 1201–19.

Stephan MA, Lega C, Penhune VB. Auditory prediction cues motor preparation in the absence of movements. NeuroImage. 2018;174:288–96. https://doi.org/10.1016/j.neuroimage.2018.03.044.

Stupacher J, Hove MJ, Novembre G, et al. Musical groove modulates motor cortex excitability: a TMS investigation. Brain Cogn. 2013;82:127–36. https://doi.org/10.1016/j.bandc.2013.03.003.

Swain JP. The concept of musical syntax. Music Q. 1995;79:281–308. https://doi.org/10.1093/mq/79.2.281.

Talamini F, Altoè G, Carretti B, Grassi M. Musicians have better memory than nonmusicians: a meta-analysis. PLoS One. 2017;12:e0186773. https://doi.org/10.1371/journal.pone.0186773.

Tarr B, Launay J, Dunbar RIM. Music and social bonding: "self-other" merging and neurohormonal mechanisms. Front Psychol. 2014;5 https://doi.org/10.3389/fpsyg.2014.01096.

Thaut M, Donald AH, editors. The Oxford handbook of music and the brain. Oxford: Oxford University Press; 2018.

Thaut M, Hoemberg V. Handbook of neurologic music therapy. Oxford University Press; 2014.

Thaut MH, Rice RR, Braun Janzen T, et al. Rhythmic auditory stimulation for reduction of falls in Parkinson's disease: a randomized controlled study. Clin Rehabil. 2019;33:34–43. https://doi.org/10.1177/0269215518788615.

Tillmann B, Janata P, Bharucha JJ. Activation of the inferior frontal cortex in musical priming. Ann N Y Acad Sci. 2003;999:209–11. https://doi.org/10.1196/annals.1284.031.

Tillmann B, Albouy P, Caclin A. Congenital amusias. In: Handbook of clinical neurology. Elsevier; 2015. p. 589–605.

Toiviainen P, Burunat I, Brattico E, et al. The chronnectome of musical beat. NeuroImage. 2020;216:116191. https://doi.org/10.1016/j.neuroimage.2019.116191.

Trainor LJ, Hannon EE. Musical development. In: The psychology of music. Elsevier; 2013. p. 423–97.
Tulving E. Episodic and semantic memory. In: Tulving E, Donaldson W, editors. Organization of memory. Academic; 1972.
Vaquero L, Hartmann K, Ripollés P, et al. Structural neuroplasticity in expert pianists depends on the age of musical training onset. NeuroImage. 2016;126:106–19. https://doi.org/10.1016/j.neuroimage.2015.11.008.
Vaquero L, Rousseau P-N, Vozian D, et al. What you learn & when you learn it: impact of early bilingual & music experience on the structural characteristics of auditory-motor pathways. NeuroImage. 2020;213:116689. https://doi.org/10.1016/j.neuroimage.2020.116689.
Vines BW, Schnider NM, Schlaug G. Testing for causality with transcranial direct current stimulation: pitch memory and the left supramarginal gyrus. Neuroreport. 2006;17:1047–50. https://doi.org/10.1097/01.wnr.0000223396.05070.a2.
Vlismas W, Malloch S, Burnham D. The effects of music and movement on mother–infant interactions. Early Child Dev Care. 2013;183:1669–88. https://doi.org/10.1080/03004430.2012.746968.
Vuust P, Ostergaard L, Pallesen KJ, et al. Predictive coding of music – brain responses to rhythmic incongruity. Cortex. 2009;45:80–92. https://doi.org/10.1016/j.cortex.2008.05.014.
Vuust P, Heggli OA, Friston KJ, Kringelbach ML. Music in the brain. Nat Rev Neurosci. 2022;23:287–305. https://doi.org/10.1038/s41583-022-00578-5.
Warren JD, Uppenkamp S, Patterson RD, Griffiths TD. Separating pitch chroma and pitch height in the human brain. Proc Natl Acad Sci USA. 2003;100:10038–42. https://doi.org/10.1073/pnas.1730682100.
Watanabe T, Yagishita S, Kikyo H. Memory of music: roles of right hippocampus and left inferior frontal gyrus. NeuroImage. 2008;39:483–91. https://doi.org/10.1016/j.neuroimage.2007.08.024.
Wilkins RW, Hodges DA, Laurienti PJ, et al. Network science and the effects of music preference on functional brain connectivity: from Beethoven to Eminem. Sci Rep. 2014;4:6130. https://doi.org/10.1038/srep06130.
Wollman I, Penhune V, Segado M, et al. Neural network retuning and neural predictors of learning success associated with cello training. Proc Natl Acad Sci USA. 2018;115:E6056. https://doi.org/10.1073/pnas.1721414115.
Yu M, Xu M, Li X, et al. The shared neural basis of music and language. Neuroscience. 2017;357:208–19. https://doi.org/10.1016/j.neuroscience.2017.06.003.
Zatorre R. Music, the food of neuroscience? Nature. 2005;434:312–5. https://doi.org/10.1038/434312a.
Zatorre RJ, Salimpoor VN. From perception to pleasure: music and its neural substrates. Proc Natl Acad Sci USA. 2013;110:10430–7. https://doi.org/10.1073/pnas.1301228110.
Zatorre RJ, Chen JL, Penhune VB. When the brain plays music: auditory–motor interactions in music perception and production. Nat Rev Neurosci. 2007;8:547–58. https://doi.org/10.1038/nrn2152.

Neurobiological Bases of Music Therapy and Music-Based Interventions

4

Enzo Grossi

Key Points

- There is a growing interest in the use of music in medicine. Music and medicine were closely linked as early as 2000 BC.
- This connection has travelled through history to reach us. In the last 80 years, science has entered the mainstream as the incredible number of scientific articles appearing in the literature shows: 37,000 scientific articles in general, of which 10,000 in the last three years, over 9000 papers on music therapy, over 4000 randomized clinical trials published, and about 900 of meta-analyses.
- Thanks to this extensive scientific literature, it has been possible to document the impact of music on brain areas. The effects have a specific molecular basis based on the activation of complex brain circuits and the release of neurochemical mediators.
- Pain is the main target of therapeutic musical intervention. Particular areas of combating pain with musical listening are cancer pain and labor in childbirth.
- A series of systematic reviews of randomized controlled trials have demonstrated the beneficial effects of music therapy in children with neuropsychiatric disorders and in adults with dementia and neurological disorders needing rehabilitation.
- The recent discipline called "Neurologic Music Therapy" uses musical exercises for the rehabilitation of upper and lower limb movement in very important diseases such as stroke, Parkinson's, and multiple sclerosis.

(continued)

E. Grossi (✉)
Villa Santa Maria Foundation, Tavernerio, CO, Italy
e-mail: enzo.grossi@bracco.com

A. Raglio (ed.), *Music and Music Therapy Interventions in Clinical Practice*, Neurocultural Health and Wellbeing,
https://doi.org/10.1007/978-3-031-88578-5_4

- At social level there is an extensive literature on the potential role of music and group singing sessions in strengthening social bonds, fostering prosocial behavior, group identity, and at the same time breaking down cultural, ethnic, or religious barriers.

4.1 Introduction

Music is part of human nature. Every human culture we know has music, which suggests that, throughout history, humans have had music as a companion in life.

The first documented traces of the use of flutes made from animal bones date back to Neanderthal man (40,000–50,000 years ago). However, it is highly probable that already 100–200,000 years ago, early hominids made musical instruments such as drums and flutes and made music cooperatively.

A flute made from the wing bone of a vulture was found in the Geißenklösterle cave in Bavaria.

It is comforting to know that during the long, cold winters of the last Ice Age, the ancestors of the people who populated present-day Germany could enjoy the uplifting music of the flute.

The healing power of sounds has been known since ancient times and is also often found in mythology.

In ancient Egypt, for example, it was normal to use music in temples to heal the sick; there are hundreds of musical references in the Bible; Aristotle in "Around the Soul" describes the soothing power of the sound of the flute; Hippocrates and Celsus played music for patients with mental illnesses.

As evidence of the concept of a strong link between music and medicine, it is interesting to note that the Chinese character for medicine is derived from that used for music, or vice versa.

This tells us that music and medicine were closely linked as early as 2000 BC (Fig. 4.1).

Today, we know that music can be considered an effective healing tool in all ages of life and in numerous clinical areas.

Important clinical studies increasingly show that sound and music stimulate and regulate emotions, attention, cognitive functions, communication, and behavior.

Sound and music foster connections between the hemispheres of the brain, stimulating and regulating emotions, attention span, cognitive functions,

Fig. 4.1 Chinese ideograms for medicine and music

藥	樂
Medicine	Music

communication, and behavior. Listening to music frequently can help reduce stress, counter chronic pain, and recover motor and neurological functions that have been damaged by a stroke or traumatic event. In the case of children on the autistic spectrum or with attention deficit and language difficulties, music is a resource for learning and relationships.

Music has among the arts the largest body of solid scientific evidence under the form of randomized controlled studies, evidence that has produced growing interest in many medical, social, and psychological fields.

Just to give a general idea, the number of randomized trials on music listening in the medical field, either direct or mediated by a music therapist in the world's top ten countries is over 1500.

Over the past three decades, modern experimental methods have been used to establish whether the beneficial effects of music are genuine and whether they are attributable to music per se, rather than to ancillary or confounding factors.

Available evidence from randomized clinical trials shows that music can elicit the secretion of neuro mediators and neuro hormones that can modulate many neurophysiological activities underlying various clinical outcomes such as pain, anxiety, stress, and depression (Chanda and Levitin 2013).

4.2 Brain and Music

Thanks to neuroimaging tools such as EEG, MEG, functional magnetic resonance imaging (fMRI) and near infrared spectroscopy (NIRS), and thanks to an extensive scientific literature, it has been possible to document the impact of music on brain areas.

It has been seen, for example, that in children, musical engagement is able to stimulate not only the auditory area, but also many other parts of the brain that have to do with sight, sensation, balance, dexterity, movement, language, emotionality, and behavior. The neurophysiological mechanisms are quite complex, and many neuroscientists are trying to reconstruct the underlying pattern of interconnections to which these effects are due.

In general, whenever one has an aesthetic experience involving any artistic form that gives a sense of pleasantness, the stress hormone cortisol "drops" as does anxiety. In the specific case of music, in the act of listening to a melody or sounds, the vibrations of the eardrum are transmitted to the cochlea, the organ of hearing, in the inner ear, and from there the acoustic nerves carry these signals to the area of the cortex responsible for receiving these stimuli, the auditory cortex, in the temporal lobe.

Here already occurs an integration of many different types of elements, which are part of music in the broadest sense, from the notes to their sequence, to harmony—to timbre, which is related to the instrument or medium that produces the note, to rhythm. When the mixture of these characteristics reaches a complexity that makes the whole thing pleasant, beautiful, we instinctively feel a sense of fulfilment. On a physiological level, what is stimulated is a center of the brain in the central cortex, which evolved with the human species and probably did not exist at the time of Homo Heidelbergensis, a hominid who lived hundreds of thousands of years ago, before Neanderthal man and

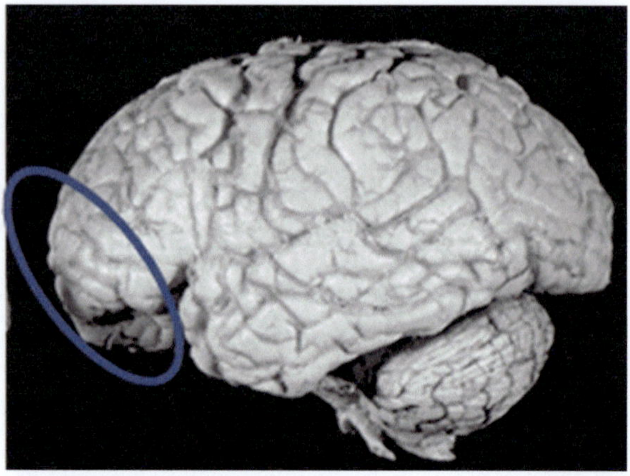

Fig. 4.2 Brain localization of beauty center in medial orbitofrontal cortex (OFC)

Homo sapiens. This center has been called the center of beauty by Semir Zeki, as it integrates sensations of various kinds that our species judges to be beautiful, be they visual, olfactory, gustatory, and even auditory (Ishizu and Zeki 2011). The stimulation of this center, which is located in the orbitofrontal cortex (Fig. 4.2), reverberates in other centers of the brain, and in particular in the basal nuclei, ancestral centers (therefore ancient at an evolutionary level) that, when activated, bring into play neuromediators, i.e., chemical substances to which we owe the various sensations of peace, contentment, and pleasantness that we experience when we appreciate beautiful music. In the brain first, and then throughout the body, molecules such as dopamine, oxytocin, serotonin, and endorphins are in fact put into circulation, each of which can interfere in various ways with anxiety, stress, and depression.

4.3 Molecular Mechanisms Underlying the Medical Effects of Music

Neurochemistry allows us to appreciate how particular neuromediators and neurohormones come into play in both salutogenic and therapeutic effects.

The most important neuromediator is dopamine to which we attribute the greatest salutogenic effects related to listening to music, such as the sensation of pleasantness, fulfilment, reward, and the classic shiver down the spine when listening to a piece of music that has specific meaning for the listener.

Numerous neuroimaging studies (PET and fMRI) attest increased blood flow when listening to music in nucleus accumbens, hippocampus, substantia nigra and ventral tegmental area (VTA), brain structures rich in dopaminergic neurons (Blood and Zatorre 2001; Brown et al. 2004; Menon and Levitin 2005; Koelsch et al. 2006; Salimpoor et al. 2011; Janata 2009).

Numerous studies show that music and singing stimulate oxytocin production, another important chemical compound which intervenes in the mechanism of action of music (Nilsson 2009; Keeler et al. 2015; Ooishi et al. 2017). This neuropeptide, produced by the hypothalamus and secreted by the pituitary gland, comes into play heavily in the phases before and after childbirth, exerting several physiological functions like promotion of maternal and paternal emotional behavior and enhancement of social relationships and empathy. Oxytocin has also anxiolytic, anti-stress, antidepressant activity (Carter et al. 2020).

Beyond salutogenic effects such as empathy, sharing, friendship, oxytocin can also modulate the pain experience. Several studies like those cited in a review published in 2015 attest its analgesic effect in acute and chronic pain (Tracy et al. 2015). Oxytocin has the potential to modulate the pain experience due to its ubiquitous involvement in central and peripheral psychological and physiological processes, and thus offers promise as a therapeutic agent.

But oxytocin has another fundamental action, i.e., attenuating the cortisol secretion, probably through an inhibition of ACTH.

A meta-analysis consisting of 18 randomized placebo-controlled studies has considered the acute effect of intranasal administration of oxytocin on the cortisol response to stressful stimuli. Overall, oxytocin administration showed a greater attenuation of the cortisol response to laboratory tasks that strongly activated the HPA axis. The effect was more robust in sick subjects than in healthy volunteers, suggesting a possible greater sensitivity to oxytocin among those with a clinical diagnosis (Cardoso et al. 2014).

Music listening enhances the release of endorphins, well-known natural hormones that stimulate opioid receptors to produce pain relief and creating a general feeling of well-being (McKinney et al. 1997). An interesting study has been carried out in preterm infants (Qiu et al. 2017). Preterm neonates undergo many painful procedures as part of their standard care in the neonatal intensive care unit. However, pain treatment is inadequate in many of these routine procedures. Sixty-two preterm neonates (gestational age of <37 weeks) were randomly assigned to either the combined music and touch intervention or standard care. In total, 3707 painful procedures were performed during their hospitalization. After 2 weeks, the serum β-endorphin concentration was higher in the experimental group than in the control group with a parallel decrease in the Premature Infant Pain Profile score.

Music listening also affects the production of the neurotransmitter serotonin (5-HT). In a recent study, Jong-In Park et al. determined the effect of music therapy in depressed children and adolescents with attention-deficit hyperactivity disorder (ADHD) (Park et al. 2023). This study is designed based on the randomization method. A total of 36 subjects participated in the experiment, consisting of an ADHD control group ($n = 18$) and ADHD music therapy group ($n = 18$). The ADHD control group received standard care, while the ADHD music therapy group received music therapy and standard care. The ADHD music therapy group received both active music therapy (improvisation) and receptive music therapy (music listening) for 50 minutes, twice a week, for 3 months: a total of 24 times. From a neurophysiological perspective, changes in depression and stress were tracked by measuring 5-HT secretion, cortisol expression, blood pressure (BP), heart rate (HR), and CDI and DHQ psychological scales. The ADHD music therapy group's 5-HT secretion increased ($p < 0.001$), whereas cortisol expression ($p < 0.001$), BP ($p < 0.001$), and HR ($p < 0.001$) decreased.

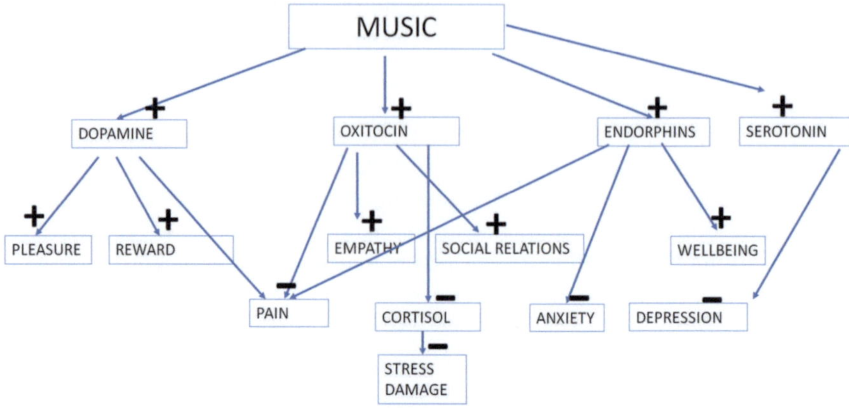

Fig. 4.3 Summary of salutogenic and therapeutic effects of music

Figure 4.3 depicts a summary of the evidence from the studies taken into consideration: Music stimulates the increase in dopamine, which on the one hand gives us feelings of well-being and on the other intervenes in the modulation of pain. The same applies to oxytocin and endorphins. The reduction of cortisol provides relief of stress damage.

In conclusion, the body of evidence on the benefit of music on pain, anxiety, stress, and depression is vast and authoritative. The effects have a well-documented molecular basis based on the activation of complex brain circuits and the release of neurochemical mediators.

4.4 Music to Counteract Pain, Anxiety, and Stress

In hospitalized patients, the most frequent causes of suffering are pain in first place, followed by psychological stress and anxiety. And it is precisely pain that is the main target of musical intervention.

Pain almost always has a well-defined somatic source, such as cancer pain. But anxiety, stress and depression often intervene on a somatic basis, amplifying the painful sensation.

Music undoubtedly has an analgesic effect. This is proven by several systematic reviews that have considered dozens of randomized studies.

The first major review was published in 2006 by the Cochrane collaboration, an organization known for the rigor of these reviews (Cepeda et al. 2006). Fifty-one studies were selected involving more than 3600 subjects, of which 1867 were exposed to music and 1796 were part of the control group.

The review showed that: (a) listening to music exerts a real analgesic effect, with a modest but significant effect size (0.5–1 units on a 0–10 scale); (b) those exposed to music have a 70% greater chance of being responsive to drug therapy; (c) the female gender responds better than the male gender; (d) live music works better than recorded music; and (e) music chosen by the patient works better than music chosen by the doctor.

As a result of listening to music, there are also significant effects on other negative correlates of pain such as nausea and vomiting, psychological distress, blood pressure, and heart rate.

A second review was published in 2021 (Bradt et al. 2021), again by the Cochrane Collaboration, which focused on the use of music in improving psychological and physical outcomes, primarily pain in subjects with cancer (Bradt et al. 2021). In this review, 81 studies with 5576 participants were considered. Most of the studies (no. 74) were conducted on adults (5306 subjects) and only seven on children (270 subjects). Forty-three studies concerned music–medicine and 38 music therapy. Overall, the comparison between music intervention and standard intervention favored the former, with superior benefits on pain, anxiety, depression, quality of life, and fatigue. In the 12 studies which considered pain as the main endpoint, the so-called effect-size was 0.67, a value which is considered important in the context of evidence-based medicine. For several outcomes, music therapy interventions delivered by a qualified music therapist led to consistent results across studies, whereas this was not the case for music medicine interventions, i.e., music listening managed and delivered by healthcare professionals.

A specific review in the pediatric field was published in 2021 (Facchini and Ruini 2021).

It is a systematic review of the literature on the application of music therapy to children and adolescents with cancer, with the aim of assessing its feasibility and benefits in terms of physical and mental health. From 462 retrieved studies, 19 were selected and included in this research, with 596 participants. These included three different types of music therapy: receptive music therapy ($n = 4$), active music therapy ($n = 9$) and the combined method of receptive and active interventions ($n = 6$). These studies indicated a significant reduction in psychological distress ($n = 9$) and an increase in well-being ($n = 8$). Eight articles evaluated effects on subjective pain and other biological parameters, with inconclusive results. In conclusion, music therapy in pediatric oncology appears to have a good feasibility and seems to exert positive effects on psychophysical health. However, some critical points emerged, such as the heterogeneity of the interventions and study designs, which still make generalizability difficult.

Patients who are candidates for surgery, in the process that takes them from the hospital bed to the operating theatre and back to the ward, suffer from different complex conditions such as anxiety, which sometimes turns into distress and pain. Listening to music can offer a great opportunity to alleviate these symptoms. A typical type of music medicine intervention may involve patients undergoing surgery listening to music before, during, and after surgery to help reduce preoperative anxiety and postoperative pain. There is a growing body of evidence showing the positive effect of these types of music medicine interventions on psychological and physiological parameters (Ginsberg et al. 2022; Spintge 2012).

A particular area of combating pain with musical listening is that of labor in childbirth.

The anxiety that women experience during labor causes general fatigue, which also makes the mother-to-be feel pain more, resulting in a vicious circle. For this reason, minimizing anxiety and pain during labor by nonpharmacological methods is very important, especially for women who refuse analgesia.

There are many noninvasive and safe methods of nonpharmacological labor pain management, such as water immersion, relaxation, acupuncture, yoga, mindfulness, and massage. However, their efficacy is unclear and is mainly based on nonrandomized studies.

In contrast, there are numerous randomized studies on the use of music in labor in childbirth, conducted mainly and interestingly in Middle Eastern and Asian countries. A meta-analysis published in 2019 collected as many as 23 of them (Corbijn Van Willenswaard et al. 2017). These studies agree that music intervention has a significant benefit over routine care for women during labor, especially primiparas, on both pain and anxiety. The use of music in the delivery room has thus become a routine technique in many gynecological centers in our country too.

4.5 Music Education and Psycho-cognitive Development

When we talk about the influence of music on cognitive development, we are referring to a vast body of evidence that collectively leads to the statement that music is good for the brain.

It is widely believed that the study of a musical instrument during childhood stimulates cognitive development, increasing a child's abilities in extramusical activities as well. Hence, the importance of including music education in school curricula starting in kindergarten and primary schools. Music and language, for example, share functional and associative areas that make a positive influence of one on the other plausible. Much scientific evidence suggests a positive influence of music training on musical domains, such as language, cognition, and executive functions. As Luisa Lopez, one of the leading scientific figures in this context, argues, we could imagine music as one of the constituents of the cognitive reserve that will be indispensable in adulthood to achieve healthy ageing (Flaugnacco et al. 2015; Mikulis et al. 2021; Aita et al. 2021).

As Sandra Trehub's pioneering research in Canada, and recently also that of Manuela Filippa and her group in Switzerland have shown, lullabies heard by young children, and even prenatally, produce a series of very significant sensory and mnemonic stimulations (Trehub et al. 2015; Filippa et al. 2020). It has been seen, for instance, that infants turn toward sounds they have already heard in utero and are more attracted to the voice of the primary caregiver, reflecting a certain innate, perhaps genetically based, mnemonic and emotional capacity toward musical sequences. Furthermore, listening to an instrumental piece or song activates both the language areas but also the motor areas of the brain, which is consistent with the common experience of a spontaneous urge to move or even dance when listening to music. In essence, music, together with reading, could be an important resource for developing both emotional and cognitive brain plasticity that can counteract possible cognitive deficits during old age.

4.6 Music Therapy in Child Neuropsychiatric and Psychiatric Settings

Music has been described as the language of emotions, as a social art and as highly rewarding. Many mental health problems, such as autism, schizophrenia, or depression, have to do with emotional problems, social relationships, and motivation. It is therefore not surprising that music has been used throughout human history to promote mental health. However, music therapy as a discipline is much younger and music therapy research is even younger.

A series of systematic reviews of randomized controlled trials have demonstrated the beneficial effects of music therapy, while highlighting the limitations of existing research.

In schizophrenia, several reviews have shown effects on negative symptoms, including emotional block, social withdrawal, and reduced motivation, documenting the growth of research, including further long-term results (Geretsegger et al. 2017; Gassner et al. 2022; Jia et al. 2020). Regarding autism, the first Cochrane review in 2006 showed an indication of effects on social interaction, a central domain of impairment in autism, however, based on very small studies. The 2022 update (Geretsegger et al. 2022) confirmed these effects, based on larger studies, but also showed considerable heterogeneity, which may be due to participants or interventions. Furthermore, the changed view of autism as a personality trait rather than a disorder has highlighted the importance of mental health outcomes and social participation.

Regarding depression, an initial Cochrane review in 2011 suggested positive effects on depressive symptoms but also highlighted methodological shortcomings and a limited scope. A subsequent update in 2017 confirmed these effects, also showing positive effects on anxiety and functioning, but still without clarity on the music therapy methods used (Aalbers et al. 2017).

In general, a growing body of research suggests that music therapy may have beneficial effects and no or few side effects. However, a growing concern is the heterogeneity of the results. Functional brain connectivity measured with fMRI is a promising methodology that is beginning to be used in the field. It may have potential as a predictive biomarker.

4.7 Music as a Life Companion for Well-being and Longevity

Ongoing research in the field of music psychology has highlighted the profound effects of listening to music on perceived well-being, quality of life, and emotions. Music can be particularly suitable for managing or regulating emotions and stress in everyday life, as it can distract and engage listeners in a variety of cognitive and emotional ways. Every time we choose a piece of music to listen to, we make a series of very sophisticated and nuanced psychological assessments of our current state of mind and the environment in which we are listening to the music.

In adolescents, music can promote the construction of personal and social identity, facilitating self-regulation, self-expression, and participation in the community. Adults often listen to music in everyday life to regulate emotions and psychophysiological functions, to evoke memories of their own experiences, to stimulate the imagination and to fantasize (Macdonald 2013). In difficult situations, such as during the Covid-19 pandemic, many people found music a resource for coping and managing their isolation (Yıldırım and Çiriş Yıldız 2022; Vinciguerra and Federico 2022). In old age, music continues to offer powerful support for improving health through cognitive stimulation, neuroprotection, and neurorehabilitation, in both healthy and impaired individuals. (Fancourt et al. 2020; Denora 2013).

A particular area of research, carried out by Liila Taruffi, a researcher in the field of music psychology at the University of Durham (Great Britain), is that of "mind-wandering," i.e., those mental experiences, which take us away from the hic et nunc (here and now) and the incessant demands of the present and the perceptual world. Although it is true that, as some studies show, mind-wandering tends to focus on autobiographical memories can make us sad (particularly for people suffering from depression), several studies based on the technique of experience sampling (in these experiments people are asked to indicate what they are thinking about while listening to music, at random intervals) show that mind-wandering is a source of positive distraction (Taruffi et al. 2017; Taruffi 2021). For example, when people in an experiment are asked to perform a memory exercise, it is seen that the number of errors is correlated with the frequency of mind-wandering. On the other hand, mind-wandering frees creativity. And the good news is that music seems to be able to help ferry our thoughts and thus modulate our mental state and functioning.

4.8 Music Therapy for Dementia and Neurological Rehabilitation

Music therapy has been shown to be effective in the field of cognitive impairment above all in reducing psycho-behavioral disorders. Indeed, the sound–music channel constitutes a privileged mediator that activates, even in cases of severe cognitive impairment, an archaic communication that allows contact with one's own emotions and constitutes an essential communicative bridge between outside and inside.

Several studies have shown that the use of sound and music has a very important value in people with dementia, because it serves to reactivate archaic, expressive but nonverbal communication (Moreno-Morales et al. 2020). In this sense, the sound–music channel helps the person with dementia to find a way to express emotions and to communicate by partly bypassing the higher cognitive functions, those most impaired by the disease. In this way, music therapy improves the quality of life of people with dementia, who have a very long perspective of the disease. But that is not all. Music therapy (through active techniques and music listening) is helpful in reducing and modulating/regulating behavioral disorders such as agitation, irritability, anxiety but also depressive symptoms. This, in turn, supports traditional care and care for the person with dementia in institutional and family settings (Raglio et al. 2018; Raglio 2017).

Sound and music also stimulate cognitive functions on which they exert an important action, especially in the early stages of dementia and mild cognitive impairment.

Another important area of application of music therapy is neurological rehabilitation.

Experiences in this field are numerous and aimed at aspects of neuromotor and cognitive rehabilitation. It has been seen that music has a very important impact on our brain areas, particularly those deputed to movement that are closely connected to the rhythmic component. This has led to the development of "Neurologic Music Therapy," which uses musical exercises for the rehabilitation of upper and lower limb movement in very important diseases such as stroke, Parkinson's, and multiple sclerosis (Raglio et al. 2017). Researchers such as Alfredo Raglio are working with advanced techniques called "sonification," for example, for the rehabilitation of the upper limb and hand, particularly after a stroke (Raglio et al. 2021). This involves providing the patient with an appropriately selected set of sonic–musical stimuli that he activates himself, with the mediation of a sensor. These stimuli are the sound representation of movements, especially from a temporal and spatial point of view. During rehabilitation, the patient performs movement that is read by the sensors and is associated with the production of sounds that acquire coherence (as they are arranged in a certain preordained sequence), in relation to the quality of movement. Through the sound he produces, the patient has feedback relative to the quality of his movement. The results obtained so far suggest that sonification sessions can be considered an effective standardized intervention for the upper limb in subacute stroke rehabilitation.

4.9 Music and Social Cohesion

There is an extensive literature on the potential role of music in strengthening social bonds (Yifan Zou and Wang 2021). In support of these theories, musical sharing has been seen to foster prosocial behavior, a shared sense of achievement, physical coordination, shared attention, shared motivation, and group identity, with increased levels of oxytocin, while at the same time breaking down cultural, ethnic, or religious barriers, e.g., with individual singing sessions, in small and large groups.

Involvement in music plays a key role in building social bonds between individuals and groups, which in turn promote health and well-being (Savage et al. 2020).

According to Steven Mithen, archaeologist and professor at the University of Reading (Great Britain), one of the pioneers of cognitive anthropology, the study of fossils and archaeological finds has helped us understand how the human mind evolved (Mithen 2009). Dancing and moving to the same rhythm have accompanied us since prehistoric times precisely because our very evolution as individuals, formed into cohesive social groups, is fundamentally linked to musicality. The use of music to build social cohesion is present in all known human societies and is deeply rooted in our evolutionary history, having emerged long before language, some 100,000 years ago. Although this phenomenon of synchronization has long been recognized and is evident in many aspects of daily life—choirs, football supporters, military bands, singing nursery rhymes with children—recent research has identified the neural mechanisms by which singing, dancing, and making music together create feelings of gratification that persist even after the communal musical activity has ceased (Janata and Parsons 2013).

4.10 Music and End of Life

The analgesic, anti-anxiety, anti-depression, and distraction properties have made the use of music listening a powerful weapon for palliative therapy in terminally ill patients.

The use of music therapy in hospices aims, on the one hand, to manage emotions, fears, anxieties, and anxieties of the disease, and on the other hand, to contribute to a better acceptance and endurance, including physical, of the disease and its treatment.

Music therapy helps the terminally ill to remember their life and promotes acceptance of death and the ability to die with dignity, comfort, and a sense of legacy.

For the terminally ill patient, the need to be listened to, acknowledged, understood, and accepted takes precedence over other needs. The unexpressed wish is to be treated as a person until death.

It is precisely for this reason that music therapy, as part of palliative care programs, is progressively entering the wards of the most avant-garde countries in this health sector.

A meta-analysis published in 2019 shows that music therapy served as an effective intervention to alleviate pain and psychological symptoms of terminally ill patients (Gao et al. 2019).

Music, a means of communication that produces emotions, takes on an even deeper significance in the management of bereavement; its use for therapeutic purposes has been recognized internationally.

Music can offer bereaved people useful options for giving reason and accepting the reality of their grief. Sometimes words are limited, or one cannot adequately express the impact that a loss causes. Hearing music or making music can help a person grieve better by, for example, bringing in personal music related to a moment experienced with the person lost. Shared listening with the group opens the possibility for the person to contact feelings, emotions, memories, thoughts, and fantasies that perhaps in no other way could have emerged with such force and intensity (Merrill et al. 2022).

4.11 Conclusions

For all the reasons that have been focused on in this chapter, it is to be hoped that music will increasingly become part of the medical armamentarium due to its effectiveness, absence of side effects and low or often zero cost.

The use of music in therapy begins with the realization that listening to and performing sounds and melodies can act on moods and emotions. Hence, the intention is to use music and sounds for rehabilitation and therapeutic purposes, in the face of pathological situations and in various clinical contexts, and not only. Music therapy, in short, takes care of the person, both those who suffer and those who are healthy but wish to improve their quality of life.

References

Aalbers S, Fusar-Poli L, Freeman RE, Spreen M, Ket JC, Vink AC, Maratos A, Crawford M, Chen XJ, Gold C. Music therapy for depression. Cochrane Database Syst Rev. 2017;11(11):CD004517. https://doi.org/10.1002/14651858.CD004517.pub3.

Aita M, De Clifford FG, Lavallée A, Feeley N, Stremler R, Rioux É, Proulx M. Effectiveness of interventions on early neurodevelopment of preterm infants: a systematic review and meta-analysis. BMC Pediatr. 2021;21(1):210. https://doi.org/10.1186/s12887-021-02559-6.

Blood AJ, Zatorre RJ. Intensely pleasurable responses to music correlate with activity in brain regions implicated in reward and emotion. Proc Natl Acad Sci USA. 2001;98:11818–23.

Bradt J, Dileo C, Myers-Coman K, Biondo J. Music interventions for improving psychological and physical outcomes in people with cancer. Cochrane Database Syst Rev. 2021;(10):CD006911. https://doi.org/10.1002/14651858.CD006911.pub4.

Brown S, et al. Passive music listening spontaneously engages limbic and paralimbic systems. Neuroreport. 2004;15:2033–7.

Cardoso C, Kingdon D, Ellenbogen MA. A meta-analytic review of the impact of intranasal oxytocin administration on cortisol concentrations during laboratory tasks: moderation by method and mental health. Psychoneuroendocrinology. 2014;49:161–70. https://doi.org/10.1016/j.psyneuen.2014.07.014.

Carter CS, Kenkel WM, MacLean EL, Wilson SR, Perkeybile AM, Yee JR, Ferris CF, Nazarloo HP, Porges SW, Davis JM, Connelly JJ, Kingsbury MA. Is oxytocin "Nature's medicine"? Pharmacol Rev. 2020;72(4):829–61. https://doi.org/10.1124/pr.120.019398.

Cepeda MS, Carr DB, Lau J, Alvarez H. Music for pain relief. Cochrane Database Syst Rev. 2006;2:CD004843. https://doi.org/10.1002/14651858.CD004843.pub2. Update in: Cochrane Database Syst Rev. 2013;10:CD004843

Chanda ML, Levitin DJ. The neurochemistry of music. Trends Cogn Sci. 2013;17(4):179–93. https://doi.org/10.1016/j.tics.2013.02.007.

Corbijn Van Willenswaard K, Lynn F, Mcneill J, Mcqueen K, Dennis CL, Lobel M. Music interventions to reduce stress and anxiety in pregnancy: a systematic review and meta-analysis. BMC Psychiatry. 2017;17(1):271. https://doi.org/10.1186/s12888-017-1432-x.

Denora T. "Time after time": a Quali-T method for assessing music's impact on well-being. Int J Qual Stud Health Well-Being. 2013;8:20611. https://doi.org/10.3402/qhw.v8i0.20611.

Facchini M, Ruini C. The role of music therapy in the treatment of children with cancer: a systematic review of literature. Complement Ther Clin Pract. 2021;42:101289. https://doi.org/10.1016/j.ctcp.2020.101289.

Fancourt D, Bhui K, Chatterjee H, Crawford P, Crossick G, Denora T, South J. Social, cultural and community engagement and mental health: cross-disciplinary, co-produced research agenda. BJPsych Open. 2020;7(1):e3. https://doi.org/10.1192/bjo.2020.133.

Filippa M, Lordier L, De Almeida JS, Monaci MG, Adam-Darque A, Grandjean D, Kuhn P, Hüppi PS. Early vocal contact and music in the NICU: new insights into preventive interventions. Pediatr Res. 2020;87(2):249–64. https://doi.org/10.1038/s41390-019-0490-9.

Flaugnacco E, Lopez L, Terribili C, Montico M, Zoia S, Schön D. Music training increases phonological awareness and reading skills in developmental dyslexia: a randomized control trial. PLoS One. 2015;10(9):e0138715. https://doi.org/10.1371/journal.pone.0138715.

Gao Y, Wei Y, Yang W, Jiang L, Li X, Ding J, Ding G. The effectiveness of music therapy for terminally ill patients: a meta-analysis and systematic review. J Pain Symptom Manage. 2019;57(2):319–29. https://doi.org/10.1016/j.jpainsymman.2018.10.504.

Gassner L, Geretsegger M, Mayer-Ferbas J. Effectiveness of music therapy for autism spectrum disorder, dementia, depression, insomnia and schizophrenia: update of systematic reviews. Eur J Pub Health. 2022;32(1):27–34. https://doi.org/10.1093/eurpub/ckab042.

Geretsegger M, Mössler KA, Bieleninik Ł, Chen XJ, Heldal TO, Gold C. Music therapy for people with schizophrenia and schizophrenia-like disorders. Cochrane Database Syst Rev. 2017;5(5):CD004025. https://doi.org/10.1002/14651858.CD004025.pub4.

Geretsegger M, Fusar-Poli L, Elefant C, Mössler KA, Vitale G, Gold C. Music therapy for autistic people. Cochrane Database Syst Rev. 2022;5(5):CD004381. https://doi.org/10.1002/14651858.CD004381.pub4.

Ginsberg JP, Raghunathan K, Bassi G, Ulloa L. Review of perioperative music medicine: mechanisms of pain and stress reduction around surgery. Front Med (Lausanne). 2022;9:821022. https://doi.org/10.3389/fmed.2022.821022.

Ishizu T, Zeki S. Toward a brain-based theory of beauty. PLoS One. 2011;6(7):e21852. https://doi.org/10.1371/journal.pone.0021852.

Janata P. The neural architecture of music-evoked autobiographical memories. Cereb Cortex. 2009;19:2579–94.

Janata P, Parsons LM. Neural mechanisms of music, singing, and dancing. In: Arbib MA, editor. Language, music, and the brain: a mysterious relationship. Cambridge, MA: MIT Press; 2013. https://doi.org/10.7551/mitpress/9780262018104.003.0013. Scholarship Online, 21 May 2015.

Jia R, Liang D, Yu J, Lu G, Wang Z, Wu Z, Huang H, Chen C. The effectiveness of adjunct music therapy for patients with schizophrenia: a meta-analysis. Psychiatry Res. 2020;293:113464. https://doi.org/10.1016/j.psychres.2020.113464.

Keeler JR, Roth EA, Neuser BL, Spitsbergen JM, Waters DJ, Vianney JM. Theneurochemistry and social flow of singing: bonding and oxytocin. Front Hum Neurosci. 2015;9:518. https://doi.org/10.3389/fnhum.2015.00518.

Koelsch S, et al. Investigating emotion with music: an fMRI study. Hum Brain Mapp. 2006;27:239–50.

Macdonald RA. Music, health, and well-being: a review. Int J Qual Stud Health Well-Being. 2013;8:20635. https://doi.org/10.3402/qhw.v8i0.20635.

McKinney CH, Tims FC, Kumar AM, Kumar M. The effect of selected classical music and spontaneous imagery on plasma beta-endorphin. J Behav Med. 1997;20(1):85–99. https://doi.org/10.1023/a:1025543330939.

Menon V, Levitin DJ. The rewards of music listening: response and physiological connectivity of the mesolimbic system. NeuroImage. 2005;28:175–84.

Merrill KJ, Catron E, Hamlin E, Calhoun J, Hastings SO. Uses and gratifications of music in bereavement: a qualitative inquiry. Omega (Westport). 2022;2:302228221121490. https://doi.org/10.1177/00302228221121490.

Mikulis N, Inder TE, Erdei C. Utilising recorded music to reduce stress and enhance infant neurodevelopment in neonatal intensive care units. Acta Paediatr. 2021;110(11):2921–36. https://doi.org/10.1111/apa.15977.

Mithen S. The music instinct: the evolutionary basis of musicality. Ann N Y Acad Sci. 2009;1169:3–12. https://doi.org/10.1111/j.1749-6632.2009.04590.x.

Moreno-Morales C, Calero R, Moreno-Morales P, Pintado C. Music therapy in the treatment of dementia: a systematic review and meta-analysis. Front Med. 2020;7 https://doi.org/10.3389/fmed.2020.00160.

Nilsson U. Soothing music can increase oxytocin levels during bed rest after open-heart surgery: a randomised control trial. J Clin Nurs. 2009;18(15):2153–61. https://doi.org/10.1111/j.1365-2702.2008.02718.x.

Ooishi Y, Mukai H, Watanabe K, Kawato S, Kashino M. Increase in salivary oxytocin and decrease in salivary cortisol after listening to relaxing slow- tempo and exciting fast-tempo music. PLoS One. 2017;12(12):e0189075. https://doi.org/10.1371/journal.pone.0189075.

Park JI, Lee IH, Lee SJ, Kwon RW, Choo EA, Nam HW, Lee JB. Effects of music therapy as an alternative treatment on depression in children and adolescents with ADHD by activating serotonin and improving stress coping ability. BMC Complement Med Ther. 2023;23(1):73. https://doi.org/10.1186/s12906-022-03832-6.

Qiu J, Jiang YF, Li F, Tong QH, Rong H, Cheng R. Effect of combined music and touch intervention on pain response and β-endorphin and cortisol concentrations in late preterm infants. BMC Pediatr. 2017;17(1):38. https://doi.org/10.1186/s12887-016-0755-y.

Raglio A. Musicoterapia e Medicina Riabilitativa: stato dell'arte e prospettive future. Editoriale [Music therapy and Rehabilitation medicine: state of the art and future perspectives. Editorial]. G Ital Med Lav Ergon. 2017;39(4):271–2. Italian

Raglio A, Zaliani A, Baiardi P, Bossi D, Sguazzin C, Capodaglio E, Imbriani C, Gontero G, Imbriani M. Active music therapy approach for stroke patients in the post-acute rehabilitation. Neurol Sci. 2017;38(5):893–7. https://doi.org/10.1007/s10072-017-2827-7.

Raglio A, Pavlic E, Bellandi D. Music listening for people living with dementia. J Am Med Dir Assoc. 2018;19(8):722–3. https://doi.org/10.1016/j.jamda.2018.05.027.

Raglio A, Panigazzi M, Colombo R, Tramontano M, Iosa M, Mastrogiacomo S, Baiardi P, Molteni D, Baldissarro E, Imbriani C, Imarisio C, Eretti L, Hamedani M, Pistarini C, Imbriani M, Mancardi GL, Caltagirone C. Hand rehabilitation with sonification techniques in the subacute stage of stroke. Sci Rep. 2021;11(1):7237. https://doi.org/10.1038/s41598-021-86627-y.

Salimpoor VN, et al. Anatomically distinct dopamine release during anticipation and experience of peak emotion to music. Nat Neurosci. 2011;14:257–62.

Savage PE, Loui P, Tarr B, Schachner A, Glowacki L, Mithen S, Fitch WT. Music as a coevolved system for social bonding. Behav Brain Sci. 2020;44:e59. https://doi.org/10.1017/S0140525X20000333.

Spintge R. Clinical use of music in operating theatres. In: MacDonald R, Kreutz G, Mitchell L, editors. Music, health, & wellbeing. Oxford University Press; 2012. p. 276–86.

Taruffi L. Mind-wandering during personal music listening in everyday life: music-evoked emotions predict thought valence. Int J Environ Res Public Health. 2021;18(23)

Taruffi L, Pehrs C, Skouras S, Koelsch S. Effects of sad and happy music on mind-wandering and the default mode network. Sci Rep. 2017;7(1):1–10.

Tracy LM, Georgiou-Karistianis N, Gibson SJ, Giummarra MJ. Oxytocin and the modulation of pain experience: Implications for chronic pain management. Neurosci Biobehav Rev. 2015;55:53–67. https://doi.org/10.1016/j.neubiorev.2015.04.013.

Trehub SE, Ghazban N, Corbeil M. Musical affect regulation in infancy. Ann N Y Acad Sci. 2015;1337:186–92. https://doi.org/10.1111/nyas.12622.

Vinciguerra C, Federico A. Neurological music therapy during the COVID-19 outbreak: updates and future challenges. Neurol Sci. 2022;43(6):3473–8. https://doi.org/10.1007/s10072-022-05957-5.

Yifan Zou I, Wang WS. Music as social bonding: a cross-cultural perspective. Behav Brain Sci. 2021;44:e95. https://doi.org/10.1017/S0140525X20001326.

Yıldırım D, Çiriş Yıldız C. The effect of mindfulness-based breathing and music therapy practice on nurses' stress, work-related strain, and psychological well-being during the COVID-19 pandemic: a randomized controlled trial. Holist Nurs Pract. 2022;36(3):156–65. https://doi.org/10.1097/HNP.0000000000000511.

Part II

The Techniques: Active Music Therapy Approaches

Proposals for Structured Active Music Therapy and Improvisation

5

Gustavo Schulz Gattino

Key Points of the Chapter

- There are different perspectives to understand active music therapy proposals based on structured and improvisational perspectives.
- The different proposals need to be adapted to the different populations, contexts, as well as goals and objectives in music therapy.
- The music and the role of the therapist directly influences the choices for structured and active proposals in music therapy.
- The active proposals need to consider different models, approaches, and orientations in music therapy.
- Structured proposals involve mainly recreational and compositional proposals.
- Improvisational proposals are focused on improvisation and spontaneous creative making.
- It is important to use different trees of decision to choose one or more appropriate active proposals.

5.1 Introduction

Music therapy practice includes a series of active proposals aimed at different populations and practice contexts. The criteria for choosing each proposal will depend on various factors such as the role of music in music therapy (Carpente and Aigen 2019), the population served (Isenberg-Grzeda 1988), the philosophical-theoretical

G. S. Gattino (✉)
Department of Communication and Psychology, Aalborg University, Aalborg, Denmark
e-mail: gattino@ikp.aau.dk

A. Raglio (ed.), *Music and Music Therapy Interventions in Clinical Practice*, Neurocultural Health and Wellbeing,
https://doi.org/10.1007/978-3-031-88578-5_5

understanding of the music therapist (Bruscia 2012), the goals and objectives of the process (Thompson 2022), and the institution where the professional works (Isenberg-Grzeda 1988). Active proposals can be organized into structured practices and practices centered on improvisation processes.

The separation between these two categories of proposals is essentially didactic since a structured practice can include a moment of improvisation, and improvisation can be structured based on the different procedures used. In this way, this organization aims to show that some proposals focus more on structure than others on improvisational processes. Structured active proposals are mainly connected to practices from behavioral music therapy (Gouveia 2024; Martin 2012, 2018), neurological music therapy, models centered on the use of the voice, and models centered on group practices in music therapy. Active improvisational practices are mainly linked to psychodynamic, music-centered, and humanistic models, as well as those centered on neurodiversity (Pickard et al. 2020) and post-capacities (Shaw 2022).

At the same time, practice perspectives can be considered "agnostic" or without a specific direction toward a model, approach, or orientation, as they are focused on using one or more music therapy methods. This is the "method-based" perspective created by Annie Heiderscheit and Nancy Jackson (2022). Similarly, it is possible to cite the perspectives on improvisation by Tony Wigram (2004), Gardstrom and Hiller (2022), the proposal by Luis Milleco Filho et al. (2001) on the use of songs in music therapy, as well as Felicity Baker's proposals regarding Songwriting (Baker 2015). This means that an active proposal can be connected to various ways of thinking but is only centered on the method used.

The term method is used here according to Kenneth Bruscia's definition (Bruscia 2014). According to this author, a method consists of using a musical experience (improvisation, composition, recreation, and receptive experiences). The recreation method is the only one that needs a direct understanding of this classification. It refers to activities in which the music therapist recreates an existing experience. Among these proposals are using musical games, singing or playing songs with the client, performing instrumental pieces, and making musical production proposals (Bruscia 2014). What will be shown in this chapter are precisely different variations of each of the active methods (improvisation, composition, and recreation), emphasizing their differences using different procedures and techniques.

By the end of this chapter, the reader will have a set of tools and guidelines to choose what best suits their practice context. The last section of this chapter proposes a decision tree to help the music therapist choose the ideal active proposal for their practice. In other words, this chapter aims to provide ideas and possibilities about the active use of music in music therapy so that music therapists have good options for making their decisions at any time in their practice, whether it is individual, group, face-to-face or via telehealth music therapy (TMT) (Clements-Cortés et al. 2023).

The terms "proposals" and "active" in the title of this chapter need to be explained before continuing with the following sections. The term "proposals" is used because there are different variations within methods (Bruscia 2014) in music therapy. The idea of the term proposals is one possible understanding of how to classify the practices in music therapy, as there are other ways of explaining what music therapists use in their practice. Some authors classify these variations as techniques (Barcellos

2022), axes of action (Schapira et al. 2007), exercises (Esposito 2016), and activities (Palazzi et al. 2019).

The term "active" refers to the client's active involvement in the music therapy sessions by playing or creating something specific. I understand that receptive methods are not considered passive since any listening activity is highly active, as it involves a conscious process involving the entire nervous system and body (Reybrouck and Van Dyck 2024). In this way, the term active is related to proactivity that involves practical participation within the session that is possible to envision. Barcellos (2022) believes that the term interactive (inter + active) is more interesting since the client experiences a relational process with the music therapist or with other participants from the music therapy process.

5.2 Theoretical Structures

The theoretical bases on which structured and improvisational proposals are based have similarities and differences—the similarities concern using variations of active methods to achieve therapeutic goals within the process. The main differences concern the understanding of the role of music in each of the proposals and the leadership process within the sessions.

The role of music is essential for all of them, as it differentiates music therapy from other therapies (Gattino 2022). However, understanding music gives rise to a particular way of seeing reality. From this reality, it is possible to describe concepts that explain the different proposals presented here (Carpente and Aigen 2019). At the same time, the role of leadership is vital to understanding structured and improvisational proposals since depending on the type of leadership (on the part of the client, on the part of the therapist, or collaborative), the therapist will choose the proposal that best fits this purpose (Carpente 2017; Gattino 2022). In addition, the type of leadership will influence the configuration of the relationships between therapist and client, giving rise to different theoretical understandings for each leadership proposal.

As explained in the introduction to this chapter, the idea here is not to construct a linear vision in which each understanding of music is necessarily linked to an active proposal. The idea here is to show that there are resonances between a proposal and a vision of music in music therapy in some directions but that each music therapist's understanding of the process can lead to a different interpretation that allows for a different association from the one presented here.

In this section, I want to emphasize the theoretical basis of each proposal from an initial understanding of the role of music and leadership and then present the main theories and thoughts underpinning each.

5.3 Theoretical Bases for Structured Active Proposals

The basic premise of structured proposals is the prior planning of music-making to achieve planned goals and objectives (Hanser 2015; Martin 2012, 2018). In this context, the music therapist understands music in two ways: as a tool or agent for changing behavior (Gattino 2022) or as a facilitator for developing relationships. Music could be separated within the music therapy process in both situations, but from different contexts.

As a tool or agent of change, music understands musical phenomena as something external and concrete that can be manipulated to produce specific results (Bonde 2007). Within this vision, music is also understood more quantitatively and measurably, where verifying aspects of duration and frequency for each musical proposal established is possible. As a tool or agent of change, music focuses on behavior and behavior change (Gouveia 2024). It is hoped that with the programmed use of music, certain behaviors can be maintained, decreased, or increased in specific situations and conditions (Lim 2023).

In the case of music as a facilitator of relationships, music is understood more subjectively. However, the focus is on relationships rather than on understanding music as the center of the process (Barcellos 2022). In this context, music serves as a way of facilitating the connection between the client and the music therapist and facilitating the client's communication and expression within this process. Music as a facilitator of relationships focuses mainly on the verbal and nonverbal dynamics present in the music therapy process but without clearly emphasizing the importance of the role of each and the influence of musical parameters in this process (Gattino 2022).

Regarding leadership, the music therapist is responsible for leading or providing the musical moments. This means that the music therapist has greater control over what is happening in the session and will create situations so the client can participate (Gattino 2022). Let me clarify that there is no value judgment about leadership on the part of the music therapist. In structured proposals, there is a different process of interaction and relationship because the flow of communication is based on a reference model to be used or followed, as suggested by the music therapist. At the same time, working in a structured way does not mean eliminating the client's creativity. Within the structures, the therapist provides, the client has a space to create something from what is proposed.

Some theories and concepts dialogue more directly with active proposals based on understanding music and leadership (Hanser 2015; Lim 2023). Only some of these concepts are applied to all structured proposal situations, which does not mean they all need to be applied together. They represent ways of understanding the concepts that structure structured proposals. These theories and concepts have their origins in some models and approaches in music therapy, of which I would highlight neurological music therapy (Thaut and Hoemberg 2014), behavioral music therapy (Lim 2023; Gouveia 2024), cognitive behavioral music therapy (Hanser 2015), and interactive music therapy by Lia Rejane Mendes Barcellos (2022). It would be impossible to list all the models and approaches that influence the theoretical thinking behind structured proposals, so I have only listed those with some critical theories and concepts that can be discussed here. The following is a list of these theories and concepts that provide an essential basis for structured proposals.

Goal- and problem-oriented focus: This concept from cognitive-behavioral music therapy originated in North America (Hanser 2015). It means the client is directed towards achieving goals and solving specific problems throughout the therapeutic process. To work on these specific focuses, the music therapist uses structured proposals.

Behavioral chains: This concept comes from behavioral music therapy and is linked to Applied Behaviour Analysis (ABA) (Lim 2023). It refers to a behavioral chain involving performing a specific series of distinct responses. Each behavior performed in the sequence modifies the environment to produce conditioned reinforcement for the previous response and, at the same time, acts as a stimulus for the following response.

Teaching musical behavior: This concept comes from behavioral music therapy and is linked to Applied Behavior Analysis (ABA). It means the development of new musical behaviors through learning musical skills can be achieved through imitation, modeling, behavioral modeling, and behavioral chains (Lim 2023).

Skills: A concept used mainly in behavioral music therapy, cognitive behavioral music therapy (Gouveia 2024), and neurological music therapy (Thaut and Hoemberg 2014); skills refer to the competencies and abilities that clients develop and use during the therapeutic process through music (AMTA 2013). In structured proposals, the music therapist learns skills through teaching, training, and guidance.

Generalization of behavior: This term originates in behavioral music therapy (Martin 2012, 2018) and neurological music therapy (Thaut and Hoemberg 2014) and concerns the transfer and transformation of what is performed musically to behaviors in the client's everyday life.

Music is an element of socialization and 'interaction' in music therapy. This term originates from Lia Rejane Barcellos's interactive music therapy (Barcellos 2022). Music can influence people's behavior, experience of time, and feelings about themselves—in terms of energy and emotion—about others and situations.

Interactive music therapy: another term from Lia Rejane Barcellos' model (2022), where the music therapist uses strategies to enhance and facilitate the building of the bond through music and interventions that can provoke the inter-actions/interactions that will contribute to the establishment of the bond. Consequently, this leads to the possibility of change, which is ultimately the main aim of therapies, and in music therapy, music can be considered a powerful tool for change.

5.4 Theoretical Bases for Active Improvisational Proposals

Improvisational proposals assume that musical experiences are focused on processes with little or no structure so that dynamics and interactions occur through events that are adjusted in real-time (Geretsegger et al. 2015). Music can be understood as a facilitator of the relationship or as the center of the process. Although many think music is always central to improvisational proposals, this is not the case within some models or approaches. For example, in some psychodynamic music therapy proposals (Benenzon 1985; Schumacher 2014), music is interpreted as a relationship facilitator.

In the context of music as the center, all interactions and experiences stem from the music itself (Aigen 2005; Carpente and Aigen 2019). Carpente and Aigen (2019) suggest that, within this perspective, music constitutes its health field. They argue that the music-centered approach emphasizes the client's ability to engage deeply and meaningfully in music-making, with the therapist playing a central role. Regarding this process being centered on music, Aigen further points out:

> (1) articulate as fully as possible the inherent value of clinically directed musical experiences; (2) create a music-centered theory based on the meaning of these experiences for the recipients of music therapy services; (3) clearly explain what makes their work therapy; and (4) emphasize that music-centered positions do not prohibit verbal interaction with clients or require performance as a clinical vehicle, but instead provide a conceptual model of practice in which verbalization is not always necessary and clinical interactions can take place outside the session room. (p. 66)

The significant difference between improvisational proposals is the understanding of collaborative or client-led leadership (Geretsegger et al. 2015). Combining an understanding of music as relational or as the center of the process and a collaborative or client-led process means that certain concepts are fundamental to underpinning these proposals. These concepts relate to the relationships developed between music therapist and client and to valuing the client as the protagonist within the music therapy process. Different models and approaches bring essential concepts to improvisational practices. Among these, I would highlight psychodynamic perspectives, music-centered perspectives (such as Nordoff-Robbins music therapy, (2006), and Aesthetic Music Therapy (Lee 2003)), vocal psychotherapy and perspectives centered on identity and social justice such as post-ableist music therapy (Shaw 2022), resource-oriented music therapy (Rolvsjord 2010) and community music therapy (Stige 2004), the latter of which does not have improvisation at its center, but instead as one of its possibilities for practice). Here are some key concepts for understanding improvisational proposals.

Facilitating musical and emotional attunement is used mainly in psychodynamic and relational approaches in general (Geretsegger et al. 2015). This concept involves the therapist matching their music to the client's behaviors, focus, and emotions, like how a caregiver interacts with a baby. This alignment creates musical moments that stimulate emotional connection.

Musical countertransference: a concept used mainly in psychodynamic approaches to music therapy (Dillard 2006). It is a relational energy exchange between the therapist and the client in the context of the music therapist, which has four strands. The phenomenon encompasses: (1) the music therapist's unconscious musical response to the client that is occurring about the music therapist's past relationship dynamics and that may become conscious over time; (2) the therapist's unconscious musical response to the client that occurs in connection with the client's past relationship dynamics; (3) a combination of both (1) and (2) occurring at the same time; and (4) an empathic musical response to the client. An empathic musical response to the client's unconscious state is associated with a strong identification with the client.

Communicative musicality is not a concept that comes from music therapy but is used in music therapy (Holck 2019). Communicative musicality consists of prelinguistic communication between the baby and the caregiver, consisting of synchronization and multimodal movement activities with temporal patterns conceived as intrinsically musical characteristics. The music therapist does not copy the relationships developed between parents and children. However, the therapist can musically amplify and strengthen primary forms of interactions, thus promoting communicative interaction and connectivity.

Integration of verbal and nonverbal communication: This concept comes from vocal psychotherapy (Austin 2009). It deals with the integration of verbal and nonverbal modes of communication. Clients can use vocalizations, sounds, and music to express emotions and experiences that are difficult to articulate verbally.

Empowerment: A concept used in resource-orientated music therapy (Rolvsjord 2010), feminist MT (Hadley and Hahna 2016), community music therapy (Stige 2004), and used in post-capacity music therapy (Shaw 2022). Rolvsjord (2010) describes three interdependent and interactive levels of empowerment: the individual, the organization, and the community. Empowerment is achieved by considering individual problems in broader social and institutional contexts, identifying and challenging oppressive conditions (external and internal), and engaging the client's resources to work on personal and social transformation from different musical experiences.

Musical interrelationship: a concept used in the Developmental Relationship-based Music Therapy Model created by Carpente (2017). This concept involves the client's creative, expressive, and communicative ability during music-making activities. This includes the initiation of musical ideas, the differentiation between their music and that of the therapist, and the reciprocal integration of musical ideas.

Coactive musical play: This concept comes from Nordoff–Robbins music therapy and concerns the involvement of the therapist and client in musical interactions that are dynamic and reciprocal (Nordoff and Robbins 2006). The therapist adapts to the client's responses, promoting shared musical experience and mutual influence.

5.5 Presentation of Active Proposals

This section presents different active proposals within the structured and improvisational context. Given the many possibilities, it was necessary to adopt some criteria to include the proposals described here. The first criterion was choosing proposals primarily based on evidence present in different quantitative, qualitative, or mixed studies relevant to music therapy. The second criterion was using proposals that do not require specific training to be applied. Some models, such as neurological music therapy and vocal psychotherapy, present specific proposals, but certification is required to apply them. The third criterion used was the clarity of the proposal presented. Some models and approaches suggest specific proposals, but there needs to be more clarity in the procedures and techniques to implement them. The last criterion adopted was the inclusion of proposals from different parts of the world, which at the same time could be adapted to the different cultures where they will be used.

The proposals presented here come from models and approaches with a specific theoretical foundation (often also aimed at a specific population) and holistic perspectives focused solely on methods. Although some of the proposals have their origins in a theoretical foundation and a specific population, I invite the reader to take a more global and flexible view, where each proposal presented can be adapted to different contexts and perspectives of music therapy practice. Adaptation is precisely the keyword for this section, as each proposal can be adapted and presented in different ways depending on the context in which it is used. At the end of the presentation of the different proposals, I present a decision tree that can help the music therapist decide which proposal or proposals best suit the situation being experienced in practice. The proposals will be described using different tables, in which I describe the names of the proposals, the authors, the perspectives from which they originated (origin), and the description of the proposal.

It is essential to make a small comment regarding the authors and the origin of the proposals. Different authors have described and used some proposals at different times or in different publications. This means some authors have described a proposal from their reality rather than using a previous publication as inspiration. This is why more than one author exists for the same proposal in specific situations. Regarding the origin of the proposals, I will only list a few since, in some cases, many authors have already described a specific proposal.

5.6 Structured Active Proposals

Structured active proposals are divided into compositional proposals, proposals, and recreational proposals. These proposals could be organized in different ways, such as the classifications by Edwards (2016) and Schapira et al. (2007). However, I have opted for Bruscia's classification (2014), not because it is the best, but because it is the best-known worldwide. Such proposals can also have an improvisational character, so in this subsection, I only want to present them in situations based on a predefined structure.

5.7 Compositional Proposals

Composition is a musical experience in which the music therapist helps the client or group create a unique musical product (Jackson and Heiderscheit 2022). This can include a song, an instrumental piece, or a multimedia musical product, which can be played or enjoyed once finalized. Compositions can be developed in one or more sessions. Within the composition, I present the following proposals in Table 5.1 below musically adapted social stories, fill-in-the-blanks, instrumental composition, musical collage, song transformation, mash-up, and composition of an original song based on a structure.

Table 5.1 Compositional proposals in music therapy

Name	Authors	Origin	Description
Social stories adapted to music	Brownell (2002, 2012, 2018)	Behavioral music therapy (mainly linked to ABA music therapy)	Stories that are narrated with a musical or sung background in which social situations are described to highlight relevant characteristics of a target behavior and provide examples of an appropriate response
Fill in the blanks	(Baker 2015)	A holistic perspective on songwriting in music therapy (Baker 2015)	The key words are "erased" from the original lyrics. The therapist's role is to involve the composer(s) in a therapeutic process that results in the identification of feelings and experiences, which are then translated into new keywords and inserted into the spaces
Instrumental composition	Bruscia (2014), Jackson and Heiderscheit (2022)	Holistic perspective on methods in music therapy (Bruscia 2014), holistic perspective on compositional methods in music therapy (Jackson and Heiderscheit 2022)	The client composes a piece of music that might consist of melody, harmony, rhythms, or any combination of these, which can then be performed on instruments
Musical collage	Baker (2015), Jackson and Heiderscheit (2022)	A holistic perspective on songwriting in music therapy (Baker 2015) holistic perspective on compositional methods in music therapy (Jackson and Heiderscheit 2022)	Music collage is a method-variation that involves the selection of sounds, songs, and music and their intentional sequencing to create a recording with a specific therapeutic focus

(continued)

Table 5.1 (continued)

Name	Authors	Origin	Description
Song transformation	Baker (2015), Jackson and Heiderscheit (2022)	A holistic perspective on songwriting in music therapy (Baker 2015) holistic perspective on compositional methods in music therapy (Jackson and Heiderscheit 2022)	The therapist assists the client in either replacing words or phrases in the original song with their own words and phrases while maintaining the melody or changing the melody and/or harmony of the original song while maintaining the original words. The result is an original song that borrows from a precomposed song but reflects the expressions of the client
Mash-up	(Baker 2015)	A holistic perspective on songwriting in music therapy (Baker 2015)	A mash-up is a composition approach in which the recordings of two or more prerecorded songs are mixed to form a new work
Composing an original song based on a structure	Baker (2015), Jackson and Heiderscheit (2022)	A holistic perspective on songwriting in music therapy (Baker 2015) holistic perspective on compositional methods in music therapy (Jackson and Heiderscheit 2022)	Lyrics and music are created from the ground up but guided by preexisting musical structures. The extent to which musical elements are borrowed and combined may vary from song creation to song creation. At the broadest level, overall forms may be drawn upon to create an original song

5.8 Recreative Proposals

"Recreation" is a broader term covering the representation, reproduction, execution, or performance of parts or all of an existing musical work, with or without an audience (Bruscia 2014). In these proposals, the client learns, sings, plays, or performs music already composed or reproduces any musical form presented as a model. The term "recreation" is used instead of "performance," as "performance" usually involves playing or singing a piece in front of an audience. Recreation proposals are described in different models, approaches, and music therapy manuals. However, they are rarely organized and categorized in the same place as described in this chapter. Of all the proposals, recreational ones are certainly the most diverse, given their variety of proposals and possibilities of use. The idea here is to present a broad spectrum that meets different goals and objectives in music therapy. The proposals presented here in Table 5.2 are modeling gestural and vocal behavior through musical performance, the performance of a song or instrumental music, the use of a color notation system for musical performance, the creation of songbooks, musical productions, musical games, and the reproduction of musical resources mediated by technology.

Table 5.2 Recreative proposals in music therapy

Name	Authors	Origin	Description
Modelling gestural behavior through musical performance	Gouveia (2024), Martin (2018) Lim (2023)	Behavioral music therapy (mainly linked to ABA music therapy) (Gouveia 2024; Martin 2018; Lim 2023)	Play a song and during its performance show models of gestures that can be repeated by the client during the musical performance
Performance of a song or instrumental music	(Bruscia 2014), Schapira et al. (2007), Millecco Filho et al. (2001)	Perspective centered on the methods of Kenneth Bruscia (2014), Music-Verbal Music Therapy (Milleco et al. 2001) and Plurimodal Music Therapy	Being the soloist or accompanist of an instrumental song being performed in the session
Using a colour notation system for musical performance	Rodrigues (2018), Gattino (2022)	Music therapy model for the deaf (Rodrigues 2018), holistic perspective on music therapy in the context of autism (Gattino 2022)	Playing or singing a song using an adapted notation system where each note to be played is represented by a specific color
Creating songbooks	Schapira et al. (2007)	Multimodal music therapy	Together with the client, create a book to include the main songs to be used in the music therapy process
Music productions	Bruscia (2014), Gattino (2022)	Kenneth Bruscia's method-centered perspective (2014), holistic perspective on music therapy in the context of autism (Gattino 2022)	The client participates in the planning and execution of a musical show, play, or drama
Musical games	Bruscia (2014), Gattino (2022)	Kenneth Bruscia's method-centered perspective (2014), holistic perspective on music therapy in the context of autism (Gattino 2022)	The client participates in musical games, such as musical questions/answers (e.g., repeats the notes heard), activities with musical circles, or activities involving toys or objects to provide musical experiences for participants (e.g., using a domino or musical card game)

(continued)

Table 5.2 (continued)

Name	Authors	Origin	Description
Reproduction of musical resources mediated by technology	Gattino (2022), Magee (2013)	Holistic perspective on music therapy in the context of autism (Gattino 2022), holistic perspective centered on the use of technology in music therapy (Magee 2013)	The client plays or sings a song with the help of a technological resource that can be an app, software, digital musical instrument, or device that facilitates their participation throughout the musical performance
Singing in harmony	Adapted from Meashey (2020)	Perspective on the use of the voice in music therapy	Using any musical phrase, introduce a musical idea in unison. Then introduce 5 min or so of harmony and then go back to unison. Through this method, clients can have the sensation of coming apart and coming back together
Toning for call and response imitation	Meashey (2020)	Perspective on the use of the voice in music therapy	Do the word toning exercise using two chords and add other phrases on one note. The therapist sings the phrase over the two-chord exercise in any metre and then the client(s) can echo the phrase

5.9 Active Improvisational Proposals

Improvisational proposals refer to those based on improvisation. However, they also include spontaneous creative processes from the flow of interaction and associative processes within the music therapy session. Many techniques and methods are specific to improvisation; some are connected to songwriting and recreational proposals. Given this large number of proposals, a careful review was necessary to include those with a broad spectrum of applications for different contexts, goals, and objectives, and at the same time, can be adapted in various ways. The proposals that will be presented include particular techniques and methods with different procedures to be applied. The improvisational proposals that will be described here in Table 5.3 are matching, free-floating dialogue, turn-taking dialogue, exaggeration, provocative technique, "once upon a time," singing by free association, musical grounding, frameworking, referential improvisation, singing and images, vocal improvisation using two or three chords, extemporizing, and creating a rap from the structure of an original song.

Table 5.3 Improvisational proposals in music therapy

Name	Authors	Origin	Description
Matching	Wigram (2004)	A holistic perspective on improvisation	Improvising music so that it is compatible with, matches, or adjusts to the client's playing style, maintaining the same rhythm, dynamics, texture, quality, and complexity of other musical elements
Free-floating dialogue	Wigram (2004)	A holistic perspective on improvisation	Making music in the middle of a continuous musical exchange dialogue-a floating dialogue. Here the participants, therapist, and client play continuously and simultaneously. In their musical and dynamic ideas, they listen and respond, without pausing during the musical process
Turn-taking dialogue	Wigram (2004)	A holistic perspective on improvisation	Making music together, where the therapist and the client play in various ways (musical or gestural) and can point to each other to take turns (changing). Turn-taking requires the therapist or client to pause and make room for each other
Exaggerate	Bruscia (1987)	A holistic perspective on improvisation	Highlighting something that is unique or stands out in a client's response or behavior, amplifying it
Frameworking	Wigram (2004)	A holistic perspective on improvisation	Creating or developing a musical structure for the client's improvisation
Provocative technique	Barcellos (2022)	Interactive music therapy	It consists of the execution [by the music therapist], through the voice or musical instruments, of a passage—sonorous, rhythmic, melodic, or harmonic of a piece of music or the lyrics of a song -, known by or from the client's culture, which becomes provocative of an attitude of closure or completeness
Once upon a time	Oldfield and Franke (2005)	Perspective centered on the use of improvisation and musical stories	This proposal allows the client to share their inner self with the therapist through improvised storytelling. The therapist uses their therapeutic skills to facilitate the child's narrative, starting with the statement: "Once upon a time..." and leaving space for the child to complete the statement

(continued)

Table 5.3 (continued)

Name	Authors	Origin	Description
Singing by free association	Schapira et al. (2007)	Multimodal music therapy	The client is asked to try to put words to music or music to words through singing
Musical grounding	Wigram (2004)	A holistic perspective on improvisation	Creating a stable song that contains musical content that can help to provide an "anchor" for the client's music
Referential improvisation	Bruscia (2014)	A holistic perspective on music therapy methods	The client improvises with a musical instrument to represent something non-musical in sound (e.g., a feeling, an idea, a title, an image, a person, an event etc.). Musical in sound (e.g., a feeling, an idea, a title, an image, a person, an event, an experience etc.), experience etc.)
Vocal improvisation using two or three chords	Meashey (2020)	Perspective on the use of voice in music therapy (Meashey 2020	Using two or three chords, play the progression repeatedly for at least 32 bars and improvise vocally
Extemporising	Wigram (2004)	A holistic perspective on improvisation	Improvising on given musical material, or as a pastiche (imitation) of a style of composition, while maintaining the musical and dynamic characteristics of the style
Create a rap from an original structure	Baker (2015)	A holistic perspective on songwriting	The composers spontaneously construct the lyrics while the music is sounding in real time

5.10 Some Reflections on the Use of the Active Proposals Presented

From the above, there are many proposals and possibilities for music therapists to use different active methods in their practice. This broad spectrum brings many advantages and concerns so that their use does not become mere experimental applications, activities to fill session time, or a direct proposal application without proper adaptation and consideration of the client's case. To facilitate the process of using the proposals presented here, I bring you two decision trees that can help the therapist.

The decision tree is a graphical representation of problems commonly used in healthcare to determine solutions to complex choices (Thompson and O'Callaghan 2013). These choices can be based on a confluence of research evidence, the preferences and needs of the client (customer or student), and the knowledge and experience of the therapist (Gattino 2022).

The first decision tree concerns the criteria for implementing an active proposal in music therapy (Box 5.1). The second decision tree aims to choose one of the three categories presented here: structured active proposals (compositional and recreational) and improvisational proposals (Box 5.2).

Box 5.1 Decision Tree to Use or Not an Active Proposal in Music Therapy
Is the client interested in participating actively by playing, singing, or creating something (partition, songbook, etc.)?

Does the therapist have experience of any active proposals that meet the client's needs?

Does the use of an active experience collaborate in any way with the goals and objectives set?

Is there any kind of scientific evidence to support the use of an active proposal intended by the music therapist?

In this first decision tree above (Box 5.1), the music therapist should consider whether he or she is adequately prepared to carry out any of the suggested proposals, whether it is essential for the client based on their needs and goals, and whether there is any critical scientific evidence. Suppose the music therapist believes it is essential to use an active experience but does not have the practical and scientific knowledge to do so. In that case, studying and preparing beforehand is essential to ensure that the best possible practices are offered. Here is a description of the second decision tree (Box 5.2).

Box 5.2 Decision Tree to Choose One or more Active Proposals
How does the therapist understand the role of music in music therapy?

Does the client have interest to compose a song or piece in structured way? (songwriting proposals).

Does the client show interest in playing and/or singing any precomposed song or piece as a soloist and/or accompanier? (Recreative proposals).

Does the client express interest in musical productions, musical games, creating songbooks or using technology or adapted systems to play/sing a song/piece? (Recreative proposals).

Does the client present interest by creating sounds and/or using words spontaneously with the musical instruments or using the voice? (improvisation proposals).

The second decision tree shows several elements to consider when deciding which active proposal to use. The different points concern the therapist and the client. On the therapist's side, the focus is on understanding music (as a tool/agent for change, as a facilitator of relationships, or as the center of the process) and on the therapist's preparedness to facilitate the different active proposals. In the case of the client, the questions address their interest in singing or playing something in a structured or spontaneous way, composing in a structured or unstructured way, and showing interest in some specific proposals (such as musical productions and games, for example).

The two trees presented here are just suggestions that can facilitate the work of music therapists in their practice. The use of decision trees is fundamental when preparing and planning sessions. One suggestion is to review these trees before and after sessions. This will help the therapist understand what is working, what needs to be changed, and what could be new in the process.

As mentioned at the beginning of the chapter, the music therapist must be aware of the influence of certain factors within their choice. Therefore, the music therapist must be clear about certain aspects to facilitate their decisions and use of different proposals. The points highlighted here are the therapist's theoretical/philosophical orientations, the client's wishes and needs, and the goals and objectives. I will not go into the role of music or goals and objectives here, as these aspects have already been included in the decision trees.

Theoretical/philosophical orientations—the music therapist must be aware of which models, approaches, and orientations are used in their practice within a vision according to the integral thinking of Kenneth Bruscia (2014). This means that the music therapist can work from a central model, approach, or orientation but can include others that are necessary in order to meet the demands and needs of the music therapy process. In this way, the theoretical and philosophical orientations that influence the music therapist's decision can change according to the changes and events within the process.

The client's wishes and needs—I see this factor as the most important of all, as the client must be empowered within the process so that their choices are a fundamental part of it and direct a large part of the proposals made in the sessions.

5.11 Final Considerations

Active proposals in music therapy present different possibilities for use and adaptation to music therapy practices. The reader of this chapter will be able to make practical use of what has been developed here, and they will also be able to add more proposals based on their experiences developed in specific contexts of practice. This chapter has also emphasized the importance of having criteria and concerns when choosing and using active proposals since it is necessary to consider the quality of each proposal presented and guarantee the client's well-being.

References

Aigen K. Music-centered music therapy. Barcelona Publishers; 2005.

American Music Therapy Association (AMTA). Professional competencies. American Music Therapy Association (AMTA); 2013. https://www.musictherapy.org/about/competencies

Austin D. The theory and practice of vocal psychotherapy: songs of the self. Jessica Kingsley Publisher; 2009.

Baker F. Therapeutic songwriting. Springer International Publishing; 2015.

Barcellos LRM. Musicoterapia interativa [Interactive music therapy]. In: Gattino G, editor. Practical and theoretical perspectives of music therapy in Brazil. Barcelona Publishers; 2022.

Benenzon R. Manual de musicoterapia [Manual of music therapy]. Trad. Clementina Nastari. Enelivros; 1985.
Bonde LO. Stages in researching the music in therapy. In: Wosch T, Wigram T, editors. Microanalysis: methods, techniques, and applications for clinicians, researchers, educators and students. Jessica Kingsley Publishers; 2007. p. 255–69.
Brownell, Mike D. Musically adapted social stories to modify behaviors in students with autism: Four case studies. Journal of music therapy 2002;39(2):117–44.
Brownell, MD, & Arbor A. Social Stories: Pairing the Story With Music and Video Modeling for Children With Autism Spectrum Disorder. In P. Kern & M. Humpal (Eds.), Early Childhood Music Therapy and Autism Spectrum Disorder. Jessica Kingsley Publishers; 2012. p. 117–129.
Brownell MD, & Schwartzberg ET. Social StoriesTM. Early Childhood Music Therapy and Autism Spectrum Disorder: Supporting Children and Their Families. Jessica Kingsley Publishers; 2018. p. 129–148.
Bruscia KE. Improvisational models of music therapy. Charles C Thomas Publishers; 1987.
Bruscia K. Reading on music therapy theory. Barcelona Publishers; 2012.
Bruscia K. Defining music therapy. Barcelona Publishers; 2014.
Carpente JA. Investigating the effectiveness of a developmental, individual difference, relationship-based (DIR) improvisational music therapy program on social communication for children with an autism spectrum disorder. Music Ther Perspect. 2017;35(2):160–74.
Carpente JA, Aigen K. A music-Centered perspective on music therapy assessment. In: McPherson GE, Silverman M, Elliott DJ, editors. The Oxford handbook of philosophical and qualitative assessment in music education. Oxford University Press; 2019. p. 243–56.
Clements-Cortés A, Pranjić M, Knott D, Mercadal-Brotons M, Fuller A, Kelly L, et al. International music therapists' perceptions and experiences in telehealth music therapy provision. Int J Environ Res Public Health. 2023;20(8):5580.
Dillard LM. Musical countertransference experiences of music therapists: a phenomenological study. Arts Psychother. 2006;33(3):208–17.
Edwards J. Approaches and models of music therapy. In: The Oxford handbook of music therapy. Oxford University Press; 2016. p. 417–27.
Esposito S. Musicoterapia para el desarrollo: 40 actividades lúdico-musicales para la estimulación neuromotora [Music therapy for development: 40 playful-musical activities for neuromotor stimulation]. Independent Production; 2016.
Gardstrom S, Hiller J. Improvisational methods of music therapy. Barcelona Publishers; 2022.
Gattino G. Music therapy and the autism spectrum: an integrative overview. Barcelona Publishers; 2022.
Geretsegger M, Holck U, Carpente JA, Elefant C, Kim J, Gold C. Common characteristics of improvisational approaches in music therapy for children with autism spectrum disorder: developing treatment guidelines. J Music Ther. 2015;52(2):258–81.
Gouveia F. Content validity of the application assessment tool for structured activities in the context of behavioral music therapy and applied behavior analysis (ABA) (Unpublished master thesis). Pablo Olavide University, Spain; 2024.
Hadley S, Hahna N. Feminist perspectives in music therapy. In: Edwards J, editor. The Oxford handbook of music therapy. Oxford Press; 2016.
Hanser S. The New Music Therapist's Handbook - 3rd Edition: Learn Essential Practices for Children, Adults and Older Adults for Music Therapy. Berklee Press; 2015.
Holck U. Communicative musicality – a basis for music therapy practice. In S. L. Jacobsen, I. N. Pedersen & L. O. Bonde (Eds.), A comprehensive guide to music therapy (2nd ed.) Jessica Kingsley; 2019. 104–111.
Isenberg-Grzeda C. Music therapy assessment: a reflection of professional identity. J Music Ther. 1988;25(3):156–69.
Jackson N, Heiderscheit A. Compositional methods of music therapy. Barcelona Publishers; 2022.
Lee CA. The architecture of Aesthetic Music Therapy. Barcelona Publishers; 2003.
Lim HA. Teaching musical skills and developing music therapy interventions. In: Handbook of applied behavior analysis: integrating research into practice. Springer International Publishing; 2023. p. 857–73.

Magee W. Indications and contraindications for using music technology with clinical populations. Music technology in therapeutic and health settings. In: Music technology in therapeutic and health setting. Jessica Kingsley Publishers; 2013. p. 83–107.

Martin L. Applied behavior analysis: introduction and practical application in music therapy for young children with autism spectrum disorder. In: Kern P, Humpal M, editors. Early childhood music therapy and autism spectrum disorder: supporting children and their families. Jessica Kingsley Publishers; 2012. p. 101–16.

Martin L. Behavioral approach: applications for children with autism spectrum disorder in music therapy practice. In: Kern P, Humpal M, editors. Early childhood music therapy and autism spectrum disorder: supporting children and their families. 2nd ed. Jessica Kingsley Publishers; 2018. p. 91–107.

Meashey K. The use of voice in music therapy. Barcelona Publishers; 2020.

Millecco Filho LA, Brandão MR, Millecco R. É preciso cantar. musicoterapia: canto e canções [Singing is needed: music therapy: singing and songs]. Enelivros; 2001.

Nordoff P, Robbins C. Creative music therapy: guide to fostering clinical musicianship. 2nd ed. Barcelona Publishers; 2006.

Oldfield A, Franke C. Improvised songs and stories in music therapy diagnostic assessments at a child and family psychiatry unit: a music therapist's and a psychotherapist's perspective. In: Songwriting: methods, techniques, and clinical applications for music therapy clinicians, educators, and students. Jessica Kingsley Publishers; 2005. p. 24–44.

Palazzi A, Meschini R, Piccinini CA. Music therapy intervention for preterm mother-baby: an intervention proposal in the neonatal ICU. Psicologia em estudo. 2019;24:e41123.

Pickard B, Thompson G, Metell M, Roginsky E, Elefant C. "It is not what is done, but why it has done": music therapists' understanding of normalization, maximization, and the neurodiversity movement. Voices: World Forum Music Ther. 2020;20(3) https://doi.org/10.15845/voices.v20i3.3110.

Reybrouck M, Van Dyck E. Is music a drug? How music listening may trigger neurochemical responses in the brain. Music Sci. 2024; https://doi.org/10.1177/1029864924123677.

Rodrigues I. As cores do som: o potencial musical do surdo [The colors of sound: the musical potential of the deaf]. Memnon; 2018.

Rolvsjord R. Resource-oriented music therapy in mental health care. Barcelona Publishers; 2010.

Schapira, D., Ferrari, K., Sánchez, V., & Hugo, M. (2007).Musicoterapia plurimodal [Plurimodal music therapy]. Adim Ediciones.

Schumacher K. Music therapy for pervasive developmental disorders, especially autism. The music in music therapy: Psychodynamic music therapy in Europe: Clinical, theoretical and research approaches. Jessica Kingsley Publishers; 2014. 107–123.

Shaw CM. An autoethnographic journey in developing post-Ableist music therapy. Voices World Forum Music Ther. 2022;22(1) https://doi.org/10.15845/voices.v22i1.3314.

Stige B. Community music therapy: culture, care, and welfare. In: Pavlicevic M, Ansdell G, editors. Community music therapy. Jessica Kingsley Publishers; 2004. p. 91–113.

Thaut M, Hoemberg V, editors. Handbook of neurologic music therapy. Oxford University Press; 2014.

Thompson G. Goal processes in music therapy practice. Jessica Kingsley Publishers; 2022.

Thompson S, O'Callaghan C. Decision-making in music therapy: the use of a decision tree. Aust J Music Ther. 2013;24:48.

Wigram T. Improvisation: methods and techniques for music therapy clinicians, educators, and students. Jessica Kingsley Publishers; 2004.

6 Songwriting Techniques in Music Therapy

Michael J. Silverman

Key Points
- Qualified music therapists can use songwriting in various settings and formats to address numerous clinical objectives.
- Clinical decision-making in songwriting can depend on contextual factors including the service users, music, structure, format and environment, clinical objectives, and the philosophical approach of the music therapist.
- Songwriting can be a powerful intervention and music therapists are uniquely qualified to prevent and safely contain and process music-induced harm unlike other practitioners who use music in therapeutic contexts.
- Music therapists conducting songwriting should practice reflexivity and emotional intelligence to maintain their wellbeing and continue developing their songwriting skills.

6.1 Introduction

Songwriting is a commonly used music therapy intervention involving the creation of music, lyrics, or music and lyrics within the context of a supportive therapeutic relationship (Baker and Wigram 2005). Songwriting has widespread therapeutic application across Europe, Australia, and the Americas (Baker et al. 2008). Qualified music therapists[1] can use songwriting in a range of clinical settings and for people

[1] I use the term "qualified music therapists" to recognize that qualifications differ by country.

M. J. Silverman (✉)
University of Minnesota, Minneapolis, MN, USA
e-mail: silvermj@umn.edu

A. Raglio (ed.), *Music and Music Therapy Interventions in Clinical Practice*, Neurocultural Health and Wellbeing,
https://doi.org/10.1007/978-3-031-88578-5_6

without music training or sophisticated musicians, in group and individual formats, within single sessions or across multiple sessions, in-person or via telehealth, as well as with children, adolescents, adults, and older adults. Pending upon the clinical context, music therapists can use various degrees of structure within songwriting to facilitate a successful compositional and therapeutic experience. Through songwriting, music therapists can empower service users[2] with creative ways to share their narratives, name their problems, explore solutions, find hope, and express themselves and their musical identities. Because of its flexibility, songwriting can address a plethora of clinical objectives based on the service users' contexts including the development of self-esteem, confidence, awareness, and clarifying and externalizing emotions (Baker et al. 2008). Songwriting can help service users develop, name, and reinforce their identities and sense of self (Baker and MacDonald 2013) and experience relief, validation, and joy (O'Callaghan and Grocke 2009; Roddy et al. 2018; Windle et al. 2020).

As service users and music therapists involved in songwriting create original compositions, an advantage of songwriting is that it can avoid previous negative musical associations. For example, people in addiction treatment may associate certain songs with past substance use. In this context, the service users and music therapist can compose a new song in a safe environment that minimizes the potential for music-induced substance craving (Silverman et al. 2023). Moreover, songwriting in this setting can empower the service users to create a future-oriented song about recovery.

6.2 Theoretical Frameworks

As a versatile music therapy intervention with widespread clinical applications, there are numerous theoretical frameworks that can help understand and explain songwriting. For the purposes of this chapter, I will focus on (1) Flow and (2) Process and product.

6.2.1 Flow in Songwriting

Songwriting can be a challenging yet rewarding task-oriented experience for service users and music therapists. As such, flow can be a way to understand and explain songwriting. Csikszentmihalyi (1975) developed the concept of flow, wherein people are immersed in a gratifying activity. While experiencing flow, people are highly focused and completely engaged in an innately rewarding task. Because of their heightened engagement, people can ignore distractions. The difficulty of the task is enough to warrant intense focus without boredom or anxiety. This highly engaged and intrinsically motivating state results in an experience where it seems that nothing else matters (Csikszentmihalyi 1990; Jackson and Csikszentmihalyi 1999).

[2] I use the general term "service users" to describe the people receiving music therapy. This term can vary by country, clinical setting, and context.

Flow is therefore considered a state of optimal experience and is accompanied by a positive affective state. Csikszentmihalyi (1990) noted that flow is characterized by nine dimensions and that each dimension represents a separate conceptual element of flow. Other researchers have found evidence supporting the concept of the nine flow dimensions (Csikszentmihalyi 1993; Jackson 1996; Jackson and Marsh 1996; Martin and Culter 2002). The nine dimensions are:

1. Challenge-skill balance: To achieve flow, there should be a balance between the challenge of the task and a person's ability.
2. Action-awareness merging: When a person is in a flow state, they experience positive emotions and are fully engaged with the task.
3. Clear goals: While experiencing flow, a person has a clear understanding of the task and is aware of how to accomplish the task.
4. Unambiguous and immediate feedback: During flow, a person receives internal or external feedback regarding their progress.
5. Concentration on the task: When in flow, a person is totally immersed in the task and extraneous thoughts and distractions are minimized.
6. Sense of control: While experiencing flow, a person has a sense of control over the task, but that sense of control is not absolute.
7. Loss of self-consciousness: During flow, a person is freed from their inner critical voice and not preoccupied with others' judgements.
8. Time transformation: While experiencing flow, a person's perception of time is altered. Some people report that time seems to stop while other people experience time as slowing down or moving quickly.
9. Autotelic experience: When in flow, the task functions as a reward and there is no expectation of an extrinsic gain. After task completion, a person feels a sense of accomplishment and purpose.

The nine dimensions of flow can occur during songwriting. Applying flow to songwriting, Silverman et al. (2016) found that flow can occur in songwriting sessions with adults with mental health and substance use conditions. In addition to the service users, Silverman and Baker (2018) discussed how flow can also occur for music therapists while composing songs with service users.

6.2.2 Process and Product

Differentiating the process from the product can provide a working theoretical framework to help describe songwriting in clinical music therapy contexts. The processes of songwriting refer to procedural aspects of songwriting. These might include brainstorming music and lyrics as well as discussing, considering, trying, and writing various ideas that may or may not be used in the song. The songwriting product refers to the finalized creation resultant of the songwriting processes. The product of therapeutic songwriting can also refer to service users' therapeutic outcomes or changes result of the songwriting (Ansdell 1995).

6.3 Techniques

Although it would be helpful for music therapy students and music therapists with less clinical experience, there is no standardized songwriting protocol for all clinical situations. The lack of a songwriting protocol highlights the idiosyncratic, dynamic, and personalized nature of therapy and songwriting. Because each song is created in a unique manner (i.e., process) and each song is idiosyncratic (i.e., product), songwriting can be an impactful personalized intervention that is contextually situated.

To augment the likelihood of a successful therapeutic songwriting experience, the music therapist will have to thoughtfully and reflexively consider the amalgamation of various factors. Figure 6.1 uses a Venn Diagram to depict contextual factors within songwriting clinical decision-making. Although the model initiates with the service users to center their importance, the music therapist will need to carefully consider all factors to determine the songwriting techniques to best ensure the service users' success. The music therapy assessment can be a helpful way to attain information regarding some factors in Fig. 6.1.

6.3.1 Service Users: Identities, Lived Experiences

Congruent with other music therapy interventions (Sears 1996), the service users represent the most consequential aspect of songwriting. As such, the music therapist will need to consider the service users' identities and lived experiences that may include but are not limited to gender identity/expression, race, ethnicity, culture,

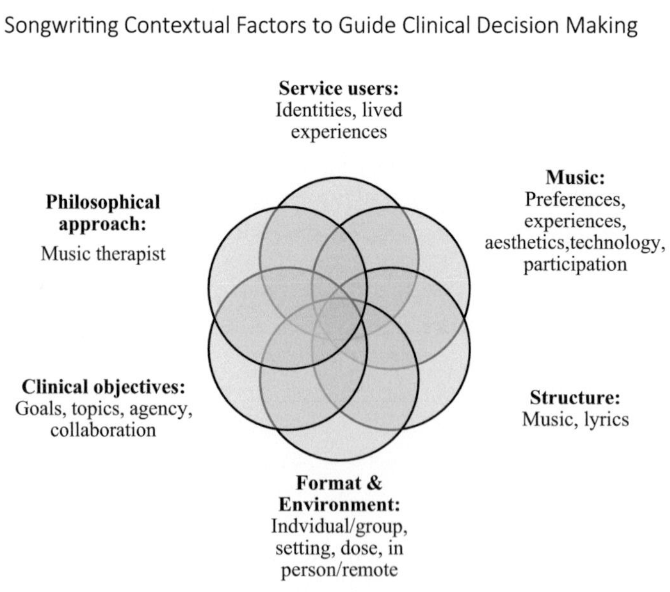

Fig. 6.1 Songwriting contextual factors to guide clinical decision-making

age, education, language, medical condition, religion, generation, and veteran status. The music therapist can learn about some of these factors during the chart review and assessment. When service users identify as belonging to communities that have been marginalized, the music therapist must be empathetic, supportive, and empowering throughout the songwriting processes. A heightened understanding of and sensitivity to service users' identities and lived experiences can augment participation, the therapeutic relationship, and therapeutic outcome (Baker 2014).

6.3.2 Music: Preferences, Experiences, Aesthetics, Technology, Participation

Music therapists will also need to consider the service users' music preferences and experiences. This can include past music experiences including participation in music ensembles, music lessons, and digital music creation. When service users have musical experience, the music therapist can empower them to participate in a strength-based manner to showcase their abilities. Moreover, songwriting in preferred genres may result in augmented engagement and outcomes. Music therapists can encourage service users who identify as visual artists to create art in their preferred medium to represent the song or songwriting experience.

Songwriting can result in musical products that are aesthetically beautiful (Rolvsjord 2005). However, the service users should ultimately decide what constitutes aesthetic beauty.[3] Although the music therapist may desire to make the musical product as aesthetically pleasing as possible, honoring service users' contributions to the song and the therapeutic processes may be more important than the terminal product. Perhaps what matters most in songwriting is the service users' meanings associated with the process and product.

Qualified music therapists can also use technology to facilitate or enhance songwriting experiences with their service users. This might include recording songs, incorporating GarageBand software (Bent et al. 2023), composing beats (Crooke 2018), changing the lyrics to existing music, and sampling. Additionally, music therapists can use music technology within improvisation to generate ideas for original compositions (Crooke and McFerran 2019). When service users are knowledgeable about music technology, music therapists can empower them to use their skills throughout the songwriting processes.

In group songwriting sessions, participation levels between service users will likely vary. Musicians may be more apt to participate while people without music experience may be more reluctant to share ideas. Some people may not enjoy or be comfortable singing (Chong 2010). In addition, the music therapist's musical abilities may inadvertently intimidate service users (Silverman 2019a). Providing service users with verbal and written options to participate can facilitate songwriting processes (Fiore 2016). As such, service users should have considerable autonomy

[3] I would argue that whatever service users create is beautiful as service users are the most important aspect of music therapy.

over their participation. Moreover, if service users are not actively participating in a group songwriting session, it does not necessarily indicate they are not benefiting from the intervention or are unengaged in the process. In the author's group-based songwriting experience, service users who verbally participate minimally often thank him and articulate that they benefited from sessions.

6.3.3 Structure: Music, Lyrics

The amount of structure within songwriting interventions can impact musical and clinical success. For example, music therapists can change some lyrics within existing songs, rewrite all lyrics to existing songs, or compose entirely new compositions. Baker (2015a), a preeminent songwriting scholar, described (1) songwriting methods that emphasize lyric creation, (2) songwriting methods that emphasize lyric and music creation, and (3) songwriting methods that emphasize music creation. In another songwriting taxonomy, Baker et al. (2009) differentiated song parodies from original songwriting. Song parody involves rewriting the words of an existing song and may be ideal in single sessions or when additional structure may facilitate songwriting processes. Original songwriting involves creating original music and lyrics. Based on the degree of musical and lyrical structure needed to be successful, Silverman (2022a, b) described three approaches to songwriting in adult mental health settings as (1) fill in the blank, (2) lyric replacement, and (3) free creation. The degree of structure is consequential as Baker and MacDonald (2013) found that greater musical autonomy during songwriting resulted in higher flow in university students and retirees. However, because music therapists often work with clinical populations, additional structure may be necessary.

Although some songwriting studies focus on aspects of lyric creation (Baker 2015b), the music within songwriting can facilitate the process and is consequential. Baker (2015b) interviewed music therapists about the music within songwriting and found that music can deliver messages and emotions, has clinical relevance, and augments self-expression. When teaching songwriting interventions to music therapy students during in-class experientials, Silverman (2022a, b) recommended to play the existing composition and to use as much music as possible (i.e., "when in doubt, play it out"). When service users get "stuck" in the composition process, music therapists can play the existing creation so service users can hear it and develop ideas. Singing the musical phrase without lyrics (i.e., singing using "la" instead of lyrics) can facilitate compositional progress. Indeed, songwriting can be challenging and requires problem solving, patience, flexibility, creativity, and compromise (Silverman 2022a, b). Using visual components such as musical notation can also facilitate songwriting interventions for service users who read music.

Music therapists can also rely upon the lyrics to facilitate songwriting. For example, brainstorming ideas and writing them on a dry erase board as a "lyric bank" may stimulate ideas. Additionally, using rhyme schemes may also help the songwriting process (i.e., "What are some words that rhyme with 'blues' that we might use to conclude this line?"). Music therapists can also number the lines and visually depict the existing lyrics to help service users discuss where lyrics may be most meaningful.

6.3.4 Format and Environment: Individual/Group, Setting, Dose, In-Person/Remote

Songwriting can occur in individual (i.e., one-on-one therapy) or group therapy formats with multiple service users. Music therapists in adult mental health settings in the United States often facilitate songwriting during group therapy (Silverman 2007, 2009). Group songwriting can augment access to treatment and may alleviate compositional pressure for service users who may be unsure of or intimated by songwriting. Specific to group settings with adults who have addictions, songwriting can also result in interpersonal connection (Bourdaghs and Silverman 2023; Silverman 2023a). However, group songwriting can limit an individual group member's musical agency and the music therapist will need to carefully consider what might be best for service users' situated context. Moreover, decisions regarding individual or group therapy may be dictated by facility policies and organizational culture.

As music therapists often practice in complex spaces that can influence the therapeutic process and relationship (Baker 2013), they will need to consider how the environment impacts songwriting. The environment can include the type of facility, the treatment dose (i.e., number of sessions), as well as the specific room where the sessions occur. For example, songwriting in open spaces may limit privacy, intimacy, and personalized topics. Baker (2013) interviewed music therapists about environmental conditions germane to songwriting and identified organizational structures, physical space, private space, and the organizational norms as factors that impact songwriting. In another example, music therapists working in acute care mental health facilities may only be able to provide single-session and group songwriting sessions (Silverman 2023b, 2024). Baker (2013) noted that sometimes music therapists modify their environments and educate staff to facilitate songwriting. However, Baker also recognized that organizational systems are not always amenable to change and music therapists may need to adapt their practices to fit the context.

Music therapists will also need to consider how the delivery model (i.e., in-person or remote) impacts songwriting. Music teletherapy may enable music therapists to make treatment more accessible for service users (Wang et al. 2023). However, music teletherapy will impact songwriting processes and products. For example, service users participating in songwriting remotely may not have access to instruments. However, remote songwriting may enable music therapists to integrate technologies such as music software, digital beat making, and word processing to facilitate songwriting.

6.3.5 Clinical Objectives: Goals, Topic, Agency, Collaboration

The music therapist will also need to consider service users' self-identified goals and reasons for attending therapy. Collaborating with, supporting, and providing service users with agency regarding clinical objectives can facilitate relational and therapeutic processes. In addition, music therapists can write songs about relevant topics germane to the service users' clinical objectives. For example, adults with anxiety and depressive conditions in a mental health facility may need to develop adaptive coping strategies. In this setting, the service users and music therapist could compose lyrics about when to use adaptive coping strategies (i.e., identifying times of augmented stress and depression) in one verse and adaptive coping strategies that can help cope with anxiety and depression in another verse. In an example of published clinical research using songwriting as an independent variable, Silverman wrote songs about stigma related to mental health conditions (verse 1) and how to cope with stigma (verse 2) with adults in an acute mental health setting (Silverman 2013) and in a substance detoxification setting (Silverman 2020). In both studies, songwriting participants had favorable results regarding stigma.

6.3.6 Philosophical Approach: Music Therapist

Based on what is best for and preferred by the service users within their situated contexts, music therapists can use various philosophical approaches to guide their songwriting interventions. For example, a music therapist working in a group setting with people who have depressive conditions might use a cognitive approach to identify and challenge cognitive distortions and maladaptive thought processes. A music therapist working individually with a person seeking insight into their relational difficulties might use a psychodynamic approach to create musical metaphors and access unconscious thoughts and repressed material. The music therapist's philosophical approach should align with the service users' values and preferences to augment the therapeutic relationship and outcomes.

6.4 Songwriting Considerations

6.4.1 Memorializing Songs

Songs created in music therapy can be meaningful for participants (Baker et al. 2016; Silverman et al. 2016) and participants may want compositions for future use and reflection. For example, in a study of mothers who had experienced childhood abuse, some participants continued to use the songs (Day et al. 2009). Anecdotally, patients have told the author that they display the song lyrics from their group compositions on their refrigerators at home or share them with their partners while hospitalized. As such, recording songs composed during music therapy can be a powerful way to memorialize the experience for service users. Music therapists recording songs should be aware of power differentials to ensure service users are emboldened to make decisions in their own best interests and obtain written approval from service users. In addition, music therapists will need to be highly cognizant of and compliant with the facility's confidentiality policies as they relate to recording. In cases wherein recording is not permitted, the music therapist can write the lyrics or notate the music and provide paper copies to service users.

Grocke et al. (2009) had music therapists facilitate songwriting with adults with mental health conditions. After composing the songs, the therapists and participants recorded them at a professional studio. In a related study, a music therapist composed both group and individual songs with adults with mental health conditions who were living in the community (Silverman 2022a, b). The music therapist and participants then recorded the songs in a professional studio and then had a CD release party wherein service users' friends and family members came to the facility to listen to and honor the compositions. Silverman then interviewed two participants and found they had positive experiences during the songwriting, recording, and CD release party.

6.4.2 Verbal Processing in Songwriting

In certain cases, service users engaged in songwriting may not be fully aware of the therapeutic objectives. As such, it is vital that music therapists and service users verbally process the intervention and reflect on how songwriting processes and products align with clinical objectives. Although music therapists may be aware of songwriting clinical objectives, these should also be explicit for service users so they can connect the clinical processes to therapeutic objectives.

6.4.3 Avoiding Appropriation in Songwriting

Music therapists may use existing songs from a variety of genres to facilitate songwriting. As such, it is important to acknowledge and honor the music genre/song and artist to avoid appropriation. For example, the current author often facilitates group blues-based songwriting with adults who have mental health conditions. As the author identifies as White and the blues genre was created by Africans and African Americans, the author verbally provides a brief history of the blues to honor it as an influential musical genre and avoid appropriation (Silverman 2022a, b).

6.4.4 Documenting and Measuring the Effects of Songwriting

Music therapists can document aspects of both the process and product of songwriting in their treatment notes. Although music therapists can include aspects of the music in service users' progress notes, it will be important to relate the music to the service users' clinical objectives for treatment team members who may not be familiar with songwriting processes or jargon. Because service users' clinical objectives will vary by their settings and contexts, music therapists can document various factors that occur throughout the arc of the songwriting including interactions with the music therapist and peers, identification of coping strategies, or motivations for treatment. In an inpatient adult mental health setting, music therapy clinicians can facilitate songwriting about coping strategies and document the coping strategies service users identified during the discussion or in the lyrics. Researchers could measure coping self-efficacy at the conclusion of the songwriting (Silverman 2019b).

Specific to meaningfulness and songwriting, Baker and MacDonald developed the Meaningfulness of Songwriting Scale (MSS; Baker and MacDonald 2013, 2014). The MSS is a psychometric inventory that measures 11 domains of meaning regarding the process and product of songwriting: achievement, arousal of emotions, associations, challenge, creativity, discovery/self-reflection, engagement, enjoyment, identity, personal value, and understanding context. These scholars have used the MSS in a variety of clinical settings and research (Baker et al. 2016).

6.4.5 Adaptations and Extensions to Songwriting

Music therapists can creatively adapt songwriting interventions to engage service users. For example, Baker (2015a, b) recommended analyzing music and lyrics to help listeners interpret the meanings of songs. As such, music therapists can facilitate song discussions and lyric analyses of songs written in therapy settings. This intervention could be used to address empathy, emotional expression, or other relevant constructs. In another example using a cognitive therapy approach, music therapists could help service users identify maladaptive thought processes within existing song lyrics and change them to rational and adaptive lyrics.

Creating therapeutic music videos can be effective interventions for adolescents and young adults (Burns et al. 2009; Robb et al. 2014). Applying therapeutic music videos to songwriting, music therapists could facilitate songwriting sessions and then collaborate with service users to make therapeutic music videos.

Table 6.1 Principles and elements of trauma-informed approaches

Principles of trauma-informed approach	Elements of trauma-informed approach
Safety	Realizes the impact of the trauma
Trustworthiness and transparency	Recognizes the signs and symptoms of trauma
Peer support	Responds by integrating knowledge about trauma into policies, procedures, and practices
Collaboration and mutuality	Resists re-traumatization
Empowerment, voice, and choice	
Cultural, historical, and gender issues	

6.4.6 Trauma-Informed Care in Songwriting

As an effective, meaningful, and powerful intervention, songwriting has the potential to access emotional content and repressed memories. The accessed content and memories can be emotionally charged. As songwriting can be powerful, musicians who are not qualified music therapists facilitating songwriting interventions with service users risk music-induced harm (Silverman et al. 2020). However, because of their comprehensive academic and clinical training (Sena Moore 2015), music therapists are uniquely qualified to help service users safely discuss content and emotions that may result from songwriting. Music therapists can incorporate trauma-informed approaches to ensure service users' safety (Lang et al. 2015; SAMSHA 2014) (Table 6.1).

6.4.7 Clinical Example of Songwriting Process and Product

I am privileged to have worked as a qualified music therapist in adult acute care mental health settings for over 25 years. This context necessitates a single-session and group-based approach. In group-based single-session songwriting, I often use the blues to facilitate the lyrical composition of two verses that focus on recovery will-power (verse 1) and recovery way-power (verse 2) based on Snyder's Hope Theory (Snyder 1994, 2002). A protocol is below, followed by a sample composition depicted in Fig. 6.2. I am grateful to the service users who shared their stories with me to compose this song. I also extend appreciation to Hannah Killmer, graduate music therapy student at the University of Minnesota, for transcribing the song.

The Recovery Blues

Music Therapy Group
arr. Hannah Killmer

Blues ♩ = 70

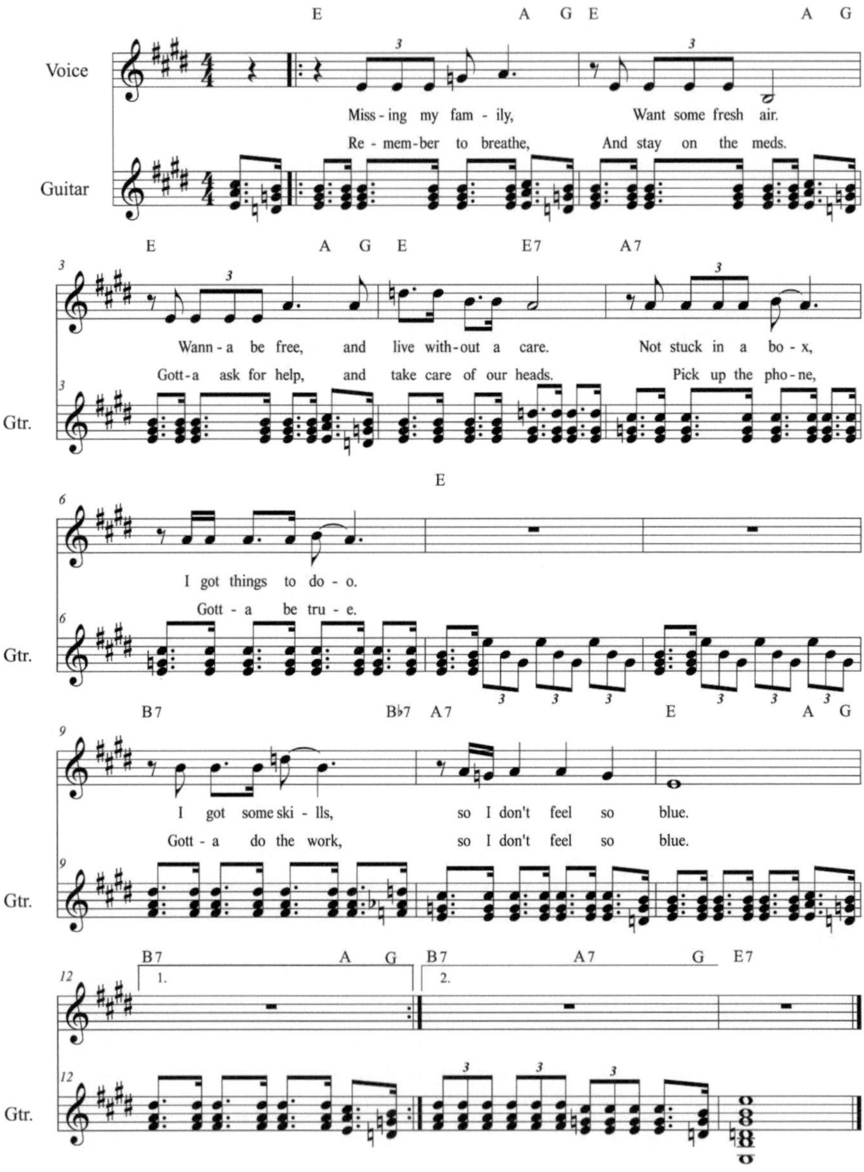
Voice
Guitar
Gtr.
Miss - ing my fam - ily, Want some fresh air.
Re - mem - ber to breathe, And stay on the meds.
Wann - a be free, and live with - out a care. Not stuck in a bo - x,
Gott - a ask for help, and take care of our heads. Pick up the pho - ne,
I got things to do - o.
Gott - a be tru - e.
I got some ski - lls, so I don't feel so blue.
Gott - a do the work, so I don't feel so blue.

Fig. 6.2 Recovery song

6.5 Group-Based Songwriting Protocol "Them Recovery Blues"

1. Introduction—blues in E (steel string acoustic guitar), each group member says name, shares favorite music genres and artists as first modeled by music therapist.
2. Introduce songwriting as today's intervention to discuss recovery motivation and pathways.
3. Introduce blues as an influential art form. State something to the effect of "…blues songwriting is about naming oppression and problems, and we'll work to address those problems and have hope for the future. I do want to first honor the blues as an amazing art form. The blues are a mix of spiritual and work songs developed by Africans and African Americans in the deep south in the 1860s. Most of the music we listen to today is derived from the blues and it is important to acknowledge the blues as an influential art form."
4. Brainstorm ideas for verse 1.
    (a) "Why might you be motivated for recovery?"
    (b) Write service users' ideas on a dry erase board and verbally reinforce service users when they share.
5. Use service users' ideas to compose lyrics in verse 1 of 12 bar blues song. Blues in E.
    (a) Use as much music as possible. Play it often so service users can hear it after each line is composed or when the group is "stuck."
    (b) Use rhyme schemes for structure and prompts.
    (c) Write lyrics on dry erase board and verbally reinforce service users when they share.
6. Brainstorm ideas for verse 2.
    (a) "What might be some things you can do to make recovery happen?"
    (b) Write service users' ideas on the dry erase board and verbally reinforce service users when they share.
7. Use service users' ideas to compose lyrics in verse 2 of 12 bar blues song.
    (a) Use as much music as possible—play it so service users can hear it after each line is composed or when group is "stuck."
    (b) Use rhyme schemes for structure and prompts.
    (c) Write lyrics on dry erase board and verbally reinforce service users when they share.
8. Play entire song to conclude session.
9. Verbally reinforce service users for their participation in the group songwriting session.
10. Verbally process the importance of motivators for recovery and pathways to recovery.
11. Ask service users if they have any questions or comments about anything they might have done in the group songwriting session.

12. Thank service users for their participation.
13. Write lyrics and make copies for service users.
14. Distribute lyric sheets to service users, thank them individually, say goodbye, collect materials, and leave the unit.

6.5.1 Reflecting on the Potential for Desensitization

After composing hundreds of songs with adults who have mental health conditions throughout my music therapy career, it felt important to reflect on these experiences. Songwriting is powerful and has the potential to engage, connect, and access consequential material in therapy settings. I remain in awe of the bravery, vulnerability, resilience, creativity, and strength of the service users with whom I am privileged to conduct songwriting interventions. Facilitating songwriting is a meaningful and humbling experience that continues to challenge me to be a better musician and therapist. I remain grateful to the service users for these experiences.

I am also fortunate to be able to bring music therapy students to clinical settings wherein they observe me conduct songwriting interventions. These experiences—along with everything the service users continue to teach me—have made me aware of the potential for desensitization. As I have written many songs with service users over the years, I am at risk of failing to adequately recognize the powerful impact of and meaning associated with songwriting. However, the students and service users continue to remind me of what a privilege it is to write songs with adults who have mental health conditions. In addition, I have had service users tell me that they remember the lyrics they composed in music therapy years later, carry the lyrics in their wallets to use as a coping strategy, or even wear composed lyrics as necklaces. I remain grateful for and humbled by these experiences.

Songwriting can be an impactful experience not only for the service users but also for the music therapist. As such, it is important to be mindful of the self and practice emotional intelligence. For music therapists to support their own health, it is vital that they are self-aware and reflexive, practice radical self-acceptance and self-care, attain regular supervision, and even participate in personal therapy.

6.6 Conclusion

Songwriting is a flexible and meaningful music therapy intervention that can successfully address numerous clinical benefits with a range of service users. Music therapists using songwriting will need to consider various factors to augment the likelihood of successful songwriting experiences. Additional research from all paradigms is warranted to better understand songwriting and increase access to songwriting interventions for music therapy service users.

References

Ansdell G. Music for life: aspects of creative music therapy with adult clients. Jessica Kingsley Publishers; 1995.

Baker FA. The environmental conditions that support or constrain the therapeutic songwriting process. Arts Psychother. 2013;40(2):230–8. https://doi.org/10.1016/j.aip.2013.02.001.

Baker FA. An investigation of the sociocultural factors impacting on the therapeutic songwriting process. Nord J Music Ther. 2014;23(2):123–51. https://doi.org/10.1080/08098131.2013.783094.

Baker FA. Therapeutic songwriting: developments in theory, methods, and practice. New York: Palgrave Macmillan; 2015a.

Baker FA. What about the music? Music therapists' perspectives on the role of music in the therapeutic songwriting process. Psychol Music. 2015b;43(1):122–39. https://doi.org/10.1177/0305735613498919.

Baker F, MacDonald RA. Flow, identity, achievement, satisfaction and ownership during therapeutic songwriting experiences with university students and retirees. Music Sci. 2013;17(2):131–46. https://doi.org/10.1177/1029864913476287.

Baker FA, MacDonald RA. Experiences of creating personally meaningful songs within a therapeutic context. Arts Health. 2014;6(2):143–61. https://doi.org/10.1080/17533015.2013.808254 .

Baker FA, Wigram T. Songwriting: methods, techniques and clinical applications for music therapy clinicians, educators and students. Jessica Kingsley Publishers; 2005.

Baker FA, Wigram T, Stott D, McFerran K. Therapeutic songwriting in music therapy: Part I: who are the therapists, who are the clients, and why is songwriting used? Nord J Music Ther. 2008;17(2):105–23. https://doi.org/10.1080/08098130809478203.

Baker FA, Wigram T, Stott D, McFerran K. Therapeutic songwriting in music therapy, Part II: comparing the literature with practice across diverse clinical populations. Nord J Music Ther. 2009;18(1):32–56. https://doi.org/10.1080/08098130802496373.

Baker FA, Silverman MJ, MacDonald RAR. Reliability and validity of the Meaningfulness of Songwriting Scale (MSS) with adults on acute psychiatric and detoxification units. J Music Ther. 2016;53:55–74. https://doi.org/10.1093/jmt/thv020.

Bent C, Wetherick D, Carr CE. 'Filling the void with melody': therapists' reflections on group songwriting using GarageBand in music therapy for adults with depression. Br J Music Ther. 2023;37(2):71–81. https://doi.org/10.1177/13594575231194304.

Bourdaghs S, Silverman MJ. An exploratory interpretivist study of how adults with substance use disorders experience peer social connectedness during recovery-oriented songwriting. Psychol Music. 2023;51(5):1440–56. https://doi.org/10.1177/03057356221146814.

Burns DS, Robb SL, Haase JE. Exploring the feasibility of a therapeutic music video intervention in adolescents and young adults during stem-cell transplantation. Cancer Nurs. 2009;32(5):E8–E16. https://doi.org/10.1002/cncr.28355.

Chong HJ. Do we all enjoy singing? A content analysis of non-vocalists' attitudes toward singing. Arts Psychother. 2010;37(2):120–4. https://doi.org/10.1016/j.aip.2010.01.001.

Crooke AHD. Music technology and the hip hop beat making tradition: a history and typology of equipment for music therapy. Voices World Forum Music Ther. 2018;18(2) https://doi.org/10.15845/voices.v18i2.996.

Crooke AHD, McFerran KS. Improvising using beat making technologies in music therapy with young people. Music Ther Perspect. 2019;37(1):55–64. https://doi.org/10.1093/mtp/miy025.

Csikszentmihalyi M. Beyond boredom and anxiety. Jossey-Bass. 1975.

Csikszentmihalyi M. Flow: the psychology of optimal experience. Harper & Row; 1990.

Csikszentmihalyi M. The evolving self. Harper & Row; 1993.

Day T, Baker FA, Darlington Y. Experiences of song writing in a group programme for mothers who had experienced childhood abuse. Nord J Music Ther. 2009;18(2):133–49. https://doi.org/10.1080/08098130903062405.

Fiore J. Analysis of lyrics from group songwriting with bereaved children and adolescents. J Music Ther. 2016;53(3):207–31. https://doi.org/10.1093/jmt/thw005.
Grocke D, Bloch S, Castle D. The effect of group music therapy on quality of life for participants living with a severe and enduring mental illness. J Music Ther. 2009;46:90–104. https://doi.org/10.1093/jmt/46.2.90.
Jackson SA. Toward a conceptual understanding of the flow experience in elite athletes. Res Q Exerc Sport. 1996;67:76–90. https://doi.org/10.1080/02701367.1996.10607928.
Jackson SA, Csikszentmihalyi M. Flow in sports: the keys to optimal experiences and performances. Human Kinetics; 1999.
Jackson SA, Marsh HW. Development and validation of a scale to measure optimal experience: the flow state scale. J Sport Exerc Psychol. 1996;18:17–35. https://doi.org/10.1123/jsep.18.1.17.
Lang JM, Campbell K, Vanderploeg JJ. Advancing trauma-informed systems for children. Farmington: Child Health and Development Institute; 2015.
Martin JJ, Culter K. An exploratory study of flow and motivation in theatre actors. J Appl Sport Psychol. 2002;14:344–52. https://doi.org/10.1080/10413200290103608.
O'Callaghan C, Grocke D. Lyric analysis research in music therapy: rationales, methods and representations. Arts Psychother. 2009;36:320–8. https://doi.org/10.1016/j.aip.2009.09.004.
Robb SL, Burns DS, Stegenga KA, Haut PR, Monahan PO, Meza J, et al. Randomized clinical trial of therapeutic music video intervention for resilience outcomes in adolescents/young adults undergoing hematopoietic stem cell transplant: a report from the Children's Oncology Group. Cancer. 2014;120(6):909–17. https://doi.org/10.1002/cncr.28355.
Roddy C, Rickard N, Tamplin J, Baker FA. Personal identity narratives of therapeutic songwriting participants following spinal cord injury: a case series analysis. J Spinal Cord Med. 2018;41(4):435–43. https://doi.org/10.1080/10790268.2017.1364559.
Rolvsjord R. Collaborations on songwriting with clients with mental health problems. In: Baker F, Wigram T, editors. Songwriting: methods, techniques and clinical applications for music therapy clinicians, educators and students. Jessica Kingsley; 2005. p. 97–115.
Sears WW. Processes in music therapy. Nord J Music Ther. 1996;5(1):33–42. https://doi.org/10.1080/08098139609477865.
Sena Moore K. Music therapy advocacy for professional recognition: a historical perspective and future directions. Music Ther Perspect. 2015;33(1):76–85. https://doi.org/10.1093/mtp.miu043.
Silverman MJ. Evaluating current trends in psychiatric music therapy: a descriptive analysis. J Music Ther. 2007;44:388–414. https://doi.org/10.1093/jmt/44.4.388.
Silverman MJ. A descriptive analysis of music therapists working with consumers in substance abuse rehabilitation. Arts Psychother. 2009;36:123–30. https://doi.org/10.1016/j.aip.2008.10.005.
Silverman MJ. Effects of music therapy on self- and experienced stigma in patients on an acute care psychiatric unit: a randomized three-group effectiveness study. Arch Psychiatr Nurs. 2013;27:223–30. https://doi.org/10.1016/j.apnu.2013.06.003.
Silverman MJ. Music therapy and therapeutic alliance in adult mental health: a qualitative investigation. J Music Ther. 2019a;56:90–116. https://doi.org/10.1093/jmt/thy019.
Silverman MJ. Music therapy for coping self-efficacy in an acute mental health setting: a randomized pilot study. Community Mental Health J. 2019b;55:615–23. https://doi.org/10.1007/s10597-018-0319-8.
Silverman MJ. Therapeutic songwriting for perceived stigma and social support in adults with substance use disorder: a cluster-randomized effectiveness study. Subst Use Misuse. 2020;55:763–71. https://doi.org/10.1080/10826084.2019.1701237.
Silverman MJ. Songwriting, professional studio recording, and a CD release party: interviews with two adults with mental health conditions. Arts Psychother. 2022a;79:101915. https://doi.org/10.1016/j.aip.2022.101915.
Silverman MJ. Music therapy in mental health for illness management and recovery. 2nd ed. Oxford University Press; 2022b.

Silverman MJ. Comparing music therapy interventions in adults with substance use disorder on a detoxification unit as measured by the group relationship: a three-group cluster-randomized study. Int J Syst Ther. 2023a; https://doi.org/10.1080/2692398X.2023.2290427.

Silverman MJ. Reconceptualizing music therapy in acute mental health settings Part I: a descriptive overview of single-session therapy. Music Ther Perspect. 2023b; https://doi.org/10.1093/mtp/miad018.

Silverman MJ. Reconceptualizing music therapy in acute mental health settings: Part II: clinical applications of single-session therapy. Music Ther Perspect. 2024; https://doi.org/10.1093/mtp/miad019.

Silverman MJ, Baker FA. Applications of flow in music therapy clinical practice and research. Approaches: an interdisciplinary. J Music Ther. 2018;10:43–51.

Silverman MJ, Baker FA, MacDonald RAR. Flow and meaningfulness as predictors of therapeutic outcome within songwriting interventions. Psychol Music. 2016;44:1331–45. https://doi.org/10.1177/030573561527505.

Silverman MJ, Gooding LF, Yinger OS. It's complicated: A theoretical model of music-induced harm. Journal of Music Therapy, 2020;57(3):251-281.https://doi.org/10.1093/jmt/thaa008.

Silverman MJ, Bourdaghs S, Abbazio J, Riegelman A. A systematic review of music-induced substance craving. Music Sci. 2023;27(1):137–75. https://doi.org/10.1177/10298649211030314.

Snyder CR. The psychology of hope: you can get there from here. Simon and Schuster; 1994.

Snyder CR. Hope theory: rainbows in the mind. Psychol Inq. 2002;13(4):249–75. https://doi.org/10.1207/S15327965PLI1304_01.

Substance Abuse and Mental Health Services Administration (SAMHSA). SAMHSA's concept of trauma and guidance for a trauma-informed approach, HHS publication No. (SMA) 14-4884. Rockville: Substance Abuse and Mental Health Services Administration; 2014.

Wang S, Cevasco-Trotter AM, Silverman MJ, Yuan SH. A narrative review of music therapy for neuropsychiatric symptoms in Alzheimer's disease and rationale for protocolized music teletherapy. Front Med. 2023;10:124825. https://doi.org/10.3389/fmed.2023.124825.

Windle E, Hickling LM, Jayacodi S, Carr C. The experiences of patients in the synchrony group music therapy trial for long-term depression. Arts Psychother. 2020;67:101580. https://doi.org/10.1016/j.aip.2019.101580.

Neurologic Music Therapy

7

Shannon K. de l'Etoile

Key Points

- Neurologic music therapy (NMT) is an evidence-based approach to research and clinical practice that has transformed the profession from a social science to a neuroscience model
- Advances in neuroscience have revealed underlying mechanisms of change, such as music induced neural plasticity, that explain the influence of music on functional, nonmusical behavior
- The Rational-Scientific Mediating Model provides a logical guide for NMT research, which the Transformational Design Model subsequently integrates into effective treatment planning
- The NMT system includes techniques to improve sensorimotor, speech and language, and cognitive-socioemotional functioning for a variety of clinical populations
- Techniques in all domains are supported by scientific evidence and theoretical models regarding the neurological, physiological, and psychological intersections of musical and nonmusical behavior

Within the United States, the music therapy profession emerged from a movement during World War II (1939–1945) in which Veterans Administration hospitals established music programs to boost soldiers' morale (Davis 2008; de l'Etoile and LaGasse 2013; LaGasse and Thaut 2012). As musicians were hired to implement

S. K. de l'Etoile (✉)
Department of Music Therapy, Frost School of Music, University of Miami, Coral Gables, FL, USA
e-mail: sdel@miami.edu

A. Raglio (ed.), *Music and Music Therapy Interventions in Clinical Practice*, Neurocultural Health and Wellbeing,
https://doi.org/10.1007/978-3-031-88578-5_7

these programs, veterans received and contributed to musical performances which promoted their social interaction and relationship building, emotional expression, and overall well-being (Koshimori and Thaut 2019; Thaut and McIntosh 2010). Thus, while beneficial, the profession was initially rooted in a social science framework that lacked clear therapeutic aims and scientific support (de l'Etoile and Roth 2019).

In the following decades, significant progress in neuroscience technology led to the development of brain imaging, motion analysis, and electromyography techniques (Illes and Bird 2006; Lu and Chang 2012; Raichle 2003, 2006, 2008; Sutherland 2001). These advances identified the neurological and biological mechanisms of music perception and experience that could be captured in real time (de l'Etoile and LaGasse 2013; LaGasse and Thaut 2012; Thaut and McIntosh 2010). By the early 1990s, accumulating evidence revealed how the human brain and body perceives, responds to, and creates music, generating two pivotal conclusions:

1. Neural structures and pathways used for music are not exclusive to music (de l'Etoile 2016; de l'Etoile and LaGasse 2013; Koelsch 2009; Thaut and McIntosh 2010). Music engages widely distributed networks that underlie numerous functional, nonmusical behaviors, including attention, memory, language, movement, emotions, and more. Therefore, musical experiences, such as music listening, singing, playing instruments, and composition, inherently activate, exercise, and strengthen brain areas also needed for nonmusical, everyday behaviors, supporting their execution.
2. Musical experiences change the brain. More recently, this phenomenon has been recognized as music induced neural plasticity. To explain, plasticity refers to the brain's capacity to adapt to complex demands by reorganizing its structure, function, and connections (Altenmüller and Schlaug 2015; Chatterjee et al. 2021). Intensive practice of a behavior along with progressive adjustments are key ingredients for plasticity that can lead to skill learning and recovery. Music serves as an effectual stimulus for plasticity, through multimodal activation of a widely distributed bi-hemispheric neuronal network that encompasses both cortical and subcortical structures (Chatterjee et al. 2021; Kraus and Chandrasekaran 2010; Piccirilli et al. 2021; Reybrouck et al. 2018; Schlaug 2001). Musical instrument playing in particular involves cognitive and motor functions, from the translation of musical symbols to the generation of bimanual movements that produce rhythmic and tonal patterns recognized as music (Hanna-Pladdy and Menken 2020). Playing an instrument well typically requires intensive, repetitive practice and use of auditory feedback for correction. Thus, music making entails repetition and fine-tuning of behaviors supported by auditory and motor brain regions as well as their interconnections (Schlaug 2009). This multisensory brain activation strengthens and optimizes existing neural pathways and helps create new connections that might not otherwise exist (Cheng et al. 2020).

Plasticity is often seen in relation to complex tasks that involve emotional arousal and activation of the brain reward system, including release of the neurotransmitter dopamine, which supports learning and memory (Altenmüller and Schlaug 2015; Chatterjee et al. 2021). Specifically, dopamine modulates long-term potentiation, a neural process that involves synapse strengthening and increased synaptic transmission, thereby enhancing plasticity at the synaptic level (Gurden et al. 2000). Music experiences are associated with significant activation within the mesocorticolimbic system which underlies reward and reinforcement (Chatterjee et al. 2021), and exposure to favorite music in particular leads to dopamine release (Ferreri et al. 2022; Zatorre and Salimpoor 2013). Music therefore serves as a powerful catalyst for neural plasticity by requiring the simultaneous use of multiple brain areas through a rewarding and dopamine-inducing experience (Chatterjee et al. 2021).

Evidence for music-induced neural plasticity originates from the observation that the brains of musicians and nonmusicians are structurally different (Chatterjee et al. 2021; Cheng et al. 2020; Hanna-Pladdy and Menken 2020; Piccirilli et al. 2021; Wan and Schlaug 2010). Intensive music training leads to long-lasting structural and functional adaptations which manifest as enhanced connectivity and network efficiency among brain regions that underlie auditory–motor control, sensory feedback, and emotional expression (Cheng et al. 2020). Most evidence of this plasticity pertains to individuals that trained musically during childhood and who continue to demonstrate differences in brain organization into adulthood (Schlaug 2015). Fortunately, the human brain remains flexible across the lifespan, supporting neural adaptation and behavioral change from music experiences at all ages (Chatterjee et al. 2021; Schlaug 2015). Moreover, data are gradually accumulating regarding the impact of short-term music training on neuroplasticity in support of functional behaviors (François et al. 2015).

These two groundbreaking conclusions have supported translational and applied research that explains how music therapy "works," thereby providing a scientific foundation for the discipline and promoting a shift from a social science model to a neuroscience model (Koshimori and Thaut 2019; LaGasse and Thaut 2012; Thaut 2005a; Thaut and McIntosh 2010). This transformational shift led to the formation of a scientifically based approach to clinical practice and research, known as Neurologic Music Therapy (NMT) through which therapists can promote focused, reliable, functional outcomes in their patients that extend beyond a general sense of well-being (Clair and Pasiali 2004; LaGasse and Thaut 2012; Thaut 2005a; Thaut and McIntosh 2010). Recognized by the World Federation of Neurorehabilitation (n.d.), NMT comprises a system of standardized therapeutic techniques for rehabilitation and development in sensorimotor, communication, and cognitive/socioemotional domains. In addition, NMT offers a theoretical model to guide research and a second, related model to support treatment planning. This chapter will review both theoretical models as well as all NMT techniques and key points of supporting evidence.

7.1 Theoretical Frameworks for Neurologic Music Therapy

To best realize and utilize the scientific evidence underlying NMT techniques, two interconnected theoretical models have been developed. The Rational-Scientific Mediating Model (RSMM) explains how research is conducted and used in support of NMT with regard to motor control, speech and language, and cognition and affect. The Transformational Design Model (TDM) describes the thought process needed for effective treatment planning, to ensure optimal therapeutic outcomes.

7.1.1 Rational-Scientific Mediating Model (RSMM)

This scientific model connects basic and applied evidence to support both research and clinical practice in NMT (Clair and Pasiali 2004; de l'Etoile 2016; de l'Etoile et al. 2012; Thaut 2000a, 2005a; Thaut et al. 2014a). Researchers should use the RSMM to explore the neurological, physiological, and psychological pathways of music perception and production and how they mediate to change behavior (de l'Etoile 2016; Thaut 2000a). The model comprises these four steps (Table 7.1):

Table 7.1 Steps of the rational-scientific mediating model (RSMM)

Step	Purpose	Example—Following a neurological approach
Step 1 Musical Response Models	Understand the neurological, physiological, or psychological mechanisms of music perception, processing, and production	What brain structures are involved in singing?
Step 2 Nonmusical parallel models	Understand the neurological, physiological, or psychological mechanisms of nonmusical behavior	What brain structures underlie speech production?
Comparative analysis	Identify a parallel process or overlap between the musical and the nonmusical behavior	What brain structures are common to both singing and speech production?
Step 3 Mediating models	Explore the immediate or short-term effect of the musical behavior on the non-musical behavior, first with a typical population, then a clinical population	What is the effect of singing on intelligible speech production in preschool-age children? What is the effective of singing on intelligible speech production in children with speech apraxia?
Step 4 Clinical research models	Conduct applied research on the long-term effect of a music intervention on a functional behavior with a clinical population	What is the long-term effect of singing in Oral Motor and Respiratory Exercises (OMREX) on intelligible speech production in children with speech apraxia?

7.1.2 Step 1 Musical Response Models

Research at this level establishes an understanding of how humans perceive, create, or respond to music. This knowledge stems from investigations of the neurological, physiological, or psychological mechanisms of a specified musical behavior within a research scenario. As an example, a researcher who ultimately wants to explore the impact of singing on speech production might ask these questions at this level: What are the brain regions and pathways that subserve singing? What are the physiological structures and processes utilized when singing? What is the developmental sequence for the acquisition of singing?

7.1.3 Step 2 Nonmusical Parallel Models

This level includes two sequential components. Initially, the target research behavior—identified as a nonmusical, functional behavior—must be investigated to clarify its underlying neurological, physiological, and perceptual systems. In the second component of this level, a comparative analysis is conducted to identify a parallel process or overlap between the musical and nonmusical behavior. If a researcher ultimately plans to examine the impact of singing impact on speech production, questions at this level might be: What brain structures are utilized in speech production? What physiological mechanisms are associated with speech production? What is the developmental sequence for speech production?

With this understanding in hand, the researcher could then realize that strong neurological parallels exist between singing and speaking, and certain brain regions are specific to each behavior; thus, singing can strengthen existing pathways or access alternative pathways to enhance speech production. In addition, the research would recognize that a well-structured singing protocol can exercise and strengthen the physiological mechanisms needed for effective speech production. These parallel processes reveal underlying mechanisms of change; that is, they explain how behavior can change in response to music. A parallel or overlapping process must be identified before proceeding to the next step, where the change mechanism can be tested.

7.1.4 Step 3 Mediating Models

At this level, research explores the short-term or immediate effects of music on the nonmusical behavior, to establish feasibility evidence for future clinical trials (Thaut et al. 2014a). Initial protocols may involve typically functioning individuals to verify the identified parallel process and to determine reference points for subsequent investigations with clinical cohorts. A researcher may first explore the impact of a short-term singing program on intelligible speech production in typically functioning preschool age children. Favorable outcomes achieved here would then support short-term explorations of singing on speech production in a clinical population, such as children with speech apraxia. Positive findings generated here would justify future research with a clinical, applied focus.

7.1.5 Step 4 Clinical Research Models

Within this final step of the RSMM, research is conducted based on evidence obtained in the first three initial stages, taking full advantage of the mechanism of change. The intention is to explore the therapeutic benefits of music, or the influence of an intensive music intervention over time on a functional behavior in a clinical population. As an example, a researcher may examine the effect of singing as part of the NMT technique Oral Motor and Respiratory Exercises (OMREXs), as applied daily for 4 weeks, on intelligible speech production in children with speech apraxia. To determine treatment efficacy, data collection should assess change over time in relation to the intervention, as well as skill maintenance through long-term follow-up.

Ultimately, the RSMM provides a scientific, logical guide for conducting research that ensures NMT techniques are evidence-based. Findings generated here are vital to demonstrating not only that NMT techniques work (i.e., do they achieve intended outcomes?) but also to explaining how NMT techniques work (i.e., what is the mechanism of change?). The importance of the basic evidence generated in steps 1 and 2 of this model cannot be overstated. If an investigator conducts clinical research without first understanding the parallel process, they may be able to produce positive outcomes, but they will not be able to explain how the results were obtained or to interpret the findings. The identified parallel process, or mechanism of change, further supports effective implementation of the intervention and an understanding of how it can be modified as needed to accommodate client needs. Ultimately, articulating the mechanism of change is essential to carrying out evidence-based, credible research that makes a meaningful contribution to the discipline.

7.2 Transformational Design Model (TDM)

This treatment planning model provides a six-step systematic approach for translating research findings from the RSMM into clinical practice (de l'Etoile 2016; Thaut 2000b, 2014a). The first three steps of the TDM are common to all therapeutic disciplines, yet the model also includes components unique to the use of music as a therapeutic medium. By following the steps below in order, clinicians will be able to engage in effective, evidence-based treatment planning, including the selection and development of the most appropriate therapeutic interventions for their clients and compelling outcome reporting (Table 7.2).

Table 7.2 Steps of the transformational design model (TDM)

Step	Purpose
Step 1 Diagnostic and functional/clinical assessment	Determine patient's medical or psychological diagnosis; assess strengths and areas of need to inform selection of the most appropriate treatment
Step 2 Development of goals and objectives	Establish broad treatment goals and corresponding, specific objectives that identify functional, nonmusical behaviors and establish measurement criteria for their improvement
Step 3 Design of Functional, non-musical therapeutic exercises and stimuli	Using knowledge of human learning, development, and rehabilitation principles, design a general therapeutic plan that will facilitate the patient's practice of the objective behavior
Step 4 Translation of Step 3 into functional therapeutic music interventions (TMIs)	Translate the general therapeutic plan into a therapeutic music intervention that uses a pleasing aesthetic experience to facilitate the objective behavior, and that is based on the best available scientific evidence regarding the impact of music on the objective behavior
Step 5 Outcome reassessment	Reassess the patient's objective behavior as in Step 1 to determine treatment effectiveness
Step 6 Transfer of therapeutic learning to functional, nonmusical, real-world applications	Provide the patient with a plan, including necessary tools and resources, to transfer therapeutic learning to daily life

7.2.1 Step 1 Diagnostic and Functional/Clinical Assessment

As the starting point of treatment for any therapeutic discipline, a thorough assessment should be conducted of the client's strengths and needs. Two types of assessment are needed, the first being diagnostic, which refers to a determination of a client's diagnoses as gained through various medical or psychological tests (Thaut 2014a). The second type is known as functional or clinical assessment, which is critical for optimal treatment selection and tracking patient progress throughout the treatment period.

7.2.2 Step 2 Development of Goals and Objectives

Based on clinical priorities identified in step 1, the NMT clinician now maps out a plan for treatment by crafting goals and objectives. A goal typically identifies a broad behavioral domain and a direction of change, such as to increase, improve, or maintain functioning. An objective is a statement that identifies a functional, measurable, nonmusical behavior related to the goal, along with measurement criteria to indicate desired frequency or duration of behavior. Objective behaviors are directly facilitated by the provided music stimulus and practiced during the NMT intervention. In addition, objective behaviors are observed and measured during therapy sessions to provide additional assessment of both client progress and the intervention itself.

7.2.3 Step 3 Design of Functional, Nonmusical Therapeutic Exercises, and Stimuli

In this step, the clinician formulates a general therapeutic plan that gives the client opportunity to practice and learn or relearn the objective behavior. The focus of this plan should remain on the client's nonmusical, objective behavior and utilize an understanding of human learning and development. Maintaining focus on the behavior without yet considering musical components of the intervention ensures a functional outcome, rather than a musical outcome. This behavioral focus also supports collaborative efforts with other disciplines who may be addressing similar treatment goals. This step of the model is critical to effective treatment planning. If omitted, the therapist is likely to provide the client with an enjoyable or entertaining music experience, but one that does not support the client in making progress toward set goals and objectives.

As one example, for a young child with speech apraxia resulting in limited speech production, the general therapeutic plan could be as follows: the client needs multiple opportunities to observe, hear, and imitate a variety of developmentally appropriate speech sounds; to gain awareness of the physical movements needed to create speech sounds; and to experience the physical, oromotor sensations associated with specific speech sounds. This nonmusical plan is based on an understanding of how children acquire the ability to produce speech sounds, by accessing and establishing underlying neural speech motor planning networks as well as strengthening oral motor musculature. By using this plan as a foundation for treatment planning, the NMT clinician will be able to design, select, and implement a therapeutic intervention that directly addresses the objective behavior of speech production.

7.2.4 Step 4 Translation of Step 3 into Functional Therapeutic Music Interventions (TMIs)

The clinician is now ready to transform the previous general therapeutic plan into an isomorphic musical experience, meaning it will follow an identical functional structure (de l'Etoile 2016; Thaut 2000b, 2014a). To ensure nonmusical, functional outcomes for the client, this translational process must take the following three components into consideration:

- Functional Logic: the TMI must serve as a direct translation of the general therapeutic plan from Step 3; that is, it must maintain an emphasis on the functional, objective behavior and the experience needed to develop or rehabilitate that behavior. In addition, the TMI must provide for repeated or sustained execution of the behavior to support lasting change. For a child with speech apraxia, the TMI should consist of musical experiences, such as singing and simple wind instrument playing, that provide multiple opportunities for the child to observe, hear, and imitate speech sounds, as well as to experience the physical movements and sensations related to those sounds.

- Musical Logic: the therapist needs to design and implement the TMI using good musical forms that provide a pleasing aesthetic experience for the client, whether presented actively (i.e., the client is actively engaged in producing the music) or receptively (i.e., the client is listening to the music). In either scenario, the client must have a rewarding perceptual experience to achieve full therapeutic benefit. The clinician should also adjust the musical complexity and intensity to accommodate the client's level of functioning, tolerance for sensory stimulation, and response capacity. In addition, careful thought should be given to the use of key musical elements in the TMI and how they are directly impacting client response. For instance, to facilitate a young child's production of speech sounds through singing, the therapist would consider pitch levels that accommodate the child's vocal range, use of simple stepwise melodic structure, and emphasis of key target sounds through rhythmic and harmonic components that provide anticipatory cues for speech movements.
- Scientific Logic: the therapist should select or design the TMI utilizing the scientific evidence generated through the RSMM. This selection process is greatly enhanced by the knowledge base that exists and that is evolving within the NMT paradigm. Thus, the therapist does not need to build the intervention "from scratch" for every session but rather, can select from a system of evidence-based NMT techniques. As one example, the use of singing as part of OMREX is supported by current research findings that identify patterns of neural and physiological activity common to both singing and speaking.

7.2.5 Step 5 Outcome Reassessment

To monitor treatment effectiveness, the therapist should reassess the client's objective behavior (Thaut 2014a), ideally using the same tools and methods from Step 1. Data can be collected during or immediately after each intervention application, or at the end of the treatment period and at periodic follow-ups. The data collection methods selected and the timing of their use will depend on the sensitivity of the measurement tool as well as the clinical setting and unique patient needs. Accurate and rigorous data capture is essential for determining and reporting treatment efficacy, as well as for continuing the process of assessment and intervention enhancement throughout the treatment period.

7.2.6 Step 6 Transfer of Therapeutic Learning to Functional, Nonmusical, Real-World Applications

To support long-term therapeutic learning, the therapist should provide the client with a transfer plan that helps them continue exercising their new behavior beyond the therapeutic setting (Thaut 2014a). The transfer plan can consist of "homework" that the client must carry out between sessions, as well as a strategy for long-term practice and connection to activities of daily living. For repetition of OMREX exercises, the therapist could create a recording of singing exercises that the client must practice on their own, with increasing levels of complexity to accommodate change over time. Using insights and skills gained from therapy, the plan could also incorporate practice of speech samples that the client must use in everyday life (i.e., at school, with siblings, etc.). The overall intent of this plan is to ensure continuation of functional gains and further optimize music-induced neuroplasticity.

7.3 Sensorimotor Training Techniques

The NMT system includes three techniques to enhance sensorimotor functioning: rhythmic auditory stimulation, patterned sensory enhancement, and therapeutic instrumental music performance. All three techniques utilize the rich interconnections between rhythm perception and motor output to facilitate improved movement outcomes (Table 7.3).

Table 7.3 NMT techniques for sensorimotor training

Technique	Treatment goals	Appropriate populations
Rhythmic Auditory Stimulation (RAS)	Overall stabilization of gait kinematics through improvements in temporal and spatial gait parameters, including cadence, velocity, stride length, and symmetry	Neurologically based gait disorders, such as stroke, Parkinson disease, traumatic brain injury, multiple sclerosis, spinal cord injury, cerebral palsy. Other issues that impact gait, including orthopedic conditions, medical or sensory disorders, aging
Patterned Sensory Enhancement (PSE)	Improved ability to carry out activities of daily living and underlying functional motor patterns through enhanced strength and endurance in upper and lower extremities, improved balance and posture, increased use of functional upper extremity movements	Neurological or orthopedic conditions, including stroke, cerebral palsy, Parkinson disease, Down syndrome; back, knee, hip, or shoulder surgery; physical recovery from surgery or illness, such as flu, cancer, or Guillain-Barré syndrome, healthy individuals
Therapeutic Instrumental Music Performance (TIMP)	Optimization of fine and gross motor skills via increased strength, endurance, range of motion of upper and lower extremities; improved bilateral coordination; enhanced speed, dexterity, and timing of movement	Neurological or orthopedic populations, such as stroke, spinal cord injury, traumatic brain injury, cerebral palsy, polio, arthritis; back, knee, hip, or shoulder surgery

7.3.1 Rhythmic Auditory Stimulation (RAS)

Rhythmic auditory stimulation (RAS) is a neurologic rehabilitation technique in which external auditory cueing is used to facilitate movements that are intrinsically and biologically rhythmic, specifically gait (Thaut and Rice 2014; Thaut 2005b). Treatment goals for RAS include improvements in the temporal components of gait, including cadence and velocity, as well as spatial parameters, such as stride length and symmetry (de l'Etoile and Roth 2019). Positive outcomes from RAS are well-documented for individuals with significant gait deficits resulting from neurologic disorders, such as stroke, Parkinson disease, traumatic brain injury, or multiple sclerosis, and data are emerging in support of RAS for patients with cerebral palsy (Janzen et al. 2022; Schaffert et al. 2019; Thaut 2015; Thaut et al. 1993; Wang et al. 2022). Based on these findings, RAS is now listed in the official stroke care guidelines of the United States Departments of Veterans Affairs and Defense (2019), as well as by the Heart and Stroke Foundation of Canada (2019) and Thaut et al. (2021). RAS can also benefit patients with gait deficits due to aging, orthopedic conditions, or other medical or sensory issues.

Drawing from the logic of the Rational-Scientific Mediating Model, the underlying therapeutic mechanism for RAS stems from a strong neurologic overlap. Many central nervous system structures involved in perceiving and responding to rhythm are also needed for the execution of gait and other functional movements, (Chen et al. 2008; Grahn and Brett 2007; Pal'tsev and El'ner 1967; Rossignol and Jones 1976). Therefore, a systematic application of rhythmic cues will engage and strengthen these structures and their connections, leading to functional, stable, and adaptive gait. The impact of this overlap can be further delineated in the following four points that specifically describe the neurophysiological effect of rhythm on the motor system:

7.3.1.1 Rhythmic Entrainment

The auditory system has an exceptional capacity for rapid and precise detection of recurring patterns in auditory cues (Felix et al. 2011; Janzen et al. 2022; Schaffert et al. 2019; Thaut 2015; Thaut et al. 2015). In addition, the human nervous system demonstrates rich interconnectivity between auditory and motor systems at the spinal cord, brain stem, subcortical, and cortical levels. These two factors support auditory motor coupling, in which central nervous system structures that support movement couple with the auditory system to drive movement patterns (Chatterjee et al. 2021; Janzen et al. 2022; Schaffert et al. 2019; Thaut and Rice 2014). Such coupling indicates that auditory neurons entrain the firing patterns of motor neurons, thereby directing the motor system to produce regulated movement patterns (Lakatos et al. 2019; Thaut 2015; Thaut et al. 2015). The result of this activity is rhythmic entrainment, the natural phenomenon whereby movement occurs at the same frequency or regularity as an external auditory cue (Thaut 2005c). When the motor system can maintain that coupling relationship over time even as the cue may fluctuate, it leads to synchronization. Entrainment of gait movements with rhythmic auditory cues promotes symmetry between the lower extremities and increased stride length as needed for greater gait velocity.

7.3.1.2 Priming of the Auditory Motor Pathway

Priming occurs when a predictable auditory cue elicits more efficient motor neuron recruitment at the spinal cord level, thereby improving muscle activation and creating a state of readiness for movement (Janzen et al. 2022; Pal'tsev and El'ner 1967; Rossignol and Jones 1976; Schaffert et al. 2019; Thaut 2015; Thaut et al. 2015). Outcomes of priming include enhanced movement quality, such as improved control and coordination. Through priming, patients are also better prepared to adapt gait patterns, as walking conditions dictate (Miller et al. 1996).

7.3.1.3 Cueing of the Movement Period

An auditory rhythmic cue comprises two important components that guide movement. First, in regard to gait movements, the audible beat cues the endpoint of the gait cycle, or the heel strike (de l'Etoile and Roth 2019). The second component is the time interval between beats, which directs and times all movements between successive heel strikes, such as weight shift, acceleration, knee trajectory during swing phase, etc. (Thaut et al. 1998). Rhythm therefore provides a continuous time reference to enhance planning and scaling of movement throughout the entire gait cycle, resulting in smoother and less variable movement trajectories and overall stabilization of the movement pattern (Janzen et al. 2022; Schaffert et al. 2019; Thaut 2015; Thaut et al. 2015).

7.3.1.4 Step-Wise Limit Cycle Entrainment (SLICE)

All moving systems have a limit cycle or preferred tempo at which they perform optimally. Most people walk at a consistent pace or tempo, which can be disrupted by disease or injury (Thaut and Rice 2014). During RAS, the therapist provides an auditory rhythmic cue that matches the patient's current limit cycle, even if it is not optimal (de l'Etoile and Roth 2019). Once gait movements entrain and kinematics stabilize, the tempo of the cue is increased in 5–10% increments, to help the patient approach premorbid limit cycles (Janzen et al. 2022; Schaffert et al. 2019; Thaut and Rice 2014).

7.3.2 RAS Clinical Protocol

RAS can be used as an immediate entrainment stimulus or as part of a long-term gait training program to regain functional movement (Schaffert et al. 2019; Thaut 2015). The protocol consists of six steps that should be conducted in order, as briefly reviewed here. For further details, see Thaut and Rice (2014).

7.3.2.1 Step 1 Assessment of Current Gait Parameters

The clinician begins by assessing step cadence, which will determine the starting tempo for the rhythmic cueing. As time and patient endurance allow, additional parameters should also be assessed, including gait velocity, stride length, and symmetry.

7.3.2.2 Step 2 Resonant Frequency Entrainment and Pre-gait Exercises

The clinician provides rhythmic auditory cueing at a tempo that matches the cadence determined in Step 1. The cue should be in duple meter to match bipedal movements and have adequate pulse clarity for effective auditory motor coupling and priming. The clinician should make decisions regarding metronome vs. music or live vs. recorded cueing based on the needs of the patient and the parameters of the clinical setting. The patient first listens and finger taps to the cue, then stands and walks to the cue. For patients who have difficulty bearing weight or initiating movement, pre-gait exercises may be necessary to address these issues prior to gait training (see next Sect. 3.10). Approximately one-third of each session is spent in resonant frequency entrainment.

7.3.2.3 Step 3 Frequency Modulation at Increments of 5–10%

If gait kinematics have stabilized at Step 2, the clinician can then increase the cue tempo by 5–10%. This step exemplifies the logic behind "SLICE" and helps the patient achieve a more functional limit cycle. Another third of each session should be devoted to frequency modulation.

7.3.2.4 Advanced Gait Exercises

If time allows and the patient is not fatigued, adaptive gait exercises are used to provide experience walking in changing scenarios. Examples include providing rhythmic cueing while the patient walks in different directions, makes sudden tempo changes, walks around obstacles, or walks on varying surfaces (i.e., carpet, tile, grass, pavement, etc.).

7.3.2.5 Fading of Rhythmic Stimulus

To help the patient with skill transfer, the rhythmic cue should be gradually faded and removed as the patient is walking. The patient should be told in advance that the cue will be withdrawn and instructed to continue walking at the pace of the cue. The final third of the session is typically devoted to fading procedures.

7.3.2.6 Reassessment of Gait Parameters

To determine progress, the clinician repeats the assessment procedures from Step 1. If the patient is fatigued or time does not allow for a full reassessment, then only step cadence should be measured.

7.3.3 Patterned Sensory Enhancement (PSE)

The technique Patterned Sensory Enhancement (PSE) uses music as a sensory cue to structure movement through both time and space, thus supporting the rehabilitation or development of motor skills (Thaut 2014a). Movements addressed through PSE may be drawn directly from activities of daily living or can emphasize the fundamental motor patterns needed for such activities, such as leaning, reaching, or grasping. While these movements tend to be discrete and nonrhythmic, they can still be cued rhythmically to facilitate repetition of cyclical motion as needed for motor learning or relearning (Thaut 2015; Thaut et al. 2015). The primary goals of PSE are to enhance physical strength and endurance of the upper and lower extremities, improve balance and posture, and increase the use of functional movements in the upper limbs (Thaut 2005b, 2014a). PSE can benefit individuals of all ages with various neurological or orthopedic conditions, with significantly positive outcomes reported for individuals with stroke or cerebral palsy (Janzen et al. 2022; Kang et al. 2020; Luft et al. 2004; Thaut et al. 2002; Wang et al. 2013). Additional effects have been noted for patients with Parkinson disease (Keenan 2011), Down syndrome (Ringenbach et al. 2014), as well as healthy adults (Ross et al. 2016).

PSE exercises provide a multidimensional sensory template to guide movement and typically involve the use of rhythmic cues, thus, the neurologic mechanisms of RAS also support this technique (Thaut 2005b, 2014a). Scientific support that is unique to PSE includes the following points:

7.3.3.1 Muscle Activation Patterns

Motor learning or relearning requires extensive movement repetition. When rhythmic cueing is used to facilitate this repetition, significant changes occur in muscle activation patterns, most likely resulting from more efficient recruitment of motor units which are the connecting points between motor neurons and muscle fibers (Monti et al. 2001; Safranek et al. 1982; Thaut et al. 1991, 1996). Observed changes include co-contraction of antagonist muscles, which indicates motor learning. Rhythmic cueing also leads to increased duration of muscle activity, more regular onset and termination of muscle activity, and repression of undesired muscle contractions that can interfere with motor learning. These changes in muscle activity effectively stabilize muscles around the joint and allow for controlled, voluntary movement.

7.3.3.2 Scaling of Movement Velocity

Carrying out activities of daily living requires the ability to adjust movement speed, even when spatial demands change (i.e., movement distance becomes longer or shorter). This ability is known as scaling of movement velocity, which is often impaired for individuals with neurologic or orthopedic conditions. With steady rhythmic cueing, these critical timing adjustments can be regained in support of functional movement (Thaut et al. 1996, 2002).

7.3.4 PSE Clinical Protocol

The implementation of PSE requires an understanding that the music is not accompanying movement, but rather, is directing and facilitating the movement (Thaut 2014a). Clinicians need to first conceptualize the target movement, paying careful attention to the overall timing of the movement, as well as components of the movement that require the most force or strength. Due to their large pitch range and capacity for dramatic dynamic changes, ideal instruments for PSE include keyboard and autoharp. Having made these important determinations, the clinician then designs a sound template to direct the movement, making best use of salient musical elements to cue the temporal, spatial, and force dynamics of the movement.

7.3.4.1 Spatial Cues

Spatial components of movement include range of motion in the horizontal and vertical planes, starting and stopping points, turning points, and movement direction. Clinicians can cue these aspects of movement using various pitch components, such as pitch range, pitch level, or pitch direction. Volume may be effectively manipulated to direct ascending versus descending movements. The use of legato versus staccato sounds determines spatial movement parameters, and harmonically, the spacing of notes within a chord (i.e., open or closed) prompts extension and flexion.

7.3.4.2 Temporal Cues

Clinicians should thoughtfully implement the rhythmic elements of beat, tempo, meter, and patterning to cue movement timing. Tempo establishes movement pace and can determine the number of repetitions in a given time period (i.e., through beats per minute). Meter communicates the temporal structure of a movement, indicating which part of the movement should be performed at a given point in time. Rhythmic patterning and accents provide effective anticipatory cues, helping patients time movement initiation. Musical form also provides a clear cue for changing movement and indicates how much time should be spent performing a movement before resting or changing to a new movement.

7.3.4.3 Force Cues

Force pertains to the type of muscle activity that is needed to carry out a movement, and ultimately determines movement intensity. Through harmonic progressions, the clinician can direct and elicit patterns of muscle tension and release. In addition, manipulations of tempo and dynamics can elicit states of motor readiness or relaxation.

7.3.5 Therapeutic Instrumental Music Performance (TIMP)

In this NMT technique, the therapist designs active instrument playing exercises for patients, to simulate and practice functional movement patterns as part of sensorimotor rehabilitation (de l'Etoile and Roth 2019; Mertel 2014a). Playing musical instruments offers numerous benefits in the rehabilitative setting, as it optimizes gross and fine motor skills, facilitates repetition of movement patterns as needed to learn or relearn functional movements, and helps patients overcome unhealthy compensation strategies. Through TIMP, patients increase strength, endurance, and range of motion, as well as improve their bilateral coordination. Additional goals include enhanced movement speed, dexterity, and timing. TIMP is appropriate for a variety of neurologic and orthopedic populations that experience paresis, weakness, or disturbed muscle tone, such as traumatic brain injury, spinal cord injury, stroke, cerebral palsy, polio, or arthritis (Altenmüller et al. 2009; Dogruoz Karatekin and

Icagasioglu 2021; Fjare 2000; Janzen et al. 2022; Mertel 2014a; Zelazny 2001), as well as any individual needing to improve functional movement.

TIMP is best implemented with musical cueing from the therapist, thereby encompassing the scientific logic that supports RAS and PSE. Therapeutic mechanisms specific to playing musical instruments include the following three constructs.

7.3.5.1 Instrument as Target

In TIMP exercises, the instrument being played is strategically positioned to provide a target for the endpoint of the patient's movement. The therapist can adjust instrument location and angle in relation to the patient's body and limb, to elicit the desired range of motion for the movement. By repeatedly contacting the target while being cued by a slightly slower tempo, the patient will experience improved muscle activation and produce a more controlled movement (Thaut et al. 1991).

7.3.5.2 Auditory Rhythmic Feedback

Playing a musical instrument creates sound which provides critical auditory feedback for the movement. This sound indicates that the desired movement has been successfully completed, and that the movement should begin again (Johnson 1989; Mertel 2014a). Consequently, auditory feedback facilitates movement repetition as needed for effective learning and rehabilitation. Further, because the feedback tends to be rhythmic in nature (i.e., producing a clear pulse), patients receive additional auditory cueing (Thaut et al. 1991).

7.3.5.3 Structured Exercise and Cortical Plasticity

Movements used to play a musical instrument within a given auditory template are well-structured and task-oriented, thereby creating the ideal environment for the establishment of new neural connections or strengthening of existing connections, specifically in auditory and motor regions (Altenmüller et al. 2009; Grau-Sanchez et al. 2013; Mertel 2014a; Pascual-Leone et al. 1993; Rojo et al. 2011). This plasticity supports movement learning and is evidenced behaviorally by increased strength and dexterity, as needed to increase movement velocity (Zelazny 2001).

7.3.6 TIMP Clinical Protocol

Similar to PSE, the design of a TIMP exercise should begin with a careful consideration of the target movement, leading to the creation of a parallel experience through instrument playing that elicits the desired trajectory, range of motion, and mechanics of the movement (Mertel 2014a). The therapist then determines if that movement can be facilitated through the traditional means, or if the instrument playing experience needs to be modified in some way, for example, through strategic instrument placement or use of adaptive mallets, etc. The patient's instrument playing should be guided by the therapist's musical cueing that determines the spatial, temporal, and force parameters of the movement. If a patient is easily distracted, disoriented, or overwhelmed, the musical cueing can be minimized to a rhythmic cue only. TIMP sessions can be provided on an individual basis, and in this case may resemble a music lesson, yet with the goal of a nonmusical outcome. Group TIMP sessions are also effective, as patients learn by observing and imitating each other (Mertel 2014a). Further, group sessions provide opportunity for patients to collectively contribute to a common musical structure and to encourage each other's rehabilitative efforts.

7.4 Speech and Language Training Techniques

The NMT system includes eight speech and language training techniques to comprehensively address the broad range of cognitive, physical, and social aspects of communication. Detailed elaborations of the scientific logic underlying each technique exceed the scope of this chapter. This section will therefore review four primary mechanisms that support the use of music in speech and language training, and subsequently provide a brief description of each technique (Table 7.4).

Table 7.4 NMT techniques for speech and language training

Technique	Treatment goals	Appropriate populations
Developmental Speech and Language Training through Music (DSLM)	Facilitation of speech production and training of basic language concepts	Speech and language delays, developmental apraxia of speech, spastic dysarthria due to cerebral palsy, autism spectrum disorder
Melodic Intonation Therapy (MIT)	Fluent language output through improvements in prosody, timing, and word use	Broca's aphasia (expressive, non-fluent aphasia), apraxia
Musical Speech Stimulation (MUSTIM)	Elicit use of non-propositional, reflexive speech	Non-fluent aphasia
Oral Motor and Respiratory Exercises (OMREX)	Improved articulatory control, increased respiratory strength, enhanced use of speech apparatus	Conditions that contribute to speech disturbances, including neurologic and sensory disorders, developmental disorders
Rhythmic Speech Cueing (RSC)	Enhanced speech rate control via improvements in speech initiation, fluency, and intelligibility	Hypokinetic dysarthria due to Parkinson disease, speech apraxia, fluency disorders
Symbolic Communication Training through Music (SYCOM)	Acquire communication behaviors of language pragmatics, speech gestures, and emotional expression	Severe language loss resulting from neurologic damage, such as stroke or traumatic brain injury; pervasive developmental disorders, including autism

(continued)

Table 7.4 (continued)

Technique	Treatment goals	Appropriate populations
Therapeutic Singing (TS)	Complement other techniques through integration of speech production skills, such as speech initiation, articulation, respiratory function	Neurologic disorders or medical conditions that impact speech production and respiratory support; aging, developmental disabilities
Vocal Intonation Therapy (VIT)	Achieve vocal control of pitch level, inflection, breath support, timbre, dynamics	Impaired vocal quality due to voice disorders, neurologic disorders, such as Parkinson disease, stroke, cerebral palsy; health conditions, including cancer, asthma, chronic obstructive pulmonary disease, medical treatments; psychological conditions, including anxiety or conversion reaction; gender affirming; cleft palate

7.4.1 Scientific Logic for Speech and Language Training Techniques

7.4.1.1 Shared Perceptual Processes

Both music and speech are complex auditory stimuli that involve the perception of specific acoustic cues, including frequency, intensity, timbre, and sound duration that unfold over time in a structured, predictable fashion for communicative purposes (François et al. 2015; Lathroum 2011; Thaut 2015). Through these shared perceptual channels, meaningful exposure to music and active engagement with music therefore enhances the perception of speech sounds.

7.4.1.2 Differential Hemispheric Processing

Within both hemispheres, certain cortical and subcortical structures and their connections are shared for both singing and speaking, while others are specific to only one behavior (Brown et al. 2004, 2006; François et al. 2015; Hanna-Pladdy and Menken 2020; Jungblut et al. 2012; Koelsch et al. 2005; Loui 2015; Patel 2014; Schön et al. 2010; Thaut 2005d, 2015). When brain functioning is impacted by injury or disease, these shared and segregated pathways provide flexible approaches to either access alternate methods for vocal output, or to promote neuroanatomical reorganization needed to regain vocal ability.

7.4.1.3 Rhythm and Timing

Mechanisms of rhythmic entrainment enhance motor control for respiration, oral motor movements, and speech rate (Barlow et al. 2004; Chatterjee et al. 2021; Haas et al. 1986; LaGasse 2013; Thaut 2015). Outcomes include significant enhancements in the timing, accuracy, and volume of speech production, as needed for intelligibility.

7.4.1.4 Physiological Overlaps

The physiological structures and processes used when singing are identical to those used for speaking, specifically within the respiratory, laryngeal, and articulatory subsystems of the vocal tract (Dayme and Vaughn 2008a, b; Rosenbaum 2009). Notably, singing involves an exaggerated use of these mechanisms, including deep inhalations and slow, regulated exhalations (Ang et al. 2017; Berlowitz and Tamplin 2013; Bonilha et al. 2009; Cheng et al. 2020; Collyer et al. 2009; Irons et al. 2010; Thaut 2015). A well-structured singing program, therefore, can engage and strengthen these physiological components, leading to more effective use of the speaking voice.

7.4.2 Developmental Speech and Language Training Through Music (DSLM)

In this technique, the clinician uses a variety of developmentally appropriate musical materials and experiences to simultaneously facilitate clear speech production and train basic language concepts (i.e., object identification) (LaGasse 2014; Schön et al. 2008; Thaut 2005d). Appropriate clinical populations include children and individuals within the developmental period who demonstrate speech and language delays, such as individuals with speech apraxia, spastic dysarthria as found in cerebral palsy, or autism spectrum disorder (Lim 2010). DSLM interventions may involve the use of singing, chanting, instrument playing, musical games, or various combinations of music, speech, and movement, as well as music, speech, and visual symbols (i.e., picture books). Through these experiences, the patient associates the perception and production of speech sounds with specific objects, actions, ideas, and events.

7.4.3 Melodic Intonation Therapy (MIT)

Melodic Intonation Therapy involves modeling and engaging the patient in melodic intoning of functional phrases while providing rhythmic, tactile input to promote fluent language output (Thaut et al. 2014b). Ideal candidates for MIT involve patients with severe Broca's aphasia (i.e., expressive, nonfluent aphasia) typically due to stroke, who demonstrate preserved language comprehension but show a disturbance in the ability to use the sounds, words, and grammar of language (Altenmüller and Schlaug 2015; Schlaug 2015; Wan et al. 2014). The melodic components of MIT provide a slower version of natural speech prosody while the rhythmic hand tapping engages a sensorimotor network that supports articulatory movements (Schlaug 2015; Schlaug et al. 2008; Thaut 2015). These two mechanisms activate the right hemisphere, thereby compensating for damaged language areas in the left hemisphere and allowing the patient to regain spoken language (Altenmüller and Schlaug 2015; Chatterjee et al. 2021; Schlaug 2015)

7.4.4 Musical Speech Stimulation (MUSTIM)

This technique utilizes overlearned musical materials, including songs, rhymes, chants, and phrases, to engage neural language networks and trigger nonpropositional, reflexive speech (Staube et al. 2008; Thaut 2014b). Appropriate populations involve patients with non-fluent aphasia who either do not have the cognitive capacity for MIT, or who have completed an MIT protocol and need to increase spontaneous speech output. MUSTIM approaches may involve presenting a well-known song phrase and omitting the final word of a lyric line (e.g., "Happy Birthday to *you*"), or prompting the patient to sing the final word of a common sentence (e.g., "Nice to meet *you*"), using a melody that follows natural speech prosody.

7.4.5 Oral Motor and Respiratory Exercises (OMREX)

Through OMREX, the patient engages in sound vocalization and wind instrument playing to improve articulatory control, increase respiratory strength, and enhance functioning of the speech apparatus (Alexander and Wagner 2012; Ang et al. 2017; Mertel 2014b). This technique benefits several clinical populations that may experience speech disturbances due to neural impairments, sensory disorders, motor aspects of speech production, or various developmental disorders. Specifically, the experiences of singing and wind instrument provide the resistance needed to strengthen inspiratory and expiratory muscles, while engaging articulatory structures (Ang et al. 2017).

7.4.6 Rhythmic Speech Cueing (RSC)

Rhythmic speech cueing is a rate control technique in which auditory rhythm is used to address speech initiation, fluency, and overall intelligibility (Mainka and Mallien 2014). Appropriate candidates for RSC include patients with hypokinetic dysarthria as found in Parkinson disease, speech apraxia, and fluency disorders (Ouellette 2015; Pilon et al. 1998; Thaut et al. 2001; Wambaugh and Martinez 2000). For patients with severely impaired speech rate, metered cueing should be provided, in which each speech syllable is cued by a steady beat (i.e., metronome click). For mildly impaired speakers, patterned cueing is recommended, which uses the rhythmic structure of natural speech patterns.

7.4.7 Symbolic Communication Training Through Music (SYCOM)

SYCOM consists of music performance exercises, such as instrumental and vocal improvisation, to train communication behaviors of language pragmatics, speech gestures, and emotional expression (Donnay et al. 2014; Thaut 2014c). This technique is recommended for patients with severe language loss due to neurologic damage, such as stroke or brain injury, or who possess some language skills but would benefit from training in pragmatics, such as individuals with a pervasive developmental disorder, like autism (Vaiouli et al. 2015). Through structured improvisation, patients can gain experience in listening and attending to others, posing questions or statements, or responding to others with appropriate sentiment.

7.4.8 Therapeutic Singing (TS)

Therapeutic singing offers a complementary approach to other speech language training techniques by promoting an integration of skills needed for effective speech production (Johnson 2014; Thaut 2005d). Through general singing activities, patients gain experience in speech and language initiation as well as articulation and respiratory function. TS is appropriate for a broad range of clinical populations, including individuals with neurologic disorders or medical conditions that impact speech and respiratory function, adults impacted by the effects of aging, or individuals with developmental disabilities. Songs should be chosen that not only have motivational qualities, but that provide opportunity for well-timed speech production and sustained breath control through long phrases.

7.4.9 Vocal Intonation Therapy

For this technique, the clinician provides vocal instruction to help the patient achieve vocal control in the areas of pitch level, inflection, breath support, timbre, and dynamics (Ang et al. 2017; Bonilha et al. 2009; Di Benedetto et al. 2009; Engen 2005; Thaut 2014d; Wade 2002; Worth 2023). VIT is effective for treating disruptions to vocal quality due to voice disorders, neurologic disorders, such as Parkinson disease, stroke, or cerebral palsy, and health issues such as asthma, cancer, or chronic obstructive pulmonary disease. Patients undergoing certain medical procedures, such as intubation or oxygen and medication treatments, also benefit from VIT. In addition, individuals facing psychological issues, like anxiety or conversion reaction, or that have a congenital disorder, such as cleft palate, are good candidates. This technique comprises vocal instruction that is customized to meet patient needs, recognizing the inherent use of vocal control in the execution of specified vocal exercises and singing instruction (Berlowitz and Tamplin 2013; Collyer et al. 2009; Irons et al. 2010, 2016).

7.5 Cognitive and Socioemotional Training Techniques

The constructs of cognition, affect, and social behavior are addressed in the third category of NMT training techniques. Cognition and affect share close neural connections and demonstrate a multifaceted, bidirectional relationship (Forgas 2008). For example, cognitive activity can determine emotions, and conversely, affect impacts how people perceive, interpret, and remember information, especially social information. These techniques are therefore designed and implemented in consideration of this complex relationship. The eight cognitive techniques are grouped into the categories of auditory attention and perception training, executive function training, and memory training. The category of psychosocial behavior training comprises two socioemotional techniques (Table 7.5).

Table 7.5 NMT techniques for cognitive and socioemotional training

Technique	Treatment goals	Appropriate populations
Auditory attention and perception training		
Musical Sensory Orientation Training (MSOT)	Promote responses in arousal, orientation, vigilance, attention	Infants, dementia, developmental disabilities, disorders of consciousness, including coma, vegetative states, post-trauma recovery
Auditory Perception Training (APT)	Enhanced auditory perception by discrimination of sounds based on timbre, duration, pitch, dynamics; encourage exploration through integration of sensory modalities	Sensory impairments, intellectual or developmental disabilities, auditory processing disorder, stroke, traumatic brain injury
Musical Attention Control Training (MACT)	Improvements in focused, sustained, selective, divided, or alternating attention	Neurologic disorders such as stroke, traumatic brain injury, dementia; developmental disorders, including autism; attention-deficit/hyperactivity disorder
Musical Neglect Training (MNT)	Direct attention to neglected visual field	Hemispatial neglect of the left visual field, resulting from right hemisphere stroke or injury
Musical executive function training		
Musical Executive Function Training (MEFT)	Enhanced executive control, through improved decision-making, problem-solving, planning, and behavior regulation	Neurologic disorders, including stroke, traumatic brain injury, post-traumatic stress disorder, attention-deficit/hyperactivity disorder, disruptive behavior disorders
Memory training		
Musical Mnemonics Training (MMT)	Improved encoding and recall of non-musical information	Memory disorders, such as learning disabilities, traumatic brain injury, multiple sclerosis, stroke
Musical Echoic Memory Training (MEM)	Promote immediate recall of sensory information to support working memory	Auditory memory dysfunction resulting from stroke; traumatic brain injury, dementia, hearing impairment with cochlear implant
Associative Mood and Memory Training (AAMT)	Support memory encoding and recall, access autobiographical memories	Neurologically based memory disorders, including traumatic brain injury, dementia of the Alzheimer's type; older adults, and terminal illness

(continued)

Table 7.5 (continued)

Technique	Treatment goals	Appropriate populations
Psychosocial behavior training		
Music in Psychosocial Training and Counseling: Mood Induction and Vectoring (MPC-MIV)	Enhanced ability to identify, process, and regulate emotions	Mood or anxiety disorders, various neurologic disorders, such as dementia, Parkinson disease, traumatic brain injury, or stroke; autism, trauma, or grief
Music in Psychosocial Training and Counseling: Social Competence Training (MPC-SCT)	Improvements in social behavior through increased self-awareness and mood enhancement	Mental illness, including mood or anxiety disorders, thought disorders, personality disorders; neurologic disorders, such as stroke, traumatic brain injury

7.5.1 Scientific Logic for Cognitive and Socioemotional Training Techniques

7.5.1.1 Neural Connections Between Music, Cognition, and Affect

The neural intersections between music, cognition, and affect are multidimensional and have the potential to facilitate a cascade of positive outcomes. Many of the neural structures and pathways that support musical behavior also underlie arousal, attention, executive function, and memory (Cuddy and Duffin 2005; de l'Etoile and Roth 2019; Heilman 2002; Koelsch 2009; Koelsch and Siebel 2005; Peretz and Zatorre 2005). Musical experiences therefore provide an opportunity to engage and fortify these neural foundations in direct support of cognitive functioning.

Music is also well-known for activating reward circuitry in the brain, leading to pleasing emotional experiences (Altenmüller and Schlaug 2015; Blood and Zatorre 2001; Chanda and Levitin 2013; Chatterjee et al. 2021; Janzen et al. 2022; Mas-Herrero et al. 2021; Menon and Levitin 2005). This musical pleasure offers affective-motivational components that facilitate communication between primitive brain reward systems and higher-order cortical regions, thereby eliciting a positive affective tone that enhances cognitive functions (Mas-Herrero et al. 2021; Thaut and Wheeler 2010; Wheeler 2014). As examples, individuals experiencing musical pleasure tend to recall more positive memories, demonstrate focused attention, engage in more efficient decision-making, and think more creatively (Bower 1981; de l'Etoile 2002a; Forgas and Matovic 2020; Lesiuk 2010a, b). The positive bias of musical pleasure also provides an inviting context for the practice of social skills, thereby establishing social interaction as a rewarding behavior.

Not only does music elicit a psychological reward but also focused music listening in particular utilizes neural structures essential for the experience and processing of a myriad of emotions, covering the spectrum from negative to positive (Blood and Zatorre 2001; de l'Etoile and LaGasse 2013; Koelsch et al. 2006; Sammler et al. 2007; Stein et al. 2007). These neural overlaps demonstrate that music can elicit authentic affective states, providing opportunities to practice appropriate forms of emotion expression and regulation. Musical experiences are also known to engage brain regions that subserve social cognition, such as the ability to understand others' intentions, which is a core feature of social interaction (de l'Etoile and LaGasse 2013; Finnigan and Starr 2010; Steinbeis and Koelsch 2009).

7.5.1.2 Musical Scaffolding

Music consists of temporally dynamic sound patterns, such as rhythm, melody, harmony, and timbre, that can be strategically utilized to direct and scaffold cognitive functions of attention, memory, and executive function (Berlyne 1971; Chatterjee et al. 2021; Conway et al. 2009; Gardiner and Thaut 2014a, b; Koshimori and Thaut 2019; Thaut et al. 2015). When thoughtfully appointed within musical experiences, such as focused music listening, instrument playing, and improvisation, these musical elements provide opportunity for continuous adaptation to a changing environment in which the unique feature of auditory feedback is used to monitor and adjust cognitive responses and social behaviors (Bodak et al. 2014; Koshimori and Thaut 2019; Thaut et al. 2015). Overall, well-designed music interventions provide the ideal medium for intensive practice of cognitive functions and social behaviors in real time as part of a rehabilitative or developmental approach to therapeutic learning.

7.5.2 Cognitive Training Techniques

7.5.2.1 Auditory Attention and Perception Training

Musical Sensory Orientation Training (MSOT)

In this technique, the clinician provides music as sensory stimulation to elicit arousal, guide orientation and vigilance, and maintain attention (de l'Etoile and Roth 2019; Gardiner 2005; Myskja 2014). Recommended populations include young infants, individuals with dementia, developmental disabilities, and disorders of consciousness, such as coma, vegetative states, or post-trauma recovery. Examples of clinical applications include playing familiar music, providing sound stimuli from instruments of different timbres, and giving patients access to corresponding haptic feedback, such as instrument vibrations.

Auditory Perception Training (APT)

This intervention uses various musical experiences to help patients identify and match specified sounds and discriminate between different sounds based on acoustic and sensory components, such as timbre, duration, pitch, dynamics, etc. (de l'Etoile and Roth 2019; Gardiner 2005; Mertel 2014c). APT can also be used to promote integration of different sensory modalities, including visual, aural, tactile, and kinesthetic. Skills gained through APT include enhanced auditory perception as needed for speech comprehension and production, and to effectively explore the environment using sensory cues (Gfeller 2016). Individuals likely to benefit from APT may have sensory impairment, intellectual or developmental disability, auditory processing disorder, stroke, or traumatic brain injury. Strategies may involve providing contrasting instrument sounds, or combining musical cues with visual cues or physical movements.

Musical Attention Control Training (MACT)

Through MACT, patients have an opportunity to practice focused, sustained, selective, divided, or alternating forms of attention (Gardiner 2005; Thaut and Gardiner 2014; Thaut et al. 2015). Appropriate populations include stroke and traumatic brain injury patients, as well as individuals with autism, attention-deficit/hyperactivity disorder, or dementia. Attention guidance may also be an effective pain management strategy. Clinical protocols involve strategic manipulation of musical elements to cue the patient's musical response. For sustained attention, the patient may play a drum on the beat for the entire duration of a song, carefully following unannounced changes in tempo and dynamics. For selective attention, the patient might sustain a rhythmic pattern on a drum, even when faced with intentional distraction by a fellow group member who is playing a contrasting pattern.

Musical Neglect Training (MNT)

MNT is the use of musical cues and stimuli to train attention in a neglected visual field as needed for safe, accurate navigation of one's environment (Abiru 2014; Bodak et al. 2014; Gardiner 2005). Ideal candidates include patients with hemispatial neglect of the left visual field due to brain injury or stroke in the right cerebral hemisphere. Clinicians provide rhythmic, melodic, and harmonic cues to guide patients' active playing of strategically arranged musical instruments, thus eliciting continuous or repeated direction of attention to the neglected visual field.

7.5.2.2 Musical Executive Function Training (MEFT)

As a stand-alone category of cognitive training techniques, MEFT addresses a myriad of functions related to executive control, including decision-making, problem-solving, planning, and inhibition of maladaptive behaviors (de l'Etoile and Roth 2019; Gardiner 2005; Gardiner and Thaut 2014a). By improving EF skills, patients are better prepared for interpersonal relationships as well as success within academic, work, and community settings. Numerous populations can benefit from MEFT, such as individuals with traumatic brain injury, stroke, attention-deficit/hyperactivity disorder, or disruptive behavior disorders (Siponkoski et al. 2020). Musical experiences, such as performance exercises, improvisation, or composition, provide the ideal medium for patients to actively practice EF skills and receive immediate feedback on their efforts (Roth 2014).

7.5.2.3 Memory Training

Musical Mnemonics Training (MMT). In MMT, the structural and motivational qualities of music are used to enhance encoding and recall of nonmusical information, such as lists of items, names, and step-wise procedures (Gardiner 2005; Gardiner and Thaut 2014b). This technique is beneficial for individuals with memory disorders, including learning disabilities, traumatic brain injury, multiple sclerosis, and stroke (Gfeller 1983; Selph 2015; Thaut et al. 2014c). Simple songs and chants are used to organize the information of interest, so that individual items can be grouped together, thereby reducing the memory load. Singing, chanting, or even listening to the musical production then provides a means to rehearse and store the information to memory for later retrieval.

Musical Echoic Memory Training (MEM). Through this technique, patients engage in immediate recall of sensory information that exists in echoic memory, or the initial stage of auditory memory creation (Thaut 2014b; Koelsch 2011). Such efforts promote the development of working memory, which is relatively more stable and slightly longer in duration than echoic memory. Recommended populations include individuals with auditory memory dysfunction due to stroke, as well as patients with traumatic brain injury, dementia, or hearing impairment with the cochlear implant. Children with autism or developmental language disorders are also likely to benefit from this technique. MEM may consist of playing a song, stopping randomly, and asking the patient to repeat the last word they heard in the song. Other examples include asking the client to discriminate between different musical sounds, or to repeat brief rhythmic or tonal patterns.

Associative Mood and Memory Training (AAMT). This technique utilizes music's mood induction capacities to activate associative mood and memory networks, thereby improving memory encoding and recall as well as accessing autobiographical memories as needed for end-of-life review and to maintain sense of self (Bower 1981; de l'Etoile and Roth 2019; de l'Etoile 2002b, 2014; Gardiner 2005; Thaut and de l'Etoile 1993). Target populations include patients with neurologically based memory disorders, such as traumatic brain injury or dementia of the Alzheimer's type, and individuals undergoing life review as part of aging and terminal illness. Clinical strategies may include focused music listening experiences to induce a mood state associated with long-term autobiographical memories.

7.5.3 Socioemotional Training Techniques

7.5.3.1 Psychosocial Behavior Training

Music in Psychosocial Training and Counseling: Mood Induction and Vectoring (MPC–MIV)

Through this intervention, the therapist facilitates musical mood induction and vectoring so that the patient experiences emotional responses with specific therapeutic significance, such as identification or processing emotions, or mood regulation (Thaut and Wheeler 2010; Wheeler 2014). Addressing these emotional competencies helps patients cope with feelings related to trauma and loss, and gain a better understanding and management of their emotions. Patients with mood or anxiety disorders are good candidates for this technique, as well as any individual having difficulty with emotional states and emotional communication, as may sometimes occur with autism spectrum disorder, dementia, Parkinson disease, stroke, or traumatic brain injury. An MIV intervention may take the form of a focused music listening exercise, in which the music initially matches the patient's current mood and then gradually shifts in emotional tone, through alteration of key elements, such as tempo, instrumentation, tonality, and energy, to help the patient achieve a more desired mood state (Starcke et al. 2021). The intervention typically also includes verbal processing to assist the patient in understanding their response to the music and how that response applies to situations outside the therapy setting.

Music in Psychosocial Training and Counseling: Social Competence Training (MPC–SCT)
This technique may also involve mood induction, which is conducted as a first step toward cognitive reorientation and behavioral reorganization (Roth 2014; Thaut and Wheeler 2010; Wheeler 2014). Through engagement in musical experiences and verbal processing, patients are guided toward healthier patterns of thinking and behaving through increased self-awareness, improved mood, and practice of social behaviors. Individuals with mental illness, such as mood, anxiety, or thought disorders, as well as personality disorders will benefit from this approach, in addition to individuals who need to improve their social competence and confidence, or who are coping with life changes due to a neurologic disorder, such as stroke or traumatic brain injury. As an SCT technique, group instrumental improvisation provides a positive context for patients to practice emotionally salient social skills of greeting, expressing, reflecting, or empathizing, in real time (Roth 2014). These experiences can be implemented at a supportive level, in which engagement in the activity itself produces the therapeutic outcome through an emphasis on overt behaviors (Wheeler 1983, 2014). For patients capable of deeper processing and insight, SCT interventions serve as a stimulus for exploring emotions and cognitive responses as needed for therapeutic change. Within this insight-oriented and reeducative focus, patients strive to better understand their emotional reactions and to gain insight into how they relate to others.

7.6 Conclusion

Fueled by progress in neuroscience that has revealed real-time responses to music in the human brain and body, the neurologic music therapy paradigm emerged and now provides a comprehensive scientific model to direct research and clinical practice in the treatment of a broad range of disorders across the life span. This evidence-based approach utilizes the neurological, physiological, and psychological components of musical behavior to produce functional, reliable outcomes in everyday, nonmusical domains. Guided by the logic of the Rational-Scientific Mediating Model, research in NMT identifies underlying mechanisms of change, so that clinicians and investigators understand how music impacts behavior and can articulate that process to patients and other healthcare professionals, thus creating greater access to clinical services. Building on that logic, the Transformational Design Model offers a systematic treatment planning approach to transform general therapeutic principles into clinically relevant music experiences that target functional behavior. The NMT system includes techniques within three domains considered fundamental to human behavior. Within the sensorimotor domain, NMT techniques maximize auditory motor coupling effects to improve gait, posture, and balance, as well as upper and lower extremity movement. Utilizing the numerous intersections between the perception and production of music, speech, and language, NMT approaches effectively train communication behavior. Finally, the cognitive and socioemotional components of musical experiences support NMT techniques for improved perception, attention, executive function, memory, and psychosocial behavior. While the depth of scientific evidence varies across these three domains, strong theoretical models further supplement NMT practice. Looking forward, the NMT approach will evolve and expand as the field of neuroscience continues to generate evidence of the critical connections between musical and nonmusical behavior.

References

Abiru M. Musical neglect training (NMT). In: Thaut MH, Hoemberg V, editors. Handbook of neurologic music therapy. Oxford University Press; 2014. p. 270–8.

Alexander JL, Wagner CL. Is harmonica playing an effective adjunct therapy to pulmonary rehabilitation? Rehabil Nurs. 2012;37(4):207–12. https://doi.org/10.1002/rnj.33.

Altenmüller E, Schlaug G. Apollo's gift: new aspects of neurologic music therapy. Prog Brain Res. 2015;127:237–52. https://doi.org/10.1016/bs.pbr.2014.11.029.

Altenmüller E, Marco-Pallares J, Münte TF, Schneider S. Neural reorganization underlies improvement in stroke-induced motor dysfunction by music-supported therapy. Ann N Y Acad Sci. 2009;1169:395–405. https://doi.org/10.1111/j.1749-6632.2009.04580.x.

Ang K, Maddocks M, Xu H, Higginson IJ. The effectiveness of singing or playing a wind instrument in improving respiratory function in patients with long-term neurological conditions: a systematic review. J Music Ther. 2017;54:108–31. https://doi.org/10.1093/jmt/thx001.

Barlow SM, Finan DS, Park S. Sensorimotor entrainment of respiratory and orofacial systems in humans. In: Maassen B, Kent RD, Peters HFM, van Lieshout PHHM, Hulstijn W, editors. Speech motor control in normal and disordered speech. Oxford University Press; 2004. p. 211–24.

Berlowitz DJ, Tamplin J. Respiratory muscle training for cervical spinal cord injury. Cochrane Database Syst Rev. 2013;7:CD008507. https://doi.org/10.1002/14651858.CD008507.pub2.

Berlyne DE. Perception. In: Aesthetics and psychobiology. Meredith Corporation; 1971. p. 96–114.

Blood AJ, Zatorre RJ. Intensely pleasurable responses to music correlate with activity in brain regions implicated in reward and emotion. Proc Natl Acad Sci USA. 2001;98:11818–23. https://doi.org/10.1073/pnas.191355898.

Bodak R, Malhotra P, Bernardi NF, Cocchini G, Stewart L. Reducing chronic visual-spatial neglect following right hemisphere stroke through instrument playing. Front Hum Neurosci. 2014;8:413. https://doi.org/10.3389/fnhum.2014.00413.

Bonilha AG, Onofre F, Vieira ML, Prado MY, Martinez JA. Effects of singing classes on pulmonary function and quality of life of COPD patients. Int J Chron Obstruct Pulmon Dis. 2009;4:1–8.

Bower GH. Mood and memory. Am Psychol. 1981;36:129–48. https://doi.org/10.1037/0003-066X.36.2.129.

Brown S, Martinez MJ, Hodges DA, Fox PT, Parsons LM. The song system of the human brain. Cogn Brain Res. 2004;20:363–75. https://doi.org/10.1016/j.cogbrainres.2004.03.016.

Brown S, Martinez MJ, Parsons LM. Music and language side by side in the brain: a PET study of the generation of melodies and sentences. Eur J Neurosci. 2006;23(May):2791–803. https://doi.org/10.1111/j.1460-9568.2006.04785.x.

Chanda ML, Levitin DJ. The neurochemistry of music. Trends Cogn Sci. 2013;17(4):179–83. https://doi.org/10.1016/j.tics.2013.02.007.
Chatterjee D, Hegde S, Thaut M. Neural plasticity: the substratum of music-based interventions in neurorehabilitation. NeuroRehabilitation. 2021;48(2):155–66. https://doi.org/10.3233/NRE-208011.
Chen JL, Penhune VB, Zatorre RJ. Listening to musical rhythms recruits motor regions of the brain. Cereb Cortex. 2008;18:2844–54. https://doi.org/10.1093/cercor/bhn042.
Cheng LK, Chiu YH, Lin YC, Li WC, Hong TY, Yang CJ, Shih CH, Yeh TC, Tseng WYI, Yu HY, Hsieh JC, Chen LF. Long-term musical training induces white matter plasticity in emotion and language networks. Hum Brain Mapp. 2020;44:5–17. https://doi.org/10.1002/hbm.26054.
Clair AA, Pasiali V. Neurologic music therapy. In: Darrow AA, editor. Introduction to approaches in music therapy. American Music Therapy Association; 2004. p. 143–58.
Collyer S, Kenny DT, Archer M. The effect of abdominal kinematic directives on respiratory behaviour in female classical singing. Logop Phoniatr Voco. 2009;34(3):100–10. https://doi.org/10.1080/14015430903008780.
Conway CM, Pisoni DB, Kronenberger WG. The importance of sound for cognitive sequencing abilities: the auditory scaffolding hypothesis. Curr Dir Psychol Sci. 2009;18(5):275–9. https://doi.org/10.1111/j.1467-8721.2009.01651.x.
Cuddy LL, Duffin J. Music, memory, and Alzheimer's disease: is music recognition spared in dementia, and how can it be assessed? Med Hypotheses. 2005;64:229–35. https://doi.org/10.1016/j.mehy.2004.09.005.
Davis WB. Music therapy: historical perspective. In: Davis WB, Gfeller KE, Thaut MH, editors. An introduction to music therapy: theory and practice. 3rd ed. American Music Therapy Association; 2008. p. 17–40.
Dayme M, Vaughn C. Articulation and expression. In: Dayme MB, Vaughn C, editors. The singing book. 2nd ed. W.W. Norton; 2008a. p. 308–18.
Dayme M, Vaughn C. Making sound. In: Dayme MB, Vaughn C, editors. The singing book. 2nd ed. W.W. Norton; 2008b. p. 292–9.
de l'Etoile SK. The effectiveness of music therapy in group psychotherapy for adults with mental illness. Arts Psychother. 2002a;29:69–78. https://doi.org/10.1016/S0197-4556(02)00139-9.
de l'Etoile SK. The effect of a musical mood induction procedure on mood state-dependent word retrieval. J Music Ther. 2002b;39:145–60. https://doi-org.access.library.miami.edu/10.1093/jmt/39.2.145.
de l'Etoile SK. Associative mood and memory training. In: Thaut MH, Hoemberg V, editors. Handbook of neurologic music therapy. Oxford University Press; 2014. p. 314–30.
de l'Etoile SK. Processes of music therapy: clinical and scientific rationales and models. In: Hallam S, Cross I, Thaut M, editors. The Oxford handbook of music psychology. 2nd ed. Oxford University Press; 2016. p. 805–17.
de l'Etoile SK, LaGasse AB. Music therapy and neuroscience: from parallel histories to converging pathways. Music Ther Perspect. 2013;31(1):6–14. https://doi.org/10.1093/mtp/31.1.6.
de l'Etoile SK, Roth EA. Music therapy. In: Rentfrow PJ, Levitin DJ, editors. Foundations in music psychology: theory and research. The MIT Press; 2019. p. 827–56.
de l'Etoile SK, Dachinger C, Fairfield J, Lathroum L. The rational-scientific mediating model (RSMM): a framework for scientific research in music therapy. Music Ther Perspect. 2012;30(2):130–40. https://doi-org.access.library.miami.edu/10.1093/mtp/30.2.130
Di Benedetto P, Cavazzon M, Mondolo F, Rugiu G, Peratoner A, Biasutti E. Voice and choral singing treatment: a new approach for speech and voice disorders in Parkinson's disease. Eur J Phys Rehabil Med. 2009;45(1):13–9.
Dogruoz Karatekin B, Icagasioglu A. The effect of therapeutic instrumental music performance method on upper extremity functions in adolescent cerebral palsy. Acta Neurol Belg. 2021;121:1179–89. https://doi.org/10.1007/s13760-021-01618-0.
Donnay GF, Rankin SK, Lopez-Gonzalez M, Jiradejvong P, Limb CJ. Neural substrates of interactive musical improvisation: an fMRI study of 'trading fours' in jazz. PLoS One. 2014;9(2):e88665. https://doi.org/10.1371/journal.pone.0088665.

Engen RL. The singer's breath: implications for treatment of persons with emphysema. J Music Ther. 2005;42:20–48. https://doi.org/10.1093/jmt/42.1.20.
Felix RA, Fridberger A, Leijon S, Berrebi AA, Magnusson AK. Sound rhythms are encoded by postinhibitory rebound spiking in the superior paraolivary nucleus. J Neurosci. 2011;31:12566–78. https://doi.org/10.1523/JNEUROSCI.2450-11.2011.
Ferreri L, Riba J, Zatorre R, Rodriguez-Fornells A. Chills, bets, and dopamine: a journey into musical reward. In: Chatterjee A, Cardillo ER, editors. Brain, beauty, & art; 2022. p. 155–60. https://doi.org/10.1093/oso/9780197513620.003.0031.
Finnigan E, Starr E. Increasing social responsiveness in a child with autism: a comparison of music and non-music interventions. Autism. 2010;14:321–48. https://doi.org/10.1177/1362361309357747.
Fjare H. Effects of keyboard exercises on the rehabilitation of the paretic hand of stroke patients. (Unpublished master's thesis). Colorado State University; 2000.
Forgas JP. Affect and cognition. Perspect Psychol Sci. 2008;3(2):87–147. https://doi.org/10.1111/j.1745-6916.2008.00067.x.
Forgas JP, Matovic D. Mood effects on humor production: positive mood improves the verbal ability to be funny. J Lang Soc Psychol. 2020;39:701–15. https://doi.org/10.1177/0261927X20917994.
François C, Grau-Sánchez J, Duarte E, Rodriguez-Fornells A. Musical training as an alternative and effective method for neuro-education and neuro-rehabilitation. Front Psychol. 2015;6:475. https://doi.org/10.3389/fpsyg.2015.00475.
Gardiner JC. Neurologic music therapy in cognitive rehabilitation. In: Thaut MH, editor. Rhythm, music, and the brain: scientific foundations and clinical applications. Routledge; 2005. p. 179–202.
Gardiner JC, Thaut MH. Musical executive function training (MEFT). In: Thaut MH, Hoemberg V, editors. Handbook of neurologic music therapy. Oxford University Press; 2014a. p. 279–93.
Gardiner JC, Thaut MH. Musical mnemonics training (MMT). In: Thaut MH, Hoemberg V, editors. Handbook of neurologic music therapy. Oxford University Press; 2014b. p. 294–310.
Gfeller KE. Musical mnemonics as an aid to retention with normal and learning disabled students. J Music Ther. 1983;20:179–89. https://doi.org/10.1093/jmt/20.4.179.
Gfeller KE. Music therapy for children and adults who are deaf or hard of hearing. In: Edwards J, editor. The Oxford handbook of music therapy. Oxford University Press; 2016. p. 225–48.
Grahn JA, Brett M. Rhythm and beat perception in motor areas of the brain. J Cogn Neurosci. 2007;19:893–906. https://doi.org/10.1162/jocn.2007.19.5.893.
Grau-Sanchez J, Amengual J, Rojo N, de las Heras MV, Montero J, Rubio F, Altenmüller E, Münte TF, RodriguezFornells A. Plasticity in the sensorimotor cortex induced by music-supported therapy in stroke patients: a TMS study. Front Hum Neurosci. 2013;7(September):494. https://doi.org/10.3389/fnhum.2013.00494.
Gurden H, Takita M, Jay TM. Essential role of D1 but not D2 receptors in the NMDA receptor-dependent long-term potentiation at hippocampal-prefrontal cortex synapses in vivo. J Neurosci. 2000;20(22):RC106. https://doi.org/10.1523/JNEUROSCI.20-22-j0003.2000.
Haas F, Distenfeld S, Axen K. Effects of perceived musical rhythm on respiratory pattern. J Appl Physiol. 1986;61:1185–91. https://doi.org/10.1152/jappl.1986.61.3.1185.
Hanna-Pladdy B, Menken M. Training-induced cognitive and neural changes in musicians: implications for healthy aging. In: Cuddy L, Belleville S, Moussard A, editors. Music and the aging brain. Elsevier Science & Technology; 2020. p. 221–43. https://doi.org/10.1016/B978-0-12-817422-7.00008-0.
Heart and Stroke Foundation of Canada. Canadian stroke best practices: rehabilitation and recovery following stroke, 6.1 balance and mobility. 2019. https://www.strokebestpractices.ca/recommendations/stroke-rehabilitation/mobility-balance-and-transfers.
Heilman KM. Emotional experience: a neurological model. In: Lane RD, Nadel L, editors. Cognitive neuroscience of emotion. Oxford University Press; 2002. p. 328–70.
Illes J, Bird SJ. Neuroethics: a modern context for ethics in neuroscience. Trends Neurosci. 2006;29(9):511–7. https://doi.org/10.1016/j.tins.2006.07.002.

Irons JY, Kenny DT, Chang AB. Singing for children and adults with bronchiectasis. Cochrane Database Syst Rev. 2010;2:CD007729. https://doi.org/10.1002/14651858.CD007729.pub2.

Irons JY, Petocz P, Kenny DT, Chang AB. Singing as an adjunct therapy for children and adults with cystic fibrosis. Cochrane Database Syst Rev. 2016;9:CD008036. https://doi.org/10.1002/14651858.CD008036.pub4.

Janzen TB, Koshimori Y, Richard NM, Thaut MH. Rhythm and music-based interventions in motor rehabilitation: current evidence and future perspectives. Front Hum Neurosci. 2022;15:789467. https://doi.org/10.3389/fnhum.2021.789467.

Johnson SB. Therapeutic use of music in upper extremity gross motor rehabilitation. (Unpublished master's thesis). Colorado State University; 1989.

Johnson SB. Therapeutic singing (TS). In: Thaut MH, Hoemberg V, editors. Handbook of neurologic music therapy. Oxford University Press; 2014. p. 185–95.

Jungblut M, Huber W, Pustelniak M, Schnitker R. The impact of rhythm complexity on brain activation during simple singing: an event-related fMRI study. Restor Neurol Neurosci. 2012;30(1):39–53. https://doi.org/10.3233/RNN-2011-0619.

Kang S, Shin JH, Kim IY, Lee J, Lee, Jeong E. Patterns of enhancement in paretic shoulder kinematics after stroke with musical cueing. Sci Rep. 2020;10:18109. https://doi.org/10.1038/s41598-020-75143-0.

Keenan EM. The immediate effect of rhythm on the timing of upper extremity movements in patients with Parkinson's disease. (Unpublished master's thesis). University of Miami; 2011.

Koelsch S. A neuroscientific perspective on music therapy. The neurosciences and music III disorders and plasticity. Ann N Y Acad Sci. 2009;1169:374–84. https://doi.org/10.1111/j.1749-6632.2009.04592.x.

Koelsch S. Toward a neural basis of music perception – a review and updated model. Front Psychol. 2011;2:110. https://doi.org/10.3389/fpsyg.2011.00110.

Koelsch S, Siebel WA. Towards a neural basis of music perception. Trends Cogn Sci. 2005;9:578–84. https://doi.org/10.1016/j.tics.2005.10.001.

Koelsch S, Fritz T, Schulze K, Alsop D, Schlaug G. Adults and children processing music: an fMRI study. NeuroImage. 2005;25:1068–76. https://doi.org/10.1016/j.neuroimage.2004.12.050.

Koelsch S, Fritz T, von Cramon DY, Müller K, Friederici AD. Investigating emotion with music: an fMRI study. Hum Brain Mapp. 2006;27:239–50. https://doi.org/10.1002/hbm.20180.

Koshimori Y, Thaut MH. New perspectives on music in rehabilitation of executive and attention functions. Front Neurosci. 2019;13:1425. https://doi.org/10.3389/fnins.2019.01245.

Kraus N, Chandrasekaran B. Music training for the development of auditory skills. Nat Rev Neurosci. 2010;11(8):599–605. https://doi.org/10.1038/nrn2882.

LaGasse AB. Influence of an external rhythm on oral motor control in children and adults. J Music Ther. 2013;50:6–24. https://doi.org/10.1093/jmt/50.1.6.

LaGasse AB. Developmental speech and language training through music (DSLM). In: Thaut MH, Hoemberg V, editors. Handbook of neurologic music therapy. Oxford University Press; 2014. p. 196–216.

LaGasse AB, Thaut MH. Music and rehabilitation: neurological approaches. In: MacDonald R, Kreutz G, Mitchell L, editors. Music, health, and wellbeing. Oxford University Press; 2012. p. 153–82. https://doi.org/10.1093/acprof:oso/9780199586974.003.0012.

Lakatos P, Gross J, Thut G. A new unifying account of the roles of neuronal entrainment. Curr Biol. 2019;29:R890–905. https://doi.org/10.1016/j.cub.2019.07.075.

Lathroum LM. The role of music perception in predicting phonological awareness in five- and six-year-old children. (Unpublished doctoral dissertation). University of Miami; 2011.

Lesiuk T. A rationale for music-based cognitive rehabilitation toward prevention of relapse in substance addiction. Music Ther Perspect. 2010a;28(2):124–30. https://doi.org/10.1093/mtp/28.2.124.

Lesiuk T. The effect of preferred music on mood and performance in a high-cognitive demand occupation. J Music Ther. 2010b;47:137–54. https://doi.org/10.1093/jmt/47.2.137.

Lim HA. Effect of 'developmental speech and language training through music' on speech production in children with autism spectrum disorders. J Music Ther. 2010;47:2–26. https://doi.org/10.1093/jmt/47.1.2.
Loui P. A dual-stream neuroanatomy of singing. Music Percept. 2015;32(3):232–41. https://doi.org/10.1525/mp.2015.32.3.232.
Lu TW, Chang CF. Biomechanics of human movement and its clinical applications. Kaohsiung J Med Sci. 2012;28:S13–25. https://doi.org/10.1016/j.kjms.2011.08.004.
Luft AR, McCombe-Waller S, Whitall J, Forrester LW, Macko R, Sorking JD, Schulz JB, Goldberg AP, Hanley DF. Repetitive bilateral arm training and motor cortex activation in chronic stroke: a randomized controlled trial. JAMA J Am Med Assoc. 2004;292:1853–61. https://doi.org/10.1001/jama.292.15.1853.
Mainka S, Mallien G. Rhythmic speech cueing (RSC). In: Thaut MH, Hoemberg V, editors. Handbook of neurologic music therapy. Oxford University Press; 2014. p. 150–60.
Mas-Herrero E, Maini L, Sescousse G, Zatorre RJ. Common and distinct neural correlates of music and food-induced pleasure: a coordinate-based meta-analysis of neuroimaging studies. Neurosci Biobehav Rev. 2021;123:61–71. https://doi.org/10.1016/j.neubiorev.2020.12.008.
Menon V, Levitin DJ. The rewards of music listening: response and physiological connectivity of the mesolimbic system. NeuroImage. 2005;28:175–84. https://doi.org/10.1016/j.neuroimage.2005.05.053.
Mertel K. Therapeutic instrumental music performance (TIMP). In: Thaut MH, Hoemberg V, editors. Handbook of neurologic music therapy. Oxford University Press; 2014a. p. 116–39.
Mertel K. Oral motor and respiratory exercises (OMREX). In: Thaut MH, Hoemberg V, editors. Handbook of neurologic music therapy. Oxford University Press; 2014b. p. 161–78.
Mertel K. Auditory perception training (APT). In: Thaut MH, Hoemberg V, editors. Handbook of neurologic music therapy. Oxford University Press; 2014c. p. 69–93.
Miller RA, Thaut MH, McIntosh G, Rice R. Components of EMG symmetry and variability in Parkinsonian and healthy elderly gait. Electroencephalogr Clin Neurophysiol. 1996;10:1–7. https://doi.org/10.1016/0013-4694(95)00209-x.
Monti RJ, Roy RR, Edgerton VR. Role of motor unit structure in defining function. Muscle Nerve. 2001;24:848–66. https://doi.org/10.1002/mus.1083.
Myskja A. Musical sensory orientation training (MSOT). In: Thaut MH, Hoemberg V, editors. Handbook of neurologic music therapy. Oxford University Press; 2014. p. 221–6.
Ouellette J. The effect of a rhythmic speech cuing protocol on speech intelligibility in patients with Parkinson's disease. (Unpublished master's thesis). University of Miami; 2015.
Pal'tsev YI, El'ner AM. Change in the functional state of the segmental apparatus of the spinal cord under the influence of sound stimuli and its role in voluntary movement. Biophysics. 1967;12:1064–70.
Pascual-Leone A, Cohen LG, Dang N, Brasil-Neto JP, Cammarota A, Hallett M. Acquisition of fine motor skills in humans is associated with the modulation of cortical motor outputs. Neurology. 1993;43:A157. (Abstract).
Patel AD. Can nonlinguistic musical training benefit the neural encoding of speech? The OPERA hypothesis. Hear Res. 2014;308:989–108. https://doi.org/10.1016/j.heares.2013.08.011.
Peretz I, Zatorre RJ. Brain organization for music processing. Annu Rev Psychol. 2005;56(February):89–114. https://doi.org/10.1146/annurev.psych.56.091103.070225.
Piccirilli M, D'Alessandro P, Elisei S. Music training as a potential neuroprotective agent. Psychiatr Danub. 2021;3(Suppl 11):44–8.
Pilon MA, McIntosh KW, Thaut MH. Auditory vs. visual speech timing cues as external rate control to enhance verbal intelligibility in mixed spastic-ataxic dysarthric speakers: a pilot study. Brain Inj. 1998;12:793–803. https://doi.org/10.1080/026990598122188.
Raichle ME. Functional brain imaging and human brain function. J Neurosci. 2003;23:3959–62. https://doi.org/10.1523/JNEUROSCI.23-10-03959.2003.
Raichle ME. Functional neuroimaging: a historical and physiological perspective. In: Cabeza R, Kingstone A, editors. Handbook of functional neuroimaging of cognition. 2nd ed. The MIT Press; 2006. p. 3–20.

Raichle ME. A brief history of human brain mapping. Trends Neurosci. 2008;32:118–26. https://doi.org/10.1016/j.tins.2008.11.001.
Reybrouck M, Vuust P, Brattico E. Music and brain plasticity: how sounds trigger neurogenerative adaptations. In: Chaban VV, editor. Neuroplasticity: insights of neural reorganization; 2018. p. 85–103. https://doi.org/10.5772/intechopen.74318.
Ringenbach SDR, Zimmerman K, Chen CC, Mulvey GM, Holzapfel SD, Weeks DJ, Thaut MH. Adults with Down syndrome performed repetitive movements fast with continuous music cues. J Motor Learn Dev. 2014;2(3):47–54. https://doi.org/10.1123/jmld.2014-0040.
Rojo N, Amengual J, Juncadella M, Rubio F, Camara E, Marco-Pallares J, Schneider S, Veciana M, Montero J, Mohammadi B, Altenmüller E, Grau C, Münte TF, Rodriguez-Fornells A. Music-supported therapy induces plasticity in the sensorimotor cortex in chronic stroke: a single-case study using multimodal imaging (fMRI-TMS). Brain Inj. 2011;25(7–8):787–93. https://doi.org/10.3109/02699052.2011.576305.
Rosenbaum DA. Speaking and singing. In: Rosenbaum DA, editor. Human motor control. 2nd ed. Elsevier; 2009. p. 323–62.
Ross JM, Warlaumont AS, Abney DH, Rigoli LM, Balasubramianiam R. Influence of musical groove on postural sway. J Exp Psychol. 2016;42(3):308–19. https://doi.org/10.1037/xhp0000198.
Rossignol S, Jones GM. Audio-spinal influence in man studied by the H-reflex and its possible role on rhythmic movements synchronized to sound. Electroencephalogr Clin Neurophysiol. 1976;41:83–92. https://doi.org/10.1016/0013-4694(76)90217-0.
Roth EA. Clinical improvisation in neurologic music therapy. In: Thaut MH, Hoemberg V, editors. Handbook of neurologic music therapy. Oxford University Press; 2014. p. 24–46.
Safranek MG, Koshland GF, Raymond G. Effect of auditory rhythm on muscle activity. Phys Ther. 1982;62(2):161–8. https://doi.org/10.1093/ptj/62.2.161.
Sammler D, Grigutsch M, Fritz T, Koelsch S. Music and emotion: electrophysiologica correlates of the processing of pleasant and unpleasant music. Psychophysiology. 2007;44:293–304. https://doi.org/10.1111/j.1469-8986.2007.00497.x.
Schaffert N, Janzen TB, Mattes K, Thaut MH. A review on the relationship between sound and movement in sports and rehabilitation. Front Psychol. 2019;10:244. https://doi.org/10.3389/fpsyg.2019.00244.
Schlaug G. The brain of musicians: a model for functional and structural adaptation. Ann N Y Acad Sci. 2001;930:281–99. PMID: 1145883.
Schlaug G. Music, musicians, and brain plasticity. In: Hallam S, Cross I, Thaut M, editors. Oxford handbook of music psychology. Oxford University Press; 2009. p. 197–207.
Schlaug G. Musicians and music making as a model for the study of brain plasticity. Prog Brain Res. 2015;217:37–55. https://doi.org/10.1016/bs.pbr.2014.11.020.
Schlaug G, Marchina S, Norton A. From singing to speaking: why singing may lead to recovery of expressive language function in patients with Broca's aphasia. Music Percept. 2008;25:315–23. https://doi.org/10.1525/mp.2008.25.4.315.
Schön D, Boyer M, Moreno S, Besson M, Peretz I, Kolinsky R. Songs as an aid for language acquisition. Cognition. 2008;106(2):975–83. https://doi.org/10.1016/j.cognition.2007.03.005.
Schön D, Gordon R, Campagne A, Magne C, Astésano C, Anton JL, Besson M. Similar cerebral networks in language, music and song perception. NeuroImage. 2010;51:450–61. https://doi.org/10.1016/j.neuroimage.2010.02.023.
Selph A. The effective of musical mnemonics on learning and recall in preschool-aged children with developmental disabilities. (Unpublished master's thesis). Colorado State University; 2015.
Siponkoski ST, Martinez-Molina N, Kuusela L, Laitinen S, Holma M, Ahlfors M, Jordan-Kilkki P, Ala-Kauhaluoma K, Melkas S, Pekkola J, Rodriguez-Fornells A, Laine M, Yinen A, Rantanen P, Koskinen S, Lipsanen J, Särkämö T. Music therapy enhances executive functions and prefrontal structural neuroplasticity after traumatic brain injury: evidence from a randomized controlled trial. J Neurotrauma. 2020;37:618–34. https://doi.org/10.1089/neu.2019.6413.

Starcke K, Mayr J, von Georgi R. Emotion modulation through music after sadness induction-the iso principle in a controlled experimental study. Int J Environ Res Public Health. 2021;18(23):12486. https://doi.org/10.3390/ijerph182312486.

Staube T, Schulz A, Geipel K, Mentzel HJ, Miltner WHR. Dissociation between singing and speaking in expressive aphasia: the role of song familiarity. Neuropsychologia. 2008;46:1505–12. https://doi.org/10.1016/j.neuropsychologia.2008.01.008.

Stein MB, Simmons AN, Feinstein JS, Paulus MP. Increased amygdala and insula activation during emotion processing in anxiety-prone subjects. Am J Psychiatry. 2007;164:318–27. https://doi.org/10.1176/ajp.2007.164.2.318.

Steinbeis N, Koelsch S. Understanding the intentions behind man-made products elicit neural activity in areas dedicated to mental state attribution. Cereb Cortex. 2009;19:619–23. https://doi.org/10.1093/cercor/bhn110.

Sutherland DH. The evolution of clinical gait analysis part I: kinesiological EMG. Gait Posture. 2001;14:61–70. https://doi.org/10.1016/s0966-6362(01)00100-x.

Thaut MH. The scientific model (R-SMM). In: A scientific model of music in therapy and medicine. IMR Press; 2000a. p. 1–24. https://lib.ugent.be/catalog/rug01:000892701.

Thaut MH. A transformational design model for functional music therapy and music medicine practice. In: A scientific model of music in therapy and medicine. IMR Press; 2000b. p. 35–9. https://lib.ugent.be/catalog/rug01:000892701.

Thaut MH. Music in therapy and medicine: from social science to neuroscience. In: Rhythm, music and the brain: scientific foundations and clinical applications. Taylor and Francis Group; 2005a. p. 113–36. https://doi.org/10.4324/9780203958827.

Thaut MH. Neurologic music therapy in sensorimotor rehabilitation. In: In MH, editor. Rhythm, music and the brain: scientific foundations and clinical applications. Taylor and Francis Group; 2005b. p. 137–64. https://doi.org/10.4324/9780203958827.

Thaut MH. Biomedical research in music. In: In MH, editor. Rhythm, music and the brain: scientific foundations and clinical applications. Taylor and Francis Group; 2005c. p. 61–84. https://doi.org/10.4324/9780203958827.

Thaut MH. Neurologic music therapy in speech and language rehabilitation. In: Thaut MH, editor. Rhythm, music, and the brain: scientific foundations and clinical applications. Routledge; 2005d. p. 165–78. https://doi.org/10.4324/9780203958827.

Thaut CP. Patterned sensory enhancement. In: Thaut IMH, Hoemberg V, editors. Handbook of neurologic music therapy. Oxford University Press; 2014a. p. 106–15.

Thaut MH. Assessment and the transformational design model (TDM). In: Thaut MH, Hoemberg V, editors. Handbook of neurologic music therapy. Oxford University Press; 2014b. p. 60–8.

Thaut CP. Musical speech stimulation. In: Thaut IMH, Hoemberg V, editors. Handbook of neurologic music therapy. Oxford University Press; 2014c. p. 146–9.

Thaut MH. Musical echoic memory training (MEM). In: Thaut MH, Hoemberg V, editors. Handbook of neurologic music therapy. Oxford University Press; 2014d. p. 311–3.

Thaut MH. The discovery of human auditory-motor entrainment and its role in the development of neurologic music therapy. Prog Brain Res. 2015;217:253–66. https://doi.org/10.1016/bs.pbr.2014.11.030.

Thaut MH, de l'Etoile SK. The effects of music on mood state-dependent recall. J Music Ther. 1993;30:70–80. https://doi.org/10.1093/jmt/30.2.70.

Thaut MH, Gardiner JC. Musical attention control training (MACT). In: Thaut MH, Hoemberg V, editors. Handbook of neurologic music therapy. Oxford University Press; 2014. p. 257–69.

Thaut MH, McIntosh GC. How music helps to heal the injured brain: therapeutic use crescendos thanks to advances in brain science; 2010. Retrieved from http://dana.org.news.cerebrum/detail.aspx?id=26122.

Thaut CP, Rice R. Rhythmic auditory stimulation (RAS). In: Thaut MH, Hoemberg V, editors. Handbook of neurologic music therapy. Oxford University Press; 2014. p. 94–105.

Thaut MH, Wheeler BL. Music therapy. In: Juslin P, Sloboda J, editors. Handbook of music and emotion. Oxford University Press; 2010. p. 819–48.

Thaut MH, Schleiffers S, Davis W. Analysis of EMG activity in biceps and triceps muscle in an upper extremity gross motor task under the influence of auditory rhythm. J Music Ther. 1991;28:64–87. https://doi.org/10.1093/JMT/28.2.64.
Thaut MH, McIntosh GC, Prassas SG, Rice RR. The effect of auditory rhythmic cuing on temporal stride and EMG patterns in hemiparetic gait of stroke patients. J Neurol Rehabil. 1993;7:9–16. https://doi.org/10.1177/136140969300700103.
Thaut MH, Brown SH, Benjamin J, Cooke JD. Rhythmic facilitation of movement sequencing: effects on spatiotemporal control and sensory modality dependence. In: Pratt RR, Spingte R, editors. Music medicine, vol. II. MMB Music; 1996. p. 104–9.
Thaut MH, Tian B, Azimi-Sadjadi MR. Rhythmic finger tapping to cosine-wave modulated metronome sequences: evidence of subliminal entrainment. Hum Mov Sci. 1998;17:839–63. https://doi.org/10.1016/S0167-9457(98)00031-1.
Thaut MH, McIntosh KW, McIntosh GC, Hoemberg V. Auditory rhythmicity enhances movement and speech motor control in patients with Parkinson's disease. Funct Neurol. 2001;16:163–72.
Thaut MH, Kenyon GP, Hurt CP, McIntosh GC, Hoemberg V. Kinematic optimization of spatiotemporal patterns in paretic arm training with stroke patients. Neuropsychologia. 2002;40:1073–81. https://doi.org/10.1016/S0028-3932(01)00141-5.
Thaut MH, McIntosh GC, Hoemberg V. Neurologic music therapy: from social science to neuroscience. In: Handbook of neurologic music therapy. Oxford University Press; 2014a. p. 1–6.
Thaut MH, Thaut CP, McIntosh K. Melodic intonation therapy. In: Thaut MH, Hoemberg V, editors. Handbook of neurologic music therapy. Oxford University Press; 2014b. p. 140–9.
Thaut MH, Peterson DA, McIntosh GC, Hoemberg V. Music mnemonics aid verbal memory and induce learning-related brain plasticity in multiple sclerosis. Front Hum Neurosci. 2014c;8(June):395. https://doi.org/10.3389/fnhum.2014.00395.
Thaut MH, McIntosh GC, Hoemberg V. Neurobiological foundations of neurologic music therapy: rhythmic entrainment and the motor system. Front Psychol. 2015;5:1185. https://doi.org/10.3389/fpsyg.2014.01185.
Thaut MH, Francisco G, Hoemberg V. Editorial: the clinical neuroscience of music: evidence based approaches and neurologic music therapy. Front Neurosci. 2021;15:740329. https://doi.org/10.3389/fnins.2021.740329.
United States Departments of Veterans Affairs and Defense. VA/DoD clinical practice guideline for the management of stroke rehabilitation; 2019. https://www.healthquality.va.gov/guidelines/Rehab/stroke/VADoDStrokeRehabCPGFinal8292019.pdf.
Vaiouli P, Grimmet K, Ruick LJ. "Bill is now singing": joint engagement and the emergence of social communication of three young children with autism. Autism. 2015;19(1):73–83. https://doi.org/10.1177/1362361313511709.
Wade LM. A comparison of the effects of vocal exercises/singing versus music-assisted relaxation on peak expiratory flow rates of children with asthma. Music Ther Perspect. 2002;20(1):31–7. https://doi.org/10.1093/mtp/20.1.31.
Wambaugh JL, Martinez AL. Effects of rate and rhythm control treatment on consonant production accuracy in apraxia of speech. Aphasiology. 2000;14:851–71. https://doi.org/10.1080/026870300412232.
Wan CY, Schlaug G. Music making as a tool for promoting brain plasticity across the life span. Neuroscientist. 2010;16(5):566–77. https://doi.org/10.1177/1073858410377805.
Wan C, Zheng X, Marchina S, Norton A, Schlaug G. Intensive therapy induces contralateral white matter changes in chronic stroke patients with Broca's aphasia. Brain Lang. 2014;136:1–7. https://doi.org/10.1016/j.bandl.2014.03.011.
Wang TH, Peng YC, Chen YL, Lu TW, Liao HF, Tang PG, Shieh JY. A home-based program using patterned sensory enhancement improves resistance exercise effects for children with cerebral palsy: a randomized controlled trail. Neurorehabil Neural Repair. 2013;27(8):684–94. https://doi.org/10.1177/1545968313491001.

Wang L, Peng JL, Xiang W, Huang YJ, Chen AL. Effects of rhythmic auditory stimulation on motor function and balance ability in stroke: a systematic review and meta-analysis of clinical randomized controlled studies. Front Neurosci. 2022;16:1043575. https://doi.org/10.3389/fnins.2022.1043575.

Wheeler BL. A psychotherapeutic classification of music therapy practices: a continuum of procedures. Music Ther Perspect. 1983;1(2):8–12. https://doi.org/10.1093/mtp/1.2.8.

Wheeler BL. Music in psychosocial training and counseling (MPC). In: Thaut MH, Hoemberg V, editors. Handbook of neurologic music therapy. Oxford University Press; 2014. p. 331–60.

World Federation for Neurorehabilitation. Neurologic music therapy. Our special interest groups; n.d. Retrieved 27 May 2014 from https://www.wfnr.co.uk/special-interest-groups/our-special-interest-groups.

Worth RS. Voice gender congruency: a case study of a young adult transgender woman's experience with voice lessons and vocal intonation therapy. (Unpublished master's thesis). University of Miami; 2023.

Zatorre RJ, Salimpoor VN. From perception to pleasure: music and its neural substrates. Proc Natl Acad Sci. 2013;110(Suppl 2):10430–7. https://doi.org/10.1073/pnas.1301228110.

Zelazny CM. Therapeutic instrumental music playing in hand rehabilitation for older adults with osteoarthritis: four case studies. J Music Ther. 2001;38:97–113. https://doi.org/10.1093/jmt/38.2.97.

Other Music-Based Approaches in Rehabilitation and Sonification Techniques

8

Daniele Molteni and Alfredo Raglio

Key Points

- Integration with standard protocols: Thanks to rhythmic entrainment and the influence on facilitation of cognitive processes such as attentional modulation and memory consolidation, music can be incorporated into conventional motor and cognitive rehabilitation protocols as a promising therapeutic integrative tool within rehabilitation for its benefits in motor and cognitive recovery.
- Technological integration: Prerecorded musical tracks could help both therapists during the training and patients in home settings or between sessions. Sonification techniques enhance rehabilitation efficacy and patient engagement.
- Neural reorganization: Music-supported therapy and sonification can promote neural plasticity, leading to improved motor function and cognitive processes such as attention, memory, and executive functions.
- Application examples: Practical applications include exercises using musical rhythms to improve coordination, strength, and mobility, and cognitive tasks that involve identifying, sequencing, and reproducing musical patterns.
- Enhanced effectiveness: Utilizing the sound–musical element can enhance the effectiveness of rehabilitation by supporting motor and cognitive tasks, thereby improving patient outcomes.

(continued)

D. Molteni (✉)
Como, Italy
e-mail: daniele.molteni@gmail.com

A. Raglio
Music Therapy Research Laboratory, Istituti Clinici Scientifici Maugeri IRCCS, Pavia, Italy
e-mail: alfredo.raglio@icsmaugeri.it

A. Raglio (ed.), *Music and Music Therapy Interventions in Clinical Practice*, Neurocultural Health and Wellbeing,
https://doi.org/10.1007/978-3-031-88578-5_8

- Increased motivation and engagement: The inclusion of music in rehabilitation programs significantly boosts patient motivation and engagement, making therapy more enjoyable and effective.
- Training for practitioners: Nonmusic therapist practitioners can effectively use music in rehabilitation with specific training focused on the operational use of instruments and techniques, even without therapist musical training. It is crucial to train physiotherapists, occupational therapists, rehabilitation specialists, and music therapists in integrating live or prerecorded musical elements into standard rehabilitation practices, even without a dedicated music therapist.
- Role of music therapists: having a music therapist on the clinical team, even on a part-time basis, can provide essential support and guidance. They can prepare materials and personalized programs for other practitioners or patients to use independently.
- Resource adaptation: implementing music therapy may require adapting the rehabilitation setting and reassessing resources, including financial considerations, to integrate a music therapist's role.
- Operational guidelines: clear operational guidelines and strategies should be developed to ensure the effective use of music in rehabilitation, fostering continuous evaluation and adaptation.

8.1 Introduction

In the context of rehabilitative practices and cognitive enhancement strategies, the incorporation of music as a therapeutic modality has gained considerable attention (Bahrami 2024). The complex interplay of rhythmic, melodic, and harmonic elements of music provides a solution for simultaneously engaging and modulating motor and cognitive functions (Gonzalez-Hoelling et al. 2024). Neuroscientific research and rehabilitation sciences have illuminated the intricate neural mechanisms underpinning music's therapeutic efficacy in motor and cognitive rehabilitation (Chen et al. 2022). Thanks to rhythmic entrainment and the influence on facilitation of cognitive processes such as attentional modulation and memory consolidation, music has emerged as a promising therapeutic integrative tool within rehabilitation contexts (Särkämö et al. 2016).

Alongside established rehabilitative interventions supported by music, particularly within the protocols of Neurologic Music Therapy (Thaut and Hoemberg 2025; Thaut et al. 2015; Lezama-Espinosa and Hernandez-Montiel 2020; Altenmüller and Schlaug 2013), literature shows how music-based interventions (live or prerecorded) can be integrated into standard practices. It is also crucial to consider the contribution of technology, particularly with sonification techniques, to enhance the quality and the effectiveness of the rehabilitation process (Reh 2024; Zatorre et al. 2007; Amad et al. 2017; Van Atteveldt et al. 2014). Sonification techniques (Nown et al. 2023;

Hermann et al. 2011) generate real-time sounds based on specific movement parameters, such as intensity and rhythm. Utilizing specialized sensors and sound synthesis algorithms, sonification provides augmented feedback, enhancing perceptual-motor coordination. With its potential to improve various aspects of motor performance, sonification is increasingly recognized as a valuable tool in rehabilitation, positively impacting planning, execution, and real-time control.

The auditory–musical element, thanks to its constitutive components, can be effectively utilized for interventions with rehabilitative purposes (Gonzalez-Hoelling 2024; Braun Janzen et al. 2022; Tramontano 2021; Särkämö 2017; Trimble and Hesdorffer 2017; Gordon et al. 2018; Altenmüller and Schlaug 2015; Schlaug 2009).

The potential rehabilitative effects of music-based interventions can impact a variety of functions—both motor and cognitive—in various neurological diseases (Altenmüller and Schlaug 2015; Kakihara et al. 2024; Thaut et al. 1999; Thaut et al. 2019; Luft et al. 2004; Schneider et al. 2005; Altenmüller et al. 2009; Grau-Sánchez et al. 2013; Thaut et al. 2001; Lim et al. 2013; Galińska 2015; Moumdjian 2017). The psychological effects and neurobiological mechanisms of these music-based interventions are rooted in shared neural systems involving reward, arousal, affect regulation, learning, and activity-driven plasticity (Wenger et al. 2017; Wan and Schlaug 2010; Sihvonen et al. 2017; Chee et al. 2024; Ghai and Ghai 2019; Magee et al. 2017).

Our neurophysiological system can react to an auditory–musical stimulus, organize itself, and modulate dynamically (Samadi et al. 2024; Huang and Qi 2025; Zhao 2024). Given these premises, music, when appropriately adapted, can be effectively integrated into rehabilitation programs addressing both motor and cognitive functions. The structural components of music (rhythm, melody, harmony, form, dynamics, timbre) can be leveraged to characterize the motor/cognitive task, functioning not merely as background but as a morphological analogy that describes and facilitates (Smith et al. 2024; Thaut 2014; Sethi et al. 2016; Scholz et al. 2016).

A concrete example is the description of movement through congruent connotative sound, which supports and assists the movement itself. An ascending gesture, such as to lift the leg, can be effectively accompanied and modulated by a series of ascending notes, thereby creating a link between the movement (from low to high in space) and the musical phrase (from low to high in pitch) (Fig. 8.1).

The goal of motor rehabilitation programs is the optimal functional recovery of one or more residual capacities (Raglio and Oasi 2015) with the objective of compensating and managing existing deficits through task-oriented practices and daily

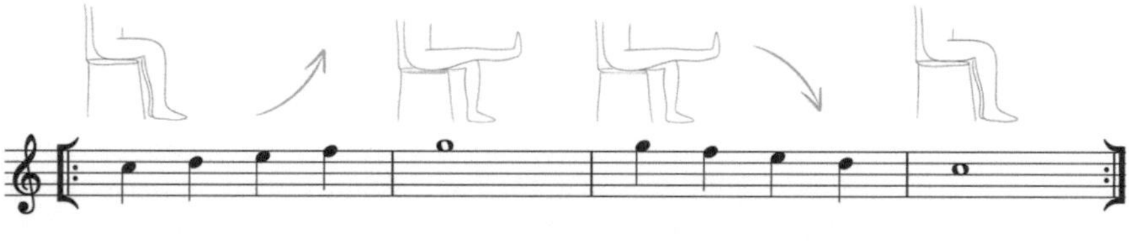

Fig. 8.1 Example of a parallel between musical trend and movement

life contexts to improve the individual's quality of life (de Dreu et al. 2012). In a rehabilitation setting, music is an adjunct element and therapeutic tool for the recovery of discrete, serial, and continuous movements of the upper and lower limbs due to its direct positive impact on motor functions (Bahrami 2024). In addition, music contributes to achieving clinical objectives by providing positive reinforcement (Della Porta et al. 2023; Gold et al. 2023), positively affecting mood (Kim et al. 2011), and enhancing executive functions (Mishra et al. 2021; Pfeiffer et al. 2024; Vik et al. 2018).

The musical element increases engagement, motivation, effort, and attention toward the required task (Smith et al. 2024; Dimitriadis et al. 2023), making the training more effective compared to standard training without music (Altenmüller et al. 2015). The combination of music with physical activity enhances its efficacy. Appropriately combining music and physical performance, even during warm-up and cool down phases, can enhance performance, reduce the perception of effort, delay fatigue, increase strength, power, endurance, and work capacity and improve arousal and mood (Terry et al. 2020; Latocha et al. 2024; Biagini et al. 2012; Eliakim et al. 2007).

In a rehabilitative framework, music is an effective support that should integrate with established training and rehabilitation protocols, determining with the clinical reference figure the most suitable phase for intervention (music can support various levels of rehabilitation even in the early stages of the process). More generally, prerecorded music, especially if self-selected and appropriately synchronized to accompany repetitive endurance tasks—such as cycling, walking, and running—can increase the distance covered and help perceive less discomfort from exercise. Music attracts attentional focus away from the exercise (Nakamura et al. 2010; Linnemann et al. 2015). Listening to music before or during exercise can also enhance positive affective valence, reduce the perception of effort, and positively influence motivation. This is crucial for maintaining adherence to the rehabilitation program, as a negative affective response to exercise can facilitate dropout (Park et al. 2023). Listening, moving to the beat, and participating in shared performances can improve mood, socialization, cognitive aspects, and other well-being indicators (Meuser 2023).

8.2 Theoretical Foundations (Motor Domain)

The use of music and its elements in rehabilitation is supported by evidence highlighting its effect on neuronal networks, in the limbic and paralimbic areas, and in brain regions involved in movement (motor cortex, supplementary motor area, cerebellum, basal ganglia, etc.). The integration of musical elements also engages emotional and motivational aspects (Raglio et al. 2021; Moumdjian et al. 2017).

Entrainment is a phenomenon where biological or brain rhythms, as well as movements and actions, synchronize and adapt to an external rhythmic element, such as a sound, a flashing light, or other periodic stimuli. Entrainment represents an innate propensity and ability of our nervous system to adapt and synchronize to rhythmic patterns, also highlighting the close correlation between an individual's movement, cognitive processes, and the surrounding environment (Schmid 2024). Neural entrainment is a fundamental mechanism underlying brain communication that "establishes an internal context for the modulation and interpretation of external signals" (Lakatos et al. 2019).

Auditory rhythmic cues, such as metrically accented music or simple isochronous metronome pulses, can promote entrainment between the auditory system and movements (Nanou et al. 2024; Gonzalez-Hoelling et al. 2024) and can thus be leveraged for the rehabilitation of motor skills.

Among the structural and constitutive elements of music, rhythm, in particular, has the fundamental ability to organize brain functions (Buzsáki 2006). This natural capability is believed to be based on the functions of temporal alignment, expectation, and prediction (Patel and Iverson 2014). According to the neural resonance theory (Large and Snyder 2009) related to the perception of musical rhythm based on a universal neural mechanism, beat, and rhythm correspond to neural rhythms that synchronize with the sound rhythm, influencing timing expectations, attention, and motor coordination.

A solid and stable link is formed between movement and stimulus, allowing the former to dynamically adjust to the latter even with potential modulations (e.g., a change in the speed of the sound stimulus can lead to an adjustment in walking cadence). Furthermore, through what is termed "forward entrainment," it is possible to retain the rhythmicity of the beat even in its absence (L'hermite and Zoefel 2023; Saberi and Hickok 2023).

The ability to perceive the beat and synchronize accordingly is a form of entrainment that establishes a solid connection between the characteristic periodicity of the rhythmic stimulus and our auditory-perceptual system (Patel 2021; Huang and Yin 2023; Grahn and Rowe 2009).

When we listen to rhythmic music, we perceive a regularity that spontaneously leads us to move in time with the music (we move, nod our head, clap our hands, or tap our foot consistently). This is a physical manifestation of a cognitive ability generated not so much on individual accents or musical beats but mentally, we continue to perceive the beat even through pauses in the music, constructing an underlying structure (Thaut and Hodges 2019).

It is important to emphasize that the true peculiarity of entrainment for rehabilitative purposes lies in its influence not only on the possibility of synchronizing movement with a beat but especially on the possibility it offers to adequately program the entire motor sequence.

The rhythmic stimulus, in fact, does not simply indicate the endpoints of the movement but provides guidance for the duration of the movement, helps regulate the timing and characteristics of the movement (such as speed, position, and trajectory).

One can thus understand the rehabilitative importance of the ability to create an expectation and predict and adapt to the development of a provided periodic reference. This means having the ability to:

- Decode the perceived musical stimulus
- Internal organization
- Gesture planning
- Execution
- Constant verification and remodulation of the effectiveness and correctness of the gesture in its temporal, spatial, force, and coordination components (in real time while performing it)
- Continuous dynamic adjustment (which is the true peculiarity)

Listening to simple rhythms with a pronounced pulse, regardless of musical training, increases activity in certain brain structures associated with motor aspects—premotor cortex, cerebellum, but particularly the basal ganglia and supplementary motor area—compared to complex stimuli or those with an undefined meter and an absent or faint pulse (Thaut and Hodges 2019; Grahn and Brett 2007).

Rhythm perception engages a network of motor areas involved in the timing and processing of musical stimuli. The basal ganglia, specifically the putamen, and the supplementary motor area appear to be particularly reactive to beat processing (Thaut et al. 2009; Thaut et al. 2014; Chen et al. 2008).

Music perceived by the listener as emotionally rewarding significantly activates the mesolimbic reward system (Salimpoor et al. 2015), which plays a key role in emotional regulation, reward, and learning, primarily mediated by dopamine and serotonin (Evers and Suhr 2000).

Auditory-motor networks, particularly the motor cortical-basal ganglia-thalamus-cortical circuit, stimulated by rhythmic stimuli, create rapid, temporally precise, and stable synchronization mechanisms between sensory input and motor output (Huang and Yin 2023). More specifically, they propose a five-stage model (1. beat detection, 2. beat continuation, 3. beat adjustment, 4. motor signal output, and 5. motor feedback) that confirms the extensive and diverse interaction between cortical and subcortical brain networks for rhythm processing, both during perception and motor execution, and the related dynamic modulation.

Brain regions involved in time perception and timing performance have also been identified through human neuroimaging studies (Kasdan et al. 2022; Huang and Yin 2023).

Music training may contribute to better motor control and could influence rehabilitation outcomes (Izbicki et al. 2023). Research comparing therapist musicians, amateur musicians, and nonmusicians found significant differences in brain structure. Musicians had increased gray matter volume in regions associated with motor and auditory processing and stronger and more integrated neural networks.

These structural differences might facilitate better outcomes in music-based neuromotor rehabilitation, with musicians potentially showing greater neuroplasticity, motor function improvements (Gaser and Schlaug 2003; Izbicki et al. 2023), and more efficient motor learning and recovery processes (Gaser and Schlaug 2003).

8.3 Theoretical Foundations (Cognitive Domain)

Cognitive rehabilitation is an intervention designed to improve cognitive processes. The ultimate goal is to enhance the patient's adaptability in a lasting and generalizable manner, allowing them to achieve the most optimal daily functioning possible.

Cognitive Processes:

- Perception: Processing of elementary sensory information conveyed by sense organs.
- Attention: Selection and filtering of surrounding stimuli.
- Memory: Encoding, storage, and retrieval of information derived from daily experiences.
- Executive Functions: A set of mental processes that help plan, organize, and control behaviors.
- Social Cognition: Processes for acquiring and interpreting the social world and modulating behaviors accordingly.

A person with cognitive function impairment faces difficulties in:

- Suppressing distractions
- Staying on task
- Switching between tasks
- Following directions
- Organizing and initiating a response
- Memory system
- Attentive system
- Executive functions system

Cognitive rehabilitation is considered a crucial treatment for improving cognitive functions in various clinical conditions. When included in combined rehabilitation programs with other forms of training, it tends to produce more significant effects (Thaut and Hodges 2019; Kukla et al. 2018; McGurk et al. 2016, 2022).

The guidelines for cognitive rehabilitation after brain injury (Jeffay et al. 2023) suggest, for individuals with executive function damage, a structured and individualized music therapy program that includes:

- Rhythm training: reproducing sequences on an instrument or the body.
- Cognitive-motor training: playing musical exercises that stimulate various types of movement on a percussion set, accompanied by a music therapist.
- Assisted instrumental training: teaching to play a melody liked by the subject on the piano with specific strategies.

Emerging evidence suggests that music, as a complex multisensory stimulus integrated into structured training programs, has specific efficacy in cognitive rehabilitation, particularly in general cognitive function, executive function, and neural changes (Ito et al. 2022; Sihvonen et al. 2017; Rajakumar and Mohan 2024; Bahrami 2024).

Music represents a complex and multidomain stimulus, involving an extensive bilateral network of temporal, frontal, parietal, cerebellar, limbic, and paralimbic brain areas associated with multiple parallel processes in cognitive, verbal, motor, and emotional domains (Särkämö and Sihvonen 2018).

Musical listening has a positive effect on cognitive performances in episodic autobiographical memory and verbal fluency in the short term. With a more structured program, it can impact general cognitive state, attention, executive functions, orientation, and remote episodic memory with long-term positive effects (Särkämö and Sihvonen 2018).

Music training can positively impact nonmusical functions such as phonological awareness, speech processing, listening skills, perceiving speech in noise, and reading (Jones 2020).

In particular, the rhythmic peculiarity of a musical stimulus (pulse, meter, and rhythm) is crucial for optimizing processes that facilitate attention and perception by modulating and synchronizing the attentional focus (Haegens and Golumbic 2018).

Rhythm is a temporal structuring and modeling process that influences perception and learning by helping to organize and segment information into more manageable units (Thaut 2010).

Exercises in melodic–rhythmic recognition and stimulation of musical and autobiographical memory can have benefits that transfer to daily life activities, thus improving quality of life, social skills, and self-esteem (London 2012).

This is because recognition abilities rely on specific brain functions that manage attention and memory networks (Zatorre and Salimpoor 2013) with overlapping areas that process memory and musical material in both the short and long term (Jacobsen et al. 2015), significantly impacting work with a reminiscence approach to one's autobiographical history (Centomo et al. 2023).

8.4 Practice: Motor Rehabilitation

8.4.1 Characteristics of Musical Patterns

An effective musical pattern for motor rehabilitation must possess specific characteristics to optimize therapeutic outcomes. Above all, consistent with the theory of entrainment, it is necessary to create rhythmic stimuli capable of inducing the perception of a clear, regular, and easily perceivable beat. Activity in motor and reward-related brain networks during music listening is associated with the groove experience, and this neural activity is linked to temporal prediction and learning (Etani et al. 2023).

The simple sequence of isochronous pulses produced by a metronome can serve as a basic but good starting point to mark the rhythm of a motor task. The most salient feature of this type of sound stimulus, known as the pulse, is the temporal regularity with which the pulses follow one another. The pulse alone can create coherence and enable the organization of movement based on the ability to adequately plan it.

The rhythm must be constant and regular to facilitate the synchronization of the patient's movements with the music. The tempo (beats per minute—BPM) should be chosen according to the patient's needs and the type of motor exercise. The music should have a well-defined structure with clear musical phrases to further support the patients as they progress through the exercise. Repetitive musical patterns facilitate the learning of movements. The use of a variety of instruments and timbres encourages the patient to maintain active interest. When opting for the use of musical pieces, consider the patient's personal preferences to increase motivation and engagement during rehabilitation.

Carefully assess and modulate complexity: more complex rhythmic patterns can be used to challenge and improve motor coordination and multitasking ability. For patients with significant difficulties, simpler rhythmic patterns are more effective to avoid confusion and frustration. The music should be adaptable to the specific needs and progress of the patient. The ability to modify the BPM, intensity, and complexity of the patterns is crucial.

Integrating these characteristics into a motor rehabilitation program can significantly enhance the effectiveness of the treatment, increasing patient motivation and facilitating the recovery of motor skills.

8.4.2 Considerations for Incrementing Musical Pattern Complexity

Given the pulse as the most basic stimulus, it is possible to gradually increase the complexity while maintaining ease of decoding for the patient. Patients are not required to have musical literacy, and clinical issues may affect sensory or cognitive aspects. By incorporating these following suggested characteristics into a motor rehabilitation program, it is possible to enhance the effectiveness of the treatment, increase patient motivation, and facilitate the recovery of motor skills.

1. Start with the expected motor/cognitive training (regardless of sound contribution)
   - Understand the correct mode of execution.
   - Determine the timing requirements (overall duration, pauses, number of repetitions, etc.).
   - Identify potential challenges for the patient (dysfunctional or incorrect movements, progressive decrease in range of motion, fatigue over the total duration, need for frequent pauses, etc.).
   - Decide whether to intervene on the rhythmicity of the gesture, range of motion (RoM), endurance, or incentive for longer duration and select the appropriate musical parameters.
2. Create the sound sequence with a balance between functionality and musicality

- Maintain the presence of the metronome pulse (i.e., clicks, woodblocks, tambourine).
- Keep the structure simple and easily decodable (repeating two–three measures may suffice).
- Use variations and a variety of timbres to encourage engagement in daily training, which can last up to 90 days.
- Consider harmonic progression, utilizing the tension-release function inherent to chords (I - IV is useful for conveying a sense of progression over time) and cadences (V - I is useful for providing a sense of rest or conclusion).
- Create aesthetically pleasing orchestrations (enhance the sequence with simple arrangements, ensuring that more complex material demands more resources for decoding).
- Priority on the pulse.
- Possible enrichment with an additional rhythmic element (percussion, drums).
- Possible enrichment with an additional harmonic element (bass, reinforcing keyboard).
- Emphasis on one functional element (Table 8.1).

At the following, some examples highlighting how music can be integrated into a rehabilitation process starting with an initial phase of sensory stimulation and then moving into exercises for functional recovery of the upper limbs, pre-gait exercises, and with an exercise of music-supported walking.

Table 8.1 Examples of possible associations between the motor tasks and music parameters, including examples of application

Motor task	Music parameters	Example of application
Incrementing the number of repetitions in the time unit	BPM Duration of the sonorous-music sequence	1. Initial Evaluation of the Parameter: The patient performs a series of repetitions in flexion-extension of the upper or lower limb accompanied by rhythmic stimulation, which can even be just the sound of a metronome set at a specific speed based on the patient's baseline frequency when performing the movement without sound support. 2. Monitoring the Number of Repetitions: The number of repetitions within the predetermined unit of time is monitored. 3. Possible Modulation Consistent with Motor Function Progress: The speed of the metronome is increased, or the duration of the exercise is lengthened, in line with motor function progress. 4. Final Reassessment of the Parameter.

(continued)

Table 8.1 (continued)

Motor task	Music parameters	Example of application
Increasing the muscle endurance (staying in a position of muscle tension against gravity for a certain amount of time)	Duration of the sonorous-music sequence	1. Initial Evaluation of the Parameter: The patient must keep the limb suspended to strengthen resistance, accompanied by supportive music that can be played live and composed to emphasize and support the phases of (i) extension from the resting position, (ii) effort position, (iii) return to the resting position. Alternatively, prerecorded sequences with similar characteristics can be used. 2. Monitoring the Duration: Monitor how long the patient can remain in the effort phase, aligning with the length of the related portion of the musical base. 3. Possible Modulation Consistent with Motor Function Progress: Extend the musical section related to the effort position or select the prerecorded base with similar characteristics. 4. Final Reassessment of the Parameter.
Increasing the Range of Motion	Melody extension (interval between the lowest and the highest pitch)	1. Initial Evaluation of the Parameter: The patient must perform extensions accompanied by a live or prerecorded musical sequence that describes the gesture by adhering to the relevant parameter (the extension of the performed or reproduced melody will reflect the amplitude reached: greater gesture amplitude = greater melody extension). 2. Monitoring the Range of Motion: The achieved Range of Motion and the related musical parameter are monitored. 3. Extending the Melody: Extend the melody consistently with the progress of motor function. 4. Final Reassessment of the Parameter.
Maintaining a steady cadence by counteracting the tendency to reduce it due to perceived fatigue	BPM Harmonic progression	1. Initial Evaluation of the Parameter: The patient must perform a cadenced movement (walking, pedaling, or repetitions of flexion-extension or abduction) with musical support that has a cadence calibrated to the previously measured base cadence. The support, live or pre-recorded, can be enriched by a harmonic progression that facilitates the patient by making the exercise more engaging (a harmonic cycle composed of 2 chords, then 3, then 4, etc., and the length of the musical phrase helps perceive the evolution of the exercise over time). 2. Monitoring and modulating: The speed of the musical support and the length of the harmonic progression are indicators to monitor and possibly modulate as motor capacity progresses. 3. Final Reassessment of the Parameter.

8.4.3 Practical Examples of Implementation Exercises for Upper Limbs

In this section, we aim to provide practical examples of how specific rehabilitative exercises can be musically characterized to enhance their effectiveness and engagement. By integrating tailored musical elements into therapy, patients can benefit from increased motivation and improved outcomes. Below are detailed examples of how music can be applied to various exercises, considering the goals, exercise specifics, timing, roles of both therapist and patient, and the characteristics for a possible useful supporting music.

Scenario 1: Sensory aspects, sensory perception, minimal fatigue resistance

Goal	Sensory aspects, sensory perception, minimal fatigue resistance
Exercise	Exploration of instruments such as rattles or drums for sensory stimulation. Simple gripping/grasping/holding/manipulating of instruments/objects (e.g., egg shakers, mallets, rattles) (Fig. 8.2).
Timing	10–15 minutes
Role of the therapist	Evaluate the motor function to be stimulated and identify the suitable instrument to stimulate sensory perception and minimal motor activity/fatigue resistance.
Role of the patient	Explore the available instruments with minimal movements, providing feedback on the tactile and auditory effects perceived.
Supporting music	Using music that creates a consistent background can be beneficial, as it provides support for integrating the patient's production. Although rhythmic pulsation is not explicitly required for the exercise, its presence can still offer a positive neurophysiological stimulus. Create a kind of continuous accompaniment with a rhythmic quality that is present but not intrusive.
Variations	(a) Extend exercise duration. (b) Increasing the weight of the instrument requires more resistance; its size or shape demands greater dexterity and fine motor skills. (c) Gradually introduce the requirement to align with the pulse, coordinating the taking, releasing, or simply touching the instrument in time.

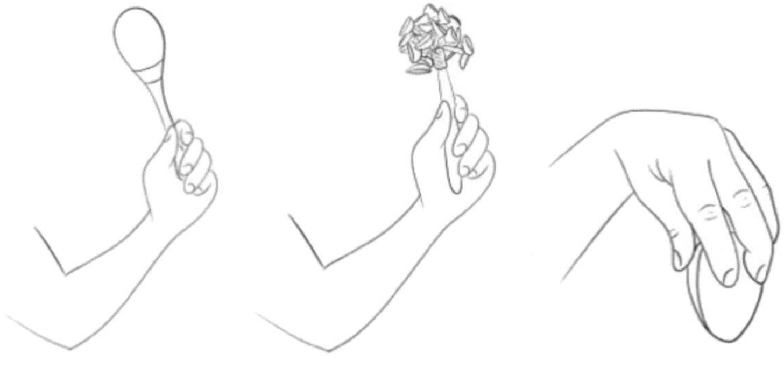

Fig. 8.2 Simple grip/hold/manipulation/grasp of an instrument

Scenario 2: Upper and lower limbs in suspension

Goal	Using music to counteract fatigue during abduction/extension and maintaining suspension
Exercise	Keep limb in suspension, against gravity
Timing	Maximum 15 minutes. Assessing the patient's fatigue and tolerance level.
Role of the therapist	Support with simple sound production the suspension phase to stimulate its longer duration. As the patient's endurance improves, the therapist can gradually increase the duration of the sound production phases, thus extending the effort period.
Role of the patient	The patient is asked to hold their limb extended while the therapist produces a continuous tone or rhythm. This tone marks the effort phase where the patient maintains the suspension. During the rest phase, the music pauses, indicating the patient can relax the limb.
Supporting music	Specifically prearranged music consisting of alternating parts appropriately calibrated to the timing of the exercise phases (effort and rest)
Detailed example	This structured musical approach can help maintaining the patient's interest, providing clear cues for timing, and effectively managing fatigue thanks to the differentiation between phases of effort and rest (Fig. 8.3). 1. Shoulder Abduction/extension and Suspension (a) Rhythmic Support: Use a clear, steady beat to provide a consistent timing cue for the shoulder abduction movement. Be sure to use an appropriate BPM to support movement that is as fluid as possible (a too slow pace might encourage a stepped movement instead of a more continuous one). Choose a pulse that is consistent with the patient's natural speed. Ask to perform the movement without the musical support and set the speed of the metronome accordingly. (b) Tensio-Distensional Alternation: Employ harmonic and rhythmic changes to emphasize periods of effort (tension) and rest (distension). For example, during the abduction phase, use chords that create tension (such as a dominant seventh chord), and during the rest phase, switch to more relaxed, resolved chords (such as a tonic chord). 2. Emphasizing Effort and Resistance (a) Effort Phase: During the abduction and holding phase, use music with a more intense, driving rhythm and tension-building harmonics. This could involve a melody/harmony that starts from the low end and arrives and stays in a higher area, increasing volume, the use of instruments with a sharper, more percussive sound (e.g., drums, staccato strings) to convey effort. (b) Rest Phase: During the rest period, switch to softer, more soothing music with harmonics that signal relaxation. Use gentle instruments (like a soft piano or legato strings) to create a more relaxed musical connotation, and convey rest. Choose resolving chords that resolve tension (such as moving from a dominant to a tonic chord). 3. Calibrated Duration for Suspension and Rest (a) Suspension Duration: Time the music to match the duration the patient is expected to hold the abduction. For example, use a segment of 10 seconds of tension music for holding the arm in suspension. (b) Rest Duration: Follow the tension segment with a rest segment of 10 seconds (or whatever duration is appropriate), using proper music to signal the transition to rest.

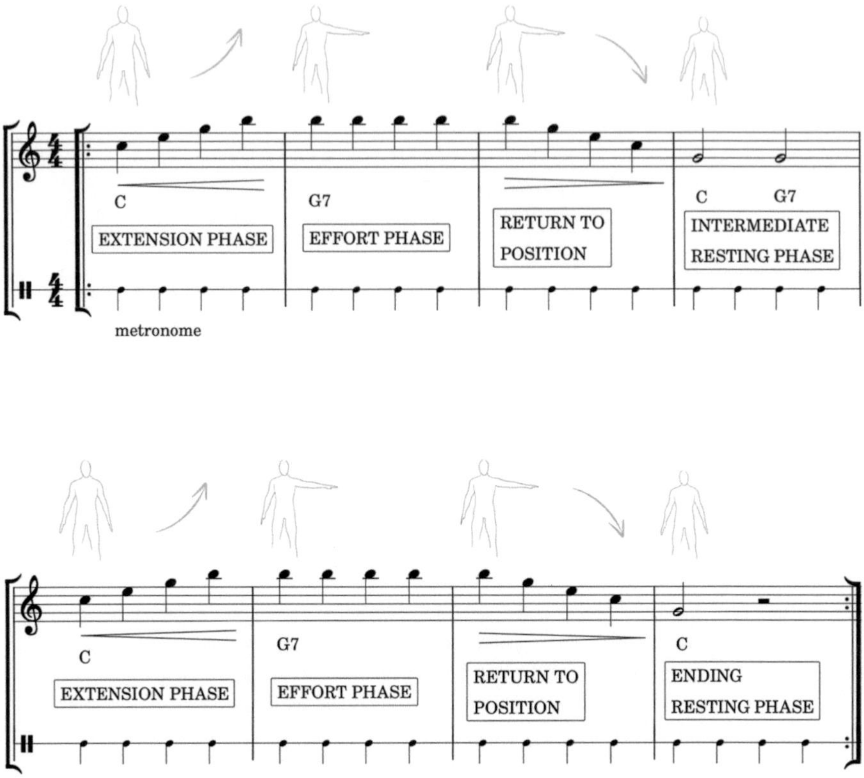

Fig. 8.3 Example of music functional to support shoulder abduction

Scenario 3: Strengthen upper extremity motor skills

Goal	Strengthen upper extremity motor skills (extension/flexion of biceps and triceps, general function, and ulnar/radial wrist deviation). Improve stability, uniformity, and regularity of gesture.
Exercise	Playing a drum with a beater
Timing	Maximum 15 minutes. Assessing the patient's fatigue and tolerance level.
Role of the therapist	Ask the patient to play a drum with a mallet, providing support as needed. If the patient is unable to grip the mallet, use a wrist brace or elastic supports to attach it to the forearm, or grips to facilitate holding it. Position the drum in the most suitable location relative to the movement being exercised or rehabilitated. Gradually vary the drum's placement by moving it farther away to increase the difficulty and further improve motor skills. Adjust the weight and type of mallet to align with the progression of rehabilitation and its objectives. Introduce variation in timbre by using maracas, rattles, bells, or egg shakers instead of the drum. Provide a simple rhythmic-harmonic accompaniment with a clear and evident pulse (using a metronome for assistance). For example, use another percussion instrument to present a simple rhythmic pattern (Fig. 8.4) or accompany with a pentatonic xylophone (emphasizing the beat, not the melody). No special musical skills are required: if the instrument is pentatonic, the resulting sound will be pleasant and consonant.

(continued)

Role of the patient	Playing the drum holding the beater and adjusting to the rhythm proposed by the therapist
Supporting music	If live accompaniment is not possible, utilize specially pre-recorded music that consists of a simple harmonic progression with a pulse and a prominent percussion instrument. This can serve as an example that the patient can easily imitate. As the training progresses, the speed and complexity of the required rhythmic pattern can be increased.

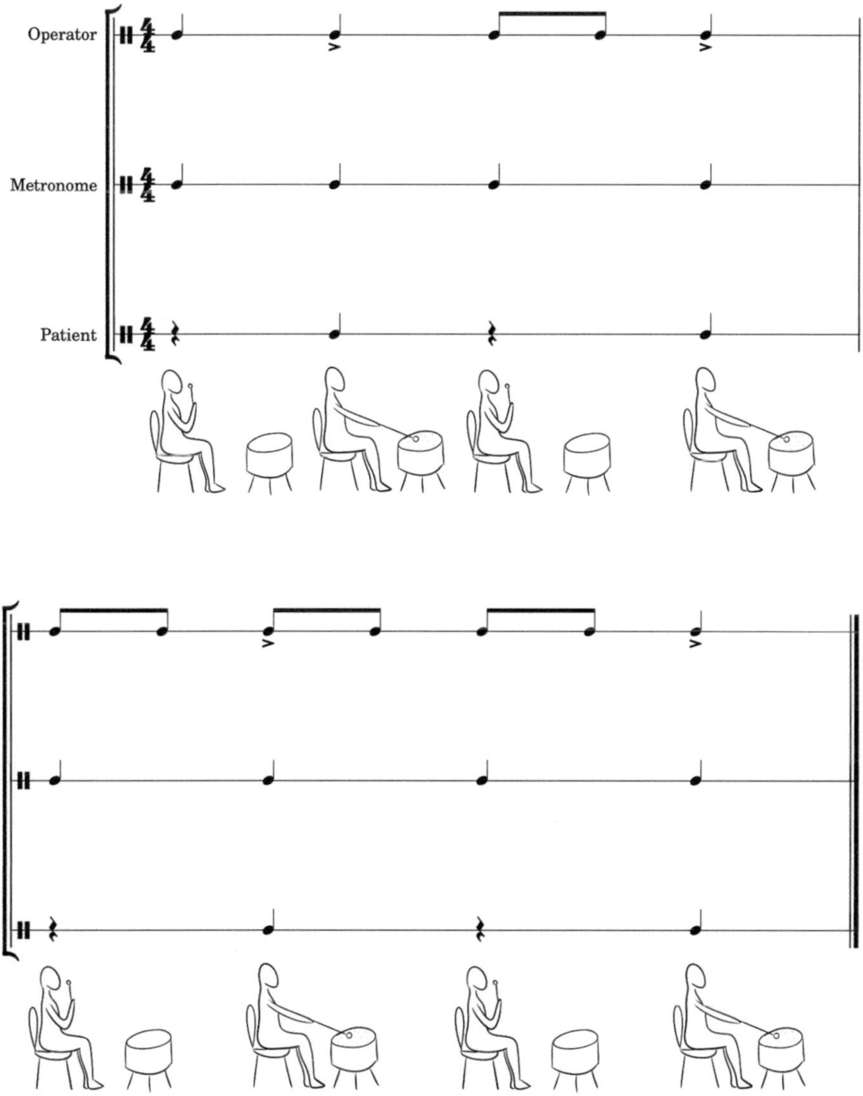

Fig. 8.4 Simple rhythmic pattern to accompany and sustain the patient who is asked to play a drum with a beater supported by a metronome too

Scenario 4: Improving upper limb fine motor function

Goal	Improving upper limb fine function.
Exercise	At the table, reach and play in a predetermined way some properly arranged target instruments (Fig. 8.5)
Timing	Maximum 15 minutes. Assessing the patient's fatigue and tolerance level.
Role of the therapist	Ask the patient, while providing support, to play the instruments arranged on the table in a manner that is functional to the identified objective: cyclically from the nearest to the farthest, alternating left and right sides, and adapting to a pulse with progressively adjustable speed. Alternatively, suggest playing a specific pattern on a metallophone: start with consecutive bars, then gradually increase the range by skipping one bar, then two, and so on. Provide a simple rhythmic-harmonic accompaniment with a clear and evident pulse (using a metronome for assistance). For example, use another percussion instrument to present a simple rhythmic pattern or accompany with a pentatonic xylophone (emphasizing the beat, not the melody). No special musical skills are required: if the instrument is pentatonic, the resulting sound will be pleasant and consonant.
Role of the patient	Play the target instruments or metallophone in the predetermined manner, adjusting to the rhythm proposed by the therapist.
Supporting music	If live accompaniment is not possible, use a specially prearranged music consisting of a simple harmonic progression with a clear beat that can suggest the sequence of alternating targets, thereby guiding the patient in the sequence to execute. As the training progresses, the speed and complexity of the required pattern can be increased.

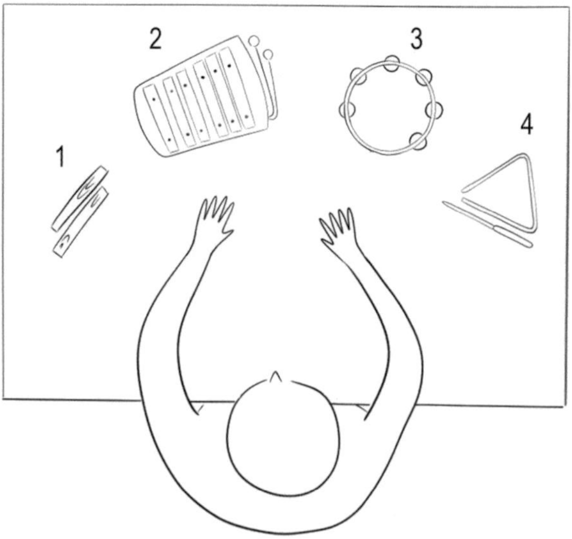

Fig. 8.5 Ask the patient to play instruments in a specific order: 1 - 2 - 3 - 4; 1 - 2 - 4; 1 - 2 - 1 - 3 - 1 - 4 ... and variations

8.4.4 Practical Implementation of Exercises for Lower Limbs and Gait

To effectively support the lower limbs and gait training process, we can start using music even in the first phase to accompany preparatory exercises by breaking down walking into more basic components, such as:

- Flexion-extension of feet and knees
- Abduction of lower limbs
- Strengthening muscle chains
- Heel–toe lifts

Music can regulate the timing of cadence and smoothness of movement, as well as counteract fatigue, which often progressively degrades performance and correctness of movement during numerous repetitions. As training progresses and motor skills consolidate, the walking exercise can be accompanied by a sound stimulus with the following characteristics:

- Evident and easily decodable rhythm: The rhythm should be clear and simple for the patient to follow without requiring specific musical skills.
- Pulse consistent with the patient's natural cadence: The tempo should match the natural walking pace of the patient.
- Structure that guides and supports walking phases: The music should help facilitate and support the different phases of walking, including stance and swing.
- Simple yet engaging musicality: To improve fatigue tolerance, the music should be simple but engaging enough to maintain the patient's interest.
- Appropriate harmonic progression: To functionally delineate the progression of the exercise over time and space, the harmonic progression should be carefully constructed.

Scenario 1: Lower limbs/pre-gait exercises

Goal	Enhance strength, coordination, and articulation of movements preparatory to walking
Exercise	Ankle flexion-extension, knee flexion-extension, hip abduction.
Timing	Maximum 20 minutes. Assessing the patient's fatigue and tolerance level.
Role of the therapist	Provide a simple rhythmic-harmonic accompaniment with a clear and evident pulse (utilizing a metronome for assistance). For instance, employ another percussion instrument to present a simple rhythmic pattern or accompany with a pentatonic xylophone (emphasizing the beat, not the melody. No special musical skills are required: if the instrument is pentatonic, the resulting sound will be pleasant and consonant). Always with the support of the metronome, accompany the extension with an ascending scale played on the pentatonic xylophone and pause on the highest note for the needed duration of the resting phase. Return to the rest position with a descending scale. Remain in the rest position for as long as necessary (the metronome still proceeds).

(continued)

Role of the patient	Perform the proposed exercise by letting the music facilitate the execution and timing of the various steps.
Supporting music	If live accompaniment is not possible, a prerecorded music with melodic fragments describing the 4 phases of the exercise may be useful, potentially supported by a simple rhythmic-harmonic loop to make the exercise more engaging and underline its evolution over time. As the training progresses, it's possible to increase the speed and/or modulate the duration of the suspension/rest phases in a functional perspective (for example, prolonging the suspension and reducing the rest).
Variation (reaching)	Position a drum or a cymbal at the point where you want the patient to achieve maximum extension and ask the patient to play it by extending the limb (the instrument serves as a target, bookend). The same strategy can be used to work on other parts, for example, placing a rattle/cymbal/plate on the ground and asking the patient to play it with the foot (toe or heel). By placing the instruments in different positions, you can act on different articulatory abilities (sideways to strengthen the lateral thigh muscles, behind for the posterior muscles, or, in both cases, in bench variations). Bilateral exercise with 2 targets on the sides of the patient, preferably of different types to make the sound more varied. Consider working on all 4 spatial directions if functional (4 instruments: in front, behind, and on both sides of the patient, in sitting or standing position). For more advanced motor skills, organize the instruments in space and, similarly to reaching at the table, arrange a sequence that the patient must follow in a sort of motor–musical path. Options for varying speed/complexity are valid, always based on a constant reassessment of progress.
Detailed example	(a) Foot and Knee Flexion-Extension: use a consistent, slow rhythm with clear beats to guide the timing of flexion and extension movements. Make sure that the melodic profile consistently follows the pattern of the gesture (from low-high in space, from low to high in pitch) (Fig. 8.6). (b) Abduction of Lower Limbs: incorporate a steady, moderate tempo with a clear pulse to help coordinate the abduction movements. Harmony could follow the gesture alternating I degree at the point of rest and V degree at the point of maximum abdication. (c) Muscle Strengthening: use rhythmic patterns that encourage endurance, with a simple harmonic progression to maintain engagement. (d) Heel-Toe Lifts: Utilize a clear, repetitive rhythm that helps the patient synchronize the heel-toe lift movements (Fig. 8.7).

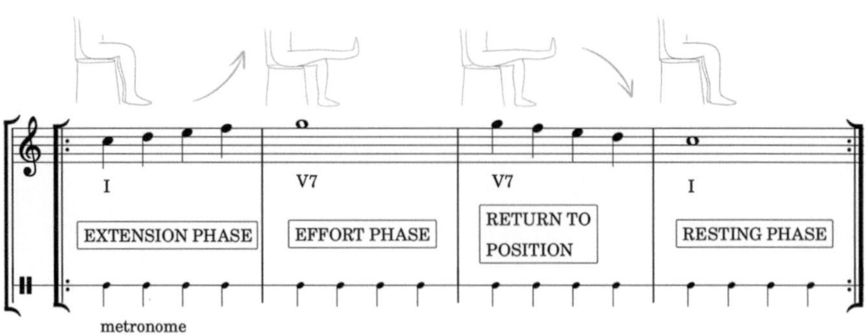

Fig. 8.6 Create congruence between melody and gesture to support the extension and return phases. Harmony can further emphasize and connote these phases by enhancing the sustain and stability of the limb during suspension

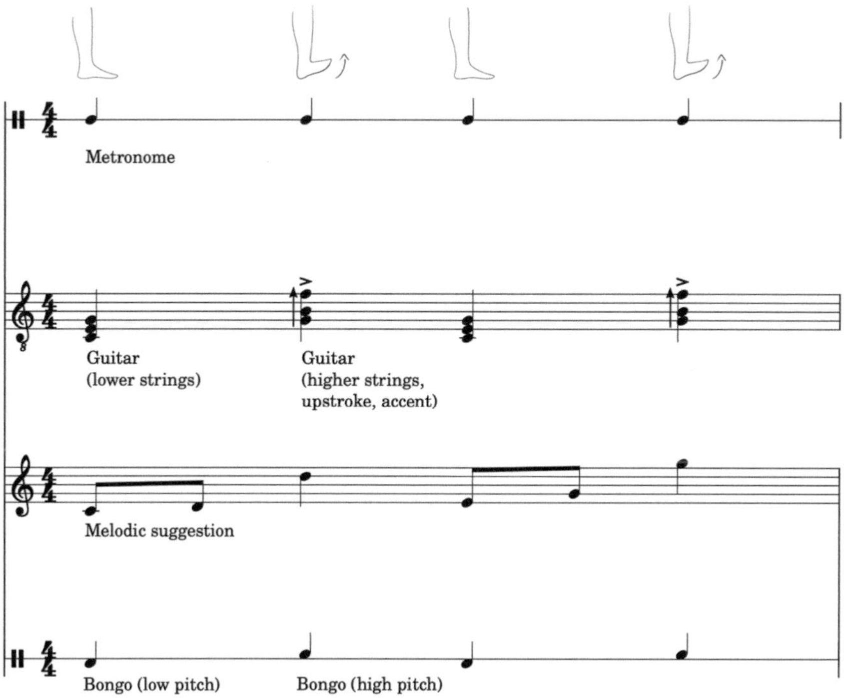

Fig. 8.7 Emphasize the supporting or lifting/raising movement component with a consistent BPM and a proper downbeat or upbeat accent (down and upstroke on a string instrument, low and high pitch on a tuned or untuned percussion)

Scenario 2: Walking exercise

Goal	Improve gait performance
Exercise	Walk with a music support.
Timing	10–20 minutes. Assessing the patient's fatigue and tolerance level.
Role of the therapist	Establish the patient's base cadence by asking the patient to walk without sound support. Set the metronome to the assessed cadence.
Role of the patient	Walk following the therapist's directions and being guided by the proposed sound stimulus.
Supporting music	The simple sound of the metronome is already an effective stimulus to regularize walking. To enrich the accompaniment, incorporate simple, repetitive rhythms and melodies that are pleasant and engaging. Use harmonic progressions that convey a sense of movement and progression. For instance, alternating between I and IV chords can provide a feeling of forward motion, while using V to I cadences can give a sense of resolution and rest (Fig. 8.8). If live accompaniment is not possible, utilize specially pre-recorded music that consists of a simple harmonic progression with a pulse and a prominent percussion instrument. This can serve as an example that the patient can easily imitate. Choose music with a clear, steady beat that matches the patient's walking cadence. For example, if the natural cadence is 60 steps per minute, select music at 60 BPM. As the training progresses, the speed and complexity of the required rhythmic pattern can be increased.

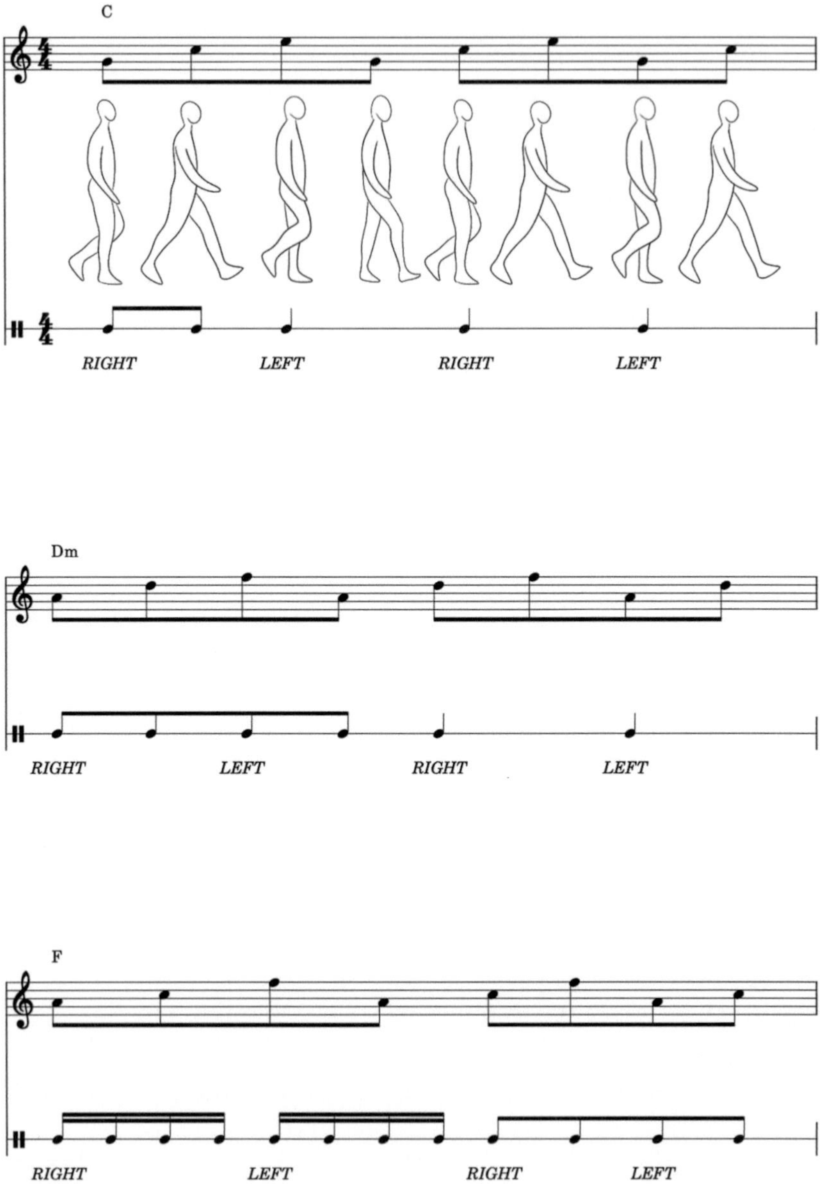

Fig. 8.8 Example of 3 different rhythmic patterns and melodic-harmonic progression conveying a sense of continuity and cyclicity

8.5 Advantages and Disadvantages of Sessions with the Presence of the Music Therapist (Sounds Produced Live During Rehabilitation)

8.5.1 Advantages

1. The presence of a music therapist allows for real-time musical material that is carefully calibrated with movements and adapts to training progress and rehabilitation goals. This ability—combined with the flexible way in which the music therapist can integrate into the rehabilitative team—contributes to a personalized approach that increases the effectiveness of therapy.
2. Close collaboration with the music therapist on the team allows physical and occupational therapists to reduce their overall workload to focus more on their specific areas of expertise.
3. The involvement of a music therapist brings greater richness and variety to the musical aspects of the rehabilitation process. This specific expertise can improve patients' experience and adherence to the pathway, making sessions more engaging and enjoyable and less monotonous—considering the main feature of repetition inherent in these types of treatments.
4. A music therapist has the ability to tailor musical interventions to the specific needs of each patient, using instruments, rhythms, and melodies that best suit the patient's abilities and rehabilitation goals.

8.5.2 Disadvantages

1. The presence of an additional specialist during rehabilitation sessions incurs extra costs, which may not be affordable for all facilities or patients.
2. The presence of multiple therapists with diverse skills requires a high level of coordination and communication to ensure interventions are mutually supportive and maximize desired outcomes. Not all physical therapists are expected to be familiar with music therapy techniques, and vice versa. A good understanding of each other's work and the potential synergy between the two fields is necessary.
3. The need for musical instruments and adequate space for music therapy sessions can pose a logistical challenge.
4. Not all patients may be open or receptive to the use of music in rehabilitation, and some may prefer more traditional approaches.

8.6 Advantages and Disadvantages of Using Prerecorded Patterns in Rehabilitation Sessions

8.6.1 Advantages

1. Training can be delivered by other appropriately trained therapists without the need for a music therapist's presence. In addition, it allows patients to perform or continue rehabilitation exercises at home, either as a follow-up after discharge or to reinforce the work between sessions.
2. Provides access to a broader range of musical materials/parameters (tones, orchestrations, rhythms, specially structured sequences).
3. Ensures precision and consistency in pulse regularity.
4. The use of prerecorded rhythmic patterns can ensure greater coherence with the movements required of the patient and uniformity in execution throughout various sessions, contributing to more stable long-term results.
5. Sessions utilizing prerecorded patterns can be more easily monitored and evaluated over time, allowing therapists to track the patient's progress and make any necessary modifications or adjustments.

8.6.2 Disadvantages

1. Less flexibility: limited ability to adapt to emergent needs during treatment sessions.
2. Therapists and patients need to become familiar with technological devices, which could be an obstacle in some cases.
3. Preparation of materials in advance is necessary, involving a wide range of parameter variations to meet diverse needs (e.g., sequences with different BPMs to accommodate training progression, sequences with varying levels of orchestral complexity to manage fatigue in decoding).
4. While the use of prerecorded patterns can ensure accuracy and consistency, it may restrict the customization of sessions according to each patient's specific needs.

8.7 Practice: Cognitive Rehabilitation/Stimulation

In addition to the theoretical foundations, this part introduces specific exercises designed to target key cognitive outcomes through music-based interventions. These exercises are structured to address various cognitive domains, providing practical tools for practitioners to integrate into their rehabilitation programs. Each exercise is tailored to stimulate specific cognitive functions (Table 8.2).

Table 8.2 Suggested music-based approach to stimulate specific cognitive functions

Cognitive domain	Suggested music-based approach
Attention	Based on the competency and training objective, ask the patient to: (i) Indicate which instrument among those present was played by the therapist. (ii) Count how many times a particular instrument is played among those present and used by the therapist. (iii) Indicate in the correct sequence the instruments played by the therapist (3 different notes on the metallophone or a certain sequence using 3 different percussion instruments). (iv) Reproduce the proposed sequence correctly as demonstrated by the therapist.
Sustained attention	The patient must play along with the therapist, but only when the therapist uses a particular instrument
Rhythmic and melodic recognition	The patient should compare short rhythmic or rhythmic-melodic sequences and say whether they are the same or not
Spatial localization	The patient should recognize whether the sound produced by the therapist is coming from the right or the left
Musical memory	The patient is asked to recall a previously unknown fragment of melody: the therapist plays a short rhythmic melodic sequence, and the patient has to play it back. As the training proceeds, also introduce a disturbing element (listening to a short known musical fragment between the proposal of the sequence and the request to repeat it back) The therapist plays a short sequence of 3 sounds with 3 different instruments. (i) Patient points to the instruments he/she heard in the correct sequence (ii) Patient replays the sequence on the instruments in the correct order
Autobiographical memory, reminiscence	Create a playlist with meaningful music from each time period of the patient's life. Listen to the playlist to stimulate memories associated with each song.
Interference sensitivity	Ask the patient to play a single stroke on a percussion when the therapist plays 2 strokes and to play 2 strokes when the therapist plays only 1 stroke (Fig. 8.9)
Inhibitory control	Ask the patient to strike once when the therapist strikes once and NOT to strike when the therapist strikes 2 times (Fig. 8.10a). The patient should NOT play on certain specific beats: PLAY – REST - PLAY – REST; PLAY - PLAY - REST - PLAY and other similar combinations (Fig. 8.10b). Patient and therapist play together but the patient should NOT play when certain conditions occur, for example: NOT to play if the therapist plays a specific instrument (e.g., drum) (Fig. 8.10c).

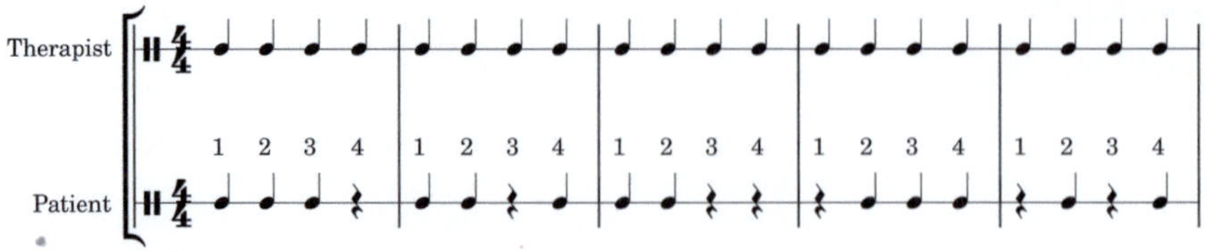

Fig. 8.9 Sample sequence for interference sensitivity training

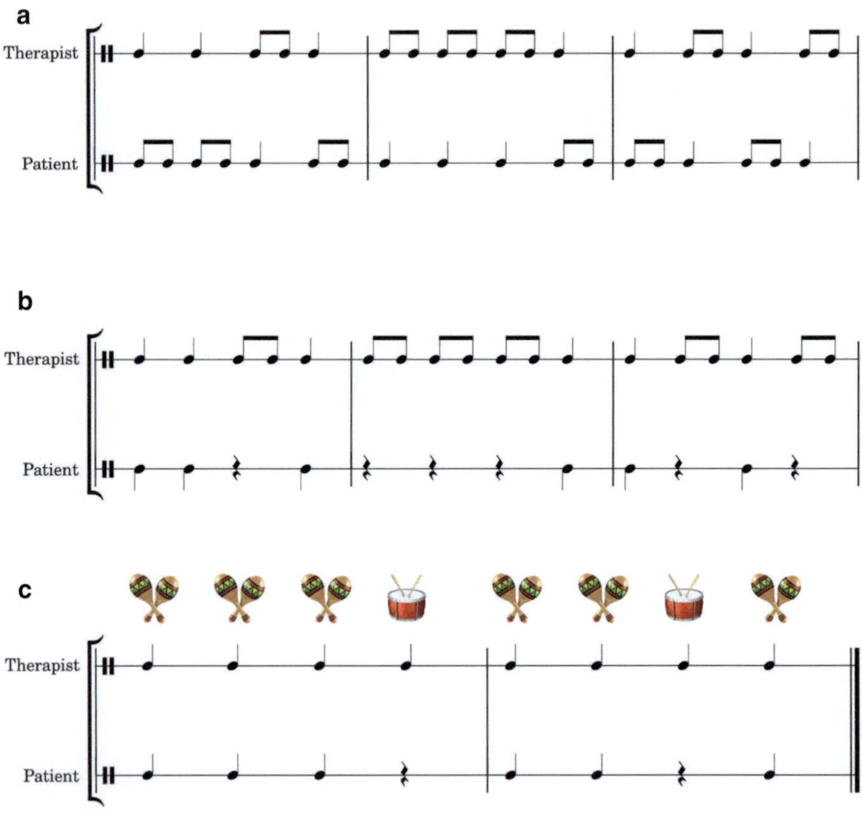

Fig. 8.10 Sample sequences for inhibitory control training

8.8 Sonification

Constant feedback is essential for providing patients with qualitative and/or quantitative information during exercise execution. This necessitates the constant presence of a therapist to ensure that movements are performed correctly and to provide support during training sessions (Corredera and Tanaka 2023). However, the repetitive nature inherent in functional recovery programs can lead to decreased interest or motivation.

Sonification is a process that converts data into sounds, allowing for the acoustic representation of information similarly to how data visualization works. In the neuromotor domain, sonification involves the real-time creation of sounds based on specific movement elements. Motor parameters are associated with sound parameters such as intensity, pitch, rhythm, and other acoustic characteristics like timbre or spatiality (Nown et al. 2022; Dubus and Bresin 2013; Spence 2011) (Table 8.3).

Sonification utilizes technologies capable of detecting specific parameters—such as spatial position, speed, force, and pressure—through specialized sensors, which then translate these into numerical data (Table 8.4). This data is processed by sound synthesis algorithms and converted into sounds. This type of feedback, where information is provided by an external mediator, is defined as extrinsic or augmented feedback.

The close correlation between the perceptual and motor systems—feedback–feedforward mechanisms—supports the use of sonification for motor rehabilitation (Reh 2024; Amad et al. 2017; Van Atteveldt et al. 2014) with the goal of improving various aspects of performance: planning, execution, and real-time control (Effenberg 2005; Schaffert 2019). Already used in sports (Agostini 2024; Schaffert 2019), sonification is increasingly recognized as a valuable resource in rehabilitation (Raglio et al. 2021), positively impacting:

- Immediate audio-motor feedback: instant feedback through sound helps patients correct movements in real-time (Peyre 2023; Schaffert et al. 2011; Yang and Hunt 2015; Dyer et al. 2015; Hossner et al. 2015; van Vugt and Tillmann 2015).
- Proprioception: the use of real-time auditory feedback shows significant benefits in improving proprioception, auditory-motor feedback can effectively compensate for damaged proprioceptive pathways, aiding the rehabilitation process. Sonification interventions promote sensorimotor learning, proprioception, and the planning and execution of movements, resulting in overall enhancements in motor performance (Ghai et al. 2018, 2019; Rodger et al. 2014; Raglio et al. 2023).
- Multimodal sensory engagement: augmented feedback enhances multimodal perception and reinforces the link between perception and action—feedback–feedforward—resulting in more efficient motor learning and performance control (Effenberg and Schmitz 2018; Castro et al. 2021; Dyer et al. 2017; Ghai et al. 2018; Oppici et al. 2020; Schaffert et al. 2019; Scholz et al. 2015; Stanton and Spence 2020).

Table 8.3 Relationship between motor parameter and musical parameter in the sonification domain

Motor parameter	Music parameter	Example
Vertical position in space	Pitch	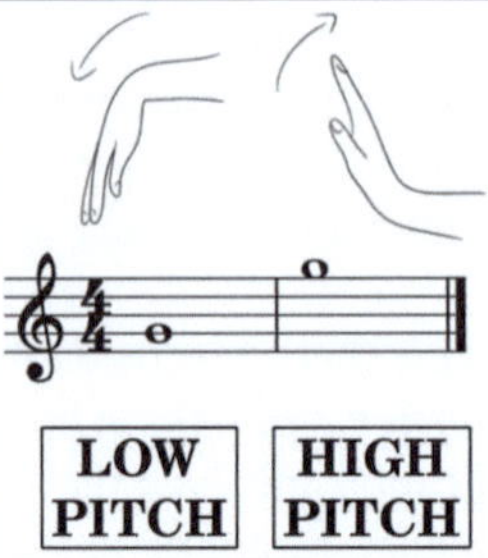
Position on the horizontal plane	Pitch and stereo panning	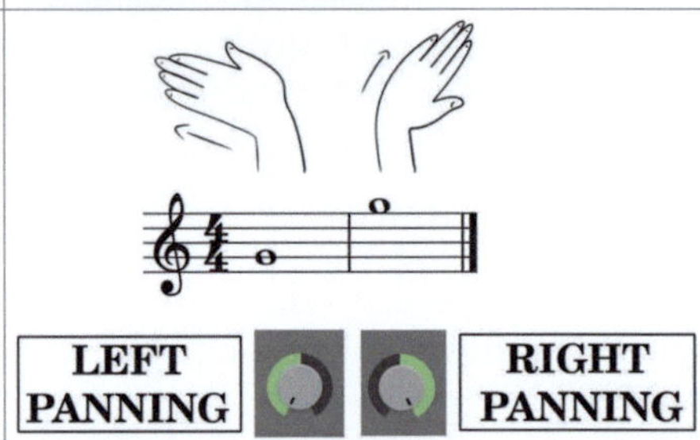
Position in space (distance from the subject)	Pitch, loudness	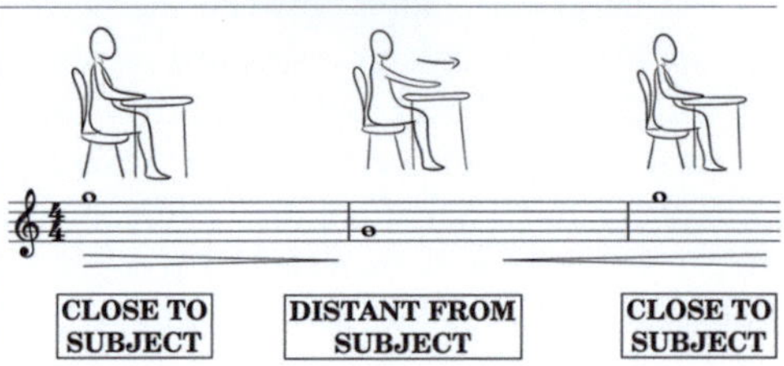
Muscle exertion	Loudness, harmony	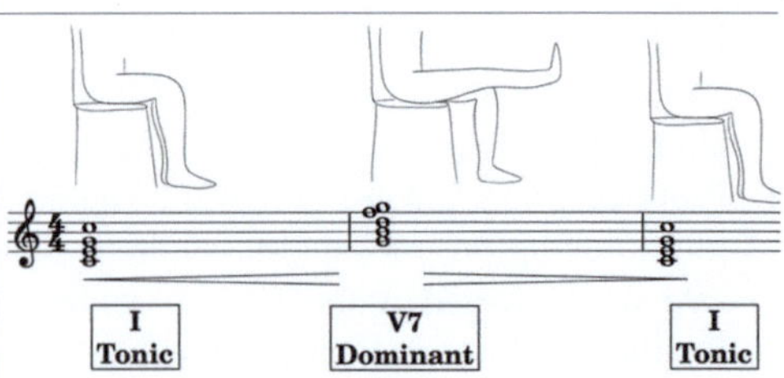
Closing/opening	Loudness, timbre, harmony	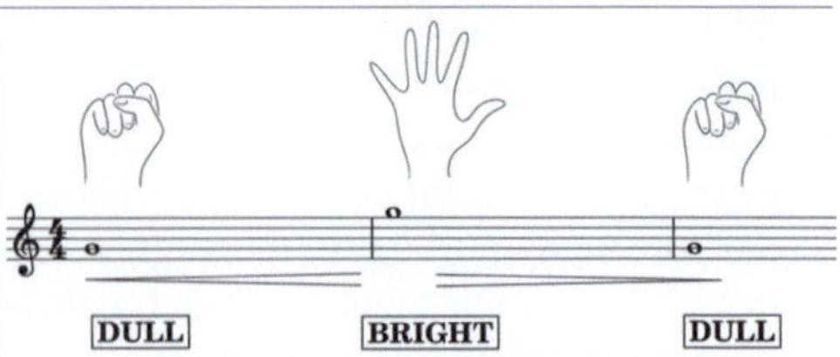

Table 8.4 Types of sensors that can be used for motion mapping

Accelerometers	Measure the acceleration of movement in one or more directions (axes).Useful for detecting speed and changes in direction.
Gyroscopes	Measure angular velocity and orientation.Useful for detecting rotations and changes in tilt.
Force and Pressure Sensors	Measure the amount of force/pressure applied.Useful for detecting pressure or effort exerted on a surface, contact, and touch intensity.
Position and Motion Sensors	Measure linear or angular position and movement. Useful for tracking position and movements of specific joints as well.

- Motivation: the presence of auditory feedback can increase patient motivation, making rehabilitation sessions more enjoyable and less monotonous (Effenberg et al. 2016; Altenmüller and Schlaug 2015).
- Motor learning: sonification can facilitate motor performance and learning (Reh 2024).
- Autonomy: immediate and intuitive feedback can, in appropriate situations, reduce the need for constant therapist supervision.

Thus, sonification enhances the overall rehabilitation process by:

- Increasing patient engagement
- Improving motor performance
- Partially reducing the assistive load on therapists

8.8.1 Example of Sonification for Upper Limb Rehabilitation: The "SonicHand" Protocol

The "SonicHand" protocol is specifically designed for the rehabilitation of upper limbs in stroke patients. This multicenter, randomized controlled study included 65 subjects who underwent five weekly sessions of either traditional motor rehabilitation or sonification-supported rehabilitation, each lasting 35 minutes, over a period of four weeks.

The study aimed to assess the effectiveness of these interventions on motor skills, fatigue, perceived pain, and quality of life (QoL). Significant improvements were observed in the experimental group, particularly in terms of enhanced motor skills, manual dexterity, and reduced perceived pain (Colombo et al. 2019; Raglio et al. 2021).

8.8.2 Example of Sonification for Gait Rehabilitation: The "SonicWalk" Protocol

The "SonicWalk" protocol targets gait rehabilitation in patients with Parkinson's disease. This preliminary, multicenter, randomized controlled study involved 19 patients who participated in 20 sessions, each lasting 30 minutes, conducted three times a week.

The study demonstrated a significant and noticeable impact of sonification treatment on balance. Training with prerecorded musical stimuli and sonification can positively influence the predictability and regularity of movement, aiding patients in better controlling and organizing their movements. The sonification component of the training may also have influenced proprioceptive aspects, enhancing movement self-perception through audio-motor feedback (Raglio et al. 2023).

Appendix: Introduction of an Alternative Graphic Mode to Standard Musical Notation

To facilitate the understanding of musical sequences without necessarily having competence in reading the musical staff, an alternative graphic mode can be considered. This alternative should be effective for the purposes in this context. The key elements to highlight are:

- The presence of the pulse
- The indication of the instrument's mode of production (on which beat to play, which specific part of the instrument to play)
- The role of the patient and the role of the therapist
- Correspondence between music and movement or cognitive task

Examples will now be given of how to graphically illustrate a musical sequence/instruction as well as how to operationally play the instruments. It is important to note that the presence of a music therapist on the team, even if not present on a daily basis, can facilitate the preparation of the instruments and these operational tools useful not only to the patients but to all involved.

Example 1 In this example, rhythmic patterns are proposed to be performed on a pair of bongos. The cue is to alternate between the 2 types of sounds offered by the instrument by synchronizing with the pulse and, progressively, make the pattern more complex by adding subdivisions. In this simple and intuitive way, it is possible to exploit different rhythmic cues that can then be declined on other types of instruments with the idea of providing both an aesthetic variation but, above all, a complexity that goes hand in hand with the consolidation of motor and cognitive skills (Table 8.5).

Example 2 This example describes the movement of the hand in the horizontal plane with a sequence of notes in the form of arpeggio. The idea is to play cyclically the sound bars that have been previously arranged in a specific order to form an arpeggio.

Table 8.5 Different rhythmic patterns on a pair of bongos

Beat (metronome)	1		2		3		4
	*		*		*		*
Pattern 1	⊙		⊙		⊙		⊙
Pattern 2	⊙		⊙		⊙	⊙	⊙
Pattern 3	⊙	⊙	⊙		⊙	⊙	⊙
Pattern 4	⊙	⊙	⊙	⊙	⊙		⊙

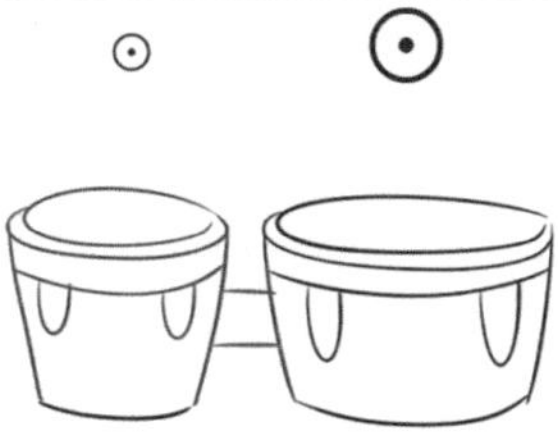

Table 8.6 Ascending and descending progression played on a metallophone/xylophone to guide the ulnar-radial deviation of the hand

Beat (metronome)	1		2		3		4		1		2		3		4	
	*		*		*		*		*		*		*		*	
Ascending and descending progression	1	2	3	4	4	3	2	1	1	2	3	4	4	3	2	1
Movement example	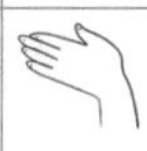		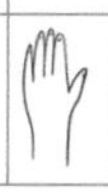		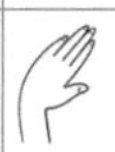		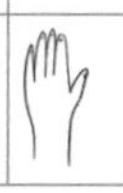		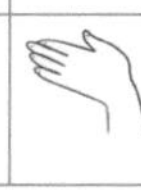		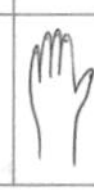		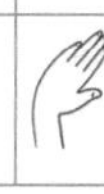		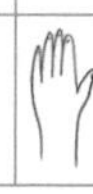	

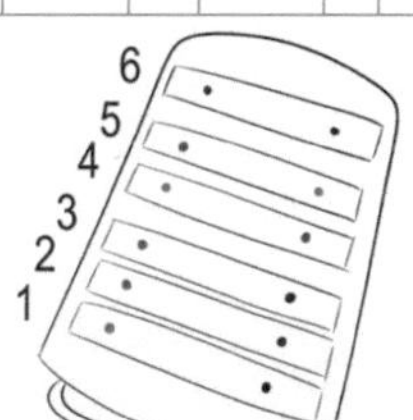

The proposed rhythmic scansion is 2 notes each pulse (it is possible to vary this mode according to specific needs if it is functional for the exercise) (Table 8.6).

Example 3 A sequence of possible patterns useful in working on the cognitive competence of inhibition is proposed here. Musically, the patient is asked not to play one or certain beats within a typical grouping of 4 (Table 8.7).

Table 8.7 Patterns for work on inhibition issues

Beat (metronome)	1	2	3	4
	*	*	*	*
Inhibition Pattern 1	⊙	⊙	⊙	
Inhibition Pattern 2	⊙	⊙		⊙
Inhibition Pattern 3	⊙	⊙		
Inhibition Pattern 4		⊙	⊙	⊙
Inhibition Pattern 5		⊙		⊙

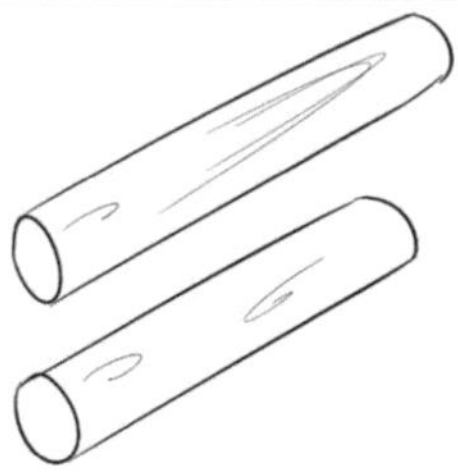

Possible Future Development: A Kit for Practicing Exercises on Your Own (Either Motor or Cognitive Domain)

Exercises should be designed with clear and simple instructions, acknowledging that the work may not be supervised by a trained therapist. The kit should specify the timing, sequence, and number of repetitions, with attention to potential issues (e.g., reduced Range of Motion due to fatigue).

The use of prerecorded sequences with suitable characteristics can be considered. Offering a margin for improvement, for instance, providing a range of prerecorded sequences with different BPMs around the patient's achieved pace and giving instructions on how to proceed (e.g., if after 5 repetitions at a speed of 70, the movement is fluid and aligned, try moving to 72 or 75).

In the cognitive domain, depending on the available technological complexity, intervention on a specific aspect—such as inhibition—can be achieved by preparing patterns that include pauses or contain a signal tone that the patient must recognize and respond to as agreed.

The verification aspect appears critical and can be entrusted to appropriate technology or a suitably trained caregiver. Considering the novelty introduced compared to standard treatments, it is useful to plan one or two training sessions to demonstrate the kit's functioning. As additional reinforcement, during therapist-led training with a specific exercise that is also included in the kit, emphasize that the patient will need to perform this exercise at home or for the next session, paying particular attention to this specific aspect, etc.

The development of a digital exercise kit for self-administered rehabilitation at home offers several advantages, including accessibility, as patients can perform the exercises independently, ensuring consistent rehabilitation by maintaining the predetermined cadence for sessions with clinical figures. It also allows for personalization, with adjustable parameters to meet individual needs and progress in functional recovery, and improves engagement. However, there are potential critical issues, such as ensuring unsupervised patient compliance, which can be addressed with clear instructions and possibly gaming elements, and addressing technology literacy issues, particularly among older adults, by simplifying the interface and providing initial training sessions.

Conclusion

Music can be effectively integrated with standard motor and cognitive rehabilitation protocols due to a solid rationale and a body of evidence attesting to its rehabilitative potential. By deepening the understanding of the sound-musical element and its components, it can be employed with awareness as an additional support for motor and cognitive tasks, enhancing effectiveness, patient motivation, and engagement. It's important to emphasize that for nonmusic therapist practitioners, while therapist musical training is not essential, specific training aimed at the operational use of instruments and techniques is crucial.

Given the need to adapt the setting and reassess resources, including financial ones, it is worth considering the possibility of having a permanent music therapist on the clinical team. As highlighted, including operational guidelines, this presence—if not guaranteed daily—can also be managed with reduced frequency, provided the necessary materials are prepared for personalized support to practices that other therapists or patients themselves will conduct autonomously, utilizing today's available technology.

The approach should focus on understanding the potential applications of the sound-musical element within specific rehabilitation processes. This involves a continuous interchange between evaluations, objectives, and strategies to ensure effective integration.

References

Agostini T, Sors F, Murgia M, et al. Enhancing perceptual—motor skills in sports: the role of ecological sounds. J Intell. 2024;12:15.

Altenmüller E, Schlaug G. Neurologic music therapy: the beneficial effects of music making on neurorehabilitation Acoust. Sci Tech. 2013;34:1.

Altenmüller E, Schlaug G. Apollo's gift: new aspects of neurologic music therapy. Prog Brain Res. 2015;217:237–52.

Altenmüller E, Marco-Pallarés J, Münte TF, et al. Neural reorganization underlies improvement in stroke-induced motor dysfunction by music-supported therapy. Ann N Y Acad Sci. 2009;1169:395–405.

Altenmüller E, Finger S, Boller F. Music, neurology, and neuroscience: evolution, the musical brain, medical conditions, and therapies, vol. 217. Netherlands: Elsevier; 2015.

Amad A, Seidman J, Draper SB, et al. Motor learning induces plasticity in the resting brain—drumming up a connection. Cereb Cortex. 2017;27:2010–21.

Bahrami S. Utilizing music therapy for enhanced recovery from neurologic disease complications. SVOA Neurol. 2024;5:7–20.
Biagini MS, Brown LE, Coburn JW, et al. Effects of self-selected music on strength, explosiveness, and mood. J Strenght Cond Res. 2012;26(7):1934–8.
Braun Janzen T, Koshimori Y, Richard NM, et al. Rhythm and music-based interventions in motor rehabilitation: current evidence and future perspectives. Front Hum Neurosci. 2022;17(15):789467.
Buzsáki G. Rhythms of the brain. Oxford: Oxford university Press; 2006.
Castro F, Osman L, Di Pino G, et al. Does sonification of action simulation training impact corticospinal excitability and audiomotor plasticity? Exp Brain Res. 2021;239:1489–1505.
Centomo F, Wyttenbach IM, Bencivenni A, et al. Music and autobiographical memory: a new experimental protocol. Psychogeriatrics. 2023;23(3):547–9.
Chee ZJ, Chang CYM, Cheong JY, et al. The effects of music and auditory stimulation on autonomic arousal, cognition and attention: a systematic review. Int J Psychophysiol. 2024;199:112328.
Chen JL, Penhune VB, Zatorre RJ. Listening to musical rhythms recruits motor regions of the brain. Cereb Cortex. 2008;18(12):2844–54.
Chen WG, Iversen JR, Kao MH, et al. Music and brain circuitry: strategies for strengthening evidence-based research for music-based interventions. J Neurosci. 2022;42(45):8498–507.
Colombo R, Raglio A, Panigazzi M, et al. The SonicHand protocol for rehabilitation of hand motor function: a validation and feasibility study. IEEE Trans Neural Syst Rehabil Eng. 2019;27(4):664–72.
Corredera JM, Tanaka A. EMG sonification as a tool for functional rehabilitation of spinal-cord injury, 2023.
de Dreu MJ, van der Wilk ASD, Poppe E, et al. Rehabilitation, exercise therapy and music in patients with Parkinson's disease: a meta-analysis of the effects of music-based movement therapy on walking ability, balance and quality of life. Parkinsonism Relat Disord. 2012;18(Suppl):1.
Dimitriadis T, Della Porta D, Perschl J, et al. Motivation and music interventions in adults: a systematic review. Neuropsychol Rehabil. 2023;21:1–30.
Dubus G, Bresin R. A systematic review of mapping strategies for the sonification of physical quantities. PLoS One. 2013;8(12):e96018.
Dyer JF, Stapleton P, Rodger MW. Sonification as concurrent augmented feedback for motor skill learning and the importance of mapping design. Open Psychol J. 2015;8(Suppl 3):192–202.
Dyer JF, Stapleton P, Rodger MW. Mapping sonification for perception and action in motor skill learning. Front Neurosci. 2017;11:254304.
Effenberg AO. Movement sonification: effects on perception and action. IEEE Multimed. 2005;12(2):53–9.
Effenberg AO, Schmitz G. Acceleration and deceleration at constant speed: systematic modulation of motion perception by kinematic sonification. Ann N Y Acad Sci. 2018;1425(1):52–69.
Effenberg AO, Fehse U, Schmitz G, et al. Movement sonification: effects on motor learning beyond rhythmic adjustments. Front Neurosci. 2016;10:195230.
Eliakim M, Meckel Y, Nemet D, et al. The effect of music during warm-up on consecutive anaerobic performance in elite adolescent volleyball players. Int J Sports Med. 2007;28(4):321–5.
Etani T, Miura A, Kawase S, et al. A review of psychological and neuroscientific research on musical groove. Neurosci Biobehav Rev. 2023;147:105522.
Evers S, Suhr B. Changes of the neurotransmitter serotonin but not of hormones during short time music perception. Eur Arch Psychiatry Clin Neurosci. 2000;250:144–7.
Galińska E. Music therapy in neurological rehabilitation settings. Psychiatr Pol. 2015;49(4):835–46.
Gaser C, Schlaug G. Brain structures differ between musicians and non-musicians. J Neurosci. 2003;23(27):9240–5.
Ghai S, Ghai I. Effects of (music-based) rhythmic auditory cueing training on gait and posture post-stroke: a systematic review & dose-response meta-analysis. Sci Rep. 2019;9(1):2183.
Ghai S, Schmitz G, Hwang TH, et al. Auditory proprioceptive integration: effects of real-time kinematic auditory feedback on knee proprioception. Front Neurosci. 2018;12:142.
Ghai S, Schmitz G, Hwang TH, et al. Training proprioception with sound: effects of real-time auditory feedback on intermodal learning. Ann N Y Acad Sci. 2019;1438(1):50–61.

Gold BP, Pearce MT, McIntosh AR, et al. Auditory and reward structures reflect the pleasure of musical expectancies during naturalistic listening. Front Neurosci. 2023;17:1209398.
Gonzalez-Hoelling S, Reig-García G, Bertran-Noguer C, et al. The effects of rhythmic auditory stimulation on functional ambulation after stroke: a systematic review. BMC Complement Med Ther. 2024;24(1):45.
Gordon C, Cobb P, Balasubramaniam R. Recruitment of the motor system during music listening: an ALE meta-analysis of fMRI data. PLoS One. 2018;13(11):e0207213.
Grahn JA, Brett M. Rhythm and beat perception in motor areas of the brain. J Cogn Neurosci. 2007;19(5):893–906.
Grahn JA, Rowe JB. Feeling the beat: premotor and striatal interactions in musicians and nonmusicians during beat perception. J Neurosci. 2009;29(23):7540–8.
Grau-Sánchez J, Amengual JL, Rojo N, et al. Plasticity in the sensorimotor cortex induced by music-supported therapy in stroke patients: a TMS study. Front Hum Neurosci. 2013;7:494.
Haegens S, Golumbic EZ. Rhythmic facilitation of sensory processing: a critical review. Neurosci Biobehav Rev. 2018;86:150–65.
Hermann T, Hunt A, Neuhoff JG. The sonification handbook, vol. 1. Berlin: Logos Verlag; 2011.
Hossner EJ, Schiebl F, Göhner U. A functional approach to movement analysis and error identification in sports and physical education. Front Psychol. 2015;6:145851.
Huang JK, Yin B. Phylogenic evolution of beat perception and synchronization: a comparative neuroscience perspective. Front Syst Neurosci. 2023;17:1169918.
Huang LZ, Qi Z. Neurobiological mechanism of music improving gait disorder in patients with Parkinson's disease: a mini review. Front Neurol. 2025;15:1502561.
Ito E, Nouchi R, Dinet J, et al. The effect of music-based intervention on general cognitive and executive functions, and episodic memory in people with mild cognitive impairment and dementia: a systematic review and meta-analysis of recent randomized controlled trials. Healthcare (Basel). 2022;10(8):1462.
Izbicki P, Mendoza T, Zaman A, et al. Differences in motor inhibition in young and older musicians and non-musicians at rest. Front Aging Neurosci. 2023;15:1230865.
Jacobsen JH, Stelzer J, Fritz TH, et al. Why musical memory can be preserved in advanced Alzheimer's disease. Brain. 2015;138(8):2438–50.
Jeffay E, Ponsford J, Harnett A, et al. INCOG 2.0 guidelines for cognitive rehabilitation following traumatic brain injury, part III: executive functions. J Head Trauma Rehabil. 2023;38(1):52–64.
Jones C. The use of therapeutic music training to remediate cognitive impairment following an acquired brain injury: the theoretical basis and a case study. Healthcare (Basel). 2020;8(3):327.
Kakihara M, Wang X, Iwasaki S, et al. The association between music performance skills and cognitive improvement in a musical instrument training program for older adults. Psychol Music. 2024; in press
Kasdan AV, Burgess AN, Pizzagalli F, et al. Identifying a brain network for musical rhythm: a functional neuroimaging meta-analysis and systematic review. Neurosci Biobehav Rev. 2022;136:104588.
Kim DS, Park YG, Choi JH, et al. Effects of music therapy on mood in stroke patients. Yonsei Med J. 2011;52(6):997–81.
Kukla M, Bell MD, Lysaker PH. A randomized controlled trial examining a cognitive behavioral therapy intervention enhanced with cognitive remediation to improve work and neurocognition outcomes among persons with schizophrenia spectrum disorders. Schizophr Res. 2018;197:400–6.
L'hermite S, Zoefel B. Rhythmic entrainment echoes in auditory perception. J Neurosci. 2023;43(39):6667–78.
Lakatos P, Gross J, Thut G. A new unifying account of the roles of neuronal entrainment. Curr Biol. 2019;29(18):R890.
Large EW, Snyder JS. Pulse and meter as neural resonance. Ann N Y Acad Sci. 2009;1169(1):46–57.
Latocha A, Jarosz J, Helbin J, et al. Will music give me power? Effects of listening to music during active and passive rest intervals on power output during resistance exercise. J Funct Morphol Kinesiol. 2024;9(1):32.

Lezama-Espinosa C, Hernandez-Montiel HL. Neuroscience of the auditory-motor system: how does sound interact with movement? Behav Brain Res. 2020;384:112535.

Lim KB, Kim YK, Lee HJ, et al. The therapeutic effect of neurologic music therapy and speech language therapy in post-stroke aphasic patients. Ann Rehabil Med. 2013;37(4):556–62.

Linnemann A, Kappert MB, Fischer S, et al. The effects of music listening on pain and stress in the daily life of patients with fibromyalgia syndrome. Front Hum Neurosci. 2015;9:434.

Luft AR, McCombe-Waller S, Whitall J, et al. Repetitive bilateral arm training and motor cortex activation in chronic stroke: a randomized controlled trial. JAMA. 2004;292:1853–1861.

Magee W, Clark I, Tamplin J, et al. Music interventions for acquired brain injury: a systematic review. Cochrane Database Syst Rev. 2017;1:CD006787.

McGurk SR, Mueser KT, Xie H, et al. Cognitive remediation for vocational rehabilitation nonresponders. Schizophr Res. 2016;175:48–56.

McGurk SR, Xie H, Bond GR, et al. Impact of cognitive remediation on the prediction of employment outcomes in severe mental illness. Schizophr Res. 2022;241:149–55.

Mishra R, Thakur M, Rani V, et al. Role of music therapy in traumatic brain injury: a systematic review and meta-analysis. World Neurosurg. 2021;148:115–23.

Moumdjian L, Sarkamo T, Leone C, et al. Effectiveness of music-based interventions on motricity or cognitive functioning in neurological populations: a systematic review. Eur J Phys Rehabil Med. 2017;53(3):466–82.

Meuser TM. Measuring music engagement in older adults: the UNE music in aging wellness scale (MAWS). Aging Ment Health. 2023;27:1887–94.

Nakamura PM, Pereira G, Papini CB, et al. Effects of preferred and nonpreferred music on continuous cycling exercise performance. Percept Mot Skills. 2010;110:257–64.

Nanou S. Rhythmic auditory stimulation in neurorehabilitation: mechanisms and clinical applications. Prog Brain Res. 2024;266:109–26.

Nown TH, Upadhyay P, Kerr A, et al. A mapping review of real-time movement sonification systems for movement rehabilitation. IEEE Rev Biomed Eng. 2022;16:672–86.

Nown TH, Upadhyay P, Kerr A, et al. A mapping review of real-time movement sonification systems for movement rehabilitation. IEEE Rev Biomed Eng. 2023;16:672–86.

Oppici L, Frith E, Rudd J, et al. A perspective on implementing movement sonification to influence movement (and eventually cognitive) creativity. Front Psychol. 2020;11:560982.

Park KS, Buseth L, Hong J, et al. Music-based multicomponent exercise training for community-dwelling older adults with mild-to-moderate cognitive decline: a feasibility study. Front Med (Lausanne). 2023;10:1224728.

Patel AD, Iverson JR. The evolutionary neuroscience of musical beat perception: the action simulation for auditory prediction (ASAP) hypothesis. Front Syst Neurosci. 2014;8:57.

Patel AD. Vocal learning as a preadaptation for the evolution of human beat perception and synchronization. Philos Trans R Soc Lond B Biol Sci. 2021;376:20200326.

Peyre I, Roby-Brami A, Segalen M, et al. Effect of sonification types in upper-limb movement: a quantitative and qualitative study in hemiparetic and healthy participants. J Neuroeng Rehabil. 2023;20:136.

Pfeiffer CF, Magee WL, Fülöp R, et al. Exploring music-based interventions for executive functioning and emotional well-being in stroke rehabilitation: a scoping review. Neurosci. 2024;5(4):565–599.

Raglio A, Oasi O. Music and health: what interventions for what results? Front Psychol. 2015;6:230.

Raglio A, Panigazzi M, Colombo R, et al. Hand rehabilitation with sonification techniques in the subacute stage of stroke. Sci Rep. 2021;11(1):7237.

Raglio A, De Maria B, Parati M, et al. Movement sonification techniques to improve balance in Parkinson's disease: a pilot randomized controlled trial. Brain Sci. 2023;13(11):1586.

Rajakumar KD, Mohan J, et al. A systematic review on effect of music intervention on cognitive impairment using EEG, fMRI, and cognitive assessment modalities. Results Eng. 2024;22:102224.

Reh J. Gait sonification for rehabilitation: adjusting gait patterns by acoustic transformation of kinematic data, 2024.

Rodger MW, Young WR, Craig CM. Synthesis of walking sounds for alleviating gait disturbances in Parkinson's disease. IEEE Trans Neural Syst Rehabil Eng. 2014;22(3):543–8.

Saberi K, Hickok G. Forward entrainment: psychophysics, neural correlates, and function. Psychon Bull Rev. 2023;30:803–21.

Salimpoor VN, Zald DH, Zatorre RJ, et al. Predictions and the brain: how musical sounds become rewarding. Trends Cogn Sci. 2015;19:86–91.

Samadi A, Rasti J, Emadi Andani M. Enhancing gait cadence through rhythm-modulated music: a study on healthy adults. Comput Biol Med. 2024;174:108465.

Särkämö T, Altenmüller E, Rodríguez-Fornells A, et al. Editorial: music, brain, and rehabilitation: emerging therapeutic applications and potential neural mechanisms. Front Hum Neurosci. 2016;10:103.

Schaffert N, Mattes K, Effenberg AO. The sound of rowing stroke cycles as acoustic feedback. In: Worall D, Wersenyi G, editors. Proceedings of the 17th International Conference on Auditory Display (ICAD); 2011 Jun 20–24; Budapest, Hungary. 2011:1–6.

Schaffert N, Janzen TB, Mattes K, et al. A review on the relationship between sound and movement in sports and rehabilitation. Front Psychol. 2019;10:412985.

Scholz DS, Rohde S, Großbach M, et al. Moving with music for stroke rehabilitation: a sonification feasibility study. Ann N Y Acad Sci. 2015;1337:69–76.

Scholz DS, Rohde S, Nikmaram N, et al. Sonification of arm movements in stroke rehabilitation–a novel approach in neurologic music therapy. Front Neurol. 2016;7:106.

Schlaug G. Part VI introduction: listening to and making music facilitates brain recovery processes. Ann N Y Acad Sci. 2009;1169:372–3.

Schmid DG. Prospects of cognitive-motor entrainment: an interdisciplinary review. Front Cogn. 2024;3:1354116.

Schneider P, Sluming V, Roberts N, et al. Structural and functional asymmetry of lateral Heschl's gyrus reflects pitch perception preference. Nat Neurosci. 2005;8(9):1241–7.

Sethi A, Stergiou N, Patterson TS, et al. Speed and rhythm affect temporal structure of variability in reaching poststroke: a pilot study. J Mot Behav. 2016;49:35–45.

Sihvonen AJ, Särkämö T, Leo V, et al. Music-based interventions in neurological rehabilitation. Lancet Neurol. 2017;16:648–60.

Smith RA, Davis N, Lagasse AB, et al. Exploring different types of music cues for arm movements in adults with Parkinson's. Music Ther Perspect. 2024;miae008.

Spence C. Crossmodal correspondences: a tutorial review. Atten Percept Psychophys. 2011;73:971–95.

Stanton TR, Spence C. The influence of auditory cues on bodily and movement perception. Front Psychol. 2020;10:507848.

Terry PC, Karageorghis CI, Curran M, et al. Effects of music in exercise and sport: a meta-analytic review. Psychol Bull. 2020;146:91–117.

Thaut CP. Patterned sensory enhancement (PSE). In Thaut M, Hoemberg V, editors. Handbook of Neurologic Music Therapy. Oxford University Press; 2014. p. 106–15.

Thaut MH, Kenyon GP, Schauer ML, et al. The connection between rhythmicity and brain function. IEEE Eng Med Biol Mag. 1999;18:101–8.

Thaut MH, Trimarchi PD, Parsons LM. Human brain basis of musical rhythm perception: common and distinct neural substrates for meter, tempo, and pattern. Brain Sci. 2014;4(2):428–52.

Thaut MH, McIntosh GC, Hoemberg V, et al. Neurobiological foundations of neurologic music therapy: rhythmic entrainment and the motor system. Front Psychol. 2015;5:1185.

Thaut MH, Stephan KM, Wunderlich G, et al. Distinct cortico-cerebellar activations in rhythmic auditory motor synchronization. Cortex. 2009;45(1):44–53.

Thaut MH, Hodges DA, editors. The Oxford handbook of music and the brain. Oxford University Press; 2019.

Thaut MH, McIntosh GC, Hoemberg V. Neurobiological foundations of neurologic music therapy: rhythmic entrainment and the motor system. Front Psychol. 2015;5:1185.

Thaut MH, Rice RR, Braun Janzen T, et al. Rhythmic auditory stimulation for reduction of falls in Parkinson's disease: a randomized controlled study. Clin Rehabil. 2019;33(1):34–43.

Thaut M, Hoemberg V. Handbook of neurologic music therapy. Oxford University Press (UK); 2025.

Tramontano M, De Angelis S, Mastrogiacomo S, et al. Music-based techniques and related devices in neurorehabilitation: a scoping review. Expert Rev Med Devices. 2021;18:733–749.

Trimble M, Hesdorffer D. Music and the brain: the neuroscience of music and musical appreciation. BJPsych Int. 2017;14:28–31.

Van Atteveldt N, Murray MM, Thut G, et al. Multisensory integration: flexible use of general operations. Neuron. 2014;81:1240–53.

van Vugt FT, Tillmann B. Auditory feedback in error-based learning of motor regularity. Brain Res. 2015;1606:54–67.

Vik BMD, Skeie GO, Vikane E, et al. Effects of music production on cortical plasticity within cognitive rehabilitation of patients with mild traumatic brain injury. Brain Inj. 2018;32:634–643.

Yang J, Hunt A. Real-time sonification of biceps curl exercise using muscular activity and kinematics. In: Proceedings of the 21st International Conference on Auditory Display (ICAD); 2015 Jul 8–10; Graz, Austria. 2015:289–293.

Wan CY, Schlaug G. Music making as a tool for promoting brain plasticity across the life span. Neuroscientist. 2010;16(5):566–77.

Wenger E, Kühn S, Verrel J, et al. Repeated structural imaging reveals non-linear progression of experience-dependent volume changes in human motor cortex. Cereb Cortex. 2017;27(5):2911–25.

Zatorre RJ, Chen JL, Penhune VB. When the brain plays music: auditory-motor interactions in music perception and production. Nat Rev Neurosci. 2007;8(7):547–58.

Zatorre RJ, Salimpoor VN, et al. From perception to pleasure: music and its neural substrates. Proc Natl Acad Sci USA. 2013;110:10430–7.

Zhao Y. Research on the mechanism of the effect of music rhythm synchronization training on biomechanics gait optimization and rehabilitation outcome. Mol Cell Biomech. 2024;21(2):390.

Part III

The Techniques: Receptive Music Therapy Approaches

Receptive Music Therapy Techniques

9

Katrina Skewes McFerran and Denise Elizabeth Grocke

Key Points

- The term receptive has many definitions, including being willing, responsive, open and prepared to consider possibilities.
- In receptive experiences, the client listens to music and responds to the experience silently, verbally, or in another modality.
- The principles of receptive music therapy include having clarity of purpose, recognising the importance of individual preferences, being willing to adjust plans, utilising repetition, making careful decisions about mode and level of the music.
- Major methods within receptive music therapy include playlist construction, song listening and lyric analysis, music and relaxation and music and imagery

9.1 Introduction

The term receptive music therapy does not signal a passive approach to therapy. Instead, it refers to the use of music listening as the key feature distinguishing it from active music making through singing or playing. In English, the term receptive has many definitions including being willing, responsive, open and prepared to consider possibilities (p. 49, McFerran and Grocke). This has two dimensions, including being open to the music, as well as trusting the relationship with the therapist.

K. S. McFerran (✉) · D. E. Grocke
The University of Melbourne, Parkville, VIC, Australia
e-mail: k.mcferran@unimelb.edu.au

A. Raglio (ed.), *Music and Music Therapy Interventions in Clinical Practice*, Neurocultural Health and Wellbeing,
https://doi.org/10.1007/978-3-031-88578-5_9

Bruscia's (2013) definition is often used to illustrate the specific therapeutic potentials and applications of receptive music therapy.

In receptive experiences, the client listens to music and responds to the experience silently, verbally, or in another modality. The music used may be live or recorded improvisations, performances, or compositions by the client or therapist or commercial recordings of music literature in various styles. The listening experience may be focused on physical, emotional, intellectual, aesthetic or spiritual aspects of the music, and the client's responses are designed according to the therapeutic purpose of the experience (p. 134–135).

However, the relative value of receptive music therapy remains contested when compared to active music therapy. This often reflects a protective attitude about professional boundaries and the frequency with which other health and well-being professionals use music listening in their practices. For example, there is a wealth of research literature investigating the value of music listening in medical settings that has been conducted by nurses, doctors and other allied health professionals. Many unwittingly refer to their techniques as music therapy, in ways that frustrate qualified music therapists who understand music therapy as a professional practice (Bunt and Stige 2014), but not a technique. But perhaps this tendency is meant to recognise the disciplinary knowledge of music therapy without transgressing professional boundaries. The English language here is complicated, since the specific procedures or techniques used by music therapists can probably be utilised by other professionals, whereas the approaches or methods of receptive music therapy should probably be reserved for music therapists. For example, in a recent review of global music therapy practices, we explained the idea of approaches in the following way (McFerran et al. 2023):

Approaches are the ways that music therapists describe their practices (the whys), often incorporating external orientations, but also incorporating reference to music-based practices and methods. Understanding of approaches directly guides the practice of music therapists, often with specific reference to workplaces, groups of people and specific needs and usually reflecting cultural, social, political influences (p. 470).

In this chapter, for example, we are writing about receptive music therapy approaches, but as part of that, specific techniques based on music listening will be outlined. In the moment of practice, these differences in vocabulary selection do not matter. However, they have had an influence on who chooses to use receptive methods in their music therapy practice.

It is anecdotally reported, for example, that some music therapy training programs in the United States do not teach receptive music therapy approaches because they argue that anyone can use music listening. It is true that music therapists must demonstrate a high level of active music making skills to be accepted into university programs. However, it is also true that some people develop excellent music listening skills without playing an instrument. These combined facts do not lead to the conclusion that music listening is unnecessary in the training of music therapists. As demonstrated in this chapter and the next (Chap. 10), specific knowledge is required to utilise music listening in therapy, and perhaps more importantly, time for music (McFerran and Grocke 2022, p. 145).

In our experience, other professionals may wish to use music listening, but often lack the time to integrate it adequately. Instead, they may hope that music playing in the background will influence a person's health or well-being, without requiring any tailoring, guidance or refinement based on individual responses. This cause-and-effect approach is not often effective, unfortunately, since individual's respond differently to the music they hear for a range of reasons. As a result, the logic of music therapists' approaches relies on models from social sciences. Gibson's (2014) ecological approach to visual perception has inspired music therapists to consider how clients appropriate the affordances of music in ways that neatly integrate active and passive engagement with music (Windsor and de Bézenac 2012). By emphasising human agency rather than mechanical application, receptive music therapy demands careful attention to aesthetic, personal and relational dimensions.

One further clarifying concept is needed about receptive music therapy approaches before explicating specific techniques. In 1999, the World Federation of Music Therapy acknowledged five models of music therapy (Wheeler et al. 2012), which included the Bonny Method of Guided Imagery and Music (GIM). Since the 1970s, training in GIM has always been open to both music therapists and non-music therapists. McFerran and Grocke (2022, p. 14–15) have compared receptive music therapy with named GIM approaches and highlighted the differences in purpose, techniques, role of therapist, skillsets, and training required, as demonstrated in Table 9.1 (McFerran and Grocke 2022, p. 14–15).

There are a range of distinctions evidenced by this comparison which are addressed in the advanced training, namely, GIM approaches require learning a prescribed set of methods that are specific to its professional practice (Jerling and Heyns 2020). The depth of work that delineates GIM is critical, however, careful music listening, the establishment of a safe and trustworthy relationship, and the ability to discuss and process what the music listening has aroused are all shared across both GIM and receptive music therapy. Further, music therapists and GIM guides might use music from the western canon, since many will be trained in both and familiar with that repertoire. Indeed, receptive music therapy techniques might also incorporate music and imagery work but will not include a deep induction focused on achieving an altered state of consciousness, or intentionally guided exploration of imagery seen as representing the unconscious (Lawes 2022). The overlap makes it easy to understand why there is some confusion about receptive music therapy approaches and where they fit in a spectrum of practices. In the following sections, we will provide clarity about several techniques that should illustrate the breadth of practice that remains even with GIM contained at one border, and music listening techniques used by other professionals at the other (Fig. 9.1).

Table 9.1 Distinctions between Receptive Music Therapy and MI/GIM approaches

	Receptive Music Therapy	Named MI/GIM Approaches
Purpose	Intentional/deep listening to music with or without imagery, using live or recorded music Inward-focused	Deep listening with intentional imagery focus Inward-focused
Methods/ techniques	Relaxation with music Music and imagery Song sharing (listening and reflecting with discussion) Music and art, e.g., music and drawing, music collage	Continuum Model (Summer) Personal MI (Scott-Moncrieff) Focused MI (Dimiceli-Mitran and Goldberg) Korta musikresor (KMR) (Wärja) Directed Music and Imagery (DMI) Music, Drawing and Narrative (MDN) (Booth)
Role of therapist	Facilitates the listening experience with a focus on intentional listening. Also, a recipient of the listening experience. May choose the music or engage the client collaboratively for music selection.	Collaboratively create playlists with the client (Continuum Model: Summer) Facilitates directive MI (Dimiceli-Mitran) Facilitates music listening with artwork (Wärja)
Skill set	Provides relaxation inductions with appropriate timing and voice tone Facilitates intentional and focused music listening that may also integrate visualisations/imagery/drawing Has knowledge of music repertoire and chooses appropriate music or engages client collaboratively to make the choice.	Has knowledge of music suitable for MI and chooses appropriate music, or engages client collaboratively to find music that matches desired imagery
Training	Training depends on the orientation of the music therapy training course. Not all courses include receptive music therapy in the curriculum. Alternative titles might be 'Music listening', 'music-assisted relaxation' and others	Additional training in Summer's Continuum Model and Wärja's KMR
Therapist qualifications	Accredited Music Therapist	No specific qualification, but training is required

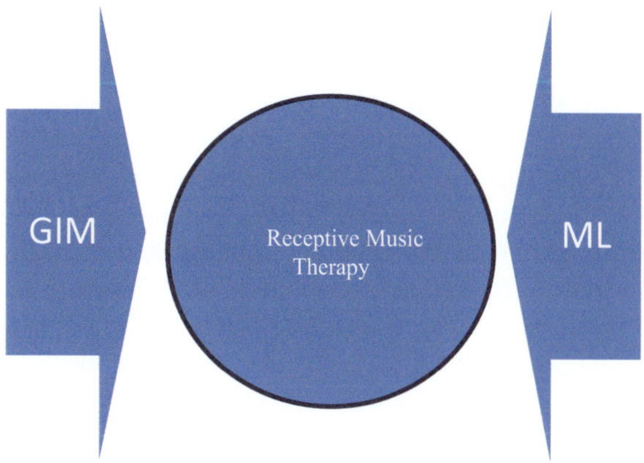

Fig. 9.1 Receptive music therapy intersections

9.2 Principles and Considerations of Receptive Music Therapy

The fundamental principles that underpin receptive music therapy approaches reflect the professional practice of music therapy broadly. Although the primary mode of musical experience is listening, there is more to be decided than what music will be listened to. The following list is one way of describing these principles (McFerran and Grocke 2022).

- Clarity about the purpose of the approach
- Understanding of people's music preferences as a primary concern
- Making ongoing adjustments as the client or group responds to the music
- Considered use of repetition rather than relying on novelty
- Awareness of individual's sensitivity to loudness
- Careful decision-making about live versus recorded performances of music for listening

Beyond broad principles of the receptive music therapy approach, the issue of music selection is probably the most important, across all techniques. Being guided by people's music preferences is fundamental, as noted above. However, there are many times when individuals or groups will benefit from the music therapist taking responsibility for selecting the music. For example:

- The person is too young to make a choice (infants and young children).
- The person is too ill or confused to make a choice (adults with severe mental illness, those living with dementia or traumatic brain injury, non-verbal people with learning disabilities and disorders).
- The person is too tired and cannot decide between two or more selections of music (in palliative care, or a person undergoing medical treatment).

- Time is short—for example, the end of the session—when there isn't enough time to collaborate on this musical decision with the person.
- It is a group session, when making a collaborative choice would take a long time (p. 32, McFerran and Grocke 2022).

There are other times when collaborative choice making between the therapist and client is more suitable. This can empower the individual, both in the moment of decision making but also in developing their own expertise to be employed in their everyday life. The dyad can reflect on different possibilities from preferred music together and examine whether some may be more healthy or unhealthy for the individual in meeting their needs. For example, selecting music that matches and mirrors the person's mood can be a powerful way of connecting with, expressing and examining different dimensions of their experience. However, when paired with pre-existing patterns of rumination and challenges in moving beyond an unhappy state, it can be helpful to consider what music might come next, once the current state has been acknowledged. This kind of therapeutic dialogue can support the person to move beyond listening to music that they like/don't like and attend to whether it is serving them in this moment.

Another form of collaborative decision making can involve the therapist providing choices between different pieces of unfamiliar music. The dyad can listen to excerpts of the music together and discuss reactions, encouraging a more intuitive approach to music selection by the individual. Once again, discussion can focus on the affordances of each piece, combined with the ways they can appropriate those potentials. This empowers people to move from passive acceptance of music that is meant to be good for them, towards music that might be helpful, or might not, depending on their personal reaction.

When making suggestions about novel music to listen to, many music therapists rely on classical western repertoire because they were trained in that genre as active musicians. This reliance on genres that are familiar to the music therapist is exemplified in the work of Margareta Wärja and Lars Ole Bonde (2014) who created a taxonomy of therapeutic music based on their experience. This included both classical music from previous centuries as well as contemporary genres such as ambient music. From there, they described supportive music as providing a secure field due to the stable and predictable nature of the music, that stays within a mood spectrum of light moods. Challenging music is more complex, with contrasts in many musical elements that can be intense and dramatic, inviting people to face more difficult feelings. In between, the authors describe music that has supportive beginnings and endings but may contain more contrasting sections, with more elaborate forms than predictable ones. The connection between purpose and musical selection is clear in these descriptions and relies on the therapist to be able to determine what is suitable for the therapeutic moment. There is no suggestion that the music has a predictable effect, just that it invites different opportunities—what De Nora (2000) describes as the affordances of different types of music.

There are some logistical affordances that can also influence the music selections made, particularly when working with groups. For example, the time available for the group to listen and process will have an impact, as will the age range of the group. The intention of the music listening activity will point towards particular music selections, as will the prevailing mood of the group and dynamics on the day. Although this has less to do with aesthetics and more to do with pragmatics, they are noteworthy. A therapist needs to be reliable in managing time and the encounters of group members. Attending to logistics can play an important role to that end, in addition to being able to guess music preferences based on age, culture and any assessments that have been completed.

Music preferences are just one part of understanding people's existing relationship with music, however. The ways that people listen to music in their everyday life can be more important in therapy than the selections themselves. Research has shown that people can use music to ruminate, intensify and isolate when their mental health is poor (McFerran and Saarikallio 2014), as well as to energise, uplift and celebrate during good times (Saarikallio et al. 2019). There is no direct relationship between particular music pieces or genres and the function that they fulfil, although once again, certain types of music afford particular responses. For example, loud, heavy and aggressive music is more often related to power issues, whereas soft, predictable and catchy tunes are more likely to represent agreeableness (North 2010).

The qualities of music afford possibilities for therapy. However, the most critical dimension is the agency of human actors as they choose which music to appropriate and for what purpose. Given the importance of commitment and intention in therapy, receptive music therapy relies on people listening to the music in a focused way to benefit from it. Since many people multi-task with music, this can require some guidance and skill development to achieve outcomes such as emotion regulation and arousal management. The following techniques all rely on the music therapist working closely with the individual or group to engage their attention to the music in an intentional way.

9.2.1 Playlist Construction

The use of playlist construction in music therapy has gained attention due to technological advances that make gathering music into carefully curated soundtracks relatively simple. Whereas previous decades required time-consuming processes of listening to the radio waiting for a preferred song to record, or manually recording from one tape to another, this feature is now established in all music streamlining platforms. This method was first delineated for therapeutic purposes by Even Ruud in Norway (1997) and extended by Dorit Amir in Israel (2011), who used the method for doing identity work, particularly in the training of music therapists. Students compiled playlists representing their personal and musical identities as illuminated in the work of Avi Gilboa who used playlists to address cultural conflicts among Israeli students of different racial backgrounds (Gilboa and Salmon 2019).

Playlist construction has also been applied in schools and mental health settings, especially with young people. Carmen Cheong-Clinch (Cheong-Clinch and McFerran 2016) explored how young people's emotional connections to music could be harnessed in therapy through playlists. Cherry Hense (Hense and McFerran 2017) further demonstrated that young people's musical identities often change with the onset of mental illness, leading to the development of methods to explore these changes through playlists.

Playlist construction has also been used in the care of older people, first documented in the early 1990s (Hanser 1990). For example, Imogen Clark et al. (2016) used playlists to promote physical exercise in cardiac patients, where the emotional connection to songs proved as important as their tempo. Playlists have also been employed to assist with activities like bathing (Ray and Fitzsimmons 2014), where therapists provide guidance on selecting and ordering tracks to optimise therapeutic outcomes.

Music therapists increasingly act as consultants in playlist construction, particularly in medical contexts. In Denmark, therapists developed software and hardware (MusicStar) allowing patients to independently select music to suit their needs (Lund et al. 2016). Although these playlists are less personalised, they still fulfil therapeutic purposes. Similar approaches have been used in emergency wards (Short and Ahern 2009) and acute neonatal care (Shoemark et al. 2015) to reduce noise and promote healing, sometimes referred to as 'ecological music therapy' or 'milieu music therapy'.

There are many ways to approach the construction of playlists in receptive music therapy, but there are a number of critical components. Being clear about the purpose of the playlist is primary, followed by the selection and then sequencing of tracks, as well as a careful review of the playlist as a whole to make adjustments.

Technique

The foundation of creating a playlist in receptive music therapy lies in identifying a clear purpose and constructing the playlist accordingly. This process must be carefully tailored to meet the specific needs of an individual or group in a particular context. Common purposes include:

- Mood management
- Emotion processing
- Life review
- Sleep promotion
- Distraction
- Relaxation
- Agitation reduction
- Identity work
- Relationship strengthening
- Orientation and focus
- Activity support

In some cases, where there are no pre-identified needs, the therapist may still consider playlists as a potential method, especially if the individual or group expresses a strong interest in music. In such scenarios, the therapist's role is to help identify a purpose before moving forward. This can be done collaboratively by asking questions like:

- How do you usually use music to make yourself feel better?
- When do you turn to music for help?
- What do you believe music is good for?
- How do you imagine music listening being useful to you?
- Are there any challenges you have that music might help with?

These questions help uncover intuitive and habitual uses of music, guiding the individual or group towards a more considered and reflective approach to their needs in music therapy.

The selection of relevant tracks can be facilitated through open-ended questions related to the purpose which prompt individuals or groups to reflect on suitable song selections. This self-reflection should be prioritised before the music therapist offers suggestions based on their knowledge of suitable music. The following illustrations may be helpful to prompt reflection.

- Mood management: What songs do you listen to in that mood? Do they match or change your mood?
- Emotion processing: What songs speak to your pain/grief/anger? Which ones reflect your feelings?
- Life review: What songs do you associate with major life events?
- Sleep promotion: What music helps you sleep? Is there a particular style you think would be helpful?
- Distraction: What tracks do you have strong associations with? What kind of music gets your attention?
- Relaxation: What music helps you relax? Have you tried relaxation to music?
- Agitation reduction: What music do you listen to when agitated? Does it help reduce your tension?
- Identity work: What songs say something about who you are? Are there performers you identify with?
- Relationship strengthening: What songs do you both like? Have you been to meaningful concerts together?
- Orientation and focus: What tracks grab your attention? What music do you find most fascinating?
- Activity support: What music complements your activity? Is there a style or speed that works best?

Sequencing the tracks is crucial and is often guided by the iso-principle, a concept introduced by Ira Altschuler (1948) which involves using music that aligns with the individual's current state and gradually transitioning towards the desire outcome. For example, in anxiety reduction, the playlist might start with a track that resonates with agitation and then move stepwise towards more peaceful music. The number of tracks depends on the intensity of the starting emotion.

After selecting and sequencing the tracks, it is essential to review the entire playlist. The playlist's overall contour will only be apparent once it is assembled. The therapist should sit with the individual or group to practice using the playlist, ensuring that all songs work well together and continue to feel appropriate. People's experiences with music are dynamic, so the therapist must remain open to adjustments. This attention to detail is critical, ensuring that the playlist serves its intended purpose while remaining adaptable to the individual's evolving needs.

In some cases, a new purpose might emerge, or the therapeutic process might prove more significant than the playlist itself. The therapist's responsibility is to evaluate the playlist's effectiveness and explain how and whether it has been helpful.

9.2.2 Song Discussion and Lyric Analysis

Shared music listening as the basis of discussion and analysis of meaning is a powerful method for advancing therapeutic objectives with clients who are able to reflect and mentalise. Without a reasonably high level of cognitive capacity, the method can be limited to concrete discussions that are more aligned with developing that capacity rather than having an insight orientation. It is the development of insight that is the focus of this method as we describe it, however.

The first references to analysing the lyrics of songs as a method in music therapy appear in the 1960s, with Becky Butler (1966) noting the affordance of music in stimulating discussion in a non-threatening manner. This was further elaborated by psychiatrist Lee Baumel (1973) who described songs as a way for patients to express themselves and connect with others. Erdonmez [Grocke] (1977) extended this technique in mental health settings, asking clients to contribute meaningful songs and facilitating discussions about their individual significance in order to foster insights. There are further references to this method during the 1980s and 1990s, with Marsha Wooten (1992) describing how clients could communicate messages through the lyrics of songs they chose. Darlene Brooks (1989) also highlighted the importance of lyrics in providing a bridge to reach patients who were not otherwise communicative. In the same year, Deborah Salmon (1989) described using familiar songs in palliative care to evoke memories and encourage self-expression. Kenneth Bruscia (1998a) described this as a way for people to explore emotions and suggested that shared listening allows for re-experiencing issues and feelings, making it a musically active process.

Since then, lyric analysis and song discussion has received minimal attention in the literature, although it underpins many of the active music therapy methods that employ song singing and playing and which often incorporate discussion. However, the focus on meaning making becomes more prominent when used as a receptive music therapy method because the attention rests more fully on the verbal processes that follow music sharing, rather than on the activities involved with singing and playing.

It is possible that this method could be more important in current times as society becomes more conscious of the identity dimensions embedded in music, as seen by emerging discussions about cultural appropriation. Playing the original artists version of a track can be more respectful than reproducing it, since the identity of the artist can get lost in this process, but it is critical in recognising cultural roots. Many authors have been pointing to the importance of recognising the cultural politics associated with songs, such as Tricia Rose's (1994) reflections on Hip-Hop is a genre rich in cultural politics and self-empowerment. Or Lie's (2015) discussions of how K-Pop blends traditional Korean music with contemporary styles, reflecting aspects of South Korean culture and making a significant contribution to the economy. Music therapists must be aware of these associations and respect the cultural meanings music holds for clients (Whitehead-Pleaux and Tan 2017), exploring them without pre-assumptions to uncover the meaning for clients or making stereotypical assumptions about their function. They must also consider whether their reproduction of a song in active music therapy diminishes the cultural meaning if they are not also representatives of that culture.

The emerging importance of using the original, recorded version of a song is not only related to the reproduction of the music. Lyrics also provide rich material for therapeutic processing as words in songs carry significant cultural meaning. For example, songs such as Kendrick Lamar's 'Alright' (Duckworth et al. 2015) or Bob Dylan's 'Blowin' in the Wind' (1963) are linked to social movements and carry messages of resistance or justice. In addition, since many major cities are now multicultural hubs home to people from a range of diverse backgrounds, it is likely that songs in languages other than the dominant one will be important for discussion. Music therapists should encourage clients to contribute songs in any language and should anticipate the possibility of this (Belgrave and Kim 2020) and be ready to translate lyrics using online technologies. The interpretation of the song's meaning can then be inspired by a full range of musical materials, rather than being limited to the therapist's capabilities.

There are many ways songs can be discussed for meaning and this usually occurs quite fluidly. However, there are a number of critical components including the selection of the song, decisions about how to listen together, the level of discussion that is then facilitated, and considerations for more or repeated listening.

Technique

In this method, it is equally common for the music therapist to select a track that is relevant to the issues that has bought the client to therapy, as it is to use their preferred music. Cora Díaz de Chumaceiro (1992) describes this process as working with 'songs of transference', akin to Sigmund Freud's concept of the 'haunting melody'. Indeed, Freud's student, Theodor Reik (1953), also suggested that the songs on the mind could be used as part of therapy because they may reveal repressed ideas and feelings that the client was not conscious of. In the psychoanalytic realm, Edith Lecourt (1998) suggested that therapists might use complementary identification, empathically selecting music relevant to the client's experience. However, when using expert-selected music, there is some risk that the therapist might project their own issues onto the music, leading Susan Gardstrom and James Hiller (2010) to issue warnings about therapists choosing or avoiding songs for personal reasons.

Whether it is expert or client selected, the music needs to be relevant to the therapeutic issues being processed. With expert selected music, that is likely to be because the lyrics describe a scenario that has shared features to the client's life such as substance use, body issues, loss and grief and many more. Whether or not the client identifies with the topic in the same way becomes the focus of the subsequent discussion, with both agreements and disagreements being useful for prompting reflections. If the client selects the music, the relevance is assumed but is usually not as clear, and may even be intentionally disguised. This would then become the thrust of the conversation, with the therapist seeking understanding about why that song was chosen for this moment in therapy. Once again, the song is not usually a direct reflection, but rather, is a prompt for diving deeply into the topic via discussion of the song.

The shared listening process is also critical to this process and should not be passed over. The therapist often must adopt a pose that makes it clear they are listening and not expecting the song to take a background role, as it normally might. This might require preparation of the other listeners, since it is uncommon for people to sit in silence listening to music when they are in the company of others. It is not usually comfortable to be too directive about quiet listening, so the ability to convey its importance is more through modelling and suggestion.

The placement of the listening technologies has an impact here too. If it is too far away, the therapist will need to anticipate the end of the song and stand up to be at the device in time to stop the music before the next song begins, for example. A quality speaker is helpful, both in symbolically emphasising the importance of hearing the music and also allowing for a more careful and detailed listening by the therapist. What the client can hear will be the focus of discussions, so this allows further depth. The volume should also always be attended to, which might require negotiation with the listener/s, since each person has a different volume of preference and what is pleasant for some, is unpleasant for others. The therapist usually attends to people's reactions throughout the song, making adjustments to volume as required. They are also noticing emotional reactions, and able to validate tears and other responses, often by passing tissues and continuing to listen. It is very common for people to cry when listening to music, and a key skill is in anticipating, normalising and supporting this natural emotional expression.

Following the listening, the therapist needs to intuit the right level of discussion to follow. Whereas some people might feel excited about discussing the meanings of the music, other people might feel vulnerable after listening—leading to a sense of being revealed. Each person responds differently to this feeling of being seen and some may be defensive while others may feel validated. In addition to reading a person's body language, the therapist might use different levels of questions to assess how safe the individual feels, both in a group or within a dyad.

Beginning with questions that focus on the music is the gentlest way to start. Inquiring about whether they liked the music and why, is one place to begin, or the artist of the music is another. This begins the encounter at the most concrete level and one which people typically remain at in everyday life. If this is comfortable, the next level of questions probes the meaning of the song. This might involve queries about the lyrics, the artists or the genre. Perhaps it is about the relevance to their current situation, or it might be about their identity more broadly, and their experience of that. Listening could also evoke non-verbal responses that could be explored, such as images or feelings. The final level is to connect the track more directly to current issues, moving from general statements to the specific. Questions such as: is there a message there for you, or for me, that you would like to hear? The movement between these levels can be fluid, but there is an overall sense of feeling into what has come up for the client and processing at a level that feels safe.

Recognising that people can feel vulnerable after sharing a song with their therapist can be thought of as the 'Killing Me Softly' (Flack 1973) phenomenon. This song names how it can be like people seeing right into our soul when we share the music that is so personally connected to our lives. The therapist cannot, of course, but it is the feeling of the client that we need to be aware of. Kenneth Bruscia (1998b) rather poetically describes this function of songs in the following way:

Songs are the ways that human beings explore emotions. They express who we are and how we feel, they bring us closer to others, they keep us company when we are alone. They articulate our beliefs and values. As the years pass, songs bear witness to our lives. They allow us to relive the past, to examine the present and to voice our dreams for the future. Songs weave the tales of our joys and sorrows, they reveal our innermost secrets, and they express our hopes and disappointments, our fears, and triumphs. They are our musical diaries. They are the sounds of our personal development. (Bruscia 1998b, p. 10).

Team members sometimes become nervous about music because of its power to evoke emotional responses, and it is sometimes banned from mental health units because of the reactions people have. The role of the music therapist can be to explain how normal it is for music to trigger emotional reactions, and remind colleagues that emotions are not bad and that the role of the therapist is to help people acknowledge and observe their emotions, rather than deny them. As demonstrated in Jennifer Bibb's research (Bibb and McFerran 2018), we may not even be privy to the reactions people are having because they may choose to manage them privately. Whilst it sounds simple to sit and listen to music with people and discuss it, the therapeutic conditions of listening carefully and caring deeply mean that it becomes very powerful very quickly. As therapists, we need to anticipate this depth in order to leverage it for therapeutic outcomes.

9.2.3 Music and Relaxation

The use of music for relaxation in therapeutic contexts varies according to the specific intention behind its application. For example, music may be introduced at the conclusion of an active music therapy session to provide a brief period of rest, during which the person is encouraged to listen passively. Alternately, Music-Assisted Relaxation (MAR) (McFerran and Grocke 2022, p. 109) may be employed to alleviate symptoms of stress, anxiety or pain, with a potential psycho-educational aim to teach individuals how to integrate music into their daily lives for symptom management. Distinctly, relaxation induction may precede the music, extending the duration of deep relaxation.

Studies have shown that a carefully prepared relaxation induction can significantly enhance the experience of listening to relaxing music, requiring skill in both the induction process and the selection of appropriate music (Clark et al. 2016; Gallagher et al. 2018; Pasiali et al. 2020). The environment for such a session, whether in a hospital bed or a comfortable chair, should be quiet, dimly lit, warm, and free from interruptions to create an ideal atmosphere for relaxation. Lighting plays a critical role, with dim or side lighting being preferable to avoid the distractions of flickering or bright lights, though some filtered light is often necessary to maintain comfort. The therapist should ensure easy access to music equipment and consider whether the client is comfortable closing their eyes, as this can deepen relaxation by minimising external distractions. The therapist's voice is also crucial, needing to be warm, calm and paced to match the client's breathing, with a consistent tone and careful sequencing of instructions to facilitate a smooth, undisturbed flow of relaxation. Adjustments should be made based on the specific needs of the group and setting, as illustrated by the use of aesthetic elements like candles and expert-selected music in a therapeutic community setting focused on mental health.

The most effective music for relaxation is often that which the client enjoys, as client preference plays a crucial role in the success of music-based interventions (Howlin and Rooney 2020; Jiang et al. 2013; Lee 2016; Tan et al. 2012). When clients are unable to communicate their preferences, music therapists typically select music based on research findings. Interestingly, Cori Pelletier's (2004) meta-analysis revealed that expert-chosen music could be more effective than client-selected music, as clients may not always be aware of the musical elements that best facilitate relaxation. Effective relaxation music is generally characterised by a slow, steady tempo, consistent rhythm, predictable melodic lines with a small range of intervals, tonal and consonant harmonic structures and minimal dynamic changes. Instrumentation typically involves strings and woodwinds, with a supportive bass line to convey a sense of security (Grocke and Wigram 2007).

Technique

When implementing relaxation techniques with patients, it is crucial to tailor the approach to individual needs and preferences, particularly in vulnerable populations such as the elderly or those recovering from cardiac surgery. Selecting music preferred by the participants can enhance the therapeutic experience. Patients who are confused or disoriented may benefit more from short, structured relaxation scripts with clear instructions, rather than those involving abstract or embodied imagery (McFerran and Grocke 2022, p. 179–191). Clients who feel vulnerable or self-conscious may struggle to close their eyes during relaxation and may need reassurance of their safety. For post-cardiac surgery patients, comfort is key, and they may require upright positioning and modified breathing instructions to avoid discomfort. Similarly, older adults with physical disabilities may need careful positioning and support to prevent pain during relaxation. For those requiring physiological support, relaxation scripts should be adapted to avoid deep breathing if it causes discomfort, and in care home settings, attention to body awareness might need to be minimised to avoid feelings of embarrassment in the presence of others.

Implementing Music-Assisted Relaxation sessions differ according to the age of the person and whether it is an individual or group session. For young children, the relaxation induction may include imagery to engage the child's attention; and the child may not close their eyes (McFerran and Grocke 2022, p. 199–201). For adults, closing their eyes should also be an option as those who have a trauma background may feel uncomfortable with the darkness.

In individual sessions, the dyad is close together, making it easier to monitor the pacing and timing of the relaxation induction, with the rise and fall of the person's breathing pattern. Whereas in a group context, the therapist needs to project their voice so that the person furthest away can still hear the invitation to relax.

The volume of the music is another consideration. In individual work, the volume can be easily managed, but in group work, it can be difficult to ensure the music is heard by all members of the group equally. Those closest to the source will hear it louder than those furthest away. The placement of the speaker/s needs attention before you begin.

At the end of the music selection, the therapist brings the individual or group back to an alert state. This is done by gently pointing out that the music has finished, and then progressively helping the individual or group members to bring their focus back to the room—listening for sounds within the room or outside of the room, then a focus on their body, and finally the invitation to open their eyes and if appropriate, stretch their limbs.

There are occasions when the intention of the MAR may be that the individual falls to sleep. When working in palliative care or with children or adults in pain, the intention of MAR may be to allow them to enjoy a restful sleep. In this instance, the therapist does not bring them back to an alert state, but instead, quietly leaves the room.

9.2.4 Music and Imagery

When discussing the use of imagery with music, it is essential to consider the role of imagination, which is fundamental to creative thinking, problem-solving and introspection. Albert Einstein ([1931] 2009) famously emphasised the importance of imagination over knowledge, viewing it as a force that stimulates progress and evolution. Similarly, Sigmund Freud ([1924] 1956) linked imagination to his technique of free association, where patients' spontaneous associations with words or images provided insights for diagnosis. Carl Jung expanded on this with his method of active imagination, encouraging patients to explore their dreams deeply, interpreting the scenes, figures, and objects to uncover deeper meanings (Jung 1959; Chodorow 1997).

The effectiveness of music imagery journeys hinges on the alignment between the music's contour and the imagery focus that has been selected. To achieve this, it is crucial to carefully listen to the entire music selection and ensure that its beginning and ending suit the intended purpose. The music should ideally mirror the imagery's progression, with its contour following the script's narrative arc. For instance, a journey along a path to a serene destination may require music with a flat yet textured contour, while ascending a mountain might call for music that builds to a broad, expansive climax. Similarly, a memory of a sunrise might be best accompanied by music that gently undulates before reaching a climactic point, mirroring the unfolding colours of dawn. Over time, building a personal library of music selections that effectively match specific imagery scripts will enhance the overall impact of the imagery journey.

Lisa Summer's (2019) Continuum Model of Group Music and Imagery (GrpMI) provides a structured approach to utilising music in group therapy across three progressive levels: supportive, re-educative and reconstructive. In the supportive phase, music fosters trust and unity among participants, helping them feel safe and connected. This phase typically uses music with minimal development to encourage focus on singular imagery. Once trust is established, the re-educative phase aims to deepen self-awareness and interpersonal understanding, using slightly more complex music to prompt introspection on personal issues. Finally, the reconstructive phase facilitates profound ego transformation and spiritual exploration through highly evocative and complex music selections. Inductions in this phase are designed to induce deep relaxation and contemplation, addressing existential or spiritual concerns. Each phase builds on the previous, progressively guiding participants through deeper levels of therapeutic engagement (Summer 2019).

In receptive music therapy, the use of music and imagery can be contraindicated for individuals who struggle to distinguish between the imagined and the real, such as those with severe mental illness. These individuals may find it challenging to engage in guided imagery, and a trial of a short imagery journey is recommended to assess its suitability for their well-being. Additionally, some individuals, particularly those with a concrete view of the world, may not see the value in imagining a special place, making structured relaxation inductions a more appropriate alternative. Resistance to creative activities like drawing to music is also common, with clients often expressing a lack of confidence in their artistic abilities. In such cases, it is essential to respect their preferences and offer alternative interventions, such as listening to music, imagery, or relaxation sessions, to support their therapeutic journey effectively.

Technique

Different techniques are used in music and imagery (MI) for diverse intentions, but the purpose is for the music to enhance the aesthetic of the image/imagery and extend its lived experience. There may be a focus on a single image, e.g. a sunset, and the addition of music extends the feeling of that memory.

A longer MI journey requires an individualised choice of music. The therapist might use a brief relaxation induction, or simply a centring of the breath before reminding the person of the image and then starting to play the music selection. It is also possible to create an individualised script by asking for descriptions of the imagery and/or feelings associated with an imagery journey—"can you describe the path?" or "how does it feel to be on that path?" The therapist writes down the description, then after the short relaxation, the therapist reads the person's own words aloud over the music as it plays.

Group MI is more complex. The group members may have a common focus for their imagery—e.g. recovery from cancer treatment. A pre-music discussion may draw out a focus image for the imagery journey—e.g. feeling an inner strength or drawing on a positive image to facilitate inner strength. Here the therapist chooses a music selection that 'best fits' the group members' foci. Sometimes group members will say the music took them to a different place or that it wasn't the best match. However, if the music is well contained, it will do no harm. A group discussion of imagery experiences often takes time, and it may be necessary to have small groups of 2–3 people sharing, rather than sharing with the whole group.

9.3 Conclusion

Receptive music therapy is one of the four main approaches in music therapy according to Bruscia's (1998a) distinctions between receptive, recreative, creative and improvisation. Due to its positioning between Guided Imagery and Music at one boundary and Music Medicine approaches at the other, it has not always received as much attention as the active methods. However, as outlined in this chapter, the approach still requires detailed consideration of techniques that draw heavily on our skills as trained therapy practitioners. A strong foundation in understanding music is necessary for music selection and capacity for ensuring safety and making careful therapeutic decisions is needed to support therapeutic outcomes. Music therapists are best placed for this task, but other practitioners have used music therapy techniques and they also need to be conscious of the careful attention to personal and emotional affordances of music listening that should be anticipated and appropriated for therapeutic outcomes.

References

Altshuler IM. The past, present, and future of musical therapy. In: Podolsky E, editor. Music therapy. New York: Philosophical Library; 1948. p. 24–35.

Amir D. "My music is me": musical presentation as a way of forming and sharing identity in music therapy group. Nord J Music Ther. 2011;21(2):176–93. https://doi.org/10.1080/08098131.2011.571279.

Baumel LN. Psychiatrist as music therapist. J Music Ther. 1973;10(2):83–5. https://doi.org/10.1093/jmt/10.2.83.

Belgrave M, Kim S. Music therapy in a multicultural context: a handbook for music therapy students and professionals. London: Jessica Kingsley Publishers; 2020.

Bibb J, McFerran KS. Musical recovery: the role of group singing in regaining healthy relationships with music to promote mental health recovery. Nord J Music Ther. 2018;27(3) https://doi.org/10.1080/08098131.2018.1432676.

Brooks DM. Music therapy enhances treatment with adolescents. Music Ther Perspect. 1989;6:77–87. https://doi.org/10.1093/mtp/6.1.37.

Bruscia KE. Defining music therapy. 2nd ed. Gilsum: Barcelona Publishers; 1998a.

Bruscia KE. The dynamics of music psychotherapy. Gilsum: Barcelona Publishers; 1998b.

Bruscia KE. Defining music therapy. Barcelona: ProQuest Ebook Central; 2013. https://ebookcentral.proquest.com/lib/unimelb/detail.action?docID=3117673

Bunt L, Stige B. Music therapy: an art beyond words. Taylor & Francis Group; 2014. ProQuest Ebook Central, https://ebookcentral.proquest.com/lib/unimelb/detail.action?docID=1682280

Butler B. Music group psychotherapy. J Music Ther. 1966;3(2):53–6. https://doi.org/10.1093/jmt/3.2.53.
Cheong-Clinch C, McFerran KS. Musical diaries: examining the daily preferred music listening of Australian young people with mental illness. J Appl Youth Stud. 2016;1(2):77–94.
Chodorow J. Jung on active imagination. Abingdon: Routledge; 1997.
Clark IN, Baker FA, Taylor NF. Older adults' music listening preferences to support physical activity following cardiac rehabilitation. J Music Ther. 2016;53(4):364–97. https://doi.org/10.1093/jmt/thw011.
DeNora T. Music in everyday life. Cambridge: Cambridge University Press; 2000.
Díaz de Chumaceiro CL. What song comes to mind? Induced song recall: transference/countertransference in dyadic music associations in treatment and supervision. Arts Psychother. 1992;19(5):325–32.
Duckworth K, Williams P, Spears M. 'Alright' [Song recorded by Kendrick Lamar]. To Pimp a Butterfly. Top Dawg/Aftermath/Interscope; 2015.
Dylan B. 'Blowin' in the wind' [Song recorded by Bob Dylan]. The Freewheelin' Bob Dylan. Columbia Records; 1963.
Einstein A. Einstein on cosmic religion and other opinions and Apho- risms. New York: Dover Publications; [1931] 2009.
Erdonmez D. [Grocke]. 'Music as a projective technique.' Proceedings of the third annual conference of the Australian Music Therapy Association, Adelaide, pp. 11–17, 1977.
Flack R. Killing me softly with his song [song]. On killing me softly. New York: Atlantic Recording Studios; 1973.
Freud S. A general introduction to psychoanalysis. New York: Washington Square Press; [1924] 1956.
Gallagher LM, Lagman R, Rybicki L. Outcomes of music therapy inter- ventions on symptom management in palliative medicine patients. Am J Hospice Palliat Med. 2018;35(2):250–7.
Gardstrom S, Hiller J. Song discussion as music psychotherapy. Music Ther Perspect. 2010;28(2):147–56.
Gibson JJ. The ecological approach to visual perception. classic ed. Psychology Press; 2014.
Gilboa A, Salman B. The roles of music in let's talk music, a model for enhancing communication between Arabs and Jews in Israel. Nord J Music Ther. 2019;28(3):256–68. https://doi.org/10.1080/08098131.2018.1533572.
Grocke D, Wigram T. Receptive methods in music therapy. London: Jessica Kingsley Publishers; 2007.
Hanser SB. A music therapy strategy for depressed older adults in the community. J Appl Gerontol. 1990;9(3):283–98. https://doi.org/10.1177/073346489000900304.
Hense C, McFerran KS. Promoting young people's musical identities to facilitate recovery from mental illness. J Youth Stud. 2017;20(8):997–1012. https://doi.org/10.1080/13676261.2017.1287888.
Howlin C, Rooney B. The cognitive mechanisms in music listening interventions for pain: a scoping review. J Music Ther. 2020;57(2):127–67. https://doi.org/10.1093/jmt/thaa003.
Jerling P, Heyns M. Exploring guided imagery and music as a well-being intervention: a systematic literature review. Nord J Music Ther. 2020;29(4):371–90. https://doi.org/10.1080/08098131.2020.1737185.
Jiang J, Zhou L, Rickson D, Jiang C. The effects of sedative and stimulative music on stress reduction depend on music preference. Arts Psychother. 2013;40:201–5. https://doi.org/10.1016/j.aip.2013.02.002.
Jung C. The archetypes and the collective unconscious. 2nd ed. London: Routledge; 1959.
Lawes MJ. On guided imagery and music (GIM) as both part of music therapy and as separate from it. Voices World Forum Music Ther. 2022;22(1) https://doi.org/10.15845/voices.v22i1.3448.
Lecourt E. The role of aesthetics in countertransference: a comparison of active versus receptive music therapy. In: Bruscia K, editor. The dynamics of music psychotherapy. Gilsum: Barcelona Publishers; 1998. p. 299–314.
Lee JH. The effects of music on pain: a meta analysis. J Music Ther. 2016;53(4):430–77. https://doi.org/10.1093/jmt/thw012.

Lie J. K-pop: popular music, cultural amnesia, and economic innovation in South Korea. University of California Press; 2015.

Lund HN, Bertelsen LR, Bonde LO. Sound and music interventions in psychiatry at Aalborg University Hospital. Sound Effect. 2016;6(1):48–68. http://www.soundeffects.dk/article/view/24912/21827

McFerran K, Grocke D. Receptive music therapy: techniques, clinical applications and new perspectives. Jessica Kingsley Publishers; 2022.

McFerran K, Saarikallio S. Depending on music to feel better: being conscious of responsibility when appropriating the power of music. Arts Psychother. 2014;41(1):89–97. https://doi.org/10.1016/j.aip.2013.11.007.

McFerran K, Chan V, Tague D, Stachyra K, Mercadal-Brotons M. A comprehensive review classifying contemporary global practices in music therapy. Music Ther Today. 2023;18(01):474–93.

North AC. Individual differences in musical taste. Am J Psychol. 2010;123(2):199–208. https://doi.org/10.5406/amerjpsyc.123.2.0199.

Pasiali V, Quick D, Hassall J, Park H. Music therapy programming for persons with eating disorders. Voices World Forum Music Ther. 2020;20(3):10.15845/voices.v20i3.2785.

Pelletier C. The effect of music on decreasing arousal due to stress: a meta-analysis. J Music Ther. 2004;41(3):192–214.

Ray KD, Fitzsimmons S. Music-assisted bathing: making shower time easier for people with dementia. J Gerontol Nurs. 2014;40(2):9–13. https://doi.org/10.3928/00989134-20131220-09.

Reik T. The haunting melody: psychoanalytic experiences in life and music. New York: Farrar, Straus & Young; 1953.

Rose T. Black noise: rap music and black culture in contemporary America / Tricia Rose. Hanover: University Press of New England; 1994.

Ruud E. Music and identity. Nord J Music Ther. 1997;6:3–13.

Saarikallio SH, Maksimainen JP, Randall WM. Relaxed and connected: insights into the emotional–motivational constituents of musical pleasure. Psychol Music. 2019;47(5):644–62. https://doi.org/10.1177/0305735618778768.

Salmon D. Partage: group-work in palliative care. In: The next step forward: music therapy with the terminally ill, proceedings from a symposium for music therapists working in palliative care. Bronx, NY: Calvary Hospital; 1989. p. 47–52.

Shoemark H, Hanson-Abromeit D, Stewart L. Constructing optimal experience for the hospitalized newborn through neuro-based music therapy. Front Hum Neurosci. 2015;9:487. https://doi.org/10.3389/fnhum.2015.00487.

Short AE, Ahern N. Evaluation of a systematic development process: relaxing music for the emergency department. Aust J Music Ther. 2009;20:3–26. Retrieved from http://ezproxy.uws.edu.au/login?url=http://search.informit.com.au/documentSummary;dn=409764338743231;res=IELHEA

Summer L. Group music and imagery therapy. In: Grocke D, editor. Guided imagery and music: the Bonny method and beyond. 2nd ed. Gilsum: Barcelona Publishers; 2019. p. 259–66.

Tan X, Yowler C, Super D, Fratianne R. The interplay of preference, familiarity and psychophysical properties in defining relaxing music. J Music Ther. 2012;49(2):15–179. https://doi.org/10.1093/jmt/49.2.150.

Warja M, Bonde LO. Music as co-therapist: towards a taxonomy of music in therapeutic music and imagery work. Music Med. 2014;6:16–27. https://doi.org/10.47513/mmd.v6i2.175.

Wheeler BL, Wagner G, Summer L, Madsen CK, Turry A, Eschen JT. Five international models of music therapy practice. Voices World Forum Music Ther. 2012;12(1) https://doi.org/10.15845/voices.v12i1.634.

Whitehead-Pleaux A, Tan X. Cultural intersections in music therapy: music, health, and the person. Barcelona Publishers; 2017. https://books.google.com.au/books?id=K9dJswEACAAJ

Windsor WL, de Bézenac C. Music and affordances. Music Sci. 2012;16(1):102–20. https://doi.org/10.1177/1029864911435734.

Wooten MA. The effects of heavy metal music on affects shifts of adolescents in an inpatient psychiatric setting. Music Ther Perspect. 1992;10(2):93–8. https://doi.org/10.1093/mtp/10.2.93.

Towards a New Model of Music Listening: The Therapeutic Music Listening

10

Alfredo Raglio

10.1 Introduction and Theoretical Background

In the realm of music therapy practice, music listening plays a pivotal role. According to a recent report by the World Federation of Music Therapy (Kern and Tague 2017), this approach constitutes approximately 47% of music therapy interventions. Receptive approaches differentiate between those grounded in psychological models, like the Bonny Method of Guided Imagery and Music (Bonny 2001; Frohne-Hagemann et al. 2015; Mc Ferran and Grocke 2022), and music listening approaches that are not explicitly tied to specific relational frameworks. The latter can be characterized as self- or experimenter-selected music listening. Such interventions (frequently defined as "music medicine" approaches), where music stands as the primary therapeutic element without a specific relational process during music listening, hold promising therapeutic potential in numerous clinical and preventive interventions (Raglio 2020). Nonetheless, in many instances, a clear therapeutic rationale and precise application protocols remain elusive.

This chapter introduces an approach referred to as Therapeutic Music Listening (TML) (Raglio 2023), centered around functional music listening. TML is designed to alleviate transient or structured symptoms, such as anxiety, stress, pain, and enhance overall well-being. It entails listening to personalized playlists created by a music therapist based on the user's clinical condition, personal information, and scientific insights, all in consideration of therapeutic objectives. The chapter seeks to systematize TML by establishing its theoretical underpinnings, application techniques, and methods of validation.

A. Raglio (✉)
Music Therapy Research Laboratory, Istituti Clinici Scientifici Maugeri IRCCS, Pavia, Italy
e-mail: alfredo.raglio@icsmaugeri.it

A. Raglio (ed.), *Music and Music Therapy Interventions in Clinical Practice*, Neurocultural Health and Wellbeing,
https://doi.org/10.1007/978-3-031-88578-5_10

Listening to music is intricately linked to the sensory processing of the acoustic elements of the musical message by the auditory system. The central nervous system comprises two auditory pathways: one that extends from the inner ear to the auditory cortex and another that connects to the reticular system, which, in turn, interfaces with the limbic and autonomic nervous systems (Boso et al. 2006). Consequently, this results in a substantial and comprehensive involvement of both cortical and subcortical regions. Music, particularly music listening, exerts profound effects at the neurochemical level as well. The neuroendocrine system, involving the hypothalamic–pituitary–adrenal axis, is engaged due to the release of corticosteroids, playing a pivotal role in stress management. The sympathoadrenal system regulates the secretion of hormones like catecholamines, adrenaline, and noradrenaline (Chanda and Levitin 2013; Finn and Fancourt 2018; Sihvonen et al. 2017).

Bernardi et al. (2009) observed how changes in rhythmic and dynamic attributes within short segments of music corresponded to alterations in physiological parameters such as heart rate, respiratory rate, blood pressure, and skin conductance. This suggests a connection between autonomic nervous system responses and music, which, through these parameter changes, might modulate the physiological responses in the music listener. Moreover, studies have revealed effects at the cardiovascular autonomic level (Koelsch and Jäncke 2015; Loomba et al. 2012; Raglio et al. 2010, 2021a, 2022) with potential implications for various clinical scenarios (Kulinski et al. 2022). Neuroimaging studies (Chan and Han 2022; Koelsch 2014) have underscored the crucial role of the limbic system in processing music information. Within the limbic system, particularly in the nucleus accumbens, opioids stimulate dopaminergic activity, releasing this neurotransmitter in the ventral tegmental area, thus participating in mediating the brain's responses to reward. This activation of systems during music processing has been instrumental in defining the neural underpinnings of music listening and the resulting satisfaction derived from it. Evidence now exists to support the existence of a mechanism whereby listening to enjoyable music leads to positive and rewarding responses (Salimpoor et al. 2011; Zatorre 2018). The reward structures activated by music in the limbic system encompass dopaminergic midbrain nuclei, ventral striatum, nucleus accumbens, amygdala, hippocampus, prefrontal, and orbitofrontal structures (Levitin and Tirovolas 2009). Musical stimuli thus trigger anticipation mechanisms for a desired stimulus, primarily mediated by dopamine but also involving other neurotransmitters like serotonin, norepinephrine, and endorphins. These mechanisms could elucidate the strong motivation for prolonged music listening, intertwined with individual experiences and cognitive processes that shape the perceived pleasure in music listening. The potential role of music in modulating limbic and paralimbic structure activity holds significant implications for its use in treating various disorders, including psychiatric or neurodegenerative conditions known to be associated with dopaminergic irregularities (Koelsch 2014).

This overview of the rationale behind the therapeutic potential of music listening paints a compelling picture that justifies its application in a range of clinical and preventative contexts. Despite the scientific insights gleaned from the literature, there's a clear call for further research to establish a more robust connection between the specifics of music listening and its clinical applications. Therefore, fostering greater collaboration and integration between professionals in clinical, psychological, neuroscientific, and music therapy fields is recommended. This interdisciplinary approach can enhance the effectiveness of interventions by making them more scientifically grounded and coherent in their application.

10.2 Applicational Fields

Areas of clinical application for music listening encompass a broad spectrum, incorporating both music therapy receptive techniques and music medicine approaches. One notable setting where music listening finds extensive utility is within hospitals, particularly as a form of music medicine. Ease of implementation during hospital stays, coupled with the transient nature of symptoms common in peri-operative setting, makes music listening a viable adjunctive therapy (Hole et al. 2015; Raglio 2019). Moreover, it proves beneficial in alleviating psychological symptoms that often accompany hospitalization, potentially mitigating the need for pharmacological interventions and even reducing hospitalization duration in some cases. Various studies indicate significant reductions in anxiety (Guétin et al. 2009; Hole et al. 2015), stress (De Witte et al. 2020; Linnemann et al. 2015; Radstaak et al. 2014; Raglio et al. 2020a), perceived pain (Chai et al. 2020; Hole et al. 2015; Lee 2021; Martin-Saavedra et al. 2018; Radstaak et al. 2018), and sleep disturbances (Cordi et al. 2019; Dickson and Schubert 2020; Jespersen et al. 2015; Kuula et al. 2020; Loewy 2020; Trahan et al. 2018) with music listening across diverse clinical scenarios. In addition, music listening has shown promise in ameliorating behavioral disorders (Gaviola et al. 2019; Gerdner 2000, 2012; Kwak et al. 2020; Maseda et al. 2018; Sakamoto et al. 2013; Särkämö et al. 2014) and enhancing cognitive function (Särkämö et al. 2008). Nonetheless, the heterogeneity in musical selections, application protocols, and outcome measures across these studies underscores the necessity for a unified approach that integrates scientific evidence with insights from music therapy, clinical practice, and neuroscience.

10.3 The Therapeutic Music Listening Approach (TML)

The approach begins with gathering anamnestic data, including personal and musical information, through a preliminary questionnaire to create an initial playlist (Appendix, Questionnaire 1). This music listening program incorporates three key elements: (a) the user's preferences, (b) the structural and parametric characteristics of music choices, and (c) therapeutic needs. While focusing on these aspects, the approach aims to address therapeutic requirements across three categories: (a) activation/stimulation, (b) relaxation/deactivation, and (c) diverting of attention, irrespective of specific medical conditions. These categories are linked to specific musical parameters, acknowledging the subjective nature of music perception while aligning with therapeutic objectives (Table 10.1). For instance, relaxation-inducing songs typically feature slow tempos (40–60 bpm), regularity, predictability, and reduced complexity, avoiding highly expressive content. Conversely, activating songs exhibit faster tempos (>60 bpm) with greater irregularities and complexities, while distracting songs contain divergent elements and high variability. The Therapeutic Musical Listening (TML) approach integrates subjective preferences with these parametric and structural characteristics, facilitating tailored interventions (Fig. 10.1).

Table 10.1 Examples of matching between music categories and therapeutic aims in various clinical conditions

Examples of clinical conditions/symptoms	Therapeutic aims/music categories	Music parameters/structures
Apathy (e.g., as a symptom of dementia) Negative symptoms (e.g., in psychiatric patients) Continuous low mood or sadness, being not motivated or having no interest in things (e.g., in depression as main diagnosis or associated to other illness) …	Activation/stimulation	Tempo: moderate to fast Melody: broad range intervals Harmonic variations/modulations: medium to high frequency Rhythmic complexity: medium to high Timbre: extensive instrumental ensemble Music progression: partial regularity
Anxiety (as main diagnosis or associated to other illness or medical conditions) (Raglio et al. 2021c) Stress (associated to medical or life conditions or in work-related stress) (Raglio et al. 2020a) Agitation, Irritability (e.g., as symptoms of dementia or as behavioral disturbances in psychiatric/neurological patients) (Raglio et al. 2015) Sleep disorders (in many clinical conditions) …	Deactivation/relaxation	Tempo: slow Melody: restrictive range of intervals Harmonic variations/modulations: low frequency Rhythmic complexity: low Timbre: solo instrument/reduced instrumental ensemble Music progression: steady
Pain (chronic and acute condition) (Raglio et al. 2023) Obsessive compulsive disorder Attention disorders …	Diverting of attention (relaxation or activation*)*	Music variations/modulations: high frequency (i.e., frequent pitch, tempo, timbre, rhythmic changes, harmonic modulations, etc.)

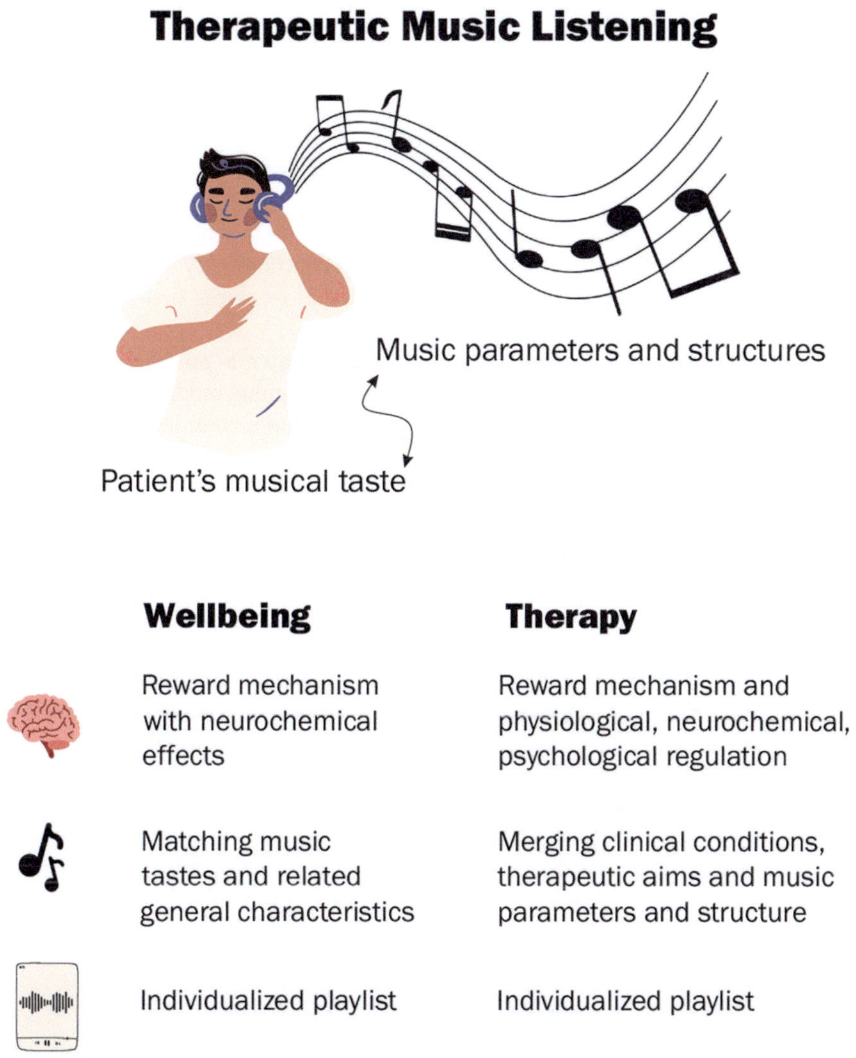

Fig. 10.1 Therapeutic Music Listening in summary

The procedure for implementing TML-based interventions involves several steps (Fig. 10.2):

1. Administering Questionnaire 1 (see the Appendix) to gather personal/clinical and musical data
2. Identifying therapeutic aims/music categories and conducting a preintervention assessment
3. Creating an individualized listening program (20–40 minutes) based on therapeutic goals and defining music tastes/parameters accordingly
4. Immediate feedback (Appendix, Questionnaire 2) to assess first music listening impact
5. Delivering the personalized listening program (after a possible adjustment depending on immediate feedback) and defining listening modalities
6. Encouraging daily listening according to agreed-upon modalities
7. Providing periodic feedback, preferably weekly
8. Adjusting the listening program based on results and treatment progression
9. Conducting a final clinical evaluation and subjective assessment at the end of treatment

This systematic approach allows for the creation and monitoring of a tailored listening program, adaptable based on treatment progress. Support from healthcare staff may be necessary, especially for patients lacking autonomy. Listening devices and modalities can be adjusted according to individual needs and clinical considerations. Clinical experience suggests sessions of 20–40 minutes, preferably with headphones, with listening frequency determined by user needs and clinical characteristics (Fig. 10.3).

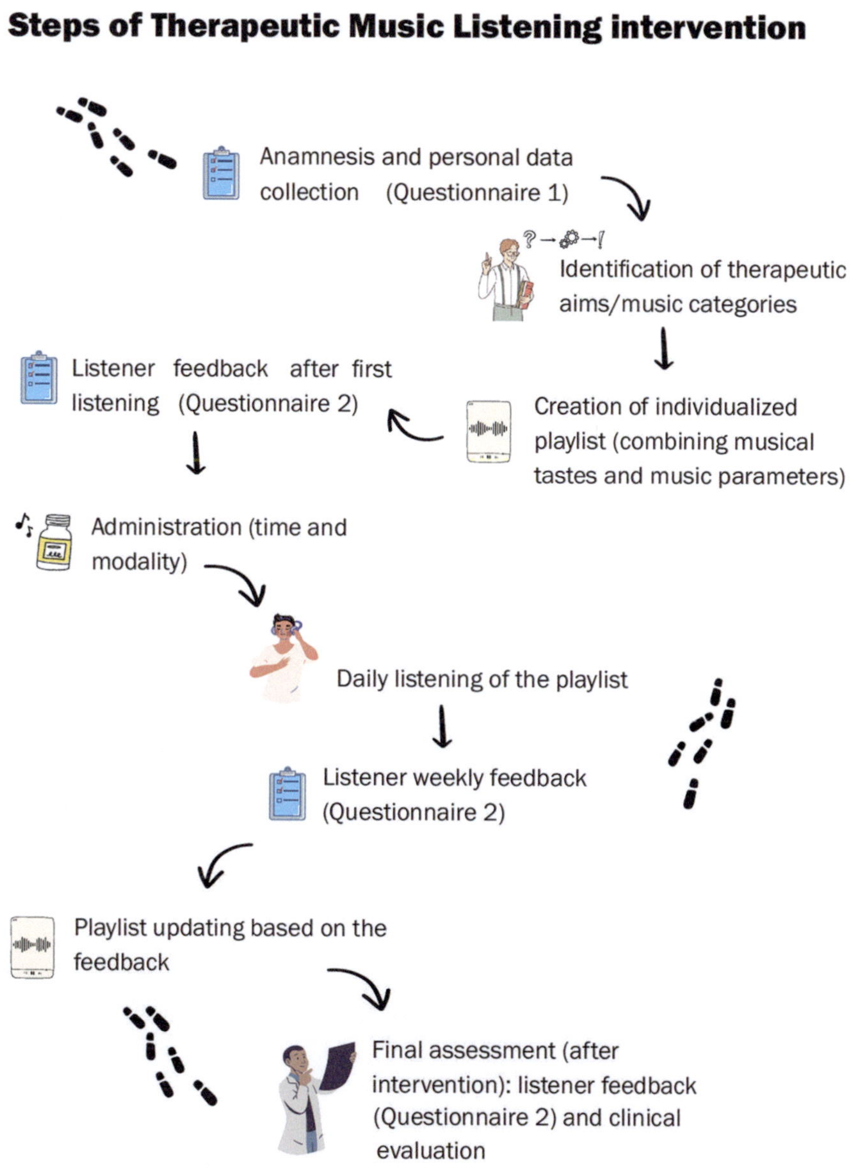

Fig. 10.2 Steps of the Therapeutic Music Listening intervention. Note: Avoid, whenever possible (especially for deactivating/relaxing playlists), songs: lyrics could divert the listener's attention or activate the listener depending on their contents

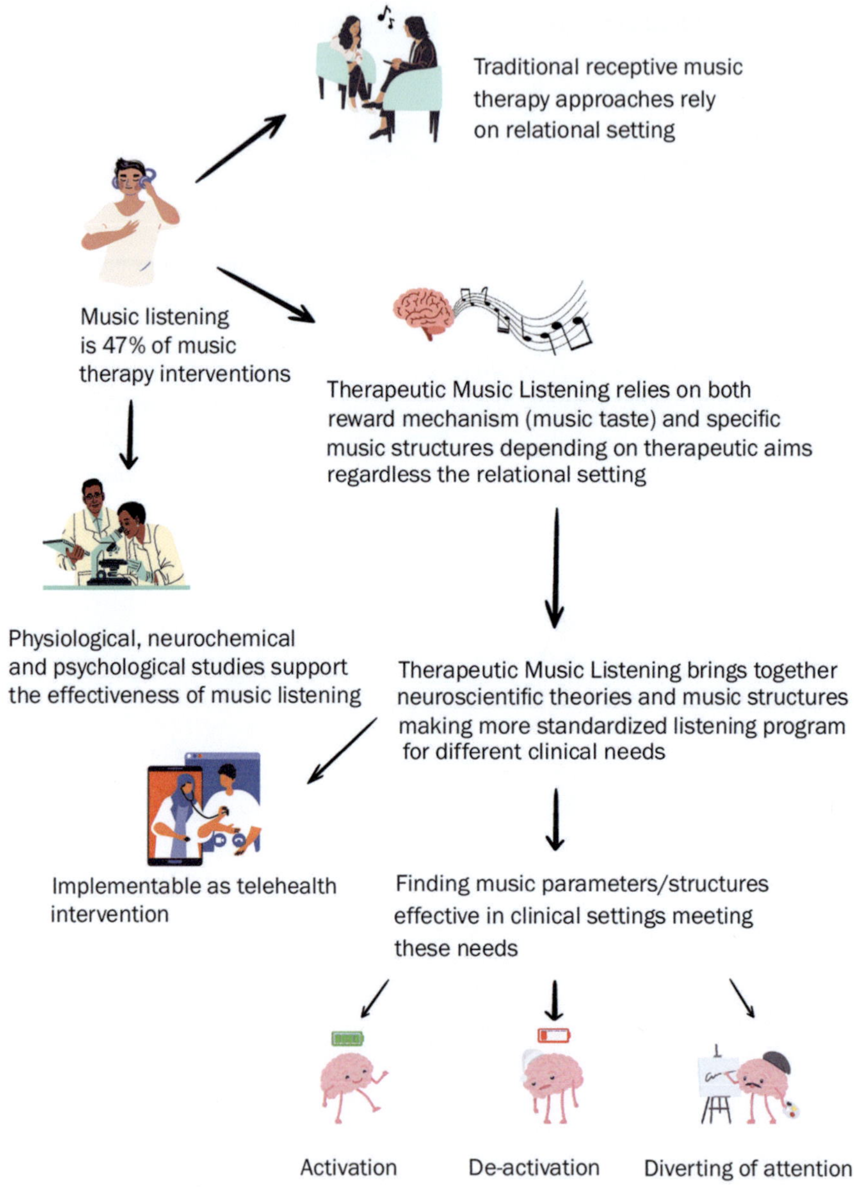

Fig. 10.3 Key points of the chapter

10.4 The Novelty in Therapeutic Music Listening

In contrast to other receptive music therapy methods like the Bonny Method of Guided Imagery and Music (Bonny 2001; Frohne-Hagemann et al. 2015), TML doesn't involve a therapist-guided introspective intervention. Instead, the therapist formulates therapeutic hypotheses based on music's potential effects and parameters, adjusting interventions over time according to patient feedback and treatment trend. This approach blends subjective music perception with specific musical parameters chosen by the therapist to achieve desired effects.

TML integrates established theoretical principles, particularly in neuroscience, regarding the relationship between preferred music and therapeutic effects, while emphasizing the importance of musical structures and parameters in therapy outcomes. This approach rejects the notion that mere musical preferences alone can suffice for therapeutic benefit, aiming for specificity in therapeutic proposals.

Identifying key musical parameters is challenging due to music's complex interaction and the subjective nature of perception. However, it's crucial to characterize music not only subjectively but also based on structural and parametric traits to better relate it to therapeutic effects (Raglio 2020). Despite efforts to understand the relationship between musical parameters and emotions, many studies lack detailed descriptions of interventions, highlighting the need for more comprehensive research.

Music psychology has contributed significantly to this area (Scherer 1995; Snowdon et al. 2019), exploring how musical preferences correlate with personality traits and cognitive styles (Anderson et al. 2021; Dobrota and Reić 2015; Eerola et al. 2016; Greenberg et al. 2015; Vuoskoski and Eerola 2011, 2017). A recent review (Reybrouck et al. 2021) suggests that emotional and cognitive processes in music listening depend on acoustic characteristics, potentially leading to mathematical models explaining the music-listener response relationship. Nevertheless, various factors, including individual, interpersonal, and external influences, can significantly impact the therapeutic outcomes of music listening interventions.

10.5 Conclusions

The presented approach aims to blend the subjective experience of music listening with a scientifically driven investigation into the connection between musical stimuli and therapeutic outcomes. The insights gained from these studies serve as a crucial foundation for future research endeavors in music listening-based treatments. This approach strives for a "modeling" of music listening characterized by quantifiable aspects, making it more objective and standardized across various clinical contexts. To achieve this, music therapy-oriented techniques for extracting musical features can be applied, enabling the development of therapeutic repertoires based on quantitatively defined musical attributes.

By leveraging Artificial Intelligence, it becomes possible to identify songs sharing similar characteristics through the quantitative assessment of musical parameters. Modern data processing techniques, such as Machine Learning and artificial neural networks, aid in defining target populations based on specific musical characteristics and uncovering hidden relationships among variables within studies. In addition, this therapeutic approach holds promise for remote delivery as a Telemedicine intervention, streamlining its application and expanding its reach to potential users, thereby presenting opportunities for widespread implementation across numerous clinical domains.

I advocate for a multidisciplinary approach to the future of music therapy, one that harmonizes musical and scientific perspectives to reinforce clinical findings derived from practice. Moreover, it's imperative to scrutinize the applicability of the methodologies outlined in this article within diverse cultural contexts. Differences in listening habits, identities, and musical structures should be taken into account when implementing these approaches elsewhere. Cultural considerations, especially regarding the impact of musical structures and parameters on individuals with varying cultural backgrounds, are essential aspects to contemplate in TML interventions.

Appendix

Questionnaire 1

(Personal/clinical data and musical anamnesis, before Therapeutic Music Listening treatment)

General and clinical information

Surname and Name:

Age:

Education:

Diagnosis:

Reported problems:

Therapeutic Aims:

Musical training:

☐ No ☐ Yes

Musical practice:

☐ No ☐ Yes

Preferred musical genre (max. 3 preferences)

☐ Pop ☐ Rock ☐ Jazz ☐ Blues

☐ Classical ☐ Folk ☐ Electronic Music ☐ Sacred Music

☐ Opera Music ☐ Movie Music ☐ Rap

☐ Ethnic/Traditional ☐ Other: ……………………………………………..

Preferred composers/songwriters/performers and pieces of music (to list 2 pieces or more):

You listen to music:

☐ Never

☐ Some time

☐ Always (daily)
You prefer:
☐ well-known pieces
☐ unknown pieces
☐ rhythmic pieces
☐ melodic pieces
☐ Slow music
☐ Fast music
Preferred musical instruments:
Music, genres, sounds, you dislike:
Why do you want a playlist?
How much do you feel you need it (from 0 to 10)?:

0 1 2 3 4 5 6 7 8 9 10

Notes:

Questionnaire 2

(after first music listening, weekly and at the end of the treatment)
Appreciation (0–10):

0 1 2 3 4 5 6 7 8 9 10

Effectiveness (0–10):

0 1 2 3 4 5 6 7 8 9 10

Pieces to replace:
Reasons:
Other remarks:
Do you feel you need to continue the treatment?
☐ No ☐ Yes
If yes, how much do you feel you need to continue the treatment (0–10)?:

0 1 2 3 4 5 6 7 8 9 10

Notes:

References

Anderson I, Gil S, Gibson C, et al. Just the way you are: linking music listening on Spotify and personality. Soc Psychol Personal Sci. 2021;2021(12):561–72.

Bernardi L, Porta C, Casucci G, et al. Dynamic interactions between musical, cardiovascular, and cerebral rhythms in humans. Circulation. 2009;119:3171–80.

Bonny HL. Music psychotherapy: guided imagery and music. Voices: a world forum for. Music Ther. 2001;10:3.

Boso M, Politi P, Barale F, et al. Neurophysiology and neurobiology of the musical experience. Funct Neurol. 2006;21:187.

Chai PR, Gale JY, Patton ME, et al. The impact of music on nociceptive processing. Pain Med. 2020;21:3047–54.

Chan MMY, Han YMY. The functional brain networks activated by music listening: a neuroimaging meta-analysis and implications for treatment. Neuropsychology. 2022;36:4–22.

Chanda ML, Levitin DJ. The neurochemistry of music. Trends Cogn Sci. 2013;17:179–93.

Cordi MJ, Ackermann S, Rasch B. Effects of relaxing music on healthy sleep. Sci Rep. 2019;9:9079.

De Witte M, Spruit A, Van Hooren S, et al. Effects of music interventions on stress-related outcomes: a systematic review and two meta-analyses. Health Psychol Rev. 2020;14:294–324.

Dickson GT, Schubert E. Music on prescription to aid sleep quality: a literature review. Front Psychol. 2020;11:1695.

Dobrota S, Reić EI. The relationship between music preferences of different mode and tempo and personality traits–implications for music pedagogy. Music Educ Res. 2015;17:234–47.

Eerola T, Vuoskoski JK, Kautiainen H. Being moved by unfamiliar sad music is associated with high empathy. Front Psychol. 2016;7:1176.

Finn S, Fancourt D. The biological impact of listening to music in clinical and nonclinical settings: a systematic review. Prog Brain Res. 2018;237:173–200.

Frohne-Hagemann I, Warja M, Pedersen IN, et al. Guided imagery & music (GIM) and music imagery methods for individual and group therapy. Jessica Kingsley Publishers; 2015.

Gaviola MA, Inder KJ, Dilworth S, et al. Impact of individualised music listening intervention on persons with dementia: a systematic review of randomised controlled trials. Australas J Ageing. 2019;39:10–20.

Gerdner LA. Effects of individualized versus classical "relaxation" music on the frequency of agitation in elderly persons with Alzheimer's disease and related disorders. Int Psychogeriatr. 2000;12:49–65.

Gerdner LA. Individualized music for dementia: evolution and application of evidence-based protocol. World J Psychiatry. 2012;2:26–32.

Greenberg DM, Baron-Cohen S, Stillwell DJ, et al. Musical preferences are linked to cognitive styles. PLoS One. 2015;10:e0131151.

Guétin S, Portet F, Picot MC, et al. Effect of music therapy on anxiety and depression in patients with Alzheimer's type dementia: randomised, controlled study. Dement Geriatr Cogn Disord. 2009;28:36–46.

Hole J, Hirsch M, Ball E, et al. Music as an aid for postoperative recovery in adults: a systematic review and meta-analysis. Lancet. 2015;386:1659–71.

Jespersen KV, Koenig J, Jennum P, et al. Music for insomnia in adults. Cochrane Database Syst Rev. 2015;8:CD010459.

Kern P, Tague DB. Music therapy practice status and trends worldwide: an international survey study. J Music Ther. 2017;54:255–86.

Koelsch S. Brain correlates of music-evoked emotions. Nat Rev Neurosci. 2014;15:170–80.

Koelsch S, Jäncke L. Music and the heart. Eur Heart J. 2015;36:3043–9.

Kulinski J, Ofori EK, Visotcky A, et al. Effects of music on the cardiovascular system. Trends Cardiovasc Med. 2022;32:390–8.

Kuula L, Halonen R, Kajanto K, et al. The effects of pre-sleep slow breathing and music listening on polysomnographic sleep measures - a pilot trial. Sci Rep. 2020;10:7427.

Kwak J, Anderson K, O'Connell VK. Findings from a prospective randomized controlled trial of an individualized music listening program for persons with dementia. J Appl Gerontol. 2020;39:567–75.

Lee JH. The effects of music on pain: a meta-analysis. J Music Ther. 2021;58:372.

Levitin DJ, Tirovolas AK. Current advances in the cognitive neuroscience of music. Ann N Y Acad Sci. 2009;1156:211–31.

Linnemann A, Ditzen B, Strahler J, et al. Music listening as a means of stress reduction in daily life. Psychoneuroendocrinology. 2015;60:82–90.

Loewy J. Music therapy as a potential intervention for sleep improvement. Nat Sci Sleep. 2020;12:1–9.

Loomba RS, Arora R, Shah PH, et al. Effects of music on systolic blood pressure, diastolic blood pressure, and heart rate: a meta-analysis. Indian Heart J. 2012;64:309–13.

Martin-Saavedra JS, Vergara-Mendez LD, Pradilla I, et al. Standardizing music characteristics for the management of pain: a systematic review and meta-analysis of clinical trials. Complement Ther Med. 2018;41:81–9.

Maseda A, Cibeira N, Lorenzo-López L, et al. Multisensory stimulation and individualized music sessions on older adults with severe dementia: effects on mood, behavior, and biomedical parameters. J Alzheimers Dis. 2018;63:1415–25.

Mc Ferran K, Grocke D. Receptive music therapy. In: Techniques clinical applications and new perspectives. 2nd ed. London: Jessica Kingsley Publishers; 2022.

Radstaak M, Geurts SA, Brosschot JF, et al. Music and psychophysiological recovery from stress. Psychosom Med. 2014;76:529–37.

Raglio A. Therapeutic use of music in hospitals: a possible intervention model. Am J Med Qual. 2019;34:618–20.

Raglio A. Therapeutic music listening as telehealth intervention. Complement Ther Clin Pract. 2020;41:101245.

Raglio A. A novel music-based therapeutic approach: the therapeutic music listening. Front Hum Neurosci. 2023;17:1204593.

Raglio A, Oasi O, Gianotti M, et al. Effects of music therapy on psychological symptoms and heart rate variability in patients with dementia. A pilot study. Curr Aging Sci. 2010;3:242–6.

Raglio A, Bellandi D, Baiardi P, et al. Effect of active music therapy and individualized listening to music on dementia: a multicenter randomized controlled trial. J Am Geriatr Soc. 2015;63:1534–9.

Raglio A, Bellandi D, Gianotti M, et al. Daily music listening to reduce work-related stress: a randomized controlled pilot trial. J Public Health. 2020a;42:e81–7.

Raglio A, Imbriani M, Imbriani C, et al. Machine learning techniques to predict the effectiveness of music therapy: a randomized controlled trial. Comput Methods Programs Biomed. 2020b;185:105160.

Raglio A, De Maria B, Perego F, et al. Effects of algorithmic music on the cardiovascular neural control. J Pers Med. 2021a;11:1084.

Raglio A, Bellandi D, Manzoni L, et al. Communication improvement reduces BPSD: a music therapy study based on artificial neural networks. Neurol Sci. 2021b;42:2103–6.

Raglio A, Oddone E, Meaglia I, et al. Conventional and algorithmic music listening before radiotherapy treatment: a randomized controlled pilot study. Brain Sci. 2021c;11:1618.

Raglio A, Maestri R, Robbi E, et al. Effect of algorithmic music listening on cardiac autonomic nervous system activity: an exploratory, randomized crossover study. J Clin Med. 2022;11:5738.

Raglio A, Bettaglio R, Manera MR, et al. Feasibility of therapeutic music listening in fibromyalgia: a randomised controlled pilot study. Neurol Sci. 2023;44:723–7.

Reybrouck M, Vuust P, Brattico E. Neural correlates of music listening: does the music matter? Brain Sci. 2021;11:1553.

Sakamoto M, Ando H, Tsutou A. Comparing the effects of different individualized music interventions for elderly individuals with severe dementia. Int Psychogeriatr. 2013;25:775–84.

Salimpoor VN, Benovoy M, Larcher K, et al. Anatomically distinct dopamine release during anticipation and experience of peak emotion to music. Nat Neurosci. 2011;14:257–62.

Särkämö T, Tervaniemi M, Laitinen S, et al. Music listening enhances cognitive recovery and mood after middle cerebral artery stroke. Brain. 2008;13:866–76.

Särkämö T, Tervaniemi M, Laitinen S, et al. Cognitive, emotional, and social benefits of regular musical activities in early dementia: randomized controlled study. Gerontologist. 2014;54:634–50.

Scherer KR. Expression of emotion in voice and music. J Voice. 1995;9:235–48.

Sihvonen AJ, Särkämö T, Leo V, et al. Music-based interventions in neurological rehabilitation. Lancet Neurol. 2017;16:648–60.

Snowdon CT, Zimmermann E, Altenmüller E. Music evolution and neuroscience. Progr Brain Res. 2019;217:17–34.

Trahan T, Durrant SJ, Müllensiefen D, et al. The music that helps people sleep and the reasons they believe it works: a mixed methods analysis of online survey reports. PLoS One. 2018;13:e0206531.

Vuoskoski J, Eerola T. The role of mood and personality in the perception of emotions represented by music. Cortex. 2011;47:1099–106.

Vuoskoski JK, Eerola T. The pleasure evoked by sad music is mediated by feelings of being moved. Front Psychol. 2017;8:439.

Zatorre RJ. Why do we love music? Cerebrum. 2018;2018:cer-16-18.

Part IV

How to Carry Out a Music-Based or Music Therapy Treatment

Music Therapy Treatment: From the Beginning to the Conclusion

11

Marta Gianotti and Alfredo Raglio

Key Points

Steps of music therapy treatment:

- *Referral* phase is the first step for a music therapy treatment. It is important to identify patients with specific needs on whom different music therapy approaches can act effectively.
- *Inclusion and exclusion criteria* are defined by clinicians and music therapists based on clinical conditions and music therapy assessment, considering the possibility to meet therapeutic goals, and suitability of music therapy approaches for their relational, emotional, physical, and cognitive abilities.
- *Therapeutic goals*, including improvement of psychological symptoms, behaviors, relationships, sensory and motor skills, cognitive abilities, psycho-physiological well-being, need to be defined before the treatment.
- *Music therapy approach* and intervention's characteristics can be defined based on therapeutic needs.
- *Qualitative and quantitative evaluations* (intra and extra-setting) should be conducted before, during and after the conclusion of the treatment.
- *The conclusion of the treatment* is predefined or depends on partial/total goals achievement (e.g., changes in behavior, mood, engagement, progress in rehabilitation, etc.).

M. Gianotti
Music Therapist, IRCCS Fondazione Don Carlo Gnocchi, Milano, Italy

A. Raglio (✉)
Music Therapy Research Laboratory, Istituti Clinici Scientifici Maugeri IRCCS, Pavia, Italy
e-mail: alfredo.raglio@icsmaugeri.it

A. Raglio (ed.), *Music and Music Therapy Interventions in Clinical Practice*, Neurocultural Health and Wellbeing,
https://doi.org/10.1007/978-3-031-88578-5_11

This chapter aims to present the steps concerning music therapy interventions and the role that the music therapist plays in these actions. It begins by highlighting the importance of the referral phase, followed by a specific evaluation period. In this phase, key elements to observe in order to make the referral more effective have been presented. Subsequently, the authors provide an overview of possible objectives that music therapy treatment aims to achieve, and the application of different music therapy approaches considering the specificity of clinical settings. A section has been dedicated to present intra and extra setting outcome measures, and finally, a part regarding the conclusion of the treatment and how to manage it. These steps, although they can be placed in a clear chronological order, are intertwined and mutually influenced, as they are conceptually dependent on each other.

11.1 Referral

Music therapy treatment generally begins with a referral from a clinician or reference figure for the patient/client.

It is important that the referrer is aware of the potential benefits of music therapy as well as any possible contraindications. At this stage, it is crucial for the music therapist to interact with the referrer regarding these aspects and possible intervention approaches. In this way, the clinical figure can be provided with the necessary information to adequately define the inclusion and exclusion criteria for music therapy, arriving at a fundamental concept: the appropriateness of the treatment. The evolution and success of an intervention can also depend on this.

There are some aspects related to referral that are common across all clinical fields. The reasons a person might be referred to music therapy can be related to difficulties encountered on the relational level, including aspects of emotional–behavioral regulation and communication management. Music therapy can also be a valuable support in the field of rehabilitation. It can, in fact, improve motor, cognitive, and linguistic functions in cases of impairment resulting from neurological conditions.

Where there are struggles or impairments in relationships, communication, or emotional regulation, music therapy can become a valuable tool to recover, reduce, or manage disorders related to these areas. Music therapy can also be a valuable support in situations of social isolation related to specific diagnoses (e.g., autism spectrum disorder, selective mutism, trauma); more generally, music therapy can be used in all situations where there is dysfunction related to an excess or deficit of a behavior or function since the sound–musical framework associated with the relational component acts as a mediator and regulator.

Referral to active/improvisational music therapy usually occurs in clinical situations where it is necessary to facilitate the patient's free self-expression, particularly in cases with significant issues related to emotion management, inhibition, or relational and communication disorders.

Music therapy can also be effective in self-affirmation and in defining one's role within a relationship, and it can help open communication channels in situations where verbal language is absent, or cognitive impairments inhibit free expression.

Some examples of relational music therapy models are those referred to Nordoff-Robbins or Benenzon models, (Nordoff and Robbins 2007; Benenzon 2008), where sound and music are used as means to create a therapeutic relationship.

If the referral is due to the need for introspective work to facilitate the expression and awareness of the patient's emotional aspects, receptive music therapy can be considered a useful approach. Among the various models (McFerran and Grocke 2022) available are, for example, the Bonny Guided Imagery and Music Model (Bonny 2002) or music listening psychodynamic approaches (De Backer 2014; Kim 2016; Wheeler 2015).

To give a practical example, receptive music therapy can be a valuable support in the psychiatric field (Lotter and van Staden 2019; Solanki et al. 2013; Paul et al. 2020) as it helps structure thoughts and works on the harmonization and internal organization of the self. In a receptive setting, music acts as a mediator and trigger for the emergence of thoughts and emotions, allowing for better intrapsychic integration. The verbal processing following musical listening, ideally guided by professionals with psychotherapeutic and psychiatric skills, integrates the therapeutic action. Moreover, in oncology, receptive music therapy can help to alleviate pain, reduce anxiety, improve mood, enhance quality of life, and provide emotional support for patients undergoing cancer treatment (Burns 2001; Stanczyk 2011; Köhler et al. 2020).

If the referral is made due to the need to reduce transient or structured psychological symptoms, achieving psycho-physiological balance, or improving a person's well-being and quality of life, Therapeutic Music Listening (Raglio 2023) (see the chapter in this volume) or music–medicine approaches can provide valuable support (Monsalve-Duarte et al. 2022; Sheikh-Wu et al. 2021).

An example of music–medicine application is in the context of dementia, where it is useful for addressing behavioral disturbances related to the condition with a view to regulation or compensation (Raglio et al. 2014; van der Steen et al. 2017). Moreover, in perioperative setting, music–medicine approach can reduce anxiety, postoperative pain and analgesia use, increasing patient satisfaction (Casarin et al. 2021; Hole et al. 2015).

If the referral is aimed at improving motor or cognitive outcomes, approaches focused on rehabilitation/stimulation supported by musical elements may be the most appropriate intervention type. For instance, Neurologic Music Therapy (Thaut and Hoember 2014) is the most widely used technique in the neurological field (e.g., Parkinson's disease, stroke, multiple sclerosis) and especially in neuromotor, linguistic, and cognitive rehabilitation concerning these clinical settings. This approach is based on tailored musical parameters aimed at rehabilitation goals (e.g., rhythm for movement, melody for language, etc.).

In rehabilitation, music-based approaches can also be used as support for movement or cognitive function, thanks to the structural elements of music (Raglio 2018).

For further details on these techniques, please refer to the dedicated chapters in this manual.

11.2 Preliminary Music Therapy Assessment and Inclusion/Exclusion Criteria

A preliminary assessment before proposing a music therapy intervention includes evaluating the patient's diagnosis, clinical history, and the compatibility of these conditions with potential music therapy interventions. Based on these evaluations, a general observation of the patient can be conducted, assessing his/her cognitive, motor, relational, and psycho-behavioral conditions.

The preliminary assessment for the relational active music therapy includes the direct observation of the patient and the connection between his/her initial condition and clinical needs. Therefore, the assessment will include:

- Motor skills, cognitive, and sensory evaluations.
- Psycho-behavioral evaluations.
- Relational attitude.

Specifically, it is recommended to propose several sessions (2–5) to verify:

- Presence in the setting: Does the patient choose to enter the room or immediately refuse entry? Does he/she stay in the setting for the established time or only partially? How long does he/she remain in the room? Do his/her behaviors change over the course of the evaluation sessions? In what direction?
- Willingness to use musical instruments: Does he/she accept or reject them? What kind of approach does he/she take towards the musical instruments? Is it immediate or gradual? Spontaneous or induced?
- Approach to nonverbal communication: Assess the patients' willingness to activate alternative communication methods to verbal communication and observe their acceptance of self-expressiveness through the sonorous–music channel. Or do patients need to use verbal communication exclusively?

The observation of these elements should be interpreted dynamically and in relation to time, the intensity of manifestations, and their possible modulation and regulation during the evaluation period.

Regarding the relational receptive music therapy approaches, it is essential to observe the patient's cognitive level and verbal communication abilities, and his/her ability to process emotional content in an abstract and symbolic manner. In addition, it is important to evaluate his/her sensitivity to the auditory–musical channel and the insight level.

For this kind of approach, it's essential for the patient to have sufficient cognitive integrity to process abstract thoughts and an adequate introspective capacity. Furthermore, the presence of acute symptoms may compromise patient compliance and treatment effectiveness.

During the assessment phase, it is also crucial to observe the patients' willingness to listen, as well as their level of attention and participation.

For music listening approach, the preliminary assessment should focus on the presence mainly of behavioral disorders or psychological symptoms (also transient symptoms) that may be sensitive to a therapeutic music listening intervention. Listening programs can also be structured to improve the patient's quality of life and increase his or her well-being. It is also important to consider the ability to ensure consistency in listening through self or assisted administration. Therefore, therapeutic music listening can be preliminarily proposed to patients who are autonomous or accompanied by constant reference figures.

For the rehabilitative music therapy approaches, the preliminary assessment should focus on the neurological impairments related to the disease. Preliminary observations should also include the patient's compliance, which must be adequate to perform the required tasks. Furthermore, the patient's willingness to participate in sessions on a frequent basis (2–3 times a week) should be evaluated. Based on the severity of the neurological damage, it will be necessary to assess the need for an intervention and its characteristics in collaboration with neurologists and/or physiatrists but also with rehabilitation therapists for defining specific rehabilitative programs.

Among the general inclusion criteria for music therapy, we find sensitivity to the auditory–musical element, the ability to adhere to the setting, the presence of a clinical condition compatible with the proposed music therapy intervention, the presence of needs related to the above-mentioned areas, and the patient's motivation. In general, as with any therapeutic treatment, the contraindication/benefit ratio must be considered for music therapy, and the potential effectiveness of the treatment should be evaluated before undertaking the music therapy intervention.

Among the exclusion criteria are the refusal or nonacceptance of the music therapy setting, a psycho-behavioral structure that is too rigid to allow real change, confirmed hypersensitivity to sound or some of its components, and acute states that could be negatively affected by excessive emotional or sensory stimulation.

Specific factors must also be considered in relation to the intervention techniques planned. For example, for active relational music therapy interventions, an exclusion criterion might be excessive resistance or refusal of direct exposure to the improvisational channel, or motor impairments that prevent the necessary movement to use instruments (e.g., in cases of tetraplegia or paralysis from brain trauma).

In receptive music therapy, exclusion criteria include the absence of verbal skills (neurological issues such as fluent and nonfluent aphasias), cognitive impairments that hinder functional verbal language, and the inability to process and symbolize emotions and thoughts abstractly (e.g., in severe intellectual disabilities). Severe attentional difficulties also constitute an exclusion criterion.

For therapeutic music listening and music medicine approaches, exclusion criteria are related to an explicit refusal of the patient or the patient's lack of sensitivity to the sound–musical element.

Within music-based rehabilitative approaches, the exclusion occurs when a patient cannot ensure their active participation in the rehabilitative process, either cognitively or motivationally. The patient's level of autonomy in performing rehabilitative exercises should also be assessed in order to define an appropriate rehabilitation program.

In some cases, a previous music training or practice could be a limiting factor, as patients might seek to relive their past musical experiences, inevitably transformed into something different from their memory. This factor could lead to frustration or create an emotional barrier that prevents the patient from using the auditory–music channel freely, without cultural or aesthetic constraints. Similarly, a preference for music does not necessarily facilitate therapy, as there is a significant gap between generic music use and the specific therapeutic application of music.

At the end of the evaluation period, the music therapist will be able to define not only the general objectives of the intervention but also the specific goals tailored to the individual referred for therapy.

11.3 Definition of Therapeutic Goals

The goals of a music therapy treatment are different and can encompass many areas. The general objectives that music therapy aims to achieve concern:

- Psychological domain.
- Behavioral Domain.
- Relational and Social Domain.
- Sensory-Motor Domain.
- Cognitive Domain.
- Physiological domain.

Music therapy can be effective in treating various psychological symptoms, including anxiety and depression. Numerous studies and research have shown that music therapy can have a positive impact on these disorders (Aalbers et al. 2017; Erkkilä et al. 2011; Lu et al. 2021; Wong et al. 2001). Music therapy is proposed preoperatively in hospitals to reduce anxiety and stress associated with surgery or hospitalization (Casarin et al. 2021; Lee et al. 2017; Wang et al. 2022).

Moreover, there is an increasing number of studies highlighting the positive impact of music therapy on psychological symptoms as stress (De Witte et al. 2022; Umbrello et al. 2019) and work-related stress (Colin et al. 2023; Raglio et al. 2020).

From a behavioral perspective, music therapy serves for regulating and modulating behaviors and emotions. For instance, in dementia, music can help reduce behavioral and psychological symptoms of dementia (BPSD) (Raglio et al. 2015, 2021a, b), and in neuropsychiatry it can be a valuable support in managing ADHD and hyperactivity (Park et al. 2023).

Music therapy can also assist in expressing and regulating emotions and facilitating relationships, for example, in autism spectrum disorders (Tsirigoti and Georgiadi 2024). It is a powerful tool for developing communicative intentionality and paving the way for communication and relationships with others. In neuropsychiatry, for example, music therapy can facilitate communicative intentionality even in nonverbal children, aiding relationships and socialization.

In rehabilitation, music therapy supports and aids the recovery of movement in the presence of conditions that impair functioning, such as Parkinson's disease or stroke (Thaut and Hoember 2014). Music therapy can positively impact the functional recovery of both upper and lower limbs, gait, balance, and motor coordination. Through rhythmic and melodic elements, music therapy can enhance the neuroplasticity required for these physical functions, supporting rehabilitation efforts in patients with motor impairments.

Cognitive aspects that can be enhanced through music therapy include language, attention, memory, executive functions, etc. For example, sound and music can promote attention and stimulate vocal production and the development of communicative and functional language (Thaut and Hoember 2014). Music therapy interventions have been shown to improve language skills in children with developmental disorders (Shi et al. 2024). Furthermore, music-based interventions have been found to enhance attention and cognitive functions (Hars et al. 2014; Särkämö et al. 2008).

From a physiological perspective, music therapy, especially music listening approaches, can help reduce heart and respiratory rates, as well as blood pressure (Chanda and Levitin 2013; Lorber and Divjak 2022), by lowering stress levels. These effects can contribute to better management of anxiety and stress, providing both emotional and physical relief.

The culmination of these aspects leads to a general improvement in quality of life, which becomes one of the primary goals of music therapy (Lin et al. 2023; Weise et al. 2018). By addressing cognitive, psychological, emotional, social, and motor domains, music therapy aims to enhance overall well-being and satisfaction with life, fostering a sense of fulfilment and empowerment in individuals undergoing therapy.

Only a few application examples related to the possible effects on the mentioned domains are reported here. In the various chapters of this textbook, you can find an extensive bibliography related to the different fields of application.

11.4 Therapeutic Contract

Before beginning music therapy treatment, it's important to inform the patient and share with him/her the details regarding the proposed treatment. The essential information to be shared includes the type of treatment, the location of sessions, the frequency and the duration of each session, the hypothesized (or already defined) duration of the treatment, and its objectives.

After sharing this information, it's necessary to ask the patient for his/her consent regarding the intervention. The manner of presentation/sharing of the intervention should be calibrated based on the type of possible interaction with the patient. In cases of cognitive or communicative impairments or in cases where patients are minors, the presence of a caregiver/family member is necessary for approval and to support the patient in the decision-making process.

11.5 Music Therapy Intervention

Music therapy intervention must consider some points regarding the therapeutic setting.

The setting should be considered not only as a physical and time space of the sessions: the setting is also a series of therapeutic rules that together create the framework of the intervention.

The size and other characteristics of the room, such as the brightness, sound insulation, etc., should be considered in addition to the temporal aspects in terms of:

- Duration of the treatment: In clinical settings, the duration of the treatments may not always be predetermined. Several factors can influence the duration, such as clinical conditions (length of patient's hospital stay, if institutionalized), economic factors (who supports the intervention).
- One study, for example, links 1–2 months music therapy treatment to a further improvement in the quality of life for people living with cancer (Li et al. 2020).

Frequently, the conclusion of the treatment will be made during the music therapy process based on the intervention evolution (see the paragraph on Conclusion of the treatment). In any case, this information should be shared with the patient and their reference figures.

- Duration of sessions: This information, like others, should be shared with the patient before starting the treatment. This data is subjected to the goals of the intervention, the patient's age and diagnosis, the severity of the disease, the type of proposed intervention (relational or rehabilitative interventions, music-based listening approaches, etc.), and whether it's an individual or group setting.
- Frequency of Sessions: It is important to determine, in relation to clinical objectives and the technique used, the frequency of music therapy sessions. In the case of rehabilitation, for example, it may be appropriate to intensify sessions up to 3 or more times a week. In the case of more "emotionally engaging" or activating interventions (receptive or improvisational music therapy), a latency period allowing asynchronous processing of the experience should be evaluated. Within this framework, the possibility of conducting cycling music therapy treatment, with wash-out periods, could be recommended, especially in the chronic diseases. This could prevent static and habituating situations (as supported by Raglio et al. 2010a, b in a music therapy study based on cycles of sessions).
- Individual or Group Session: Generally, group settings are favoured where needs related to sharing, socialization, and the needing not to expose the patient to an excessively intense relationship. The strategies adopted by the music therapist should consider the idea of the individual within a group, thus enhancing the relationship among participants by reinforcing each individual's resources. Conversely, individual settings allow for the deepening of objectives related to the individual's needs, enabling the adoption of specific strategies to explore the themes emerging from the objectives and the therapeutic relationship.

11.6 Process and Outcomes Evaluations

The monitoring within and outside the setting is a fundamental aspect of the therapeutic process, not strictly linked to the direction of the therapy evolution but also to make it more effective and personalized. Monitoring the process is already a way to collect data of clinical and research interest. Therefore, it is necessary to be aware of the method of assessment before starting of music therapy intervention to implement all conditions to make the monitoring effective and functional.

Intra-setting evaluations refer to all procedures aimed at verifying the progress of music therapy process observing dynamics and behaviors occurring during the sessions and through the treatment.

Evaluation tools include:

- Descriptive protocols: At the end of each session, the music therapist writes a report in chronological order, drawing main dynamics and behaviors observed during the session. Music therapists can describe verbal and nonverbal responses as accurately and neutrally as possible (noninterpretative way), evaluating them as positive or negative, considering clinical aspects and the consistency with music stimuli. Descriptive protocols can also include personal impressions, emotional feedback, and free associations, which are important for a global evaluation of the treatment and for a possible supervision.
- Structured tools: The music therapist may utilize a structured observation based on quantitative parameters or specific evaluation scales for music therapy intervention, choosing the tool that best suits the technique used, the clinical intervention context, and the level of detail requested but also the aims of the evaluations (e.g., Music Therapy Session Assessment Scale by Raglio et al. 2017 can be considered an example of this type of assessment concerning active music therapy approach). Other similar evaluation scales require observing the session later, through the sessions videorecording (e.g., Music Therapy Rating Scale by Raglio et al. 2011).
- Supervision: Supervision is an important moment that indirectly monitors the process by acting on the therapist's therapeutic strategies. The supervision can be crucial for modifying and regulating any dysfunctional therapist actions and/or to support the interpretation of the process. Supervision can be based on the therapist's reports, descriptive protocols, evaluation scales, or audio/video materials.

For extra-setting evaluations, we define all procedures aim at verifying the progress of treatment from a clinical perspective. The choice of extra-setting evaluation tools is linked to the clinical condition, the established clinical objectives, but also the patient's level of compliance. Normally, extra-setting evaluation is carried out by a clinician with whom it is important to share the expected results to identify the most appropriate outcome measures and tools.

Team meetings are another useful tool for extra-setting monitoring: a multidisciplinary perspective can help the music therapist and the team both to verify the effect of the treatment and to exchange information reciprocally concerning the patient.

Short-term evaluations may be important to evaluate the immediate effects of the treatment and parameters most sensitive to the early stages of therapeutic intervention; long-term evaluations are instead useful to verify the patient's changes over time. Long-term evaluations may also include follow-up evaluations planned after the end of the music therapy treatment aimed at verifying the maintenance of results obtained.

Another type of monitoring concerns the field of research in music therapy. These evaluations can include more objective outcome measures such as physiological parameters (e.g., heart and respiratory rate, oxygen saturation, blood pressure) (Lee et al. 2017; Parizek et al. 2023; Raglio et al. 2010a, b, 2022), biomarkers (e.g., salivary and plasma cortisol, salivary α-amylase detection) (Sliwka et al. 2021; Wong et al. 2021), or neuroimaging (e.g., functional magnetic resonance imaging, fMRI) (Pauwels et al. 2014; Raglio et al. 2016). This type of assessment is usually supported also by strong research methodologies that provide valuable insights of physiological and neurobiological effects of music therapy interventions, contributing to a deeper understanding of music therapy mechanisms in various clinical contexts.

11.7 The Conclusion of Music Therapy Treatment

The most natural factor determining the conclusion of treatment is the achievement of the predefined aims in relation to the patient's clinical change potential. When music therapy treatment can be considered concluded, it is advisable to continue the intervention for a limited period of time to consolidate and stabilize the changes and then to gradually conclude the intervention.

Another factor that can determine the end of music therapy treatment is the patient's self-disengagement (loss of motivation, appearance of personal or organizational problems) or the changes in his/her clinical and health conditions. In this case, and in the case of an institutionalized patient, worsening of clinical conditions requires their management and related pharmacological support (for example, bedridden, acute psychiatric episodes, etc.).

If such conditions are irreversible, the conclusion of treatment can be discussed; however, if they are temporary, a potential continuation of treatment can be reconsidered, adjusting therapeutic objectives if necessary. It is important to always consider the benefit of music therapy treatment for the patient and balance both the achievement of objectives and the potential effect of interruption.

However, the timing of conclusion should always be shared with the patient, caregivers, and relevant figures, and adequately prepared in advance to allow the patient to process the discontinuation of the intervention.

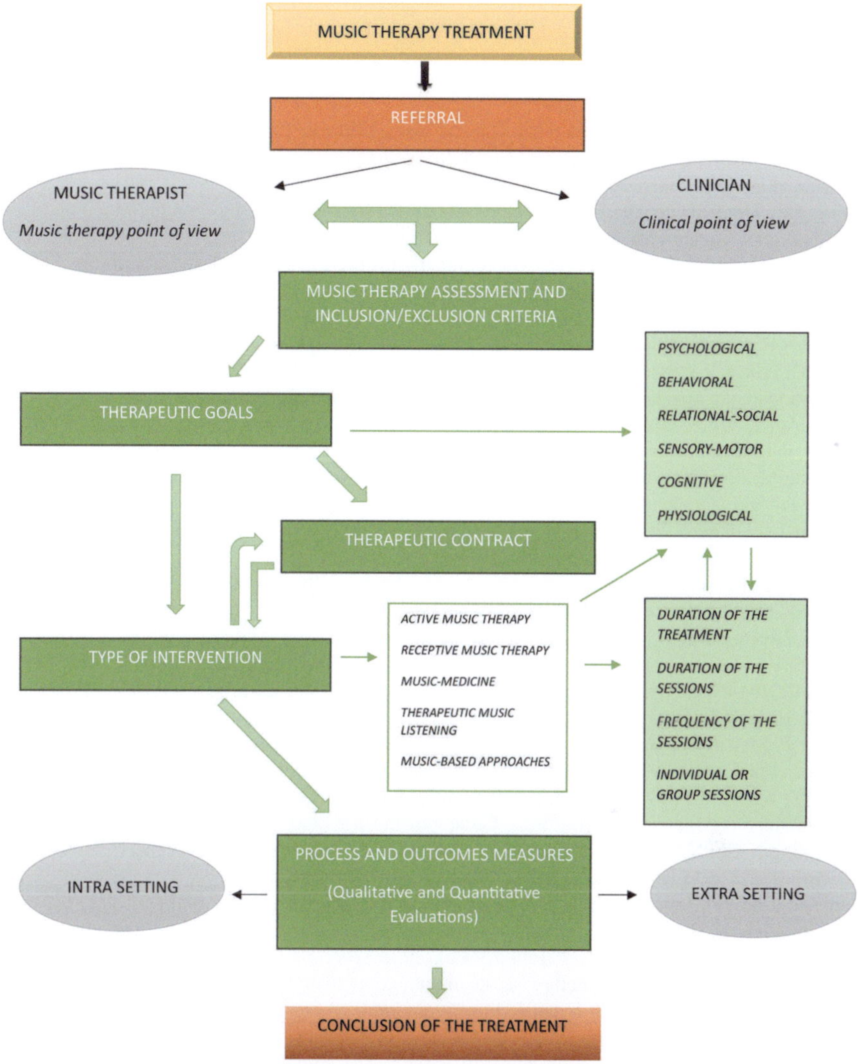

Fig. 11.1 Flow chart of Music therapy treatment: from referral to conclusion

Understanding the interplay between clinical conditions, treatment goals, therapeutic techniques, and the treatment setting is essential for making informed decisions about concluding a music therapy intervention. This comprehensive evaluation helps ensure that the conclusion of the treatment is both timely and beneficial for the individual receiving therapy (Fig. 11.1).

References

Aalbers S, Fusar-Poli L, Freeman RE, et al. Music therapy for depression. Cochrane Database of Syst Rev. 2017;11(11):CD004517.
Benenzon RO. La nueva musicoterapia. Buenos Aires: Editorial Lumen; 2008.
Bonny HL. Music and consciousness: The evolution of guided imagery and music. New Braunfels: Barcelona Publishers; 2002.
Burns DS. The Effect of the Bonny Method of Guided Imagery and Music on the Mood and Life Quality of Cancer Patients. J Music Ther. 2001;38(1):51–65.
Casarin J, Cromi A, Sgobbi B, et al. Music therapy for preoperative anxiety reduction in women undergoing total laparoscopic hysterectomy: a randomized controlled trial. J Minim Invasive Gynecol. 2021;28(9):1618–24.
Chanda ML, Levitin DJ. The neurochemistry of music. Trends Cogn Sci. 2013;17(4):179–93.
Colin C, Prince V, Bensoussan JL, et al. Music therapy for health workers to reduce stress, mental workload and anxiety: a systematic review. J Public Health. 2023;45(3):e532–41.
De Backer J, editor. The music in music therapy: Psychodynamic music therapy in Europe: clinical, theoretical and research approaches. London: Jessica Kingsley Publishers; 2014.
de Witte M, da Silva Pinho A, Stams G, et al. Music therapy for stress reduction: A systematic review and meta-analysis. Health Psychol Rev. 2022;16(1):134–59.
Erkkilä J, Punkanen M, Fachner J, et al. Individual music therapy for depression: randomised controlled trial. Br J Psychiatry. 2011;199:132–9.
Hars M, Herrmann FR, Gold G, et al. Effect of music-based multitask training on cognition and mood in older adults. Age Ageing. 2014;43:196–200.
Hole J, Hirsch M, Ball E, et al. Music as an aid for postoperative recovery in adults: a systematic review and meta-analysis. Lancet. 2015;386(10004):1659–71.
Kim J (2016) Psychodynamic music therapy. Voices World Forum Music Ther 16(2). https://doi.org/10.15845/voices.v16i2.2312
Köhler F, Martin ZS, Hertrampf RS, et al. Music therapy in the psychosocial treatment of adult cancer patients: a systematic review and meta-analysis. Front Psychol. 2020;11:2095.
Lee WP, Wu PY, Lee MY, et al. Music listening alleviates anxiety and physiological responses in patients receiving spinal anaesthesia. Complement Ther Med. 2017;31:8–13.
Li Y, Xing X, Shi X, et al. The effectiveness of music therapy for patients with cancer: a systematic review and meta-analysis. J Adv Nurs. 2020;76(5):1091–281.
Lin TH, Liao YC, Tam KW, et al. Effects of music therapy on cognition, quality of life, and neuropsychiatric symptoms of patients with dementia: a systematic review and meta-analysis of randomized controlled trials. Psychiatry Res. 2023;329:115498.
Lorber M, Divjak S. Music therapy as an intervention to reduce blood pressure and anxiety levels in older adults with hypertension: a randomized controlled trial. Res Gerontol Nurs. 2022;15(2):85–92.
Lotter C, van Staden W. Verbal affordances of active and receptive music therapy methods in major depressive disorder and schizophrenia-spectrum disorder. Arts Psychother. 2019;64:59–65.
Lu G, Jia R, Liang D, et al. Effects of music therapy on anxiety: a meta-analysis of randomized controlled trials. Psychiatry Res. 2021;304:114137.
McFerran K, Grocke D. Receptive music therapy: techniques, clinical applications and new perspectives. 2nd ed. London: Jessica Kingsley Publishers; 2022.
Monsalve-Duarte S, Betancourt-Zapata W, Suarez-Cañon N, et al. Music therapy and music medicine interventions with adult burn patients: a systematic review and meta-analysis. Burns. 2022;48:510–21.
Nordoff P, Robbins C. Creative music therapy: a guide to fostering clinical musicianship. New Braunfels: Barcelona Publishers; 2007.
Parizek D, Visnovcova N, Hamza Sladicekova K. Effect of selected music soundtracks on cardiac vagal control and complexity assessed by heart rate variability. Physiol Res. 2023;72:587–96.

Park JI, Lee IH, Lee SJ, et al. Effects of music therapy as an alternative treatment on depression in children and adolescents with ADHD by activating serotonin and improving stress coping ability. BMC Complement Ther. 2023;23(1):73.

Paul N, Lotter C, van Staden W. Patient reflections on individual music therapy for a major depressive disorder or acute phase schizophrenia spectrum disorder. J Music Ther. 2020;57(2):168–92.

Pauwels EKJ, Volterrani D, Mariani G, et al. Mozart, music and medicine. Med Princ Pract. 2014;23(5):403–12.

Raglio A. Music and neurorehabilitation: yes, we can! Funct Neurol. 2018;33(4):173–4.

Raglio A, Bellelli G, Traficante D, et al. Efficacy of music therapy treatment based on cycles of sessions: a randomised controlled trial. Aging Ment Health. 2010a;14(8):900–4.

Raglio A, Oasi O, Gianotti M, et al. Effects of music therapy on psychological symptoms and heart rate variability in patients with dementia: a pilot study. Curr Aging Sci. 2010b;3(3):242–6.

Raglio A, Traficante D, Oasi O. The evaluation of music therapy process in the intersubjective perspective: the music therapy rating scale. Pragmat Obs Res. 2011;2:19–23.

Raglio A, Filippi S, Bellandi D, et al. Global music approach to persons with dementia: evidence and practice. Clin Interv Aging. 2014;6(9):1669–76.

Raglio A, Bellandi D, Baiardi P, et al. Effect of active music therapy and individualized listening to music on dementia: a multicenter randomized controlled trial. J Am Geriatr Soc. 2015;63(8):1534–9.

Raglio A, Galandra C, Sibilla L, et al. Effects of active music therapy on the normal brain: fMRI based evidence. Brain Imaging Behav. 2016;10(1):182–6.

Raglio A, Gnesi M, Monti MC, et al. The Music Therapy Session Assessment Scale (MT-SAS): validation of a new tool for music therapy process evaluation. Clin Psychol Psychother. 2017;24(6):O1547–61.

Raglio A, Bellandi D, Gianotti M, et al. Daily music listening to reduce work-related stress: a randomized controlled pilot trial. J Public Health. 2020;42(1):e81–7.

Raglio A, Bellandi D, Manzoni L, et al. Communication improvement reduces BPSD: a music therapy study based on artificial neural networks. Neurol Sci. 2021a;42:2103–6.

Raglio A, Castelli M, Manzoni L, Vico F. What happens if algorithmic music meets medicine. G Ital Med Lav Ergon. 2021b;43(4):379–81.

Raglio A, Maestri R, Robbi E, et al. Effect of algorithmic music listening on cardiac autonomic nervous system activity: an exploratory, randomized crossover study. J Clin Med. 2022;11(19):5738.

Raglio A. A novel music-based therapeutic approach: the Therapeutic Music Listening. Front Hum Neurosci. 2023;17:1204593.

Särkämö T, Tervaniemi M, Laitinen S, et al. Music listening enhances cognitive recovery and mood after middle cerebral artery stroke. Brain. 2008;131(Pt 3):866–76.

Sheikh-Wu SF, Kauffman MA, Anglade D, et al. Effectiveness of different music interventions on managing symptoms in cancer survivors: a meta-analysis. Eur J Oncol Nurs. 2021;52:101968.

Shi Z, Wang S, Chen M, et al. The effect of music therapy on language communication and social skills in children with autism spectrum disorder: a systematic review and meta-analysis. Front Psychol. 2024;15:1336421.

Sliwka A, Kaszuba M, Piliński R, et al. The comparison between pulmonary rehabilitation with music therapy and pulmonary rehabilitation alone on respiratory drive, cortisol level and asthma control in patients hospitalized with asthma exacerbation. J Asthma. 2021;58(10):1367–76.

Solanki MS, Zafar M, Rastogi R. Music as a therapy: role in psychiatry. Asian J Psychiatr. 2013;6(3):193–9.

Stanczyk MM. Music therapy in supportive cancer care. Rep Pract Oncol Radiother. 2011;16(5):170–2.

Thaut M, Hoember V. Handbook of neurologic music therapy. Oxford: Oxford University Press; 2014.

Tsirigoti A, Georgiadi M. The efficacy of music therapy programs on the development of social communication in children with autism spectrum disorder: a systematic review. Educ Sci. 2024;14:373.

Umbrello M, Sorrenti T, Mistraletti G, et al. Music therapy reduces stress and anxiety in critically ill patients: a systematic review of randomized clinical trials. Minerva Anestesiol. 2019;85(8):886–98.

van der Steen JT, van Soest-Poortvliet MC, van der Wouden JC, et al. Music-based therapeutic interventions for people with dementia. Cochrane Database Syst Rev. 2017;5(5):CD003477.

Wang R, Huang X, Wang Y, et al. Non-pharmacologic approaches in preoperative anxiety, a comprehensive review. Front Public Health. 2022;10:854673.

Weise L, Jakob E, Töpfer NF, et al. Study protocol: individualized music for people with dementia – improvement of quality of life and social participation for people with dementia in institutional care. BMC Geriatr. 2018;18(1):313.

Wheeler BL, editor. Music therapy handbook. New York: The Guilford Press; 2015.

Wong HLC, Lopez-Nahas V, Molassiotis A. Effects of music therapy on anxiety in ventilator-dependent patients. Heart Lung. 2001;30(5):376–87.

Wong MM, Tahir T, Wong MM, et al. Biomarkers of stress in music interventions: a systematic review. J Music Ther. 2021;58(3):241–77.

Part V

Fields of Application

Music Therapy and Music-Based Interventions in Neurology and Neurological Rehabilitation

12

Eckart Altenmüller

Key Points

- Music therapy and music-based interventions in neurology and neurological rehabilitation are efficient.
- They take advantage from music-induced neuroplasticity and from music's ability to relieve stress.
- Music can induce powerful biographic memories and thus reduce anxiety and improve quality of life in dementia.
- Music-supported therapy after stroke leads to neuroplastic changes in sensorimotor-auditory networks of the cerebral cortex.
- In aphasia, melodic intonation therapy with singing of phrases and thus augmenting prosodic transitions, reducing speech rate, and emphasizing rhythmic elements is frequently beneficial.
- Music-supported therapy in Parkinson's disease activates rhythmic oscillators in the basal ganglia and supports motivation. It improves stride length and speed of gait.
- Individualized music therapy in neurodegenerative disorders improves quality of life in patients and caregivers.
- Music therapy needs to be more strongly included among the non-pharmacological therapies in neurological disorders.

E. Altenmüller (✉)
Institute of Music Physiology and Musicians' Medicine (IMMM), University of Music, Drama and Media, Hanover, Germany
e-mail: eckart.altenmueller@hmtm-hannover.de

A. Raglio (ed.), *Music and Music Therapy Interventions in Clinical Practice*, Neurocultural Health and Wellbeing,
https://doi.org/10.1007/978-3-031-88578-5_12

12.1 Introduction and Definitions

The healing powers of music have been recognized for thousands of years. In early shamanistic societies, illness was viewed as originating from magico-religious forces or from the breaking of taboos (for review, see Bunt 2014) and music was considered to be efficacious in exorcising disease and healing wounds. Greek Philosophers, such as Plato, ascribed music powerful effects and it is notable that Apollo, the god of the healing powers and of science, was also the patron of music and the arts, referring to the close relationships between these disciplines (Thaut 2015). It was not until the second half of the nineteenth century—at a time when scientific medicine was becoming established—that research into the effects of music on mental disease began (Horden 2000). The term "music therapy" was introduced a century later, when mechanisms underlying the healing effects of music began to be systematically studied (Thaut 2015). While music's efficacy for the treatment of psychiatric conditions such as anxiety and depression was an early consideration, the application of music to treat neurological conditions began in earnest in the 1980s. A key development in this regard was the establishment, by the German–American music therapist and researcher, Michael Thaut, of a subdiscipline of music therapy termed "Neurologic Music Therapy" comprising "music-supported therapy in neuro-rehabilitation" (Thaut and Hoemberg 2014).

In this chapter, we define *"Music therapy and music-based interventions" as clinical, evidence-based interventions using music to improve motor, sensory, cognitive, and emotional functions following central nervous injury and/or degeneration.* The underlying scientific paradigm is music-induced functional brain plasticity, reinforced by motivational factors linked to music listening and music making. In contrast, "music therapy" is defined as "the clinical and evidence-based use of music interventions to accomplish individualized goals within a therapeutic relationship by a qualified professional who has completed an approved music therapy program" (https://www.musictherapy.org/about/ AMTA). In this definition, the emphasis is on the therapeutic relationship and the specific qualifications of music therapists, such as combining psychotherapeutic expertise with practical musical skills. These may be constituents of music-supported therapy in neurorehabilitation, but also enable trained music therapists to apply music in many other clinical settings, such as psychiatric diseases, neurodevelopmental disorders, genetic disorders, and palliative care. Therefore, "music therapy" has many more indications and its professional application would require a far more comprehensive treatment than this chapter permits.

12.2 Neurobiological Foundations of Music Interventions

Music is one of the richest human emotional, sensorimotor, and cognitive experiences. It involves listening, watching, feeling, moving and coordinating, remembering, and expecting musical elements. It is frequently accompanied by strong emotions resulting in joy, happiness, and bittersweet sadness or even in overwhelming bodily reactions like tears in the eyes or shivers down the spine. Correspondingly, many cortical and subcortical brain regions are involved in music-listening and music-making activities (for reviews see: Altenmüller and Furuya 2017; Stewart 2008).

Primary and secondary regions in the cerebral cortex are critical for any conscious perception of sensory information, be it auditory, visual, or somatosensory. However, music also influences and changes activity in multisensory and motor integration regions in frontal, parietal, and temporo-occipital brain regions (Bangert et al. 2006). The frontal lobe is involved in the guidance of attention, in planning and motor preparation, in integrating auditory and motor information, and in specific human skills such as imitation and empathy (Haslinger et al. 2005). Multisensory integration regions in the parietal lobe and temporo-occipital areas integrate different sensory inputs from the auditory, visual, and somatosensory system into a combined sensory impression; it is this multisensory brain representation which constitutes the typical musical experience (Brown et al. 2015). The basal ganglia and the cerebellum also play a critical role in musical experience. Basal ganglia are crucial for motor learning, timing, and emotional integration, whereas the cerebellum is important not only for motor coordination but also plays an important role in various cognitive tasks especially when they include demands on timing (Paquette et al. 2017). Typically, basal ganglia and cerebellum are activated in rhythm processing or tapping in synchrony with an external pacemaker such as a metronome (Nozaradan et al. 2017). Finally, the emotional network, subserved by the limbic system, is crucial for the emotional perception of music and therefore for an individual's motivation to listen to or to engage in any musical activity (Salimpoor et al. 2009, for a review on this topic: Wan and Schlaug 2010).

12.3 Musical Training Induces Brain Plasticity

During the past three decades, brain imaging has provided important insights into the enormous capacity of the human brain to adapt, via neural plasticity, to complex demands in healthy individuals of all ages. Plasticity can include morphological change, as in the generation of new synapses and new neurons as well as functional change, where the strength of synaptic connections can be altered (for a review see Belzung and Wigmore 2013). Long-term training and the accompanying development of expertise characterize numerous domains (sports, music, and chess to name a few) (Ericsson and Smith 1991). Since this chapter focuses on the potential for rehabilitation to draw on aspects of music making, this section emphasizes the adaptations that have been found to accompany the development of expertise in high-level musicians.

Briefly summarizing (but see Altenmüller and Schlaug 2013 and Criscuolo et al. 2022): comparison of the brain anatomy of skilled musicians with that of nonmusicians shows that prolonged instrumental practice leads to an enlargement of the hand area in the motor cortex (Amunts et al. 1997). Furthermore, Gaser and Schlaug (2003) could demonstrate enhancement of grey matter density in cortical sensorimotor regions, auditory regions, the left dorsolateral prefrontal cortex, and in the cerebellum in professional instrumentalists as compared to nonmusicians and amateurs. These adaptations of brain structures are accompanied by behaviorally relevant improvements of fine finger coordination and two-point discrimination abilities (Ragert et al. 2003), enhanced auditory working memory (Schneider et al. 2002), and precision of timing (Furuya et al. 2015). Interestingly, musicians who start early, before the age of seven, do not display these structural adaptations of the brain at least in the sensorimotor cortices and the callosal fibers; however, they seem to have an "early optimized network," which allows superior performance of motor tasks without enlarged anatomical structures (Steele et al. 2013; Vaquero et al. 2016). This phenomenon is termed "Metaplasticity." It refers to neural changes that are induced by activity in early age and that persist and optimize subsequent brain adaptations (Altenmüller and Furuya 2016). In contrast, later starters, after age seven do show the abovementioned structural adaptations accounting for the effects observed in many morphological brain imaging studies (e.g., Bangert and Schlaug 2006; Gärtner et al. 2013).

In addition to focusing on structural measures such as grey matter density, several studies have investigated measures that related to structural connectivity between brain regions. Using diffusion tensor imaging (DTI)—a technique that allows for the reconstruction of white matter tracts and the characterization of their microstructural status using diffusivity measures, such as fractional anisotropy (FA)—Bengtsson and her colleagues (Bengtsson et al. 2005) and more recently Rueber et al. (2015) found structural differences in the corticospinal tract, particularly in the posterior limb of the internal capsule, between musicians and nonmusicians as well as within musicians' groups (keyboard players compared to string players). Halwani et al. (2011)—also using DTI—reported differences in macrostructure and microstructure of the arcuate fasciculus (AF)—a prominent white-matter tract connecting temporal and frontal brain regions—between singers, instrumentalists, and nonmusicians. Thus, structural changes to white matter tracts are not only altered by musical training per se, but by the precise sensorimotor demands of the type of musical training (according to instrument) and—as has been shown in behavioral tests, these morphological adaptations can also be accompanied by faster reaction times and improved coordination (2017).

The above findings serve to illustrate the potential for musical training to result in structural and functional adaptations across a number of different brain areas and their connections. It is relevant to note that such changes are not only restricted to individuals who have undergone musical training over a period of years but have also been observed through longitudinal studies incorporating relatively short periods of training (e.g., Hyde et al. 2009; Stewart et al. 2003). Furthermore, these changes are not restricted to children or adolescents but apply also for seniors. In the largest longitudinal study on 156 senior novices, half of them receiving one-year weekly piano instruction and two hours weekly homework, and half of them participating in a course, aiming at deepening music-listening behaviors and understanding of music we could demonstrate remarkable signs of plasticity with respect to reduced grey matter loss in temporal and limbic brain areas and improved connectivity, specifically in auditory-motor networks (Worschech et al. 2022; Jünemann et al. 2023).

Given that active music-based rehabilitation involves multiple components analogous to training and music learning (i.e., iterated practice of movements coupled with auditory feedback and extensive cognitive processing), it is reasonable to suggest that some of the principles of music training-induced plasticity can be usefully exploited through the use of music-supported therapy in neurorehabilitation.

It should be noted that patients who are receiving music-supported therapy are not only *producing* aspects of music through their movement, they are also *perceiving* the music they produce (in addition to any live or recorded accompaniment that may be part of the protocol). The perception of music can elicit powerful feelings of pleasure, and studies have shown that such experiences (most dramatically seen during musical 'shivers' down the spine) strongly activate the dopaminergic mesolimbic system (for a review see Zatorre 2015). Dopamine release has been shown to have demonstrable effects on the strength of synaptic connections (Wickens et al. 2003). In a similar vein, music's anxiolytic properties are well known (see Nilsson 2008 for a review) and responses to music can produce measurable cardiovascular and endocrine responses, indicated by reduced serum cortisol levels and inhibition of cardiovascular stress reactions (Okada et al. 2009; Bradt et al. 2013). In animal models, prolonged stress can have maladaptive effects on neuroplasticity, such as dendritic atrophy, synapse loss, and decreased hippocampal neurogenesis (Radley et al. 2015), while elevated cortisol levels in patients with acute stroke correlate with increased infarct volume, and increases the risk of depression, poor prognosis, and fatal outcome (Douven et al. 2017). Hence, bearing in mind that that music is perceived as well as produced in music-support therapy, it may be that the potential of music to evoke both pleasure and reduce anxiety may confer particular benefits for sensorimotor learning and plasticity, though this remains to be empirically tested.

12.4 Music-Supported Motor Therapy in Upper Limb Dysfunction in Stroke Patients

In a comprehensive review, we identified seven controlled studies that evaluated the efficacy of music as an add-on therapy in stroke rehabilitation (Sihvonen et al. 2017). In these studies, training of finger dexterity of the paretic hand was done using either a piano-keyboard or, for wrist movements, drum-pads tuned to a c-major scale. Furthermore, in one study sonification of proximal arm movements was applied (see below for details). These patients had never played a musical instrument before. The main outcome measures were standard motor tests (e.g., Fugl-Meyer assessment [FMA], Box and Block test [BBT], Nine-hole Pegboard test [NHPT], Action Research Arm Test [ARAT], Arm-Paresis Score [APS], for review see Lindmark 1988). Furthermore, mood, cognitive performance, quality of life (QoL), and speech abilities were often also assessed. In upper extremity paresis, music-supported therapy (MST) aiming at rehabilitation of fine motor hand skills was first systematically investigated by Schneider et al. (2007). The setting included initially eight drum pads digitally set up to produce piano sounds and the drums forming a major scale. Patients had to tap with the paretic hands on the drum pads. As the patients progressed from tapping single sounds to well-known simple melodies, such as children songs or the "Ode to Joy," they were transferred to a digital keyboard and had to perform individuated finger movements on the keyboard, again stepwise including technically more demanding melodies, i.e., more complicated sequences of finger flexions and extensions. To prevent spasticity, it was helpful to support the paretic forearm of the patients.

The superiority of the music group (MG) over fine motor training without music (TG) and over conventional physiotherapy (PT) was evident after intervention containing five 30-minute sessions per week for three weeks. Scoring of the BBT improved by 14 in the MG (2 TG, 1.8 PT), NHPT by 1,2 (TG = 0.2, PT, 0.15), ARAT by 9 (TG 1.2, PT 2.3), and APS by 2,4 (TG 1, PT 0.8). In order to obtain a measure of statistical significance, the effect sizes were determined using Cohen's *d*. In the literature, effect sizes of 0.2 are considered small, effect sizes of 0.4–0.6 moderate, and effect sizes above 0.8 large. In the music group, effect sizes concerning improvements in behavioral tests varied between 0.66 and 0.34. In both control groups effect sizes were very small, with values between 0.01 and 0.14. The beneficial effect seen in the music group can be specifically attributed to the musical component of the training rather than the motor training per se, since patients practicing with mute instruments remained inferior to the music group. Here, FMA was applied before and after 20 sessions of either music-supported therapy on a keyboard or equivalent therapy without sound. FMA scores of the motor functions of the upper limb improved by 16 in the music group and by 5 in the control group, both improvements being statistically significant although to a lesser degree in the control group ($p = 0.02$ vs. $p = 0.04$) (Tong et al. 2015).

Regarding the neurophysiological basis of behavioral improvement, it was demonstrated that patients undergoing music-supported therapy not only regained their motor abilities at a faster rate but also improved in timing, precision, and smoothness of fine motor skills as well as showing increases in neuronal connectivity between sensorimotor and auditory cortex assessed by means of EEG-coherence measures (Altenmüller et al. 2009; Schneider et al. 2010). The establishment of an auditory-sensorimotor co-representation can therefore be suggested to be an important prerequisite to these improvements (see Fig. 12.1).

The importance of establishing an audio-sensorimotor co-representation in rehabilitation is corroborated by findings from a patient who underwent music-supported training 20 months after suffering a stroke. Along with clinical improvement, fMRI follow-up demonstrated activation of motor and premotor areas, when listening to simple piano tunes, thus providing additional evidence for the establishment of an auditory-sensory motor co-representation due to the training procedure (Rojo et al. 2012). In a larger group of 20 chronic stroke patients, an increase in motor cortex excitability following a four-week intervention with the same method was demonstrated using transcranial magnetic stimulation (TMS). These changes were accompanied by marked improvements of fine motor skills (Amengual et al. 2013). The authors argue that the increased excitability demonstrated by the enlargement of MEP amplitudes might be explained by an increase of the strength of synaptic transmission rather than a reduction in the threshold of the membrane potential. These results are coherent with previous studies demonstrating the effects on the

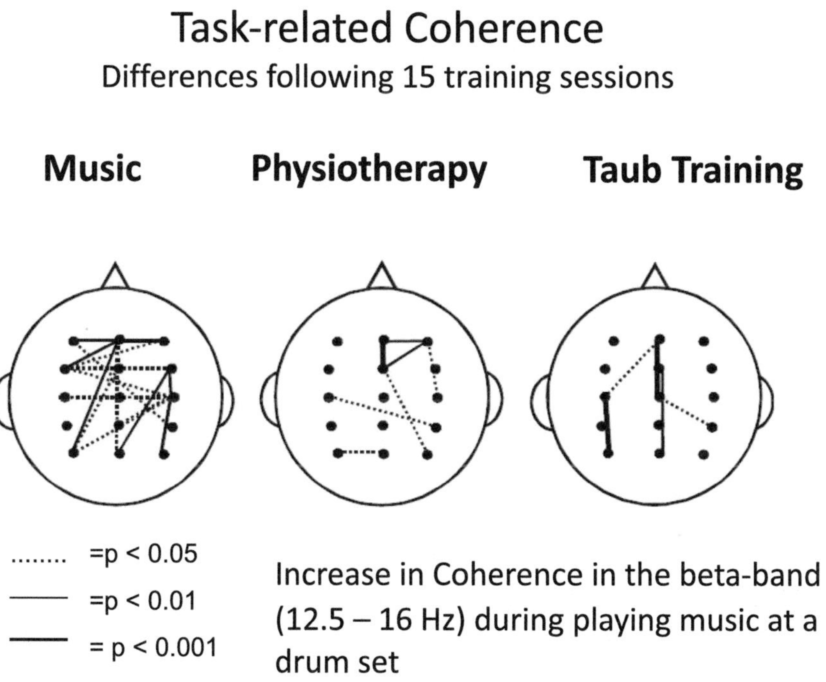

Fig. 12.1 Topographic task-related coherence maps for the Music group compared to the physiotherapy control group without sound and the fine motor training according to the principles auf Taub during self-paced arm movements for the drum pad condition in the beta band (12,5–16 Hz). Statistically significant increases in task-related coherence during the motor performance after 3 weeks and 15 sessions of music supported therapy on sonified drum pads are displayed

modulation of the strength of synaptic plasticity within the motor cortex during the learning of new skill (Pascual-Leone 1995).

However, the situation in chronic stroke patients seems to be more complex. Fujioka and colleagues (Fujioka et al. 2018) could demonstrate, in a 10-week-long randomized controlled trial (RCT), including 14 patients with music-supported therapy (MG) and 14 patients with conventional physiotherapy (CG), that both groups only showed minor improvements. As behavioral measures, the Chedoke McMaster Stroke Assessment (CMSA) and the ARAT were applied. The former improved by 0.2 in both, the MG and CG group, and the ARAT score improved by 0.2 in the MG and by 0.05 in the CG. As expected, effect sizes according to Cohen's *d* were very small, between 0.15 and 0.25, and the music group showed merely a tendency toward better performance in the ARAT-test ($p = 0.08$) as compared to the control group. However, the music group performed significantly better in the trail-making test indicating an improvement in cognitive flexibility and furthermore showed enhanced social and communal participation in the Stroke Impairment Scale and in the PANAS (Positive and Negative Affect Schedule, Watson et al. 1988), again lending support to the prosocial effects of music. In another, shorter, RCT with an intervention of only four weeks, Grau Sanchez and colleagues (2018) demonstrated no superiority on fine motor skills in the music group as compared to a control group, but also an increase in general QoL as assessed by the Profile of Mood states (POMS, MG: 7–4, CG: unchanged) (Curran et al. 1995) and the stroke specific QoL questionnaire, MG: 180–185, unchanged in the CG (Alonso et al. 1995).

During the Corona Pandemic, enriched music-supported therapy (eMST) was introduced. This consisted of a 10-week program of home-based musical training doing three weekly individual self-training sessions using an APP (eMST-App) and one weekly group music therapy led by a music therapist on ZOOM. In an RCT involving 58 chronic stroke patients (26 Verum, 32 Controls), the eMST protocol demonstrated superior outcomes in the motor improvement of upper-limb mobility and—importantly—greater improvements in emotional well-being as compared to a purely motor training program (Segura et al. 2024).

As a further development, movement sonification therapy is promising (Scholz et al. 2015). Gross movements of the arm are transformed into discrete sounds, providing continuous feedback in a melodic way, tuned to a major scale (i.e., patients could use movements of their paretic arms as a musical instrument, see Fig. 12.2). Here, sound perception could substitute for defective proprioception. Sonification therapy reduced joint pain in the Fugl-Meyer pain subscale (MG difference to CG by −10; $d = 1.96$) and improved smoothness of movement ($d = 1.16$)

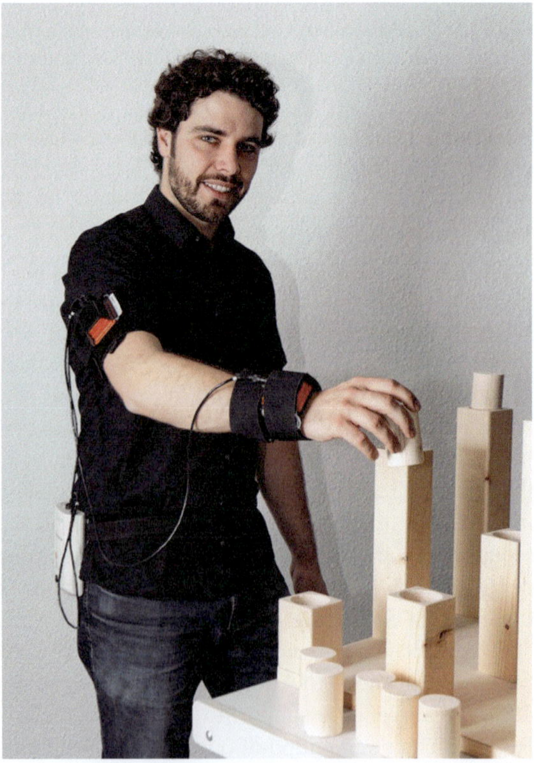

Fig. 12.2 Sonification of arm-movements. The device contains a movement sensor applied to the forearm and upper arm (Xsense [(R)]) and allows to transform movements into music coding the vertical axis into pitch, the horizontal axis into timbre and the z-axis into loudness. This way, the paretic arm is transformed into a simple musical instrument, allowing to "move" tunes. (With permission of Prof. Dr. Scholz)

more than movement therapy without sound (Scholz et al. 2016; Nikmaram et al. 2019). These positive results were confirmed in a large RCT by Raglio et al. (2021).

Summarizing effects for the rehabilitation of the upper limb after stroke, music-supported training is undoubtedly efficient and seems to be more helpful than functional motor training using no auditory feedback, but otherwise similar fine motor training. With respect to the underlying mechanisms, a number of open questions still remain. First, the role of motivational factors must be clarified. From the patients' informal descriptions of their experience with the music-supported training, it appears that this was highly enjoyable and a highlight of their rehabilitation process, regardless of the form of auditory stimulation, be it piano tones, or sonification of movement with other timbres. Thus, as already explored in the first part of this chapter, motivational and emotional factors might have contributed to the success of the training program (Särkämö et al. 2008; Chang et al. 2020).

Another issue is related to the auditory feedback mechanisms. Up to now it has not been clarified whether any auditory feedback (e.g., simple beep tones) would have a similar effect on fine motor rehabilitation or whether explicit musical parameters such as a sophisticated pitch and time structure are prerequisites for the success of the training. This has to be addressed in a study comparing the effects of musical feedback compared to simple acoustic feedback. With respect to the latter, according to a study by Thaut et al. (2002), simple rhythmic cueing with a metronome significantly improves the spatiotemporal precision of reaching movements in stroke patients.

Furthermore, it is not clear whether timing regularity and predictability are crucial for the beneficial effect of music-supported therapy using tapping on drum pads or playing on a keyboard. Although it has been argued that the effectiveness of this therapy relies on the fact that the patient's brain receives time-locked auditory feedback with each movement, new results challenge this viewpoint. Van Vugt et al. (2016) studied 15 patients in early stroke rehabilitation with no previous musical background. They learned to play simple finger exercises and familiar children's songs on the piano. The participants were assigned to one of two groups: in the *normal* group, the keyboard emitted a tone immediately at keystroke, in the *delay* group, the tone was delayed by a random time interval between 100 and 600 ms. To assess recovery, standard clinical tests such as the nine-hole-pegboard test and index finger tapping speed and regularity were used. Surprisingly, patients in the delay group improved in the nine-hole-pegboard test (time to complete difference—5.63; Cohen's $d = 0.64$), whereas patients in the normal group did not (time to complete—2.11). In finger tapping rate and regularity, both groups showed improvements (reduction of inter-tap-interval in the music group from 396 to 333 ms, albeit to a lesser degree than in the normal group (from 398 to 292, Cohen's d between 0.32 and 0.29). The normal group showed reduced depression whereas the delay group did not. Thus, music-supported therapy even with a randomly delayed keyboard can improve motor recovery after stroke, possibly because patients in the delayed feedback group implicitly learn to be independent of the auditory feedback and therefore outperform those in the normal condition when auditory feedback is not available.

Future research should address the long-term sustainability of improvements and strive to optimize the length and number of training sessions, according to patients' needs and preferences. Most probably, a client-tailored treatment algorithm considering the severity of impairment, psychological status, and motivational drive will be most efficient.

12.5 Music-Supported Motor Therapy in Rehabilitation of Gait in Stroke Patients

With respect to *gait and lower limb malfunction*, simple rhythmic cueing with either a metronome or another sound-producing device has been applied. Since this is related to musical timing, we subsume this method under music-supported motor therapy, although pitches and timbres are not varied and therefore important musical parameters are not included in this form of rehabilitation strategy. Furthermore, it is hypothesized that the mechanisms of action are more related to temporal organization of motor output and less to the emotional and motivational aspects of motor rehabilitation. Thus, rhythmic auditory cueing (RAC) may act on cerebellar and basal ganglia networks involved in the timing of movement organization. In a study by Thaut et al. (2007), a three-week training program for hemiparetic stroke patients reported an increase in gait speed for the rhythmic cueing group by 129%, while conventional physiotherapy resulted in an 88% increase. Stride length increased by 66% (vs. 46%), cadence by 54% (vs. 22%), and walking symmetry by 39% (vs. 20%). Another group reported that rhythmic cueing increased stride length by 18% (vs. 0%), reduced asymmetry by 58% (vs. 20%), increased gait speed by 27% (vs. 4%), and increased length of foot contact to surface by 28% (vs. 11%) (Schauer and Mauritz 2003). In a meta-analysis, positive effects of music on gait velocity and stride length have been confirmed (Yoo and Kim 2016): Analyzing a total of 10 randomized or clinical controlled trials with 356 individuals included, large effect sizes were reported concerning walking velocity (increase in RAC vs control by 0,3 m/s; Hedges's $g = 0.98$), cadence (increase in steps per minute by 9 steps in RAC vs. control; Hedges's $g = 0.84$), and stride length (increase in RAC vs control by 5 cm 0.76). Additional subgroup analysis demonstrated that although the type of rhythmic cueing and stage of stroke did not lead to statistically substantial group differences, the effect sizes and heterogeneity values in each subgroup implied differences in treatment effect, depending on loudness, timbre, and sound structure of the rhythmic cueing. Recent progress was reached by an autonomous rehabilitation system that combines the closed-loop control of music with real-time gait analysis to fully automate patient-tailored walking rehabilitation. Specifically, the mechanism of action of auditory-motor entrainment was applied to induce targeted changes in the post-stroke gait pattern and obtain more symmetry in the walking pattern. This led to remarkable improvements in 10 individuals with chronic post-stroke hemiparesis (Collimore et al. 2023)

12.6 Music in the Rehabilitation of Aphasia: Melodic Intonation Therapy

While the close links between music and movement make motor rehabilitation an obvious avenue for music-supported rehabilitation, recovery of language can also benefit from a music-supported approach. Aphasia is a common and devastating complication of stroke or other brain injuries that results in the loss of ability to produce and/or comprehend language. It has been estimated that between 24% and 52% of acute stroke patients have some form of aphasia if tested within 7 days of their stroke; 12% of survivors still have significant aphasia at 6 months after stroke (63).

Based on clinical observations that patients with severe nonfluent aphasia can sing lyrics better than they can speak the same words, an intonation-based therapy called Melodic Intonation Therapy (MIT) was first developed by Albert and colleagues in the 1970s of the last century (Albert et al. 1973; Sparks and Holland 1976) and recently further elaborated by the Gottfried Schlaug and colleagues (Schlaug et al. 2010; Wan et al. 2010). The two unique components of MIT are first the intonation of words and simple phrases using a melodic contour that follows the prosody of speech, and second the rhythmic tapping of the left hand that accompanies the production of each syllable and serves as a catalyst for fluency. Thus, MIT emphasizes melody and contour and engages a sensorimotor network of articulation on the unaffected (usually right) hemisphere through rhythmic tapping.

To date, studies using MIT have produced positive outcomes in patients with nonfluent aphasia. These outcomes range from improvements on the Boston Diagnostic Aphasia Examination (BDAE; Goodglass and Kaplan 1983), to improvements in articulation and phrase production (increase in syllable production/minute after 40 sessions in the MIT group by 200% group vs. 120% in the CG; Bonakdarpour et al. 2000; Wilson et al. 2006) after treatment. The effectiveness of this intervention is further demonstrated in a study that examined the transfer of language skills to untrained contexts. Schlaug et al. (2008) compared the effects of MIT with a control intervention (speech repetition) on picture naming performance and measures of propositional speech. After 40 daily sessions, both therapy techniques resulted in significant improvement on all outcome measures, but the extent of this improvement was far greater for the patient who underwent MIT compared to the one who underwent the control therapy. These positive effects were also confirmed by Raglio et al. (2016) as well as in an enlarged treatment program, including breathing and awareness exercises (Jungblut and Aldridge 2004). A recent comprehensive meta-analysis of 22 RCTs (Popescu et al. 2022) found progress on validated tests mainly from gains in repetition tasks rather than other domains of verbal expression, such as everyday communication ability. Interestingly, effect sizes for non-RCT data decreased with number of months post-stroke, suggesting confounding through spontaneous recovery. Deviation from the original MIT protocol did not systematically alter benefit from treatment.

The therapeutic effect of MIT is also evident in neuroimaging studies that show reorganization of brain functions. MIT resulted in increased activation in a right-hemisphere network involving the premotor, inferior frontal, and temporal lobes (Schlaug et al. 2009), as well as increased fiber number and volume of the arcuate fasciculus in the right hemisphere (Wan et al. 2014) suggesting an increased audio-motor connectivity of the right hemisphere; these findings demonstrate that intensive therapies such as MIT—when applied over a longer period of time in chronic stroke patients—can induce functional and structural brain changes in a right hemisphere vocal-motor network, and these changes are related to speech output improvements.

The mechanisms underlying the recovery-enhancing effects of MIT are not completely clear. Four possible mechanisms by which MIT's therapeutic effect is achieved have been discussed (for details, see Wan and Schlaug 2010): (1) *reduction of speed* to approximately one syllable/sec, which may specifically engage right hemisphere perceptual and perception-action coupling, since the right hemisphere has been shown to integrate sensory information over a larger time window than the left hemisphere (Abrams et al. 2008; Poeppel 2003); (2) *syllable lengthening* that isolates/emphasizes individual phonemes even as they remain part of the continuously voiced words/phrases; and (3) *"chunking"* that not only combines prosodic information with meaningful content to facilitate production of longer, more fluent phrases, but has also been shown to lead to more right than left hemisphere activation in healthy subjects (Ozdemir et al. 2006; Meyer et al. 2002). Given that patients with right hemisphere lesions have greater difficulty with global processing tasks (e.g., melody and contour processing) than those with left hemisphere lesions (Peretz 1990; Schuppert et al. 2000). It is possible that the melodic element of MIT does indeed engage the right hemisphere, particularly the right temporal lobe, more than therapies that do not make use of tonal information or melodic contour, and again intervention that would integrate information over a larger timescale favoring right over left hemispheric processing (Abrams et al. 2008). The fourth mechanism—*Left hand-tapping (one tap/syllable, one syllable/sec.)*—is likely to play an important role in engaging a right-hemispheric, sensorimotor network capable of providing an impulse for verbal production in much the same way that a metronome has been shown to serve as a "pacemaker" when rhythmic motor activities prime and/or entrain sensorimotor networks (Thaut et al. 1999; Thaut and Abiru 2010). In addition, research suggesting that hand movements and articulatory movements may share neural correlates (Meister et al. 2003) further supports the notion that hand-tapping is critically important for facilitating the coupling of sounds to orofacial and articulatory actions (Lahav et al. 2007). Since concurrent speech and hand use occurs in daily life, and gestures are frequently used to emphasize/accompany important and/or elusive concepts in speech, rhythmic hand movements, in synchrony with articulatory movements, may have similarly beneficial effects on speech production and in particular in relearning of speech-motor functions after a stroke.

12.7 Music-Supported Therapy in Rehabilitation of Other Neurological Disorders

12.7.1 Parkinson's Disease

Rhythmic auditory cueing as a means to improve gait in Parkinson's disease (PD) has been scientifically investigated for the last 20 years (Thaut et al. 1996), while the positive effects of dancing on locomotion and balance in PD patients were recognized more recently (Hackney and Earhart 2009). Generally, the majority of the studies on music-supported therapy in Parkinson's disease have used music to improve mobility and gait parameters. In a review, effect sizes (Cohen's *d*) of the peer reviewed published interventions were calculated (Sihvonen et al. 2017): the most coherent and clinically significant beneficial effect on motor symptoms in PD was produced by dancing. Compared to the control group, both tango and waltz/foxtrot intervention groups improved in balance (Berg Balance Scale between +2 and +5; Cohen's $d = 2.98$, $d = 3.17$, respectively), 6-minute walk test (+98 m vs +24 m; $d = 2.50$, $d = 2.24$), and backward stride length (+14 cm vs. +6 cm; $d = 2.19$, $d = 1.96$). Furthermore, dancing also improved overall mobility ($d = 2.50$) (Hackney et al. 2007). In a smaller study, tango improved balance (d=2.18) (Hackney and Earhart 2009). These positive effects have been confirmed by a meta-analysis (de Drieu et al. 2012). Bearing a close analogy to dancing, music therapy with rhythmic movements improved mobility, and gait training synchronized to music resulted in improved velocity (by 0, 2 m/s; $d = 2.64$), stride time (by 0, 21 s; $d = 1.76$), and cadence (by 0, 17 m; $d = 2.16$) compared to the control group. Other studies equally reported a reduction in PD-specific motor symptoms ($d = 0.50$) (de Bruin et al. 2010; Pohl et al. 2013).

Huang et al. (2024) recently published a meta-analysis of 38 original studies involving 1486 participants. Rhythmically cued exercise interventions demonstrated superior effects on motor function compared to exercise therapy without rhythm (standardized mean difference [SMD] = −0.31). However, no significant improvements were observed in cognition and mental state. Overall, significant improvements were observed in motor examination, balance, walking velocity, step length, and stride length following rhythmically cued exercise interventions. No significant improvements were observed in freezing of gait and cadence. The authors conclude that rhythmically cued exercise interventions are effective in improving motor function in the early to middle stages of Parkinson's disease. Interestingly, more than 10 weeks of intervention yielded better results.

Summarizing, the reviewed evidence suggests that dancing and music-based interventions that synchronize movement to music can be beneficial in the maintenance of motor performance in this slowly progressing disease, at least in a significant percentage of patients at an early to middle stage of disease progression. In all of the studies reviewed, the follow-up period was too short to allow conclusions on the long-term effects of music interventions. The effects of music on the autonomic disturbances in PD have not been addressed in controlled studies. Rhythmical use of musical stimulus most probably compensates for the failing control by the extrapyramidal system and enhances the audio perception and movement synchronization (e.g., Cha et al. 2014). The perceived rhythm in music activates the neural circuits involved in motor actions and acts as an external cue for movement thus replacing the impaired internal timing function in PD. The use of music as stimulus may be more effective than auditory stimulation without music (e.g., metronome beat) in gait rehabilitation, as shown in stroke (Thaut et al. 2007). This might also explain the positive effects of dancing in PD. Furthermore, the improvement in motor control and decrease in disease-specific symptoms could in turn improve the QoL. However, according to a new study, it seems that there are "responders" and nonresponders with respect to both, response to musical cueing and to improvement of QoL (Benoit et al. 2014; Cochen De Cock et al. 2018). One of the sources of this variability could be individual musical preferences and listening habits; however, this has not been addressed in the abovementioned studies. In this regard, Simone dalla Bella et al. (2018) convincingly argue in a review that rhythmic auditory cueing needs to be individualized according to the patient's preferences, the stage of motor impairment, and the perceptual capabilities of the individual.

12.7.2 Multiple Sclerosis

Multiple sclerosis is the most common severe neurological disease of the young adult population and manifests as a wide range of neurological deficiencies, including severe motor impairments and sensory deficits. Treatments aim to ameliorate the function after flare-up of an MS-episode or preventing new episodes, mostly acting via modulation of the autoimmune responses and anti-inflammatory effects. Two randomized controlled studies have addressed the effect of musical interventions in alleviating the manifestations of MS. In one study, the effect of keyboard playing (audible vs. mute) in hand functionality was investigated (Gatti et al. 2015). The audible keyboard playing improved the subjective functional use of the hand significantly in the audible keyboard group (ABILHAND assessment 2,3 to 3,5 vs 2,2, to 2,3; $d = 0.60$ vs. $d = 0.32$); however, fine motor abilities assessed objectively with the nine-hole pegboard test improved in both groups (MG: 57 to 30 vs. CG 37 to 28). A feasibility study on MS patients with gait problems found rhythmic auditory cueing to be effective in decreasing double-support time, the effect size being large (from 54 s to 112 s; $d = 0.72$) (Conklyn et al. 2010). While decreased double-support time may reflect improved dynamic balance, none of the other gait parameters differed from controls. The only available meta-analysis by Lopes and Keppers (2021) confirmed in 253 patients suffering MS that music-based therapies, such as rhythmic auditory cueing, playing musical instruments, and that music-based interventions were better than conventional therapy or no intervention, with regard to gait parameters (double support time and walking speed), fatigue level, fatigability, coordination, dexterity, balance, walking endurance, lower extremity functional strength, emotional status, and pain. Regarding mental fatigability and memory, however, the data were conflicting.

12.7.3 Epilepsy

Epilepsy was treated with music in only one RCT ($N = 73$) (Bodner et al. 2012). Patients were exposed to Mozart's music periodically every night for a year and a significant 17% reduction in seizure frequency was detected during the study period. In addition, a 16% reduction in seizure frequency persisted for one year. While no other RCTs on adult population have been published, a meta-analysis of 12 studies including both pediatric and adult patients indicated that 85% of the patients responded favorably to music, the average reduction in interictal epileptic activity being 31% and 24% during and after the listening period, respectively (Dastgheib et al. 2014). Definite conclusions cannot be drawn, since all but two studies lacked a separate control group. In terms of underlying mechanism, it is hypothesized that exposure to patterned auditory stimuli provides an excitatory stimulation of the cortex, which may reduce epileptiform activity.

12.8 Music-Supported Therapy in Dementia

Since ancient times, music in connection with lyrics was used as support for memory formation, be it in religious rites, memorization of heroic saga, or songs important for group identity. Indeed, biographical memories can be enriched and consolidated with music, probably due to tight linkages of biographical events and music to the limbic emotional system (Sheldon and Donahue 2017). With respect to neurophysiological mechanisms, it could be demonstrated that musical training can induce functional plasticity in the human hippocampus (Herdener et al. 2010) which provides a possible motivation for considering the effects of music-supported therapy in memory loss due to dementia.

In our review, we identified altogether 16 RCTs on persons with dementia ($n = 1048$, Sihvonen et al. 2017). Mostly neuropsychiatric and behavioral symptoms, such as anxiety, and agitation, depression, cognitive status as well as QoL, were assessed and improved. Those studies specifically addressing cognitive elements (reminiscence, attention training) or physical exercise improved overall cognitive performance (measured by MMSE) of patients with dementia compared to standard care in four studies published by three separate groups ($d = 0.47$–0.76) (Ceccato et al. 2012; Chu et al. 2014; Särkämö et al. 2014, 2015). In addition, improved performance in these music interventions was reported for tests measuring attention and executive functions, orientation, and verbal or episodic memory (Särkämö et al. 2015). In one RCT, caregiver-implemented singing was also found to enhance working memory, especially in mild dementia and also to reduce caregiver burden (Särkämö et al. 2014). On the contrary, no significant changes in cognitive performance were observed for group-based music. In this trial, a cooking intervention in persons with moderate-severe dementia was included as a control for musical activities and similarly did not yield any effects on cognitive performance (Narme et al. 2014). This "negative" result was confirmed in a meta-analysis on six studies with 330 dementia patients (Fusar-Poli et al. 2018).

The cognitive benefits of musical activities such as singing or playing an instrument in the early stages of dementia may be related to enhanced cognitive reserve, the utilization of alternative networks and cognitive strategies to cope with advancing pathology (Hall et al. 2009). Overall, the effects of musical interventions in dementia may be driven by the comfort and emotional safety induced by familiar music, which can temporarily overcome the confusion and disorientation by anchoring attention on a positive familiar stimulus in an otherwise confusing environment. As mentioned above, familiar music is also imbued with personal emotions, which can trigger autobiographical memories and help to restore a sense of identity for a while (Ismail et al. 2018).

12.9 Music-Supported Therapy in Rehabilitation of Disorders of Consciousness

Disorders of consciousness (DOC) may frequently be observed among early neurological rehabilitation patients (Heinz and Rollnik 2015): altogether 83% of hypoxic encephalopathy patients suffer from DOC on admission and less than one out of five comatose subjects regain consciousness during rehabilitation. Alarmingly, there is only little evidence for the effectiveness of DOC rehabilitation interventions with music (Lancioni et al. 2022).

DOC are subdivided into coma, unresponsive wakefulness syndrome (UWS),—previously known as vegetative state (VS)—and minimally conscious state (MCS). Coma is characterized by a state of deep, unarousable unconsciousness and may be graded based on the absence or presence of reflexive responses to stimuli, such as present or absent eye-opening to strong painful stimuli (Rollnik and Altenmüller 2014). In UWS, despite open eyes and existing reflex behavior, patients are completely unresponsive (e.g., absence of command following) (Bodard et al. 2013). Patients in MCS exhibit some signs of consciousness, such as command following (even if inconsistent), visual pursuit, localization to noxious stimulation, and appropriate responses to emotional stimuli without being able to functionally communicate (Teasdale and Jennett 1974).

It has been hypothesized that comatose patients might suffer from a condition of "environmental deprivation" (LeWinn and Dimancescu 1978). Viewed in this context, patients might benefit from stimulation of all five sensory pathways and thus enhancing the rate and degree of recovery from coma. The concept of "enriched environment" inspires therapeutic approaches using sensory stimulation in neurological early rehabilitation (Lippert-Grüner et al. 2007). Preferred music as therapeutic auditive intervention has recently been used in a few studies in patients with UWS or MCS (O'Kelly et al. 2013; Castro et al. 2015). A neurophysiological and behavioral study compared electroencephalogram (EEG), heart rate variability, respiratory, and behavioral responses of 20 healthy subjects with 21 individuals with UWS or MCS (O'Kelly et al. 2013). Healthy subjects and patients were presented with live music chosen according to their musical preferences. Furthermore, improvised music entrained to respiration (procedures typically used in music therapy) was applied, and recordings of disliked music, white noise, and silence. The ANOVA results indicated a range of significant responses across healthy subjects corresponding to arousal and attention in response to preferred music including concurrent increases in respiratory rate with globally enhanced EEG power spectra responses across frequency bandwidths. While physiological responses were heterogeneous across patient cohorts, significant post hoc EEG amplitude increases for stimuli associated with preferred music were found for frontal midline theta in six UWS and four MCS patients and frontal alpha in three UWS and four MCS subjects. Furthermore, behavioral data showed a significantly increased blink rate for preferred music within the UWS cohort. Two UWS patients exhibited concurrent changes across measures indicative of discriminatory responses to both music therapy procedures.

In another recent study, 13 DOC patients were examined using bedside EEG while listening to preferred music (Castro et al. 2015). Event-related potentials to the patient's first name were recorded after either preferred music (music condition) or a continuous sound (control condition). The cerebral response to the patient's first name was more frequently observed in the music than in the control condition. Furthermore, the presence or absence of a discriminative response in the music condition seemed to be associated with a favorable or unfavorable outcome after six months. The authors suggested that preferred music might boost cognition in DOC. To the best of our knowledge, psychophysiological reactions like heart rate, blood pressure, or respiration frequency changes have not been examined as of yet. Taken together, the rehabilitative potential of music therapy in patients with coma, UWS, or MCS in neurological early rehabilitation merits further investigation. In a recent Cochrane review, the authors conclude that music interventions may be beneficial and first results are encouraging. Controlled trials are strongly encouraged to improve the evidence-base of music as a therapeutic tool in neurological early rehabilitation patients with DOC (Magee et al. 2017).

12.10 Conclusion and Outlook

The research of the last two decades reviewed in this chapter demonstrates that music exposure and active musical training can be a strong stimulant for neuroplastic adaptations and behavioral improvements following brain injury or degenerative processes. Making music including singing and dancing leads to a strong coupling of perception and action mediated by sensory, motor, and multimodal brain regions and affects either in a top-down or bottom-up fashion important relay stations in the brainstem and thalamus. Furthermore, listening to music and making music provokes motions and emotions, increases between-subject communications and interactions, and—mediated via neurotransmitters such as serotonin and dopamine—is experienced as joyous and rewarding through activity changes in amygdala, ventral striatum, and other components of the limbic system. Making music makes rehabilitation more enjoyable and can remediate impaired neural processes or neural connections by engaging and linking nondamaged brain regions.

As with other interventions, music-supported therapy in neurorehabilitation needs to be grounded within a neurobiological understanding of how and why particular brain systems could be affected. The efficacy of these still-experimental interventions should be assessed quantitatively and in an unbiased way. Here, researchers have started the journey toward a sound neuroscientific basis for music-based interventions, which—not unexpectedly—yielded in some instances controversial results. The studies reviewed here—mostly randomized clinical trials—are important steps in establishing neurologic music therapy that might have the power to enhance brain recovery processes by exploiting neuroplasticity.

What is urgently needed are larger RCTs demonstrating the assumed specific value of musical interventions based on the aforementioned neurobiological mechanisms. In order to transcend the effects of novelty or motivation, randomized controlled music therapy trials will need to include nonmusic-related control activities with similar motivational power and novelty. Furthermore, in these trials, well-defined patient groups, stratified with respect to musical expertise, music-listening behaviors, premorbid health and cognitive status and timepoint of onset of therapies after the lesion have to be recruited. In order to gain more information on the sustainability of interventions long-term follow-ups, studies are necessary. Finally, novel biomarkers, may help to recruit patients based on their initial potential for reactive neurobiological recovery, for example, by assessing neurophysiological parameters, such as resting state connectivity of brain regions (Winters et al. 2018). Collecting this information may allow clinicians to better predict which patients will benefit from which aspects of neurologic-based music therapy and provide a more personalized rehabilitation strategy.

Acknowledgements Parts of this Review Article are based on previous reviews on similar topics, published together with Aleksi Sihvonen and colleagues in Lancet Neurology in 2017 and with Prof. Lauren Stewart 2020 in the "Oxford Textbook of Neurorehabilitation, edited by Volker Dietz and Nick S. Ward.

References

Abrams DA, Nicol T, Zecker S, Kraus N. Right-hemisphere auditory cortex is dominant for coding syllable patterns in speech. J Neurosci. 2008;28:3958–65.

Albert ML, Sparks RW, Helm NA. Melodic intonation therapy for aphasia. Arch Neurol. 1973;29:130–1.

Alonso J, Prieto L, Anto JM. The Spanish version of the SF-36 Health Survey (the SF-36 health questionnaire): an instrument for measuring clinical results. Med Clin (Barc). 1995;104:771–6.

Altenmüller E, Furuya S. Brain plasticity and the concept of Metaplasticity in skilled musicians. Adv Exp Med Biol. 2016;957:197–208. https://doi.org/10.1007/978-3-319-47313-0_11.

Altenmüller E, Furuya S. Apollos gift and curse: making music as a model for adaptive and maladaptive plasticity. e-Neuroforum. 2017;23(2):57–75.

Altenmüller E, Schlaug G. Neurobiological aspects of neurologic music therapy. Music Med. 2013;5:210–6.

Altenmüller E, Schneider S, Marco-Pallares PW, Münte TF. Neural reorganization underlies improvement in stroke induced motor dysfunction by music supported therapy. Ann N Y Acad Sci. 2009;1169:395–405.

Amengual JL, Rojo N, Veciana de las Heras M, Marco-Pallarés J, Grau J, Schneider S, et al. Sensorimotor plasticity after music-supported therapy in chronic stroke patients revealed by transcranial magnetic stimulation. PLoS One. 2013;8:e61883. https://doi.org/10.1371/journal.pone.0061883.

Amunts K, Schlaug G, Jäncke L, Steinmetz H, Schleicher A, Dabringhaus A, et al. Motor cortex and hand motor skills: structural compliance in the human brain. Hum Brain Mapping. 1997;5:206–15.

Bangert M, Schlaug G. Specialization of the spezialized in features of external brain morphology. Eur J Neurosci. 2006;24:1832–4.

Bangert M, Peschel T, Rotte M, Drescher D, Hinrichs H, Schlaug G, et al. Shared networks for auditory and motor processing in professional pianists: evidence from fMRI conjunction. NeuroImage. 2006;30:917–26.

Belzung C, Wigmore P. Neurogenesis and neuroplasticity. Heidelberg: Springer; 2013.

Bengtsson SL, Nagy Z, Skare S, Forsman L, Forssberg H, Ullen F. Extensive piano practicing has regionally specific effects on white matter development. Nat Neurosci. 2005;8:1148–50.

Benoit CE, Dalla Bella S, Farrugia N, Obrig H, Mainka S, Kotz SA. Musically cued gait-training improves both perceptual and motor timing in Parkinson's disease. Front Hum Neurosci. 2014;8:494. https://doi.org/10.3389/fnhum.2014.00494.

Bodard O, Laureys S, Gosseries O. Coma and disorders of consciousness: scientific advances and practical considerations for clinicians. Semin Neurol. 2013;33:83–90.

Bodner M, Turner RP, Schwacke J, Bowers C, Norment C. Reduction of seizure occurrence from exposure to auditory stimulation in individuals with neurological handicaps: a randomized controlled trial. PLoS One. 2012;7(10):e45303.

Bonakdarpour B, Eftekharzadeh A, Ashayeri H. Preliminary report on the effects of melodic intonation therapy in the rehabilitation of Persian aphasic patients. Iranian J Med Sci. 2000;25:156–60.

Bradt J, Dileo C, Potvin N. Music for stress and anxiety reduction in coronary heart disease patients. Cochrane Database Syst Rev. 2013;12:CD006577.

Brown RM, Penhune VB, Zatorre R. Expert music performance: cognitive, neural, and developmental bases. In: Altenmüller E, Finger S, Boller F. (eds.) music, neurology and neuroscience. Evolution, the musical brain, medical conditions, and therapies. Prog Brain Res. 2015;2017:57–86.

Bunt L. Music therapy, Second Edition, An Art beyond words. Oxford: Routledge; 2014.

Castro M, Tillmann B, Luauté J, Corneyllie A, Dailler F, André-Obadia N, Perrin F. Boosting cognition with music in patients with disorders of consciousness. Neurorehabil Neural Repair. 2015;29:pii: 1545968314565464. [Epub ahead of print].

Ceccato E, Vigato G, Bonetto C, Bevilacqua A, Pizziolo P, Crociani S, et al. STAM protocol in dementia: a multicenter, single-blind, randomized, and controlled trial. Am J Alzheimers Dis Other Dement. 2012;27(5):301–10.

Cha Y, Kim Y, Hwang S, Chung Y. Intensive gait training with rhythmic auditory stimulation in individuals with chronic hemiparetic stroke: a pilot randomized controlled study. NeuroRehabilitation. 2014;35(4):681–8. https://doi.org/10.3233/NRE-141182.

Chang MC, Park SW, Lee BJ, Park D. Relationship between recovery of motor function and neuropsychological functioning in cerebral infarction patients: the importance of social functioning in motor recovery. J Integr Neurosci. 2020;19(3):405–11. https://doi.org/10.31083/j.jin.2020.03.175.

Chu H, Yang CY, Lin Y, Ou KL, Lee TY, O'Brien AP, Chou KR. The impact of group music therapy on depression and cognition in elderly persons with dementia: a randomized controlled study. Biol Res Nurs. 2014;16(2):209–17.

Cochen De Cock V, Dotov DG, Ihalainen P, Bégel V, Galtier F, Lebrun C, et al. Rhythmic abilities and musical training in Parkinson's disease: do they help? NPJ Parkinsons Dis. 2018;4:8. https://doi.org/10.1038/s41531-018-0043-7. eCollection 2018

Collimore AN, Roto Cataldo AV, Aiello AJ, Sloutsky R, Hutchinson KJ, Harris B, Ellis T, Awad LN. Autonomous control of music to retrain walking after stroke. Neurorehabil Neural Repair.

2023;37(5):255–65. https://doi.org/10.1177/15459683231174223. Epub 2023 Jun 5. PMID: 37272500; PMCID: PMC10272623

Conklyn D, Stough D, Novak E, Paczak S, Chemali K, Bethoux F. A home-based walking program using rhythmic auditory stimulation improves gait performance in patients with multiple sclerosis: a pilot study. Neurorehabil Neural Repair. 2010;24(9):835–42.

Criscuolo A, Pando-Naude V, Bonetti L, Vuust P, Brattico E. An ALE meta-analytic review of musical expertise. Sci Rep. 2022;12(1):11726. https://doi.org/10.1038/s41598-022-14959-4. PMID: 35821035; PMCID: PMC9276732

Curran SL, Andrykowski MA, Studts JL. Short Form of the Profile of Mood States (POMS-SF). Psychol Assess. 1995;7:80–3.

Dalla Bella S, Dotov D, Bardy B, Cochen de Cock V. Individualization of music-based rhythmic auditory cueing in Parkinson's disease. Ann N Y Acad Sci. 2018;1423:308–17.

Dastgheib SS, Layegh P, Sadeghi R, Foroughipur M, Shoeibi A, Gorji A. The effects of Mozart's music on interictal activity in epileptic patients: systematic review and meta-analysis of the literature. Curr Neurol Neurosci Rep. 2014;14(1):420,013-0420-x.

de Bruin N, Doan JB, Turnbull G, Suchowersky O, Bonfield S, Hu B, Brown LA. Walking with music is a safe and viable tool for gait training in Parkinson's disease: the effect of a 13-week feasibility study on single and dual task walking. Parkinsons Dis. 2010;2010:483530.

de Drieu MJ, van der Wilk AS, Poppe E, Kwakkel G, van Wegen EE. Rehabilitation, exercise therapy and music in patients with Parkinson's disease: a meta-analysis of the effects of music-based movement therapy on walking ability, balance and quality of life. Parkinsonism Relat Disord. 2012;18(Suppl 1):S114–9.

Douven E, Köhler S, Rodriguez MMF, Staals J, Verhey FR, Aalten P. Imaging markers of post-stroke depression and apathy: a systematic review and meta-analysis. Neuropsychol Rev. 2017;27:202–19. https://doi.org/10.1007/s11065-017-9356-2.

Ericsson KA, Smith J, editors. Toward a general theory of expertise: prospects and limits. Cambridge University Press; 1991.

Fujioka T, Dawson DR, Wright R, Honjo K, Chen JL, Chen JJ, et al. The effects of music-supported therapy on motor, cognitive, and psychological functions in chronic stroke. Ann N Y Acad Sci. 2018;1423:264–74.

Furuya S, Oku T, Miyazaki F, Kinoshita H. Secrets of virtuoso: neuromuscular attributes of motor virtuosity in expert musicians. Sci Rep. 2015;2015(5):15750. https://doi.org/10.1038/srep15750.

Fusar-Poli L, Bieleninik Ł, Brondino N, Chen XJ, Gold C. The effect of music therapy on cognitive functions in patients with dementia: a systematic review and meta-analysis. Aging Ment Health. 2018;22(9):1097–106. https://doi.org/10.1080/13607863.2017.1348474. Epub 2017 Jul 10

Gärtner H, Minnerop M, Pieperhoff P, Schleicher A, Zilles K, Altenmüller E, Amunts K. Brain morphometry shows effects of long-term musical practice in middle-aged keyboard players. Front Psychol. 2013;4:636. https://doi.org/10.3389/fpsyg.2013.00636.

Gaser C, Schlaug G. Brain structures differ between musicians and non-musicians. J Neurosci. 2003;23:9240–5.

Gatti R, Tettamanti A, Lambiase S, Rossi P, Comola M. Improving hand functional use in subjects with multiple sclerosis using a musical keyboard: a randomized controlled trial. Physiother Res Int. 2015;20(2):100–7.

Goodglass H, Kaplan E. Boston diagnostic aphasia examination. 2nd ed. Philadelphia: Lea & Febiger; 1983.

Hackney ME, Earhart GM. Effects of dance on movement control in Parkinson's disease: a comparison of Argentine tango and American ballroom. J Rehabil Med. 2009;41(6):475–81.

Hackney ME, Kantorovich S, Levin R, Earhart GM. Effects of tango on functional mobility in Parkinson's disease: a preliminary study. J Neurol Phys Ther. 2007;31(4):173–9.

Hall CB, Lipton RB, Sliwinski M, Katz MJ, Derby CA, Verghese J. Cognitive activities delay onset of memory decline in persons who develop dementia. Neurology. 2009;73(5):356–61.

Halwani GF, Loui P, Rüber T, Schlaug G. Effects of practice and experience on the arcuate fasciculus: comparing singers, instrumentalists, and non-musicians. Front Psychol. 2011:2. https://doi.org/10.3389/fpsyg.2011.001561.

Haslinger B, Erhard P, Altenmüller E, Schroeder U, Boecker H, Ceballos-Baumann AJ. Cogn Neurosci. 2005;17:282–93.

Heinz UE, Rollnik JD. Outcome and prognosis of hypoxic brain damage patients undergoing neurological early rehabilitation. BMC Res Notes. 2015;8:243. https://doi.org/10.1186/s13104-015-1175-z.

Herdener M, Esposito F, di Salle F, Boller C, Hilti CC, Habermeyer B, Scheffler K, Wetzel S, Seifritz E, Cattapan-Ludewig K. Musical training induces functional plasticity in human hippocampus. J Neurosci. 2010;30(4):1377–84. https://doi.org/10.1523/JNEUROSCI.4513-09.2010.

Horden P. Music as medicine: the history of music therapy since antiquity. Aldershot: Ashgate Publishing Ltd.; 2000.

Huang X, Dong K, Gan C, Xu Z, Lei D, Dong X, Liu H, Chen X. Effect of rhythmically cued exercise interventions on functions in patients with Parkinson disease: a meta-analysis. Phys Ther. 2024;104(3):pzad158. https://doi.org/10.1093/ptj/pzad158.

Hyde KL, Lerch J, Norton A, Forgeard M, Winner E, Evans AC, et al. Musical training shapes structural brain development. J Neurosci. 2009;2009(29):3019–25.

Ismail S, Christopher G, Dodd E, Wildschut T, Sedikides C, Jones RW, et al. Psychological and mnemonic benefits of nostalgia for people with dementia. J Alz Dis. 2018;65:1327. https://doi.org/10.3233/JAD-180075.

Jünemann K, Engels A, Marie D, Worschech F, Scholz DS, Grouiller F, Kliegel M, Van De Ville D, Altenmüller E, Krüger THC, James CE, Sinke C. Increased functional connectivity in the right dorsal auditory stream after a full year of piano training in healthy older adults. Sci Rep. 2023;13(1):19993. https://doi.org/10.1038/s41598-023-46513-1. PMID: 37968500; PMCID: PMC10652022

Jungblut M, Aldridge D. The musictherapy intervention SIPARI with chronic aphasics – research findings. Neurologie Rehabil. 2004;10(2):69–78.

Lahav A, Saltzman E, Schlaug G. Action representation of sound: audiomotor recognition network while listening to newly acquired actions. J Neurosci. 2007;27:308–14.

Lancioni GE, Singh NN, O'Reilly MF, Sigafoos J, Desideri L. Behavioral intervention approaches for people with disorders of consciousness: a scoping review. Disabil Rehabil. 2022;44(24):7677–92. https://doi.org/10.1080/09638288.2021.1985634. Epub 2021 Oct 6. PMID: 34613851

LeWinn EB, Dimancescu MD. Environmental deprivation and enrichment in coma. Lancet. 1978;2:156–7.

Lindmark B. Evaluation of functional capacity after stroke with special emphasis on motor function and activities of daily living. Scand J Rehab Med Suppl. 1988;21:1–40.

Lippert-Grüner M, Maegele M, Pokorný J, Angelov DN, Svestková O, Wittner M, Trojan S. Early rehabilitation model shows positive effects on neural degeneration and recovery from neuromotor deficits following traumatic brain injury. Physiol Res. 2007;56:359–68.

Lopes J, Keppers II. Music-based therapy in rehabilitation of people with multiple sclerosis: a systematic review of clinical trials. Arq Neuropsiquiatr. 2021;79(6):527–35. https://doi.org/10.1590/0004-282X-ANP-2020-0374. PMID: 34320057; PMCID: PMC9394567

Magee WL, Clark I, Tamplin J, Bradt J. Music interventions for aquired bran injury. Cochrane Database Syst Rev. 2017;15:255. https://doi.org/10.1002/14651858.

Meister IG, Boroojerdi B, Foltys H, Sparing R, Huber W, Topper R. Motor cortex hand area and speech: implications for the development of language. Neuropsychologia. 2003;41:401–6.

Meyer M, Alter K, Friederici AD, Lohmann G, von Cramon DY. fMRI reveals brain regions mediating slow prosodic modulations in spoken sentences. Hum Brain Mapping. 2002;17:73–88.

Narme P, Clement S, Ehrle N, Schiaratura L, Vachez S, Courtaigne B, et al. Efficacy of musical interventions in dementia: evidence from a randomized controlled trial. J Alzheimers Dis. 2014;38(2):359–69.

Nikmaram N, Scholz DS, Großbach M, Schmidt SB, Spogis J, Belardinelli P, Müller-Dahlhaus F, Remy J, Ziemann U, Rollnik JD, Altenmüller E. Musical Sonification of arm movements in stroke rehabilitation yields limited benefits. Front Neurosci. 2019;13:1378. https://doi.org/10.3389/fnins.2019.01378. PMID: 31920526; PMCID: PMC6933006

Nilsson U. The anxiety-and pain-reducing effects of music interventions: a systematic review. AORN J. 2008;87(4):780–807.

Nozaradan S, Schwartze M, Obermeiner C, Kotz SA. Specific contributions of basal ganglia and cerebellum to the neural tracking of rhythm. Cortex. 2017;95:156–68.

O'Kelly J, James L, Palaniappan-Taborin J, Fachner J, Magee WL. Neurophysiological and behavioral responses to music therapy in vegetative and minimally conscious states. Frontiers Hum Neurosci. 2013;7:884.

Okada K, Kurita A, Takase B. Effects of music therapy on autonomic nervous system activity, incidence of heart failure events, and plasma cytokine and catecholamine levels in elderly patients with cerebrovascular disease and dementia. Int Heart J. 2009;50:95–110.

Ozdemir E, Norton A, Schlaug G. Shared and distinct neural correlates of singing and speaking. NeuroImage. 2006;33:628–35.

Paquette S, Fujii S, Schlaug G. The cerebellum's contribution to beat interval discrimination. NeuroImage. 2017;163:177–82. https://doi.org/10.1016/j.neuroimage.2017.09.017.

Pascual-Leone A. Reorganization of cortical motor outputs in the acquisition of new motor skills. Electroencephalogr Clin Neurophysiol. 1995;97:25–2.

Peretz I. Processing of local and global musical information by unilateral brain-damaged patients. Brain. 1990;113:1185–205.

Poeppel D. The analysis of speech in different temporal integration windows: cerebral lateralization as "asymmetric sampling in time". Speech Comm. 2003;41:245–55.

Pohl P, Dizdar N, Hallert E. The Ronnie Gardiner rhythm and music method – a feasibility study in Parkinson's disease. Disabil Rehabil. 2013;35(26):2197–204.

Popescu T, Stahl B, Wiernik BM, Haiduk F, Zemanek M, Helm H, Matzinger T, Beisteiner R, Fitch WT. Melodic Intonation Therapy for aphasia: a multi-level meta-analysis of randomized controlled trials and individual participant data. Ann N Y Acad Sci. 2022;1516(1):76–84. https://doi.org/10.1111/nyas.14848. Epub 2022 Aug 2. PMID: 35918503; PMCID: PMC9804200

Radley J, Morilak D, Viau V, Campeau S. Chronic stress and brain plasticity: mechanisms underlying adaptive and maladaptive changes and implications for stress-related CNS disorders. Neurosci Biobehav Rev. 2015;58:79–91.

Ragert P, Schmidt A, Altenmüller E, Dinse HR. Superior tactile performance and learning in professional pianists: evidence for meta-plasticity in musicians. Eur J Neurosci. 2003;19(2):473–8.

Raglio A, Oasi O, Gianotti M, Rossi A, Goulene K, Stramba-Badiale M. Improvement of spontaneous language in stroke patients with chronic aphasia treated with music. Int J Neurosci. 2016;126(3):235–42. https://doi.org/10.3109/00207454.2015.1010647. Epub 2015 Jun 10

Raglio A, Panigazzi M, Colombo R, Tramontano M, Iosa M, Mastrogiacomo S, Baiardi P, Molteni D, Baldissarro E, Imbriani C, Imarisio C, Eretti L, Hamedani M, Pistarini C, Imbriani M, Mancardi GL, Caltagirone C. Hand rehabilitation with sonification techniques in the subacute stage of stroke. Sci Rep. 2021;11(1):7237. https://doi.org/10.1038/s41598-021-86627-y. PMID: 33790343; PMCID: PMC8012636

Rojo N, Amengual J, Juncadella M, Rubio F, Camara E, Marco-Pallares J, et al. Music-Supported Therapy induces plasticity in the sensorimotor cortex in chronic stroke: a single-case study using multimodal imaging (fMRI-TMS). Brain Inj. 2012;2012(25):787–93.

Rollnik JD, Altenmüller E. Music in disorders of consciousness. Front Neurosci. 2014;8:190. https://doi.org/10.3389/fnins.2014.00190.

Rueber T, Lindenberg R, Schlaug G. Differential adaptation of descending motor pathways in musicians. Cereb Cortex. 2015;25(6):1490–8. https://doi.org/10.1093/cercor/bht331.

Salimpoor VN, Benovoy M, Longo G, Cooperstock JR, Zatorre RJ. The rewarding aspects of music listening are related to degree of emotional arousal. PLoS One. 2009;16(4):e7487. https://doi.org/10.1371/journal.pone.0007487.

Särkämö T, Tervaniemi M, Laitinen S, Forsblom A, Soinila S, Mikkonen M. Music listening enhances cognitive recovery and mood after middle cerebral artery stroke. Brain. 2008;131:866–76.
Särkämö T, Tervaniemi M, Laitinen S, Numminen A, Kurki M, Johnson JK, Rantanen P. Cognitive, emotional, and social benefits of regular musical activities in early dementia: randomized controlled study. Gerontologist. 2014;54(4):634–50.
Särkämö T, Laitinen S, Numminen A, Kurki M, Johnson JK, Rantanen P. Clinical and demographic factors associated with the cognitive and emotional efficacy of regular musical activities in dementia. J Alzheimers Dis. 2015;49(3):767–81.
Schauer M, Mauritz K. Musical motor feedback (MMF) in walking hemiparetic stroke patients: randomized trials of gait improvement. Clin Rehabil. 2003;17(7):713–22.
Schlaug G, Marchina S, Norton A. From singing to speaking: why patients with Broca's aphasia can sing and how that may lead to recovery of expressive language functions. Music Percept. 2008;25:315–23.
Schlaug G, Marchina S, Norton A. Evidence for plasticity in white-matter tracts of patients with chronic Broca's aphasia undergoing intense intonation-based speech therapy. Ann N Y Acad Sci. 2009;2009(1169):385–94.
Schlaug G, Norton A, Marchina S, Zipse L, Wan CY. From singing to speaking: facilitating recovery from nonfluent aphasia. Future Neurol. 2010;5:657–65.
Schneider P, Scherg M, Dosch HG, Specht HJ, Gutschalk A, Rupp A. Morphology of Heschl's gyrus reflects enhanced activation in the auditory cortex of musicians. Nat Neurosci. 2002;5:688–94.
Schneider S, Schönle PW, Altenmüller E, Münte TF. Using musical instruments to improve motor skill recovery following a stroke. J Neurol. 2007;254:1339–46.
Schneider S, Münte TF, Rodriguez-Fornells A, Sailer M, Altenmüller E. Music supported training is more efficient than functional motor training for recovery of fine motor skills in stroke patients. Music Percept. 2010;27:271–80.
Scholz DS, Rohde S, Großbach M, Rollnik J, Altenmüller E. Moving with music for stroke rehabilitation: a sonification feasability study. Ann N Y Acad Sci. 2015;1337:69–76.
Scholz DS, Rohde S, Nikmaram N, Brückner HP, Großbach M, Rollnik JD, Altenmüller EO. Sonification of arm movements in stroke rehabilitation – a novel approach in neurologic music therapy. Front Neurol. 2016;7:106. https://doi.org/10.3389/fneur.2016.00106. eCollection 2016
Schuppert M, Münte TF, Wieringa BM, Altenmüller E. Receptive amusia: evidence for cross-hemispheric neural networks underlying music processing strategies. Brain. 2000;123:546–59.
Segura E, Grau-Sánchez J, Cerda-Company X, Porto MF, De la Cruz-Puebla M, Sanchez-Pinsach D, Cerquides J, Duarte E, Palumbo A, Turry A, Raghavan P, Särkämö T, Münte TF, Arcos JL, Rodríguez-Fornells A. Enriched music-supported therapy for individuals with chronic stroke: a randomized controlled trial. J Neurol. 2024;271:6606. https://doi.org/10.1007/s00415-024-12570-3. Epub ahead of print. PMID: 39112892.
Sheldon S, Donahue J. More than a feeling: emotional cues impact the access and experience of autobiographica memories. Mem Cogn. 2017;45:731–44.
Sihvonen AJ, Särkämö T, Leo V, Tervaniemi M, Altenmüller E, Soinila S. Music-based interventions in neurological rehabilitation. Lancet Neurol. 2017;16(8):648–60. https://doi.org/10.1016/S1474-4422(17)30168-0. Epub 2017 Jun 26. Review
Sparks RW, Holland AL. Method: melodic intonation therapy for aphasia. J Speech Hear Dis. 1976;1976(41):287–97.
Steele CJ, Bailey JA, Zatorre RJ, Penhune VB. Early musical training and white-matter plasticity in the corpus callosum: evidence for a sensitive period. J Neurosci. 2013;33:1282–90.
Stewart L. Do musicians have different brains. Clin Med. 2008;8:304–8.
Stewart L, Henson R, Kampe K, Walsh V, Turner R, Frith U. Brain changes after learning to read and play music. NeuroImage. 2003;20:71–83.
Teasdale G, Jennett B. Assessment of coma and impaired consciousness. A practical scale. Lancet. 1974;2:81–4.

Thaut M. Music as therapy in early history. In: Altenmüller E, Finger S, Boller F, editors. Music, neurology and neuroscience. Evolution, the musical brain, medical conditions, and therapies, vol. 217. Prog Brain Res; 2015. p. 143–57.

Thaut MH, Abiru M. Rhythmic auditory stimulation in rehabilitation of movement disoders: a review of current research. Music Percept. 2010;27:263–9.

Thaut M, Hoemberg V. Handbook of neurologic music therapy. Oxford: Oxford University Press; 2014.

Thaut MH, McIntosh GC, Rice RR, Miller RA, Rathbun J, Brault JM. Rhythmic auditory stimulation in gait training for Parkinson's disease patients. Mov Disord. 1996;11(2):193–200.

Thaut MH, Kenyon GP, Schauer ML, McIntosh GC. The connection between rhythmicity and brain function. IEEE Eng Med Biol Mag. 1999;18:101–8.

Thaut MH, Kenyon GP, Hurt CP, McIntosh GC, Hoemberg V. Kinematic optimization of spatiotemporal patterns in paretic arm training with stroke patients. Neuropsychologia. 2002;2002(40):1073–81.

Thaut MH, Leins AK, Rice RR, Kenyon GP, Argstatter H, Fetter M, et al. Rhythmic auditory stimulation improves gait more than NDT/Bobath training in near-ambulatory patients early poststroke: a single-blind, randomized trial. Neurorehabil Neural Repair. 2007;21(5):455–9.

Tong Y, Forreider B, Sun X, et al. Music-supported therapy (MST) in improving post-stroke patients' upper-limb motor function: a randomised controlled pilot study. Neurol Res. 2015;37(5):434–40.

van Vugt FT, Kafczyk T, Kuhn W, Rollnik JD, Tillmann B, Altenmüller E. The role of auditory feedback in music-supported stroke rehabilitation: a single-blinded randomised controlled intervention. Restor Neurol Neurosci. 2016;34(2):297–311. https://doi.org/10.3233/RNN-150588.

Vaquero L, Hartmann K, Ripolles P, Rojo N, Sierpowska J, François C, et al. Structural neuroplasticity in expert pianists depends on the age of musical training onset. NeuroImage. 2016;126:106–19. https://doi.org/10.1016/j.neuroimage.2015.11.008.

Wan CY, Schlaug G. Music making as a tool for promoting brain plasticity across the life-span. Neuroscientist. 2010;16:566–77.

Wan CY, Rueber T, Hohmann A, Schlaug G. The therapeutic effects of singing in neurological disorders. Music Percept. 2010;27:287–95.

Wan CY, Zheng X, Marchina S, Norton A, Schlaug G. Intensive therapy induces contralateral white matter changes in chronic stroke patients with Broca's aphasia. Brain Lang. 2014;136:1–7.

Watson D, Clark LA, Tellegen A. Development and validation of brief measures of positive and negative affect: the PANAS scales. J Pers Soc Psychol. 1988;54:1063–70.

Wickens JR, Reynolds JN, Hyland BI. Neural mechanisms of reward-related motor learning. Curr Opin Neurobiol. 2003;13(6):685–90.

Wilson SJ, Parsons K, Reutens DC. Preserved singing in aphasia: a case study of the efficacy of the melodic intonation therapy. Music Percept. 2006;24:23–36.

Winters C, Kwakkel G, van Wegen EEH, Nijland RHM, Verbeek JM, Meskers CGM. Moving stroke rehabilitation forward. The need to change research. NeuroRehabilitation. 2018;43:19–30. https://doi.org/10.3233/NRE-172393.

Worschech F, Altenmüller E, Jünemann K, Sinke C, Krüger THC, Scholz DS, Müller CAH, Kliegel M, James CE, Marie D. Evidence of cortical thickness increases in bilateral auditory brain structures following piano learning in older adults. Ann N Y Acad Sci. 2022;1513(1):21–30. https://doi.org/10.1111/nyas.14762. Epub 2022 Mar 15. PMID: 35292982

Yoo GE, Kim SJ. Rhythmic auditory cueing in motor rehabilitation for stroke-patients: systematic review and meta-analysis. J Music Ther. 2016;53(2):149–77.

Zatorre RJ. Musical pleasure and reward: mechanisms and dysfunction. Ann N Y Acad Sci. 2015;1337:202–11. https://doi.org/10.1111/nyas.12677.

Music Therapy and Music-Based Intervention in Psychiatry

13

Laura Fusar-Poli and Pierluigi Politi

Key Points

- Mental disorders affect a large part of the population worldwide with variable levels of severity and functional impairment.
- Music exerts beneficial effects on the psychological and physiological states associated with mental disorders, as supported by neuroscientific research.
- Music therapy and music-based interventions have demonstrated to improve the symptoms of several mental disorders, including depression, schizophrenia, post-traumatic stress disorder, sleep disorders, and substance use disorders.
- Music may represent a promising viable, free-of-cost, complementary therapeutic tool in psychiatry.
- Research on music therapy and music-based interventions for some psychiatric disorders, such as anxiety disorders, obsessive-compulsive disorder, and eating disorders, is still scarce.
- Future studies should evaluate the long-lasting effects of music therapy and music-based interventions.

13.1 Introduction

Music has always held a special place in our lives, forming an integral part of human culture for millennials, transcending barriers of language and geography. The Ancient Greek philosopher Plato (428–347 BC) said, "Music gives a soul to the

L. Fusar-Poli (✉) · P. Politi
Department of Brain and Behavioral Sciences, University of Pavia, Pavia, Italy
e-mail: laura.fusarpoli@unipv.it

A. Raglio (ed.), *Music and Music Therapy Interventions in Clinical Practice*, Neurocultural Health and Wellbeing,
https://doi.org/10.1007/978-3-031-88578-5_13

universe, wings to the mind, flight to the imagination and life to everything." Plato considered that music played in different modes would arouse different emotions (West 1992).

In the realm of psychiatry, music-based interventions have garnered increasing attention as complementary therapeutic approaches, offering unique benefits for individuals grappling with various mental health conditions (Golden et al. 2022). The therapeutic use of music encompasses a wide range of activities, from passive listening to active participation, including music therapy (MT), music-assisted relaxation, and community music-making (Robb et al. 2011).

Whether we passively listen to our favorite songs or actively engage in music-making by singing or playing instruments, music can have a profound influence on our well-being. The mechanisms by which music exerts its therapeutic effects are multifaceted. The rhythmic and melodic elements of music can facilitate nonverbal communication (Shim 2007), emotional expression (Juslin 2013), and social connection (Koelsch 2013), making it particularly valuable in therapeutic settings where traditional verbal communication may be challenging. The evidence of music's effects on core mental health variables is readily apparent in our growing understanding of music's biological foundations. For instance, neuroimaging studies have revealed that music activates multiple brain regions involved in emotion, memory, and motor control, suggesting a robust neurobiological foundation for its therapeutic potential (Chan and Han 2022; Koelsch 2014). Critically, these foundations provide a rational basis for standardizing and expanding psychiatric applications and benefits of music (Boso et al. 2006; Bowling 2023). Moreover, music-based interventions offer a culturally sensitive approach to mental health care, allowing for the incorporation of patients' musical preferences and cultural backgrounds into their treatment plans (Roy and Dowd 2010). This personalization fosters a greater sense of agency and comfort, which can enhance therapeutic rapport and treatment adherence (Ramirez-Melendez 2023).

In this chapter, we will provide a summary of the evidence regarding the effects of MT and music-based interventions in the field of mental health. In each section, we will start with a description of each mental disorder, discuss the potential mechanisms of action, and finally synthesize the literature findings on the applications of music as a therapeutic tool for the specific condition.

13.2 Music Therapy and Music-Based Intervention for Depressive Disorders

13.2.1 Depressive Disorders

Clinical depression is a common mental disorder that affects more than 300 million people worldwide (Lim et al. 2018; Marcus et al. 2012). Depression is characterized by core symptoms of persistent low mood, diminished interest, loss of pleasure, and lack of energy, along with other symptoms such as sleep disturbance, appetite and weight disturbance, poor concentration, psychomotor changes, and feelings of guilt, worthlessness, and low self-esteem (American Psychiatric Association 2013). Depressive disorders may be comorbid with a wide array of other psychiatric and medical conditions (Smith et al. 2014).

Depressive symptoms can become chronic and recurrent and can lead to substantial impairment in an individual's ability to function in everyday life (Marcus et al. 2012). At its worst, depression can lead to suicide, and it has been linked to approximately 800,000 cases of suicide per year (World Health Organization 2021).

Depending on the quality and quantity of symptoms and the degree of functional impairment, depression can present at different levels of severity (American Psychiatric Association 2013). According to the severity level, guidelines may indicate psychological (e.g., cognitive behavioral therapy and interpersonal psychotherapy), pharmacological (e.g., antidepressants) treatment strategies, or a combination of both. Complementary therapies (e.g., exercise, light therapy, biofeedback, and MT) are also indicated (Lam et al. 2024).

13.2.2 How the Intervention Might Work

MT and music-based interventions may act on depression and related symptomatology through different mechanisms. It is well-known that depression is often accompanied by difficulties in emotion regulation. In this regard, music may represent an effective strategy to modulate emotions and moods, either as a self-therapeutic tool or with the help of a professional (Saarikallio et al. 2013; Maratos et al. 2011). Additionally, music may enable the depressed person to express emotions by creating musical sounds and structures (Punkanen et al. 2011).

Also, the act of playing musical instruments requires purposeful physical movement. The role of physical activity in alleviating depressive symptoms is well-recognized (Singh et al. 2023). In the case of music, this is not simply a matter of getting people moving, but also of enabling people to experience themselves as physical beings (Maratos et al. 2011).

Finally, music listening and music making are social, pleasurable, and meaningful activities. Trials of MT interventions have shown high levels of engagement with patient groups who are traditionally difficult to engage. The social function of music has been extensively discussed, particularly in group music-making (Koelsch 2013). In the case of MT and music-based interventions, patients may create a musical relationship with the therapist as well as other patients, in the case the intervention is conducted in a group. This may in turn enable the person with depression to experience and gain insight into relational and emotional problems by talking about the musical dialogue (Odell-Miller 1995).

Depression and anxiety are frequently co-occurring (Xin et al. 2015). In active MT, synchronization and attuned musical expression can modulate levels of anxiety (Trondalen 2016). In receptive MT, listening enables the patient to focus, relax, experience, and share experiences, and leads to reduced anxiety, particularly when involving adjunctive activities performed while listening, such as relaxation, meditation, movement, drawing, or reminiscence (Edwards 2016).

From a biological point of view, the capacity of rhythm to entrain activity in broad auditory-motor networks and simultaneously increase positive affect has also been hypothesized to account for a significant proportion of the benefits of musical treatments for anxiety and depression. Specifically, engaging these brain networks with high-groove rhythms may provide an efficient way to disrupt maladaptive patterns of neural activity associated with negative affect and self-focused negative rumination (Hamilton et al. 2015; Moberly and Watkins 2008).

13.2.3 Clinical Findings

The efficacy of MT and music-based interventions have been extensively studied in randomized clinical trials as well as longitudinal observational studies. The most up-to-date Cochrane meta-analysis on the topic included nine randomized controlled trials (RCTs) or controlled clinical trials (CCTs) comparing MT versus treatment as usual (TAU), psychological therapies, pharmacological therapies, other therapies, or different forms of MT for improving depression (Aalbers et al. 2024; Aalbers et al. 2017). Findings showed that MT was superior to treatment as usual in improving not only depressive symptoms but also anxiety and functioning. Conversely, no evidence of superiority was found for quality of life (Aalbers et al. 2017). However, functioning and quality of life, which are important domains to measure in psychiatric practice, were evaluated in one study only (Erkkilä et al. 2011).

More recently, a larger meta-analysis including 55 RCTs evaluating the efficacy of MT and music medicine revealed that both interventions exhibited a significant reduction in depressive symptoms compared with the control group, with music medicine exhibiting a stronger effect. Among the specific methods, efficacy was stronger for recreative MT and increasingly weaker for guided imagery and music, music-assisted relaxation, music and imagery, improvisational music therapy, and music and discussion. MT and music medicine both exhibited stronger effects in the short- and medium-term compared with longer durations of the intervention periods (Tang et al. 2020).

Other reviews have focused on the efficacy of music interventions on depressive symptoms in specific age groups or special populations. As for children and adolescents, a recent review (Belski et al. 2022) reported that four out of six RCTs (total sample = 428) favored MT for improvement of depressive symptoms at short- and intermediate-term follow-ups compared to control. Nevertheless, the authors underlined the extreme heterogeneity and flaws of the currently available literature.

A meta-analysis focused on older patients with depression reported that MT may improve depression, anxiety, cognitive ability, and blood pressure (Wang et al. 2023). Interestingly, longer durations of treatment were associated with better therapeutic effects (Wang et al. 2023). Similarly, Dhyppayom et al. (Dhippayom et al. 2022) reviewed the RCTs of music interventions in participants aged ≥60 years. Music interventions were classified based on the theme, intensity, and provider/platform. The authors acknowledged active MT for more than 60 minutes/week as the most effective music intervention to alleviate depression in older adults. Nevertheless, music medicine by listening to music of participants' own preference >60 minutes/week was acknowledged as an alternative approach in settings with limited resources (Dhippayom et al. 2022).

Table 13.1 Summary of the key findings on the efficacy of music therapy and music-based interventions for depression and schizophrenia spectrum disorders

Depression	
Mechanisms of action	**Findings**
Emotion regulation Physical activity Social engagement Relaxation	MT and MBI are effective in improving depressive and anxiety symptoms, and functioning, in adults with clinical depression MT appears useful to treat depression in children and adolescents, although the evidence available is heterogeneous MT and MBI improve depression, anxiety, cognitive ability, and blood pressure in older adults with depression, with better effects for longer and more intense treatment periods MT improves depressive symptoms in women with post-partum depression although the beneficial effects are not long-lasting
Schizophrenia spectrum disorders	
Mechanisms of action	**Findings**
Nonverbal communication Emotional expression Social engagement	MT improves total symptoms, negative symptoms (e.g., diminished emotional expression), depressive symptoms, social functioning, and quality of life General functioning is improved only with high-frequency interventions MT and MBI do not improve positive psychotic symptoms (e.g., delusions and hallucinations) MT may exert a beneficial effect on cognition MBI appear useful also in acute settings

Legend: *MBI* music-based interventions, *MT* music therapy

Finally, some studies have focused specifically on post-partum depression. A longitudinal study reported that the frequency of listening to music during pregnancy was associated with higher levels of well-being and reduced symptoms of postnatal depression in the first three months after birth. However, the beneficial effects disappeared by 4–6 months after birth. These results appeared to be particularly strong among women with lower levels of well-being and high levels of depression at baseline (Fancourt and Perkins 2018). These findings are in line with a meta-analysis specifically focused on the efficacy of MT for women with post-partum depression. The analysis included four studies involving 763 patients and showed that MT had a significant effect on depressive symptoms compared to the control group (Yang et al. 2019).

A summary of the key findings is reported in Table 13.1.

13.3 Music Therapy and Music-Based Intervention for Schizophrenia Spectrum Disorders

13.3.1 Schizophrenia Spectrum Disorders

Schizophrenia spectrum disorders are a group of conditions characterized by a variety of severe symptoms interfering with a person's "relationship with reality," including delusions, hallucinations, disorganized thinking, speech and behavior, and negative symptoms (e.g., diminished emotional expression or avolition). According to the main psychiatric diagnostic manuals, schizophrenia spectrum disorders are schizotypal personality disorder, delusional disorder, brief psychotic disorder, schizophreniform disorder, schizophrenia, schizoaffective disorder, substance/medication-induced psychotic disorder, psychotic disorder due to another medical condition, catatonia, other specified schizophrenia spectrum and other psychotic disorder, and unspecified schizophrenia spectrum and other psychotic disorders (American Psychiatric Association 2013).

The prevalence of schizophrenia spectrum disorders has been estimated at around 2.5% of the general population, with schizophrenia (i.e., the most chronic and impairing psychotic disorder) having a lifetime prevalence of around 1% (Chang et al. 2017). Schizophrenia typically occurs during adolescence or early adulthood, while childhood and late-life onset forms are rare. More specifically, the modal age of onset is between 18 and 25 for men and between 25 and 35 for women, with a second peak occurring around menopause (American Psychiatric Association 2013). Of note, the risk for comorbid mental and physical disorders (Halstead et al. 2024; Salari et al. 2024) and mortality rates for all causes, natural causes, and unnatural causes (Correll et al. 2022) in patients with schizophrenia are higher than those in the general population. On average, schizophrenia is associated with 10–25 years of potential life-years lost (Tanskanen et al. 2018; Crump et al. 2013).

Guidelines indicate antipsychotic medications as the first-line therapeutic option for schizophrenia spectrum disorders (Barnes et al. 2019). Psychosocial interventions, such as family psychoeducation, cognitive behavioral therapy, cognitive remediation, and individual placement and support for employment are also suggested (Solmi et al. 2023).

13.3.2 How the Intervention Might Work

Music is naturally considered a powerful nonverbal communication tool. Some people with, or without, mental health problems may prefer a medium for communication and expression other than verbal language. Words are often too specific, for example, in defining nuanced, ambivalent, or uncertain emotions or conditions. Based on this, people who struggle to express their thoughts and emotions through words may benefit from nonverbal interventions such as music or MT due to their unique qualities (Solli 2008; Fusar-Poli et al. 2017). From the patients' perspective, improving musical skills and resources through MT may positively affect many aspects of daily life (Ansdell et al. 2010).

Patients experiencing the negative symptoms of schizophrenia (e.g., social withdrawal, expressive deficits, or affective flattening) may find it difficult to translate into words such experiences and emotions when talking to a conventional therapist (Millan et al. 2014). Indeed, it has been suggested that music-evoked emotions might have a peculiar profile in patients with schizophrenia spectrum disorders, which would be also associated with symptom severity (Abe et al. 2017). Music as a medium of therapy addresses issues related to emotion and social interaction and is described as motivating. Therefore, it has been speculated earlier (e.g., Mössler et al. 2011) that it may be particularly well-suited to the treatment of negative symptoms, such as affective flattening and bluntness, poor social interaction, and a general lack of interest.

From a neurobiological point of view, research has demonstrated that music interventions may increase functional connectivity in the right middle temporal gyrus (Yang et al. 2018) and the insular cortex (He et al. 2017), thus improving the patients' psychiatric symptoms through normalizing the salience and sensorimotor networks.

13.3.3 Clinical Findings

A Cochrane meta-analysis (Geretsegger et al. 2017) including 18 studies including 1215 participants examined the effects of MT over the short-, medium-, and long-term, with treatment dosage varying from 7 to 240 sessions. It demonstrated that MT plus standard care—compared to standard care alone—improved general mental health, negative symptoms of schizophrenia, and social functioning. No effects were observed for general functioning or positive symptoms of schizophrenia. Interestingly, the strongest effects were found in studies that provided long-term, high-frequency music therapy (Geretsegger et al. 2017). This is in line with an earlier review specifically focused on the dose-effect relation in MT (Gold et al. 2009). Effects on social functioning were in favor of MT in the short-, medium-, and long-term, with effect sizes ranging from medium to large. Results for cognitive functioning were mixed, with some scales suggesting benefit and others suggesting no effect. The effects on general functioning were significant and large for "high-dose" music therapy, both in the medium term and in the long term, while low-dose music therapy did not affect general functioning. Overall, these results suggest that MT may affect social functioning more quickly than general functioning. This appears plausible, given the focus of especially active MT on social interaction. Effects of MT on general functioning likely require more sessions and more time (Geretsegger et al. 2017).

More recently, Jia et al. (2020) found that adjunct MT significantly improved total symptoms, negative symptoms, depression symptoms, and quality of life compared with the control group (Jia et al. 2020). Again, MT did not appear to significantly affect positive symptoms (Jia et al. 2020).

Interestingly, music interventions may ameliorate neglected and difficult-to-treat symptoms of schizophrenia spectrum disorders, such as cognitive impairments. A recent scoping review has reported that MT interventions seem to improve different cognitive areas, including attention, executive function, language, memory, and processing speed (Stone and Short 2024).

Finally, some studies were specifically focused on the acute phases of psychotic disorders, showing that MT improved general psychiatric symptoms in hospitalized patients (Volpe et al. 2018; Metzner et al. 2018; Morgan et al. 2011).

A summary of the key findings is reported in Table 13.1.

13.4 Music Therapy and Music-Based Intervention for Anxiety Disorders

13.4.1 Anxiety Disorders

Anxiety is a common emotional state biologically rooted in the original fight-or-flight response. It is characterized by tension, worry and/or fear, and physical changes, such as rapid heartbeat, shortness of breath, nausea, and vomiting that may occur as a reaction to stress and worries about future or current events (American Psychiatric Association 2013). Studies have shown that many individuals experience subclinical anxiety symptoms during their lifetime (Haller et al. 2014). Even if these symptoms do not reach the diagnostic threshold, they can still cause significant suffering and impairment (Bosman et al. 2019; Barlow and Campbell 2000).

When quantitatively exaggerated, anxiety becomes pathological. The DSM-5 chapter on anxiety disorders comprises separation anxiety disorder, selective mutism, specific phobia, social anxiety disorder (social phobia), panic disorder, agoraphobia, generalized anxiety disorder, substance/medication-induced anxiety disorder, and anxiety disorder due to another medical condition. It has been estimated that around 4% of the general population worldwide suffer from at least one anxiety disorder (Metrics, Evaluation 2021), even though in the real clinical world these categories are frequently comorbid.

The main treatments for anxiety disorders are psychotherapy (e.g., cognitive behavioral therapy), psychotropic medications, (e.g., antidepressants and benzodiazepines), or a combination of both (Bandelow et al. 2017).

13.4.2 How the Intervention Might Work

Music can exert its influence on the hypothalamic-pituitary-adrenal (HPA) axis, a fundamental component of the body's stress response system. This effect can potentially lead to a decrease in the levels of stress hormones, including cortisol, contributing further to a sense of tranquillity and emotional well-being (Kreutz et al. 2012).

Additionally, music interventions operate by engaging the brain's intricate network of emotional and sensory pathways. When individuals are exposed to soothing melodies and rhythmic patterns, their brains respond by releasing neurotransmitters such as dopamine and serotonin (Chanda and Levitin 2013). Neurochemicals play a pivotal role in promoting relaxation and reducing stress, contributing to a noticeable decrease in heart rate and blood pressure (Koelsch and Jäncke 2015; Loomba et al. 2012).

13.4.3 Clinical Findings

To our knowledge, only one pilot longitudinal study has specifically focused on a population of patients affected by anxiety disorder, namely generalized anxiety disorder (GAD). The study revealed that MT was effective in significantly reducing both self-reported anxiety and depressive symptoms in participants (Gutiérrez and Camarena 2015).

Conversely, a large amount of studies have focused on anxiety as a transdiagnostic clinical dimension. In 2020, De Witte and colleagues (de Witte et al. 2020) performed two multilevel meta-analyses of 104 RCTs to assess the strength of the effects of music interventions on both physiological and psychological stress-related outcomes, and to test the potential moderators of the intervention effects. Results showed that music interventions had an overall significant effect on stress reduction in both physiological (e.g., heart rate, blood pressure, and hormonal levels) and psychological (e.g., restlessness, anxiety, and nervousness) outcomes. Larger effects were found on heart rate compared to blood pressure and hormone levels (de Witte et al. 2020).

A meta-analytic review by Lu et al. (Lu et al. 2021) included 32 studies to evaluate the efficacy of MT on anxiety as a transdiagnostic dimension. MT significantly reduced anxiety compared to the control group at post-intervention, but not at follow-up. Subgroup analyses conducted dividing the studies by age (<60 vs. ≥60 years old), country (developed vs. developing), and number of sessions (<12 vs. ≥12 sessions) also revealed significant post-treatment effects of MT (Lu et al. 2021).

Other important studies have focused on specific populations at risk for anxiety disorders, such as people affected by medical illnesses. For instance, music interventions may have a large anxiety-reducing effect in adults with cancer (Bradt et al. 2021), more specifically when receiving chemotherapy (Nguyen et al. 2022), with no significant difference between patient-selected music and researcher-selected music, recorded music, and live music. Of note, a length of 15–20 min/session and offering immediately before chemotherapy were more effective on anxiety than that of 30–45 min and delivering during chemotherapy (Nguyen et al. 2022). Also, perioperative music interventions have been shown to improve anxiety in people undergoing surgery (Kühlmann et al. 2018; Hole et al. 2015; Bradt et al. 2013; van der Heijden et al. 2015).

A summary of the key findings is reported in Table 13.2.

Table 13.2 Summary of the key findings on the efficacy of music therapy and music-based interventions for anxiety, post-traumatic stress disorder, and obsessive-compulsive disorder

Anxiety	
Mechanisms of action	**Findings**
Effect on the stress response system Decrease in blood pressure and heart rate	One pilot study reported improvements in anxiety and depressive symptoms in patients with generalized anxiety disorders MBI have a significant effect on anxiety as a dimension in both physiological (e.g., heart rate, blood pressure, and hormonal levels) and psychological (e.g., restlessness and nervousness) outcomes Music may be helpful in reducing anxiety in specific at-risk populations, such as people undergoing chemotherapy or surgery
Obsessive-compulsive disorder	
Mechanisms of action	**Findings**
Anxiety reduction Emotion regulation Improvement of cognitive flexibility Social support	Two studies reported that music listening may improve obsessions, compulsions, as well as depression and anxiety symptoms
Post-traumatic stress disorder	
Mechanisms of action	**Findings**
Emotion regulation Anxiety reduction Social connections Decrease in arousal levels	MT and MBI may improve PTSD symptoms comparably to active control groups Guided imagery music (GIM) has shown some effectiveness on refugees, military veterans, and abused women, with significant changes in physiological measures of autonomic dysregulation

Legend: *MBI* music-based interventions, *MT* music therapy, *PTSD* post-traumatic stress disorder

13.5 Music Therapy and Music-Based Intervention for Obsessive-Compulsive Disorder

13.5.1 Obsessive-Compulsive Disorder

Obsessive-compulsive disorder (OCD) is a chronic mental health condition characterized by persistent, intrusive thoughts (obsessions) and repetitive behaviors or mental acts (compulsions) that individuals feel driven to perform. These obsessions and compulsions can significantly interfere with daily functioning and cause considerable distress. Common obsessions include fears of contamination, aggressive impulses, and concerns about symmetry, while compulsions often involve excessive cleaning, checking, counting, or arranging. The prevalence of OCD is estimated to be around 1–3% of the general population (American Psychiatric Association 2013).

Treatment typically includes cognitive-behavioral therapy (CBT), particularly exposure and response prevention (ERP) (Reid et al. 2021) and medications, such as selective serotonin reuptake inhibitors (SSRIs) (Pittenger and Bloch 2014),

13.5.2 How the Intervention Might Work

One way music-based interventions help is by reducing anxiety, a common comorbidity in OCD that often exacerbates obsessive and compulsive behaviors. Listening to calming music can lower cortisol levels and induce relaxation, making it easier for individuals to manage stress and reduce the severity of their symptoms (Khalfa et al. 2003).

Furthermore, MT can assist in emotional regulation and provide a nonverbal outlet for expressing complex emotions. Individuals with OCD often experience intense feelings of fear and guilt related to their obsessions and compulsions (Mavrogiorgou et al. 2024). Through activities like songwriting, improvisation, and musical expression, patients can explore and articulate these emotions in a safe and structured environment. This process can help decrease the emotional burden of OCD and improve overall emotional well-being.

In addition to emotional benefits, music interventions can also engage cognitive processes in beneficial ways. Structured musical activities, such as learning to play an instrument or engaging in rhythmic exercises, can enhance concentration and cognitive flexibility, potentially counteracting the rigid thought patterns typical in OCD (Gruner and Pittenger 2017). Cognitive-behavioral MT, which integrates cognitive-behavioral techniques with music-based activities, can directly target maladaptive thought patterns and behaviors by combining musical engagement with therapeutic exercises (Hanser 2015).

Group MT sessions can provide social support and reduce feelings of isolation, which are often experienced by individuals with OCD (Timpano et al. 2014).

13.5.3 Clinical Findings

Literature has reported cases of musical obsessions in OCD patients (Pfizer and Andrade 1999; Orjuela-Rojas and Rodríguez 2018). Individuals with OCD also appear more sensitive to tense music and have an increased desire for harmony in music (Truong et al. 2021). Nevertheless, to our knowledge, only two studies have specifically tested the efficacy of music interventions in people with OCD. Abdulah et al. (Abdulah et al. 2019) investigated the effect of listening to selected music tracks like relaxing music, sleep music, and meditation in OCD with a control group under standard treatment only. Patients in the music group had significantly less severe obsessive and compulsive symptoms (Abdulah et al. 2019). Similarly, another study (Shiranibidabadi and Mehryar 2017) investigated the use of receptive music therapy, which consisted of listening to selected tracks of Iranian classical music followed by discussions with experienced psychiatrists, in 30 patients with OCD, compared with standard treatment. Also in this case, the music group showed a greater decrease in the total obsessive scores, with significant differences for checking and slowness, but not for washing or responsibility. Additionally, MT exhibited a greater reduction in depressive and anxiety symptoms (Shiranibidabadi and Mehryar 2017). Findings are summarized in a recent review (Truong et al. 2021).

A summary of the key findings is reported in Table 13.2.

13.6 Music Therapy and Music-Based Intervention for Post-traumatic Stress Disorder

13.6.1 Post-Traumatic Stress Disorder

Post-traumatic stress disorder (PTSD) is characterized by an inability to recover from a reaction to stress by one month following exposure to a traumatic event (American Psychiatric Association 2013). Symptoms can include re-experiencing the event, intrusive memories of the event, prolonged emotional distress and physiological reactivity after exposure to trauma-related stimuli, avoidance of trauma-related thoughts and external reminders, negative alterations in mood and cognition (e.g., anhedonia, constricted affect, social detachment, persistent negative trauma-related emotions, and beliefs), and alterations in arousal and reactivity (e.g., hyperarousal, irritable and aggressive behavior, and exaggerated startle response) (American Psychiatric Association 2013). In a large epidemiological study conducted in the United States, 60% of men and 51% of women experienced at least one traumatic event in their lifetime, with 8% experiencing PTSD (Kessler et al. 2013). Even though many individuals who experience trauma do not meet the full criteria for PTSD, many trauma-exposed individuals still experience residual post-traumatic stress symptoms that negatively impact their quality of life as well as increased risk for other mental health conditions such as depression and problematic substance use (Thomas et al. 2010; Campbell et al. 2007).

PTSD is usually managed with specific psychotherapies, such as trauma-focused cognitive behavioral therapy or Eye Movement Desensitization and Reprocessing (EMDR) (Wright et al. 2024). Selective serotonin reuptake inhibitors (SSRIs), specifically paroxetine and sertraline, are also suggested as pharmacological therapy (Hoskins et al. 2021).

13.6.2 How the Intervention Might Work

MT may offer a more accessible and less stigmatizing therapeutic option for treating many reactions to stress, including PTSD. The therapeutic effects of music therapy for PTSD may involve social, cognitive, and neurobiological mechanisms (Landis-Shack et al. 2017). For example, music is frequently used as a grounding method in psychotherapy to manage emotions linked with intrusive or unsettling reminders (Carr et al. 2012). Similar to other mental disorders, also in PTSD, music interventions, especially if conducted in a group, may boost social connections and alleviate isolation, consequently enhancing emotional well-being and reducing avoidant behaviors (Koelsch 2013). As reported in the sections above, MT and music-based interventions have been proven to reduce stress and anxiety in other clinical populations.

From a biological perspective, experimental studies indicate that music can increase the production of dopamine and endorphins, decrease cortisol levels, and increase cerebral blood flow to areas correlated with pleasing behaviors, consequently attenuating fear, sadness, co-occurring depression and anxiety, and over-arousal and amplifying experiences of pleasure and reward (Boso et al. 2006). Thus, music has the potential to act on the circuitry of the brain involved in the autonomic dysregulation associated with PTSD (Wang et al. 2024).

13.6.3 Clinical Findings

A recent systematic review summarized the findings of 14 studies evaluating the effect of music-based interventions for PTSD, of which mostly were feasibility studies. A decrease in PTSD symptoms was reported by a large majority of the included trials (13 out of 14), including those using passive listening rather than the traditional MT format of therapist-led interventions (Wang et al. 2024).

Another meta-analysis of nine studies focused specifically on the effectiveness of MT (Ma et al. 2024), finding that post-treatment PTSD symptom scores were significantly lower in the MT group than the inactive control group, but comparable between the MT group and the active control group. The retention rates did not differ significantly between the MT group and both control groups. These results suggest that MT may be useful in relieving PTSD symptoms, but its therapeutic effect is comparable to that of standard psychotherapy (Ma et al. 2024).

Guided imagery music (GIM) is a specific method based on the assumption that it is indeed possible to select the most appropriate music for the patient, depending on the therapist's understanding of the patient's needs (Beck et al. 2018). GIM has shown some effectiveness on different groups of individuals suffering from PTSD, such as refugees (Beck et al. 2018), military veterans (Story and Beck 2017), and abused women (Rudstam et al. 2022). Interestingly, Rudstam et al. (2023) reported that measurements of heart rate, heart rate variability, inter-beat differences, and electrodermal reactivity showed significant changes indicating decreased arousal during trauma script after treatment and an improvement of vagal function in the treatment group. Significant treatment-related reductions were found in symptoms of PTSD, re-experiencing, and avoidance. The changes pre- to post-treatment in heart rate reactivity and self-rated PTSD symptoms correlated significantly (Rudstam et al. 2023).

A summary of the key findings is reported in Table 13.2.

13.7 Music Therapy and Music-Based Intervention for Sleep Disorders

13.7.1 Sleep Disorders

Sleep disorders are distressing and disabling conditions affecting a significant proportion of the general population, with a prevalence estimated at around 10–48% (Ferrie et al. 2011).

Paradoxically, sleep disorders are usually defined and diagnosed based on daytime distress and/or functional impairment as a consequence of bad quality, timing, and amount of sleep. Primary and commonly diagnosed sleep disorders are organized in the DSM-5 into three major categories: insomnia, hypersomnia, and arousal disorder (American Psychiatric Association 2013). Insomnia is the most common sleep disorder, with a recent prevalence in the past year which has been estimated at around 30% of the adult population. Chronic insomnia—defined by difficulties in falling asleep, maintaining sleep, and early morning awakening and coupled with daytime consequences such as fatigue, attention deficits, and mood instability (Riemann et al. 2015)—is complained by 10% of adults (Ferrie et al. 2011). Of note, sleep–wake disorders are often a co-occurrent manifestation of different medical or mental health conditions.

Medical conditions frequently associated with sleep–wake disorders are, for instance, lung disease, gastroesophageal reflux, chronic renal disease, chronic pain, infectious diseases, menopause, and cancer (Parish 2009). Of note, disrupted sleep might be a contributory causal factor in the occurrence of major types of mental health disorders. It is argued that insomnia and other mental health conditions not only share common causes but also show a bidirectional relationship, with typically the strongest pathway being disrupted sleep as a causal factor in the occurrence of other psychiatric problems (Freeman et al. 2020).

Sleep disturbances are thus broad, transdiagnostic issues. Treatments for sleep disorders may involve the management of potential underlying medical causes as well as behavioral, psychological, and pharmacological therapeutic options, depending on the type of disorder and functional impairment. As for medications, benzodiazepines are frequently used to treat insomnia, even though their long-term use may lead to a withdrawal syndrome with rapid eye movement (REM) rebound. Other agents for insomnia include sedating antidepressants and over-the-counter sleep products (sedating antihistamines). Melatonin is also suggested as a treatment option (Riemann et al. 2017).

13.7.2 How the Intervention Might Work

The use of music as a therapeutic tool for sleep has been documented since antiquities. Indeed, music can be either a potent stimulator or can be also used to soothe and sedate. In the Old Testament of the Bible, there were a few accounts of spirits tormenting Saul, resulting in David playing the lyre and strumming a soothing tune. As a result, Saul was relieved from his terror, as the music prompted the evil spirits to leave his tormented body, so he could rest with ease (Friedmann 2013).

These most basic essential music elements (i.e., melody, harmony, rhythm, meter, and timbre) of music might serve their integrated prowess. As a result, programmers, musicians, and therapists seeking to invoke sleep responses using music would likely include decisions related to content and genre within these combined elements (Delle Monache et al. 2022).

Increased arousal levels in the cognitive, emotional, and physiological domains may represent both predisposing and perpetuating factors for sleep disturbances (Mainieri et al. 2021). For this reason, music that, as previously reported, has been shown to regulate arousal and stress, may act as a complementary tool for the treatment of insomnia and, more broadly, sleep disorders.

Overall, literature has identified six potential mechanisms of action of music on sleep: (1) relaxation, where music encourages physiological or psychological relaxation; (2) distraction, where music acts as a focal point to distract from inner stressful thoughts; (3) entrainment, synchronization of biological rhythms to beat structures in music; (4) masking, obscuring noxious background noise with music; (5) enjoyment, listening to preferred, emotionally relatable, or pleasant music; and (6) expectation, individuals cultural beliefs around music (Dickson and Schubert 2019).

13.7.3 Clinical Findings

Music interventions seemed to offer clear advantages for adults with primary insomnia. In fact, according to meta-analytic evidence (Feng et al. 2018), insomnia symptoms—measured using the Pittsburgh Sleep Quality Index (PSQI) scores—improved more with music interventions rather than standard care, with patients ranking listening to music as the best means of intervention. For overall sleep quality, only music-associated relaxation was statistically more effective than the standard treatment. In terms of sleep onset latency, music-associated relaxation and listening to music had significant advantages. Listening to music and music with exercise displayed a tendency to improve sleep efficiency. According to the authors, listening to music and music-associated relaxation are probably the best options to consider in the application of music intervention (Feng et al. 2018).

Results were confirmed by a recent Cochrane systematic review reporting that music listening improved sleep quality measured with the PSQI in the music groups (Jespersen et al. 2022). However, no clear difference was found in the effects of listening to music on insomnia severity and sleep interruption, and low-certainty evidence that, compared to no treatment or treatment as usual, listening to music may reduce problems with sleep-onset latency, total sleep time, and sleep efficiency (Jespersen et al. 2022).

Other studies reported more specific beneficial effects of music in older adults (Wang et al. 2016, 2021; Petrovsky et al. 2021), people with dementia (Mu et al. 2022), and hospitalized patients (Jespersen et al. 2023; Kakar et al. 2021).

A summary of the key findings is reported in Table 13.3.

Table 13.3 Summary of the key findings on the efficacy of music therapy and music-based interventions for sleep disorders, substance use disorders, and eating disorders

Sleep disorders	
Mechanisms of action	**Findings**
Decrease in arousal levels Relaxation Distraction Synchronization with biological rhythms	MBI improve overall sleep quality, but it might be less effective in improving insomnia severity and sleep interruption sleep-onset latency, total sleep time, and sleep efficiency MBI appear effective in special populations, such as older adults, people with dementia, and hospitalized patients
Substance use disorders	
Mechanisms of action	**Findings**
Emotion regulation Decrease in substance craving due to dopamine release Awareness of maladaptive coping styles and interpersonal patterns Effect on co-occurrent mental disorders	MT increases motivation for change and improves short-term mental health outcomes, but long-term effects have not been addressed Effects of MT may vary according to specific MT type and participant characteristics No clear evidence of MT on depression, motivation to stay sober/clean, and anxiety The combination with psychoeducation may reduce stress, increase self-efficacy, and prevent relapses
Eating disorders	
Mechanisms of action	**Findings**
Stress reduction Emotional expression Awareness of own's body Social interaction	MBI are useful in improving mood regulation, emotional Well-being, and management of meal-related distress Vodcast (video podcast) interventions are associated with healthful eating Relaxing music may help reducing anxiety around eating The majority of studies have focused on anorexia and bulimia, while there is a lack of research on binge eating disorder.

Legend: *MBI* music-based interventions, *MT* music therapy

13.8 Music Therapy for Substance Use Disorders

13.8.1 Substance Use Disorders

Substance use disorders (SUD) may be defined as the use of one or more psychoactive substances, medically prescribed or not (e.g., alcohol, cannabis, cocaine, opioids, and anti-anxiety drugs), in a manner that results in continued use despite significant substance-related problems in areas of the person's cognitive, behavioral, physiological, or social functioning (American Psychiatric Association 2013). Problematic substance use is a widespread issue and related high-risk behavior has a negative impact on individuals, families, and global public health. The burden of problematic substance use on systems such as healthcare, criminal justice, and unemployment/welfare is substantial. It has been estimated that approximately 35.6

million people worldwide experienced drug use disorder in 2018, amounting to 0.62% of the adult population (aged 15–64 years) (Johnson et al. 2022).

Treatment of SUD must meet the complex biopsychosocial needs of the person involved and thus must be multidisciplinary in nature. Treatment programs may include psychosocial therapies—including individual, family, or group counseling—medications to reduce substance withdrawal or for comorbid mental and physical disorders as well as residential facility programs for detoxification and rehabilitation (Rosenthal et al. 2022).

13.8.2 How the Intervention Might Work

Music interventions have a direct neurobiological impact on areas of the brain implicated in substance use, including emotion regulation and reward (Cournoyer Lemaire et al. 2021). They also indirectly impact substance use behavior by supporting social engagement, improving coping skills, and increasing motivation for treatment.

People with SUD demonstrate dysfunction in emotion regulation, such as dampened inhibition of intense affects and abnormal emotional reactions to emotional stimuli in line with neuroimaging findings showing changes in emotion-related brain areas (Wilcox et al. 2016; O'Daly et al. 2012). Indeed, people with SUD often use substances as a strategy for coping with difficult emotions. Music therapists understand and utilize the various ways that music induces emotions thus enabling the development of a broader and more flexible array of strategies for coping with emotions, which in turn can lead to increased motivation and sustained engagement in the therapeutic music process. (Koelsch et al. 2015; Koelsch 2014; Hakvoort et al. 2020).

Importantly, music that provokes peak experiences stimulates neural reward and emotion systems similar to those that are activated by (illicit) drug use (Blood and Zatorre 2001), which can result in dopamine release (Salimpoor et al. 2011). As music provides a means of promoting positive mood states (Koelsch 2014), it may consequently buffer against the risk of relapse that is associated with negative mood states (Koob 2013). Importantly, individuals with SUD can experience a decrease in substance craving after listening to songs they identify as helping them stay clean/sober, but they may also experience an increase in substance craving after listening to songs they identify as making them want to use substances (Short and Dingle 2016). Thus, important aims of music interventions, especially when conducted by a trained professional such as in the case of MT, within substance use treatment include gaining awareness of healthy and unhealthy uses of music, and understanding how context impacts perception of the music (Hohmann et al. 2017).

Music-based interventions and MT conducted in group settings enable participants to become aware of maladaptive coping and interpersonal patterns. Participants who have difficulty forming relationships with others may find that music offers a nonverbal means of being with and relating to others with tangible social and interpersonal benefits. Expansion of positive social experiences through MT can be an essential factor in increasing motivation for continued treatment.

Finally, as a large number of people with SUD also have co-occurring mental health disorders, the broader effects of music interventions on mental health may have relevance in the context of SUD treatment.

13.8.3 Clinical Findings

Rigorous evidence syntheses from Cochrane suggest that MT reduces craving, increases motivation for change, and improves short-term mental health outcomes, but long-term effects have not been addressed (Ghetti et al. 2022). Effects of MT may vary according to specific MT type (e.g., active, listening, and combined), but also according to participant characteristics such as SUD type, age, gender, or minority status. However, no clear evidence was found of a beneficial effect on depression, motivation to stay sober/clean, and anxiety (Ghetti et al. 2022).

Interestingly, a recent RCT suggested that the combination of psychoeducation with music intervention effectively reduced stress, increased self-efficacy, and prevented relapses in people with SUD (Kayaoğlu and Şahin 2022).

A summary of the key findings is reported in Table 13.3.

13.9 Music-Based Interventions for Eating Disorders

13.9.1 Eating Disorders

Eating disorders (ED) are complex mental health conditions characterized by abnormal eating habits that negatively affect a person's physical and emotional well-being. These disorders include anorexia nervosa, bulimia nervosa, and binge-eating disorder. Individuals with eating disorders may experience intense fear of gaining weight, distorted body image, and a compulsive need to control food intake, leading to severe nutritional deficiencies and health complications (American Psychiatric Association 2013).

Treatment typically involves a multidisciplinary approach, including psychological therapy, nutritional counseling, and medical intervention, aimed at restoring healthy eating patterns and addressing underlying emotional issues (Treasure et al. 2020).

13.9.2 How the Intervention Might Work

One of the primary effects of music-based interventions is the reduction of anxiety and stress, which are commonly experienced by individuals with eating disorders (Kerr-Gaffney et al. 2018). This stress reduction can in turn alleviate some of the intense emotional distress that often accompanies eating disorders, creating a more supportive environment for therapeutic work (Meule et al. 2021).

Moreover, MT can enhance emotional expression and processing, which is crucial for individuals with eating disorders who might struggle to articulate their feelings or understand their emotional triggers (Romero-Mesa et al. 2021; Westwood et al. 2017). Engaging in music-making activities, such as playing instruments, singing, or composing music, allows individuals to express emotions in a nonverbal way, facilitating deeper emotional exploration and release. This can help patients identify and address underlying psychological issues contributing to their disorder, such as trauma, low self-esteem, or perfectionism.

In addition to emotional benefits, music-based interventions can also improve physical health outcomes. For example, incorporating movement and dance into MT can promote body awareness and a more positive relationship with one's body. This is particularly beneficial for individuals with eating disorders, who often experience distorted body image and discomfort with their physical selves (Ahrberg et al. 2011). Dance and movement therapy can encourage body positivity, improve coordination and strength, and foster a more mindful and appreciative connection with the body.

Social interaction and support are other critical aspects of music-based interventions. Group music therapy sessions can provide a sense of community and belonging, reducing feelings of isolation that many individuals with eating disorders experience (Meneguzzo et al. 2024b; Makri et al. 2022). The collaborative nature of making music in a group setting encourages social bonding, enhances communication skills, and builds a support network that can be pivotal in the recovery process.

13.9.3 Clinical Findings

A recent review has summarized the evidence on MT (five studies), music medicine (four studies), and other music-based interventions (seven studies) in individuals with anorexia nervosa, bulimia nervosa, binge eating disorder, or other ED. The interventions examined varied widely but were reported to be generally associated with improved mood regulation, emotional well-being, and management of meal-related distress. Vodcast (video podcast) interventions were associated with healthful eating in non-inpatient populations (Chang et al. 2023).

Similarly, Testa and colleagues (2020) performed a systematic review of 16 studies involving a total of 3792 participants with ED or at risk for ED. In inpatients with anorexia nervosa, listening to classical music was beneficial to food consumption. Singing in a group reduced post-prandial anxiety in anorexia nervosa inpatients and outpatients. Vodcasts which also included positive visual or autobiographical stimuli helped bulimia nervosa patients with anxiety and body image perception. Songwriting and sessions with a Body Monochord helped with the processing of therapeutically relevant topics in anorexia. Watching music videos, however, reinforced body dissatisfaction, drive for thinness, bodyweight concerns, preoccupation with physical appearance in pre-teenage and teenage girls, and drive for muscularity in adolescent boys (Testa et al. 2020).

Of note, the majority of studies included in the two aforementioned reviews mainly included studies involving participants with anorexia and bulimia nervosa, while there is a lack of research on binge eating disorder.

Research has also shown that listening to calming music before and after meals can help reduce anxiety around eating, making the process less daunting for individuals with anorexia nervosa or bulimia nervosa. For instance, in a recent study, women diagnosed with ED were exposed to three randomized music conditions (i.e., no music, focus piano music, and pop music) over two weeks. Results showed that the absence of music led to an increase in uneaten food and the presence of eating rituals during mealtimes. Significantly, only silence during mealtime reduced positive emotional states, while background music maintained positive emotions. No specific differences emerged between the two types of music (focus piano and pop)(Meneguzzo et al. 2024a).

A summary of the key findings is reported in Table 13.3.

13.10 Conclusion

Music is a widespread, culture-free medium for people to communicate with others and express themselves outside of the verbal language. Music-based interventions have emerged as effective complementary treatments in psychiatry, demonstrating significant benefits across a range of mental health conditions.

Indeed, clinical applications of music in psychiatric settings have been demonstrated to reduce anxiety and depression symptoms by facilitating emotional expression and regulation, increase engagement in treatment, reduce agitation, and contribute to better overall outcomes. Music may also facilitate patients to learn and develop musical talents; this process could improve their confidence/self-esteem, coping mechanisms, mood, cognitive functioning, social functioning, and improve mental health. Group sessions have been particularly effective in fostering social connections and providing a sense of community, which is crucial for individuals experiencing isolation due to their mental health conditions. The versatility and adaptability of music-based interventions make them suitable for diverse patient populations, including those for whom traditional verbal therapies may be less effective.

Importantly, when conducted by trained professionals, music-based interventions can be tailored to individual preferences and needs, making them highly adaptable. This flexibility allows therapists to design interventions that resonate deeply with each patient, enhancing engagement and effectiveness. Various forms of engagement in musical experiences are systematically and intentionally employed to trigger specific neurological, biological, psychological, and social mechanisms through a culturally sensitive approach that aligns with patients' preferences and backgrounds.

In therapeutic and clinical settings, music can represent an option that is viable, low-cost, and free from side effects. Music-based interventions are not intended to be an alternative to other treatments, but may instead support key elements of traditional interventions, such as being engaging and enjoyable, providing social context, and increasing structure and predictability. Indeed, some music therapists incorporate principles from existing psychotherapeutic models (Chwalek and McKinney 2015; Dingle et al. 2008) and, conversely, newer therapeutic models (e.g., mindfulness) incorporate music into their practice (Tang et al. 2012). It is not yet possible to disentangle which aspects of music interventions best synergize with or strengthen standard pharmacological and psychosocial practices, but this will be possible with better reporting standards and quality experimental design. The integration of music-based interventions into a comprehensive treatment plan can provide a holistic approach to addressing the biopsychosocial aspects of mental disorders.

At present, the quantity and quality of evidence on music-based interventions for specific psychiatric conditions is still low. More methodologically stringent studies with larger sample sizes are needed to confirm the efficacy and acceptability of music-based interventions in psychiatry, either in combination with standard treatment or alone. Future research should also evaluate long-term effects as well as the lasting effects after the intervention is discontinued. As the field of music-based interventions in psychiatry continues to evolve, it is essential to integrate rigorous research, clinical expertise, and patient-centered approaches to fully harness the healing potential of music.

Overall, the integration of music-based interventions into psychiatric care represents a promising avenue for enhancing therapeutic outcomes in mental health. This chapter underscores the importance of continued research and clinical innovation to fully leverage the healing potential of music in psychiatry.

References

Aalbers S, Fusar-Poli L, Freeman RE, Spreen M, Ket JC, Vink AC, et al. Music therapy for depression. Cochrane Database Syst Rev. 2017;11(11):CD004517. https://doi.org/10.1002/14651858.CD004517.pub3.

Aalbers S, Fusar-Poli L, Freeman RE, Spreen M, Ket JC, Vink AC, et al. Music therapy for depression: a Cochrane review. BJPsych Adv. 2024;30(2):72.

Abdulah DM, Miho Alhakem SS, Piro RS. Effects of music as an adjunctive therapy on severity of symptoms in patients with obsessive-compulsive disorder: randomized controlled trial. Nord J Music Ther. 2019;28(1):27–40.

Abe D, Arai M, Itokawa M. Music-evoked emotions in schizophrenia. Schizophr Res. 2017;185:144–7.

Ahrberg M, Trojca D, Nasrawi N, Vocks S. Body image disturbance in binge eating disorder: a review. Eur Eat Disord Rev. 2011;19(5):375–81.

American Psychiatric Association. Diagnostic and statistical manual of mental disorders: DSM-5. 5th ed. Arlington: American Psychiatric Association; 2013.

Ansdell G, Davidson J, Magee WL, Meehan J, Procter S. From "This F*** ing life" to "that's better"… in four minutes: an interdisciplinary study of music therapy's "present moments" and their potential for affect modulation. Nord J Music Ther. 2010;19(1):3–28.

Bandelow B, Michaelis S, Wedekind D. Treatment of anxiety disorders. Dialogues Clin Neurosci. 2017;19(2):93–107. https://doi.org/10.31887/DCNS.2017.19.2/bbandelow.

Barlow DH, Campbell LA. Mixed anxiety-depression and its implications for models of mood and anxiety disorders. Compr Psychiatry. 2000;41(2):55–60.

Barnes TRE, Drake R, Paton C, Cooper SJ, Deakin B, Ferrier IN, et al. Evidence-based guidelines for the pharmacological treatment of schizophrenia: updated recommendations from the British Association for Psychopharmacology. J Psychopharmacol. 2019;34(1):3–78. https://doi.org/10.1177/0269881119889296.

Beck BD, Messel C, Meyer SL, Cordtz TO, Søgaard U, Simonsen E, et al. Feasibility of trauma-focused guided imagery and music with adult refugees diagnosed with PTSD: a pilot study. Nord J Music Ther. 2018;27(1):67–86.

Belski N, Abdul-Rahman Z, Youn E, Balasundaram V, Diep D. Review: the effectiveness of musical therapy in improving depression and anxiety symptoms among children and adolescents – a systematic review. Child Adolesc Mental Health. 2022;27(4):369–77. https://doi.org/10.1111/camh.12526.

Blood AJ, Zatorre RJ. Intensely pleasurable responses to music correlate with activity in brain regions implicated in reward and emotion. Proc Natl Acad Sci. 2001;98(20):11818–23.

Bosman RC, Ten Have M, de Graaf R, Muntingh AD, van Balkom AJ, Batelaan NM. Prevalence and course of subthreshold anxiety disorder in the general population: a three-year follow-up study. J Affect Disord. 2019;247:105–13.

Boso M, Politi P, Barale F, Emanuele E. Neurophysiology and neurobiology of the musical experience. Funct Neurol. 2006;21(4):187.

Bowling DL. Biological principles for music and mental health. Transl Psychiatry. 2023;13(1):374.

Bradt J, Dileo C, Shim M. Music interventions for preoperative anxiety. Cochrane Database Syst Rev. 2013;6:CD006908.

Bradt J, Dileo C, Myers-Coffman K, Biondo J. Music interventions for improving psychological and physical outcomes in people with cancer. Cochrane Database Syst Rev. 2021;10(10):CD006911. https://doi.org/10.1002/14651858.CD006911.pub4.

Campbell DG, Felker BL, Liu C-F, Yano EM, Kirchner JE, Chan D, et al. Prevalence of depression–PTSD comorbidity: implications for clinical practice guidelines and primary care-based interventions. J Gen Intern Med. 2007;22:711–8.

Carr C, d'Ardenne P, Sloboda A, Scott C, Wang D, Priebe S. Group music therapy for patients with persistent post-traumatic stress disorder–an exploratory randomized controlled trial with mixed methods evaluation. Psychol Psychother Theory Res Pract. 2012;85(2):179–202.

Chan MM, Han YM. The functional brain networks activated by music listening: a neuroimaging meta-analysis and implications for treatment. Neuropsychology. 2022;36(1):4.

Chanda ML, Levitin DJ. The neurochemistry of music. Trends Cogn Sci. 2013;17(4):179–93.

Chang WC, Wong CSM, Chen EYH, Lam LCW, Chan WC, Ng RMK, et al. Lifetime prevalence and correlates of schizophrenia-Spectrum, affective, and other non-affective psychotic disorders in the Chinese adult population. Schizophr Bull. 2017;43(6):1280–90. https://doi.org/10.1093/schbul/sbx056.

Chang EX, Brooker J, Hiscock R, O'Callaghan C. Music-based intervention impacts for people with eating disorders: a narrative synthesis systematic review. J Music Ther. 2023;60(2):202–31. https://doi.org/10.1093/jmt/thac018.

Chwalek CM, McKinney CH. The use of Dialectical Behavior Therapy (DBT) in music therapy: a sequential explanatory study. J Music Ther. 2015;52(2):282–318. https://doi.org/10.1093/jmt/thv002.

Correll CU, Solmi M, Croatto G, Schneider LK, Rohani-Montez SC, Fairley L, et al. Mortality in people with schizophrenia: a systematic review and meta-analysis of relative risk and aggravating or attenuating factors. World Psychiatry. 2022;21(2):248–71.

Cournoyer Lemaire E, Loignon C, Bertrand K. A critical scoping review about the impact of music in the lives of young adults who use drugs. Drug Alcohol Rev. 2021;40(1):135–54. https://doi.org/10.1111/dar.13136.

Crump C, Winkleby MA, Sundquist K, Sundquist J. Comorbidities and mortality in persons with schizophrenia: a Swedish national cohort study. Am J Psychiatry. 2013;170(3):324–33. https://doi.org/10.1176/appi.ajp.2012.12050599.

de Witte M, Spruit A, van Hooren S, Moonen X, Stams GJ. Effects of music interventions on stress-related outcomes: a systematic review and two meta-analyses. Health Psychol Rev. 2020;14(2):294–324. https://doi.org/10.1080/17437199.2019.1627897.

Delle Monache S, Jia D, Kamphuis D, Özcan E, editors. Exploring profiling and personalisation in sleep music design: towards conceptualising musical sleep aids for hospital use. Proceedings of the 17th International Audio Mostly Conference; 2022.

Dhippayom T, Saensook T, Promkhatja N, Teaktong T, Chaiyakunapruk N, Devine B. Comparative effects of music interventions on depression in older adults: a systematic review and network meta-analysis. EClinicalMedicine. 2022;50:101509. https://doi.org/10.1016/j.eclinm.2022.101509.

Dickson GT, Schubert E. How does music aid sleep? Literature review. Sleep Med. 2019;63:142–50. https://doi.org/10.1016/j.sleep.2019.05.016.

Dingle GA, Gleadhill L, Baker FA. Can music therapy engage patients in group cognitive behaviour therapy for substance abuse treatment? Drug Alcohol Rev. 2008;27(2):190–6. https://doi.org/10.1080/09595230701829371.

Edwards J. The Oxford handbook of music therapy. Oxford University Press; 2016.

Erkkilä J, Punkanen M, Fachner J, Ala-Ruona E, Pöntiö I, Tervaniemi M, et al. Individual music therapy for depression: randomised controlled trial. Br J Psychiatry. 2011;199(2):132–9. https://doi.org/10.1192/bjp.bp.110.085431.

Fancourt D, Perkins R. Could listening to music during pregnancy be protective against post-natal depression and poor wellbeing post birth? Longitudinal associations from a preliminary prospective cohort study. BMJ Open. 2018;8(7):e021251. https://doi.org/10.1136/bmjopen-2017-021251.

Feng F, Zhang Y, Hou J, Cai J, Jiang Q, Li X, et al. Can music improve sleep quality in adults with primary insomnia? A systematic review and network meta-analysis. Int J Nurs Stud. 2018;77:189–96.

Ferrie JE, Kumari M, Salo P, Singh-Manoux A, Kivimäki M. Sleep epidemiology—a rapidly growing field. Oxford University Press; 2011. p. 1431–7.

Freeman D, Sheaves B, Waite F, Harvey AG, Harrison PJ. Sleep disturbance and psychiatric disorders. Lancet Psychiatry. 2020;7(7):628–37.

Friedmann JL. Music in biblical life: the roles of song in ancient Israel. McFarland; 2013.

Fusar-Poli L, Rocchetti M, Garda M, Politi P. 'Aut'-sider: the invisible talent of Simona Concaro. Epidemiol Psychiatr Sci. 2017;26(2):119–21.

Geretsegger M, Mössler KA, Bieleninik Ł, Chen XJ, Heldal TO, Gold C. Music therapy for people with schizophrenia and schizophrenia-like disorders. Cochrane Database Syst Rev. 2017;5

Ghetti C, Chen XJ, Brenner AK, Hakvoort LG, Lien L, Fachner J, et al. Music therapy for people with substance use disorders. Cochrane Database Syst Rev. 2022;5 https://doi.org/10.1002/14651858.CD012576.pub3.

Gold C, Solli HP, Krüger V, Lie SA. Dose–response relationship in music therapy for people with serious mental disorders: systematic review and meta-analysis. Clin Psychol Rev. 2009;29(3):193–207.

Golden TL, Tetreault E, Ray CE, Kuge MN, Tiedemann A, Magsamen S. The state of music-based interventions for mental illness: thought leaders on barriers, opportunities, and the value of interdisciplinarity. Community Ment Health J. 2022;58(3):487–98.

Gruner P, Pittenger C. Cognitive inflexibility in obsessive-compulsive disorder. Neuroscience. 2017;345:243–55.

Gutiérrez EOF, Camarena VAT. Music therapy in generalized anxiety disorder. Arts Psychother. 2015;44:19–24. https://doi.org/10.1016/j.aip.2015.02.003.

Hakvoort L, de Jong S, van de Ree M, Kok T, Macfarlane C, de Haan H. Music therapy to regulate arousal and attention in patients with substance use disorder and posttraumatic stress disorder: a feasibility study. J Music Ther. 2020;57(3):353–78. https://doi.org/10.1093/jmt/thaa007.
Haller H, Cramer H, Lauche R, Gass F, Dobos GJ. The prevalence and burden of subthreshold generalized anxiety disorder: a systematic review. BMC Psychiatry. 2014;14:1–13.
Halstead S, Cao C, Høgnason Mohr G, Ebdrup BH, Pillinger T, McCutcheon RA, et al. Prevalence of multimorbidity in people with and without severe mental illness: a systematic review and meta-analysis. Lancet Psychiatry. 2024;11(6):431–42. https://doi.org/10.1016/s2215-0366(24)00091-9.
Hamilton JP, Farmer M, Fogelman P, Gotlib IH. Depressive rumination, the default-mode network, and the dark matter of clinical neuroscience. Biol Psychiatry. 2015;78(4):224–30. https://doi.org/10.1016/j.biopsych.2015.02.020.
Hanser S. Cognitive-behavioral approaches Music therapy handbook 2015. p. 161–171.
He H, Yang M, Duan M, Chen X, Lai Y, Xia Y, et al. Music intervention leads to increased insular connectivity and improved clinical symptoms in schizophrenia. Front Neurosci. 2017;11:744. https://doi.org/10.3389/fnins.2017.00744.
Hohmann L, Bradt J, Stegemann T, Koelsch S. Effects of music therapy and music-based interventions in the treatment of substance use disorders: a systematic review. PLoS One. 2017;12(11):e0187363.
Hole J, Hirsch M, Ball E, Meads C. Music as an aid for postoperative recovery in adults: a systematic review and meta-analysis. Lancet. 2015;386(10004):1659–71.
Hoskins MD, Bridges J, Sinnerton R, Nakamura A, Underwood JF, Slater A, et al. Pharmacological therapy for post-traumatic stress disorder: a systematic review and meta-analysis of monotherapy, augmentation and head-to-head approaches. Eur J Psychotraumatol. 2021;12(1):1802920.
Jespersen KV, Pando-Naude V, Koenig J, Jennum P, Vuust P. Listening to music for insomnia in adults. Cochrane Database Syst Rev. 2022;8:CD010459.
Jespersen KV, Hansen MH, Vuust P. The effect of music on sleep in hospitalized patients: a systematic review and meta-analysis. Sleep Health. 2023;9(4):441–8.
Jia R, Liang D, Yu J, Lu G, Wang Z, Wu Z, et al. The effectiveness of adjunct music therapy for patients with schizophrenia: a meta-analysis. Psychiatry Res. 2020;293:113464.
Johnson K, Pinchuk I, Melgar MIE, Agwogie MO, Salazar Silva F. The global movement towards a public health approach to substance use disorders. Ann Med. 2022;54(1):1797–808.
Juslin PN. From everyday emotions to aesthetic emotions: towards a unified theory of musical emotions. Phys Life Rev. 2013;10(3):235–66.
Kakar E, Venema E, Jeekel J, Klimek M, van der Jagt M. Music intervention for sleep quality in critically ill and surgical patients: a meta-analysis. BMJ Open. 2021;11(5):e042510.
Kayaoğlu K, Şahin Altun Ö. The effect of combined cognitive-behavioral psychoeducation and music intervention on stress, self-efficacy, and relapse rates in patients with alcohol and substance use disorders: a randomized controlled trial. Perspect Psychiatr Care. 2022;58(3):968–77. https://doi.org/10.1111/ppc.12884.
Kerr-Gaffney J, Harrison A, Tchanturia K. Social anxiety in the eating disorders: a systematic review and meta-analysis. Psychol Med. 2018;48(15):2477–91. https://doi.org/10.1017/S0033291718000752.
Kessler RC, Sonnega A, Bromet E, Hughes M, Nelson CB. Posttraumatic stress disorder in the National Comorbidity Survey. Fear and anxiety. Routledge; 2013. p. 22–34.
Khalfa S, Bella SD, Roy M, Peretz I, Lupien SJ. Effects of relaxing music on salivary cortisol level after psychological stress. Ann N Y Acad Sci. 2003;999(1):374–6.
Koelsch S. From social contact to social cohesion—the 7 Cs. Music Med. 2013;5(4):204–9.
Koelsch S. Brain correlates of music-evoked emotions. Nat Rev Neurosci. 2014;15(3):170–80.
Koelsch S, Jäncke L. Music and the heart. Eur Heart J. 2015;36(44):3043–9.
Koelsch S, Jacobs AM, Menninghaus W, Liebal K, Klann-Delius G, von Scheve C, et al. The quartet theory of human emotions: an integrative and neurofunctional model. Phys Life Rev. 2015;13:1–27. https://doi.org/10.1016/j.plrev.2015.03.001.
Koob GF. Addiction is a reward deficit and stress surfeit disorder. Front Psych. 2013;4:72.

Kreutz G, Murcia CQ, Bongard S. Psychoneuroendocrine research on music and health: an overview. In: Music, health, and wellbeing. Oxford University Press; 2012. p. 457–76.

Kühlmann AYR, de Rooij A, Kroese LF, van Dijk M, Hunink MGM, Jeekel J. Meta-analysis evaluating music interventions for anxiety and pain in surgery. Br J Surg. 2018;105(7):773–83. https://doi.org/10.1002/bjs.10853.

Lam RW, Kennedy SH, Adams C, Bahji A, Beaulieu S, Bhat V, et al. Canadian Network for Mood and Anxiety Treatments (CANMAT) 2023 Update on Clinical Guidelines for Management of Major Depressive Disorder in Adults: Réseau canadien pour les traitements de l'humeur et de l'anxiété (CANMAT) 2023: Mise à jour des lignes directrices cliniques pour la prise en charge du trouble dépressif majeur chez les adultes. Can J Psychiatry. 2024:7067437241245384. https://doi.org/10.1177/07067437241245384.

Landis-Shack N, Heinz AJ, Bonn-Miller MO. Music therapy for posttraumatic stress in adults: a theoretical review. Psychomusicology. 2017;27(4):334–42. https://doi.org/10.1037/pmu0000192.

Lim GY, Tam WW, Lu Y, Ho CS, Zhang MW, Ho RC. Prevalence of depression in the community from 30 countries between 1994 and 2014. Sci Rep. 2018;8(1):2861.

Loomba RS, Arora R, Shah PH, Chandrasekar S, Molnar J. Effects of music on systolic blood pressure, diastolic blood pressure, and heart rate: a meta-analysis. Indian Heart J. 2012;64(3):309–13.

Lu G, Jia R, Liang D, Yu J, Wu Z, Chen C. Effects of music therapy on anxiety: a meta-analysis of randomized controlled trials. Psychiatry Res. 2021;304:114137. https://doi.org/10.1016/j.psychres.2021.114137.

Ma YM, Yuan MD, Zhong BL. Efficacy and acceptability of music therapy for post-traumatic stress disorder: a systematic review and meta-analysis of randomized controlled trials. Eur J Psychotraumatol. 2024;15(1):2342739. https://doi.org/10.1080/20008066.2024.2342739.

Mainieri G, Loddo G, Provini F. Disorders of arousal: a chronobiological perspective. Clocks Sleep. 2021;3(1):53–65.

Makri E, Michopoulos I, Gonidakis F. Investigation of loneliness and social support in patients with eating disorders: a case-control study. Psychiatry International. 2022;3(2):142–57.

Maratos A, Crawford MJ, Procter S. Music therapy for depression: it seems to work, but how? Br J Psychiatry. 2011;199(2):92–3.

Marcus M, Yasamy MT, van Ommeren MV, Chisholm D, Saxena S. Depression: a global public health concern. 2012.

Mavrogiorgou P, Becker S, Juckel G. Guilt and shame in patients with obsessive-compulsive disorders. Psychopathology. 2024:1–11. https://doi.org/10.1159/000537996.

Meneguzzo P, Baron E, Marchesin S, Andretta AM, Nalesso L, Stella S, et al. Tuning in to recovery: influence of music on emotional well-being during mealtime in inpatient facilities for eating disorders. J Eat Disord. 2024a;12(1):7. https://doi.org/10.1186/s40337-024-00970-9.

Meneguzzo P, Terlizzi S, Maggi L, Todisco P. The loneliness factor in eating disorders: implications for psychopathology and biological signatures. Compr Psychiatry. 2024b;132:152493.

Metrics IoH, Evaluation. Global health data exchange (GHDx) 2021.

Metzner S, Jaeger U, Masuhr O, Olschewski U, Gräfe E, Böske AC, et al. Forms of attunement during the initial stages of music therapy for patients with acute psychosis-a multicentre clinical study. Nord J Music Ther. 2018;27(5):360–80.

Meule A, Richard A, Schnepper R, Reichenberger J, Georgii C, Naab S, et al. Emotion regulation and emotional eating in anorexia nervosa and bulimia nervosa. Eat Disord. 2021;29(2):175–91.

Millan MJ, Fone K, Steckler T, Horan WP. Negative symptoms of schizophrenia: clinical characteristics, pathophysiological substrates, experimental models and prospects for improved treatment. Eur Neuropsychopharmacol. 2014;24(5):645–92.

Moberly NJ, Watkins ER. Ruminative self-focus and negative affect: an experience sampling study. J Abnorm Psychol. 2008;117(2):314–23. https://doi.org/10.1037/0021-843x.117.2.314.

Morgan K, Bartrop R, Telfer J, Tennant C. A controlled trial investigating the effect of music therapy during an acute psychotic episode. Acta Psychiatr Scand. 2011;124(5):363–71. https://doi.org/10.1111/j.1600-0447.2011.01739.x.

Mössler K, Chen X, Heldal TO, Gold C. Music therapy for people with schizophrenia and schizophrenia-like disorders. Cochrane Database Syst Rev. 2011;12

Mu CX, Lee S, Boddupalli S, Meng H. Effects of music interventions on sleep in people with dementia: a systematic review. Dementia. 2022;21(6):2053–71.

Nguyen KT, Xiao J, Chan DNS, Zhang M, Chan CWH. Effects of music intervention on anxiety, depression, and quality of life of cancer patients receiving chemotherapy: a systematic review and meta-analysis. Support Care Cancer. 2022;30(7):5615–26. https://doi.org/10.1007/s00520-022-06881-2.

O'Daly OG, Trick L, Scaife J, Marshall J, Ball D, Phillips ML, et al. Withdrawal-associated increases and decreases in functional neural connectivity associated with altered emotional regulation in alcoholism. Neuropsychopharmacology. 2012;37(10):2267–76. https://doi.org/10.1038/npp.2012.77.

Odell-Miller H. Why provide music therapy in the community for adults with mental health problems? Br J Music Ther. 1995;9(1):4–10.

Organization WH. Suicide worldwide in 2019: global health estimates. 2021.

Orjuela-Rojas JM, Rodríguez ILL. The stuck song syndrome: a case of musical obsessions. Am J Case Rep. 2018;19:1329.

Parish JM. Sleep-related problems in common medical conditions. Chest. 2009;135(2):563–72.

Petrovsky DV, Ramesh P, McPhillips MV, Hodgson NA. Effects of music interventions on sleep in older adults: a systematic review. Geriatr Nurs. 2021;42(4):869–79.

Pfizer N, Andrade C. Isolated musical obsessions. Indian J Psychiatry. 1999;41(1):77–8.

Pittenger C, Bloch MH. Pharmacological treatment of obsessive-compulsive disorder. Psychiatr Clin. 2014;37(3):375–91.

Punkanen M, Eerola T, Erkkilä J. Biased emotional preferences in depression: decreased liking of angry and energetic music by depressed patients. Music Med. 2011;3(2):114–20.

Ramirez-Melendez R. Personalizing music interventions. Neurocognitive music therapy: intersecting music, medicine and technology for health and well-being. Springer; 2023. p. 83–9.

Reid JE, Laws KR, Drummond L, Vismara M, Grancini B, Mpavaenda D, et al. Cognitive behavioural therapy with exposure and response prevention in the treatment of obsessive-compulsive disorder: a systematic review and meta-analysis of randomised controlled trials. Compr Psychiatry. 2021;106:152223.

Riemann D, Nissen C, Palagini L, Otte A, Perlis ML, Spiegelhalder K. The neurobiology, investigation, and treatment of chronic insomnia. Lancet Neurol. 2015;14(5):547–58.

Riemann D, Baglioni C, Bassetti C, Bjorvatn B, Dolenc Groselj L, Ellis JG, et al. European guideline for the diagnosis and treatment of insomnia. J Sleep Res. 2017;26(6):675–700. https://doi.org/10.1111/jsr.12594.

Robb SL, Carpenter JS, Burns DS. Reporting guidelines for music-based interventions. J Health Psychol. 2011;16(2):342–52.

Romero-Mesa J, Peláez-Fernández MA, Extremera N. Emotional intelligence and eating disorders: a systematic review. Eat Weight Disord. 2021;26(5):1287–301. https://doi.org/10.1007/s40519-020-00968-7.

Rosenthal A, Ebrahimi C, Wedemeyer F, Romanczuk-Seiferth N, Beck A. The treatment of substance use disorders: recent developments and new perspectives. Neuropsychobiology. 2022;81(5):451–72. https://doi.org/10.1159/000525268.

Roy WG, Dowd TJ. What is sociological about music? Annu Rev Sociol. 2010;36(1):183–203.

Rudstam G, Elofsson UO, Söndergaard HP, Bonde LO, Beck BD. Trauma-focused group music and imagery with women suffering from PTSD/complex PTSD: a randomized controlled study. Eur J Trauma Dissociat. 2022;6(3):100277.

Rudstam G, Elofsson UOE, Söndergaard HP, Beck BD. Psychophysiological assessment of trauma-focused group music and imagery therapy for women with PTSD or CPTSD using script-driven imagery. A randomised controlled study. European. J Trauma Dissociation. 2023;7(4):100353. https://doi.org/10.1016/j.ejtd.2023.100353.

Saarikallio S, Nieminen S, Brattico E. Affective reactions to musical stimuli reflect emotional use of music in everyday life. Music Sci. 2013;17(1):27–39.

Salari N, Maghami N, Ammari T, Mosafer H, Abdullahi R, Rasoulpoor S, et al. Global prevalence of metabolic syndrome in schizophrenia patients: a systematic review and meta-analysis. J Prev (2022). 2024;45 https://doi.org/10.1007/s10935-024-00798-8.

Salimpoor VN, Benovoy M, Larcher K, Dagher A, Zatorre RJ. Anatomically distinct dopamine release during anticipation and experience of peak emotion to music. Nat Neurosci. 2011;14(2):257–62.

Shim S-Y, editor. Personal experiences of non-verbal communication through musical dialogue (clinical improvisation). Voices: A World Forum for Music Therapy; 2007.

Shiranibidabadi M, Mehryar A. "Music therapy as an adjunct to standard treatment for obsessive compulsive disorder and co-morbid anxiety and depression: a randomized clinical trial": Corrigendum; 2017.

Short AD, Dingle GA. Music as an auditory cue for emotions and cravings in adults with substance use disorders. Psychol Music. 2016;44(3):559–73.

Singh B, Olds T, Curtis R, Dumuid D, Virgara R, Watson A, et al. Effectiveness of physical activity interventions for improving depression, anxiety and distress: an overview of systematic reviews. Br J Sports Med. 2023;57(18):1203–9. https://doi.org/10.1136/bjsports-2022-106195.

Smith DJ, McLean G, Martin D, Martin JL, Guthrie B, Gunn J, et al. Depression and multimorbidity: a cross-sectional study of 1,751,841 patients in primary care. J Clin Psychiatry. 2014;75(11):4205.

Solli HP. "Shut up and play!" Improvisational use of popular music for a man with schizophrenia. Nord J Music Ther. 2008;17(1):67–77.

Solmi M, Croatto G, Piva G, Rosson S, Fusar-Poli P, Rubio JM, et al. Efficacy and acceptability of psychosocial interventions in schizophrenia: systematic overview and quality appraisal of the meta-analytic evidence. Mol Psychiatry. 2023;28(1):354–68. https://doi.org/10.1038/s41380-022-01727-z.

Stone T, Short A. Can music therapy help adults with schizophrenia improve their cognitive skills? A scoping review. Issues Ment Health Nurs. 2024;45(1):55–65. https://doi.org/10.1080/01612840.2023.2266851.

Story KM, Beck BD. Guided imagery and music with female military veterans: an intervention development study. Arts Psychother. 2017;55:93–102.

Tang YY, Yang L, Leve LD, Harold GT. Improving executive function and its neurobiological mechanisms through a mindfulness-based intervention: advances within the field of developmental neuroscience. Child Dev Perspect. 2012;6(4):361–6. https://doi.org/10.1111/j.1750-8606.2012.00250.x.

Tang Q, Huang Z, Zhou H, Ye P. Effects of music therapy on depression: a meta-analysis of randomized controlled trials. PLoS One. 2020;15(11):e0240862. https://doi.org/10.1371/journal.pone.0240862.

Tanskanen A, Tiihonen J, Taipale H. Mortality in schizophrenia: 30-year nationwide follow-up study. Acta Psychiatr Scand. 2018;138(6):492–9. https://doi.org/10.1111/acps.12913.

Testa F, Arunachalam S, Heiderscheit A, Himmerich H. A systematic review of scientific studies on the effects of music in people with or at risk for eating disorders. Psychiatr Danub. 2020;32(3–4, 334):–45. https://doi.org/10.24869/psyd.2020.334.

Thomas JL, Wilk JE, Riviere LA, McGurk D, Castro CA, Hoge CW. Prevalence of mental health problems and functional impairment among active component and National Guard soldiers 3 and 12 months following combat in Iraq. Arch Gen Psychiatry. 2010;67(6):614–23.

Timpano KR, Çek D, Rubenstein LM, Murphy D, Schmidt NB. Exploring the association between obsessive-compulsive symptoms and loneliness: consideration of specificity and gender. J Cogn Psychother. 2014;28(4):264–73.

Treasure J, Duarte TA, Schmidt U. Eating disorders. Lancet (London, England). 2020;395(10227):899–911. https://doi.org/10.1016/s0140-6736(20)30059-3.

Trondalen G. Resource-oriented bonny method of guided imagery and music (R-oGIM) as a creative health resource for musicians. Nord J Music Ther. 2016;25(1):5–31.

Truong TPA, Applewhite B, Heiderscheit A, Himmerich H. A systematic review of scientific studies and case reports on music and obsessive-compulsive disorder. Int J Environ Res Public Health. 2021;18(22) https://doi.org/10.3390/ijerph182211799.

van der Heijden MJ, Oliai Araghi S, van Dijk M, Jeekel J, Hunink MM. The effects of perioperative music interventions in pediatric surgery: a systematic review and meta-analysis of randomized controlled trials. PLoS One. 2015;10(8):e0133608.

Volpe U, Gianoglio C, Autiero L, Marino ML, Facchini D, Mucci A, et al. Acute effects of music therapy in subjects with psychosis during inpatient treatment. Psychiatry. 2018;81(3):218–27.

Wang Q, Chair SY, Wong EML, Li X. The effects of music intervention on sleep quality in community-dwelling elderly. J Altern Complement Med. 2016;22(7):576–84.

Wang C, Li G, Zheng L, Meng X, Meng Q, Wang S, et al. Effects of music intervention on sleep quality of older adults: a systematic review and meta-analysis. Complement Ther Med. 2021;59:102719.

Wang M, Wu J, Yan H. Effect of music therapy on older adults with depression: a systematic review and meta-analysis. Complement Ther Clin Pract. 2023;53:101809. https://doi.org/10.1016/j.ctcp.2023.101809.

Wang CC, Emrich M, Rives H, Ovalles A, Wright D, Wyka K, et al. Music interventions for posttraumatic stress disorder: a systematic review. J Mood Anxiety Disord. 2024;6:100053. https://doi.org/10.1016/j.xjmad.2024.100053.

West ML. Ancient Greek music. Clarendon Press; 1992.

Westwood H, Kerr-Gaffney J, Stahl D, Tchanturia K. Alexithymia in eating disorders: systematic review and meta-analyses of studies using the Toronto Alexithymia Scale. J Psychosom Res. 2017;99:66–81. https://doi.org/10.1016/j.jpsychores.2017.06.007.

Wilcox CE, Pommy JM, Adinoff B. Neural circuitry of impaired emotion regulation in substance use disorders. Am J Psychiatry. 2016;173(4):344–61. https://doi.org/10.1176/appi.ajp.2015.15060710.

Wright SL, Karyotaki E, Cuijpers P, Bisson J, Papola D, Witteveen A, et al. EMDR v. other psychological therapies for PTSD: a systematic review and individual participant data meta-analysis. Psychol Med. 2024:1–9.

Xin L-M, Chen L, Ji Z-P, Zhang S-Y, Wang J, Liu Y-H, et al. Risk factors for anxiety in major depressive disorder patients. Clin Psychopharmacol Neurosci. 2015;13(3):263.

Yang M, He H, Duan M, Chen X, Chang X, Lai Y, et al. The effects of music intervention on functional connectivity strength of the brain in schizophrenia. Neural Plast. 2018;2018:2821832. https://doi.org/10.1155/2018/2821832.

Yang WJ, Bai YM, Qin L, Xu XL, Bao KF, Xiao JL, et al. The effectiveness of music therapy for postpartum depression: a systematic review and meta-analysis. Complement Ther Clin Pract. 2019;37:93–101. https://doi.org/10.1016/j.ctcp.2019.09.002.

The Importance of Music in Children's Development

14

Luisa Lopez

Key Points

- This chapter emphasized the role of music from an early age, considering the developmental milestones of musical abilities, from the basic elements of pitch and timing to consonance preferences and memory.
- The discussion is framed in the concept of critical periods for development and plasticity.
- A clarification is then provided about the use of music therapy and music training in the scientific literature, and how best practices can take advantage of both approaches.
- The case for the appropriateness of music intervention is explored in language and reading disorders such as dyslexia, executive functions, and, in particular, ADHD, as well as social and communication disorders, particularly ASD.

14.1 Introduction

Children are exposed to sounds and rhythms that can significantly influence their cognitive, emotional, social, and physical growth from the earliest stages of life. Music is not just a form of entertainment; it plays a vital role in changing the developmental trajectory of various skills and abilities crucial for a child's overall well-being.

L. Lopez (✉)
Fondazione Mariani, Milano, Italy

Casa di Cura Villa Immacolata, Viterbo, Italy
e-mail: lopez@uniroma2.it

A. Raglio (ed.), *Music and Music Therapy Interventions in Clinical Practice*, Neurocultural Health and Wellbeing,
https://doi.org/10.1007/978-3-031-88578-5_14

In June 2014, Nati per la Musica[1] released its Manifesto, "Good Music Practices Help Children Grow," a strong and forceful call for those involved in childcare and education-teachers, healthcare providers, administrators, and those in charge of ministerial educational programs and extracurricular activities to promote the use of good and early music practices, both in the family and at school.

Early signatories and supporters of the Manifesto include Elisa, Riccardo Muti, Paolo Fresu, José Antonio Abreu, Daniel Barenboim, Antonio Pappano, and American neuroscientist Nina Kraus (crf. Box 14.1).

Box 14.1 Manifesto, "Good Music Practices Help Children Grow"—Nati per la Musica. With Permission from Centro Salute del Bambino, Trieste

Effects of Musical Activity

1. Interacting musically from an early age promotes the development of interaction and communication skills.
2. Musical experience develops attention, memory, and language.
3. Sharing musical experiences promotes sociability.
4. The child actively and positively involved in a musical context learns with pleasure, creates and invents, and is motivated to learn.
5. Among musical activities, singing is particularly useful in promoting communicative exchange between parent and child and promotes affective attunement in the early stages of life.
6. Music making since early childhood is helpful throughout life.

Helpful Tips for Parents and Children

1. Respect a sound ecology in home environments by reducing constant and invasive noises (e.g., background television) as much as possible.
2. Enhance the child's spontaneous singing, his ability to produce sounds with various objects, and his movement in the presence of music.
3. Encourage his spontaneous curiosity about objects and instruments that produce sounds.
4. Make available to the child and encourage the exploration of a wide range of objects (including everyday objects) that produce sounds: shaking, tapping, and rubbing objects.
5. Find moments in the day (even short ones) in which to listen to music and sing along with the child.
6. Avoid having the child listen only to "children's" music, and propose a good variety of music.

(continued)

[1] www.natiperlamusica.org

Box 14.1 (continued)

Suggestions for Kindergartens and Preschools

1. Respect a sound ecology of learning environments by reducing constant and invasive noises (e.g., music always on in the background).
2. Observe, value the child's singing, and guide the child to expressive use of the voice.
3. Give the child the opportunity to produce sounds and music from the earliest months of life, valuing sound stimuli and sound productions of which the child is a user and active creator.
4. Educate the child to listen to the surrounding environment and soundscape.
5. Promote the child's enjoyment of the most significant musical proposals from various European and non-European cultures.

The use of music in children's development is multifaceted, offering benefits that span across cognitive, emotional, social, and physical domains. Incorporating music into a child's daily routine, whether through listening, singing, dancing, or playing instruments, can significantly contribute to their overall growth and well-being. As such, music should be seen not just as an extracurricular activity but as an integral part of a child's development.

14.2 Music in Prenatal Life

The earliest reports on the impact of music during the first months of pregnancy (Kisilevsky et al. 2004) show that exposure to music during pregnancy can have various effects on both the developing fetus and the expectant mother. Fetuses begin to develop auditory capabilities around the 25th week of gestation. By the third trimester, they can hear external sounds, including music.

The sounds in utero transform due to the presence of the amniotic fluid and the interference of maternal sounds so that higher frequencies are more attenuated. In comparison, lower frequencies can penetrate more effectively. As a result, fetuses are more likely to hear lower pitched sounds, such as bass frequencies, rather than high-pitched sounds.

The fetus may more easily detect musical sounds with lower frequencies compared to those with higher frequencies.

Sounds outside the womb are also attenuated in intensity by approximately 20–30 decibels when they reach the fetus. Due to these filtering effects, music heard in utero may sound more muffled and less distinct, with less clarity in pitch and timbre compared to how the mother hears it. Nevertheless, studies have shown that fetuses can respond to music through changes in heart rate and movement. (Kisilevsky et al. 2004).

14.3 The Development of Musical Abilities in Early Infancy

In a series of experiments, the researchers led by the late scientist Sandra Trehub showed that infants can remember and recognize familiar tunes and rhythms. After hearing a melody just a few times—sometimes as few as three—infants aged 5–10 months recognize transpositions of that melody (where the pitches are altered but the intervals, i.e., the distances in frequency, are maintained) as familiar, and/or similar to the original melody. However, when the sequence of internal tones is rearranged or a single tone is altered, especially if it changes the melody's contour (the pattern of rising and falling pitches), infants perceive the melody as new. The pitch contour seems to be the most relevant aspect and can drive the detection of change in a melody. (Chang and Trehub 1977; Trehub and Hannon 2006). Furthermore, when manipulating consonance and dissonance, for both adults and infants, consonance played a more crucial role than interval width in determining the perceived similarity of harmonic intervals (Schellenberg and Trainor 1996). The studies that explored infant's preference initially favored consonance as the main determinant of infants' preferences (Trainor and Heinmiller 1998) but later revisited the evidence manipulating the exposure, and thus concluding that familiarity seems more relevant in determining infants' preference (Plantinga and Trehub 2014).

Based on studies by Kisilevski and Hepper, it is known that besides recognizing and responding to musical themes they heard in the womb, human fetuses and newborns can retain information about the rhythmic structure of external sounds over short periods (Kisilevsky et al. 2004; Hepper 1991).

This knowledge comes most likely from exposure to natural rhythms in their fetal environment (mother's heartbeat and respiration, or rhythms perceived while being bounced during the mother's daily activities, such as walking, dancing, and pacing) (Hepper 1991; Ullal-Gupta et al. 2013). The evidence of actual implicit learning coming from this experience is scarce, but indirect evidence can be found in evoked potential studies (Winkler et al. 2009).

14.4 Critical Periods

The fact that infants seem to have a very natural ease with musical features and show early learning of complex sound environments leads to the hypothesis that such stimuli might have a role in developing other functions such as language, sensorimotor integration, social, and emotional skills.

When referring to such learning possibilities, it is important to consider critical periods that are "the time window(s) during which the effect of experience on brain development is unusually profound and can strongly modulate the neural circuits." In contrast, sensitive periods are time windows in which changes may still occur in response to stimuli but they have less impact on the stability of learning. This ability decreases with age (cfr Ismail et al. 2017). The implication of such a notion has been a search for the best possible combination of time and kind of exposure to stimuli capable of producing the most positive changes.

There has been development in behavioral, pharmacological, electrical/magnetic, and cell-based neuromodulation.

In 2005, Laurel Trainor reviewed the basic aspects of critical periods for music. She concluded that basic aspects like tonotopic map formation and absolute pitch perception are more clearly linked to critical periods than more complex aspects such as harmony and musical composition (Trainor 2005). There is evidence, for example, that childhood musical practice enhances brainstem auditory responses, yielding stronger signal-to-noise ratios for musical signals. (Barrett et al. 2013) While early exposure to music and intensive practice play significant roles in shaping musical abilities, the extent to which critical periods influence higher level musical expertise remains unclear.

The reopening of plasticity windows could also be responsible for findings of long-term effects of music practice even after the typical critical and sensitive periods have closed.

Whether these interconnections between music and plasticity could be helpful for a wider range of application remains to be explored. It seems reasonable considering that Hensch and Bilimoria proposed that disruption of a critical period due to disease or abnormal experiences in one brain region might disturb the synchronization of critical periods in other connected regions. Similarly, if one critical period is abnormally shortened or extended, it could prematurely trigger or delay the onset of others. They concluded that researchers need to focus on finding ways to provide efficient stimulation (Hensch and Bilimoria 2012).

14.5 Music Intervention: Music Training and Music Therapy

In the scientific literature, whenever music is quoted in relation to child development, there might be some confusion about the actual kind of intervention being analyzed. Music therapy and training may involve music but have distinct purposes, methods, and outcomes.

The primary goal of music therapy is therapeutic, using clinical and evidence-based music interventions to achieve individualized outcomes such as enhancing emotional well-being, cognitive function, physical health, or social interaction. It is often integrated into treatment plans for conditions like anxiety, depression, autism, but also Alzheimer's cognitive decline, chronic pain, and physical rehabilitation, with a focus on healing and well-being rather than musical skill development.

Music therapy is conducted by certified therapists with specialized training in both music and clinical interventions, while music training is led by music teachers or instructors who focus on imparting musical knowledge and skills, without the need for therapeutic expertise.

Teaching methods can be more complex when working with typically developing children, as long as the child is willing to participate. In this case, it is crucial to select the appropriate method based on the child's age and the program's objectives. It is also important to consider the duration of the program and the child's compliance with instructions.

Therapy, on the other hand, is a term reserved for situations involving special needs, whether temporary (e.g., during surgery, delivery, or hospitalization) or related to developmental or acquired disabilities. Therapy interventions can involve various methods or models, such as receptive music therapy (focused on listening and processing experiences) and active music therapy (focused on activation, improvisation, and observation of musical production).

In the context of therapy and training, it is possible to combine the two approaches based on specific intervention goals. For example, music therapy can help explore emotions and music training can be adapted for individuals with special needs. Evaluation of efficacy is crucial for rehabilitation and is an essential consideration in music therapy, where the patient's interaction and participation, the use of musical instruments, and their voice are assessed.

The separation between training and therapy in musical activities has become less clear as we learn more about their potential benefits. While some differences still exist in recent papers, there is significant overlap in the kilds of professionals who deliver these activities and the possible goals and results. A recent review of the use of music in treating pediatric patients noted that there are different types of music-based interventions. These include music medicine, provided by healthcare professionals, and music therapy, which credentialed music therapists offer. Additionally, other music-based interventions can be provided by healthcare professionals, musicians, teachers, caregivers, and others. (Stegemann et al. 2019).

14.6 The Case of Music and Language and Reading

Music and language share common processes throughout development, connected to physical features of both signals in the pitch structure (melody, scales, harmony, and tonality) and temporal structure (duration, rhythm grouping, meter, and timing). These processes are also connected to socially and emotionally relevant characteristics that boost some aspects of both (shared attention, eye contact, turn-taking, and shared emotions) before even reaching actual communication.

Steven Pinker, in 1997, defined music as something that "confers no survival advantage … I suspect music is auditory cheesecake, an exquisite confection crafted to tickle the sensitive spots of at least six of our mental faculties"[2] (Pinker 2009). Starting from this famous statement, there have been opposite opinions in defense of either music or language. As Patel correctly pointed out in the chapter on evolution of his book "Music Language and the Brain," one has to prove the importance of music in shaping evolution, so Pinker was not being dismissive of the importance of music in itself, but rather on the evidence that its appearance had indeed changed the course of human evolution as language did (Patel 2008).

[2] 1. Language, 2. Auditory scene analysis, 3. Emotional calls, 4. Habitat selection, 5. Motor control, 6. Something else. Something that explains how the whole is more than the sum of the parts.

Whatever the outcome of these ongoing discussions, for the purpose of this chapter, it is noteworthy that evidence points toward a mutual advantage of music and language during development.

Two proposals addressing cross-domain plasticity focus on how musical training impacts auditory attention and working memory, both crucial for speech processing. Besson et al. (2011) and Strait and Kraus (2011) argue that musical training enhances these cognitive functions, improving speech comprehension, particularly in challenging environments like noisy settings. Neuroimaging studies support the idea that music and speech processing share cortical mechanisms for auditory attention and working memory, highlighting the interconnectedness of these domains.

While both proposals agree on the benefits of musical training for auditory processing, their emphasis differs. Strait and Kraus (2011) suggest a reciprocal interaction between cognitive and sensory processes, where cognitive enhancements from musical training shape the nervous system's auditory responses. This perspective challenges the traditional view of auditory processing as a bottom-up process, proposing that training-induced cortical changes also influence subcortical structures. On the other hand, Besson et al. (2011) focus on how increased sensitivity to acoustic features through music training could lead to sharper phonological representations in long-term memory, potentially benefiting language processing and addressing deficits such as those seen in dyslexia.

The OPERA Hypothesis, first proposed by neuroscientist Aniruddh Patel in 2011, explores the connection between music and language processing in the brain. This hypothesis suggests that musical training can enhance linguistic abilities through overlapping neural processes, which he terms "shared resources" (Patel 2011).

Box 14.2 OPERA Hypothesis, Patel 2011. With Permission from Prof. Aniruddh Patel

Key Components of the Opera Hypothesis

Overlap: Music and language processing involve shared brain regions, particularly in the auditory and motor systems. These overlaps include pitch, rhythm, and timing, which are crucial in both domains.

Precision: Musical training demands higher precision in processing these shared elements than language, which can lead to the enhancement of these cognitive functions.

Emotion: Music often engages emotional processing more intensely than language, potentially enhancing memory and learning.

Repetition: The repetitive nature of musical practice strengthens the neural pathways involved in these shared processes, leading to improvements in language skills.

Attention: Focused attention on sound is a key part of musical training; together with Emotion and Repetition, this promotes neural plasticity in sound processing networks.

Patel's Opera Hypothesis posits that these five factors explain why individuals with musical training often show superior language-related abilities, such as better pitch perception in speech, improved reading skills, and more effective auditory memory.

In 2014 Patel expanded the OPERA hypothesis, taking into account both views coming from Strait and Kraus and Besson et al. and stating that besides the obvious sensory involvement, the cognitive demands linked to music training drive adaptive plasticity in speech processing networks. He considered that evidence of overlapping brain networks supports the idea that both music and language share a sensory or cognitive process (e.g., the encoding of waveform periodicity or auditory working memory). In his view, music imposes greater demands on this process compared to speech. And finally, music activates neural plasticity through emotion, repetition, and focused attention (Patel 2014).

14.7 Music and Dyslexia

The evidence supporting the effectiveness of musical interventions in dyslexia rehabilitation allows music and music therapy (clinical-rehabilitative, educational-preventive, and therapeutic) to be applied within an Evidence-Based Education (EBE) framework. This approach uses research findings and intervention criteria recognized as Evidence-Based Practice (EBP) within the EBE movement, extending this methodology to the field of music (Chiappetta Cajola and Rizzo 2016; Kern 2010).

While the biological foundations of dyslexia have garnered the attention of many researchers, exploring each theory in depth is beyond the scope of this discussion. However, it is necessary to present key elements to demonstrate the theoretical plausibility of a cause-effect relationship between low-level deficits in perception or motor skills and reading difficulties. These elements help clarify the theoretical assumptions underlying the project called ReMus: Rhythm and Music to Rehabilitate Reading Disorders (Flaugnacco et al. 2014, 2015).

A key distinction exists between the single-deficit hypothesis and the multi-factorial-deficit hypothesis (Pennington et al. 2012; Ramus and Ahissar 2012). The first suggests that reading disorders are primarily caused by phonological awareness deficits (Ramus et al. 2003). In contrast, the second emphasizes that phonological awareness deficits result from disrupted biological systems influenced by both genetic and environmental factors (Peterson and Pennington 2012). Various theories have focused on visual and auditory deficits (e.g., magnocellular theory, auditory processing deficit), highlighting the role of temporal processing in dyslexia. Goswami (2011, 2014, 2015) and other researchers have proposed that temporal processing deficits may contribute to unifying these theories, laying the foundation for using music to improve auditory attention, phonological awareness, and reading.

International research frequently reports a correlation between musical abilities and reading disorders. In typically developing children, pitch perception has been positively linked to phonological awareness and reading skills (Anvari et al. 2002). This has been further confirmed in comparisons between dyslexic and amusic individuals (Loui et al. 2011). Additionally, the ability to synchronize to a beat correlates with reading and auditory attention skills (Thomson and Goswami 2008; Tiernay and Kraus 2013). In the ReMus project, rhythm synchronization was also related to reading abilities and phonological awareness (Flaugnacco et al. 2014).

In children with dyslexia, the rhythmic-temporal dimension is particularly challenging, indicating difficulty discriminating rapid acoustic changes, duration, rhythm, meter, and sound attack time. Dyslexic children often display deficits in analyzing temporal structures and struggle with tasks involving tapping (keeping the beat) and synchronization (Overy 2003; Thomson and Goswami 2008; Tiernay and Kraus 2013). These challenges suggest a broader difficulty in processing the temporal aspects of sound.

Nina Kraus observed that musical training enhances the ability of subcortical structures to respond accurately to external auditory stimuli, suggesting it is a fundamental physiological marker underlying general synchronization skills (Kraus and Chandrasekaran 2010). Synchronization and tapping abilities improve with musical training and are proportional to years of practice. Like other learned skills, these abilities have critical periods where experience is more likely to enhance performance (Bailey and Penhune 2012; Thompson et al. 2015).

In a meta-analysis Gordon and collaborators showed that music activities had variable effects on phonological and metalinguistic awareness, with outcomes linked to the amount of musical training (Gordon et al. 2015). The authors hypothesized that musical training may gradually impact reading skills, initially enhancing auditory discrimination, thus improving metalinguistic abilities, and eventually supporting reading skills. She noted, however, the large variability in the studies, including differences in language, control group activities, and lack of information on participants' verbal IQ and socioeconomic status. The Italian ReMus project controlled for these variables in its sample of 48 children aged 8–11 with dyslexia. This study compared the effects of musical versus painting training. Both groups improved in self-esteem, reading speed, and behavior, but musical training showed specific significant effects. The music group performed better in reading pseudowords accuracy, ($p = 0.016$), text accuracy ($p = 0.038$), and phoneme blending ($p = 0.004$) besides rhythmic reproduction ($p = 0.0018$). Musical training also improved working memory ($p = 0.01$) and auditory attention ($p = 0.0037$). Meanwhile, the painting group excelled in visuospatial reasoning ($p = 0.02$). These findings highlight the unique benefits of musical training for dyslexia.

Bruce Pennington, in 2011, distinguished between process-based therapies, which target underlying sensory or motor processes to treat learning disorders indirectly, and performance-based therapies, which directly address the symptoms. He outlined that demonstrating evidence is generally easier for performance-based therapies (e.g., improving reading by having the child read) than for process-based ones (e.g., training rhythm to improve reading), nevertheless, nonconventional therapies can be considered evidence-based if they meet four critical theoretical criteria (Pennington 2011).

The four key principles, according to Pennington, could be summarized as follows: a disorder in higher cognitive functions and instrumental skills is caused by either a low-level perceptual or motor deficit or a higher level deficit affecting representation and access to these functions. Training improves low- or high-level skills, with the transfer effect showing that enhancing low-level processes also improves higher level cognitive abilities. Parents, educators, and professionals need to seek evidence of effectiveness for both therapy types. More programs have been developed to aid in the rehabilitation of dyslexia. Habib et al. (2016) created a set of musical exercises that engage sensory (visual, auditory, and somatosensory) and motor systems simultaneously, focusing on rhythmic perception and production, along with comprehensive training of different aspects of the musical auditory signal. They found improvements in both linguistic and nonlinguistic variables. Several authors have proposed that musical interventions should complement traditional remedial approaches. Cancer and Antonietti in their literature review suggest that interventions focused on music and auditory processing should also incorporate phonological and reading-related activities. Integrating decoding tasks into music or auditory-based exercises would improve the transfer of benefits to reading performance (Cancer and Antonietti 2022).

14.8 The Case of Music and Executive Functions

In an entertaining article on neuromyths, MacDonald et al. (2017) uncovered a hard-to-die bias toward the idea that music increases reasoning abilities in children. Such a notion became very popular in the 1990s because of the finding by Rauscher and Shaw on the short-term advantages of music listening on visual-spatial skills (Rauscher et al. 1993). Schellenberg and Hallam, in their subsequent experiment, explained why such claims could not be confirmed (Schellenberg and Hallam 2005). Still, since 2004, Schellenberg started a series of studies to understand if long-term training could promote increased intellectual abilities. He showed encouraging results in the cognitive evaluations of children taking music lessons for 1 year compared to an active group taking drama lessons and a passive control group (Schellenberg 2004). Nevertheless, as Schellenberg himself pointed out, such differences would be flattened subsequently, and he concluded that some other factor might probably contribute to so many correlational findings that emerge in the literature. One possible mediator of the observed changes is the increased ability to apply some core processes to problem-solving, defined as executive functions (EF). According to Adele Diamond, EFs are "a family of top-down mental processes needed when you have to concentrate and pay attention." In 2013, she defined three core EFs: "inhibition, which includes self-control (behavioral inhibition) and interference control (selective attention and cognitive inhibition), working memory (WM), and cognitive flexibility (also called set shifting, mental flexibility, or mental set shifting and closely linked to creativity)" (Diamond 2013).

Among the cognitive abilities, the EF is the one for which "an impact of music training makes the most intuitive sense. After all, playing music requires self-regulation, flexibility, attention, inhibitory control, and planning and implementation of goal-directed behaviors" (Schellenberg and Lima 2024). The results of the literature review, according to Schellenberg, are not conclusive in this respect. Notwithstanding the previous remarks, there has been an encouraging growth of better-designed studies, so one could expect more solid evidence supporting the idea of music reinforcing focused attention and inhibitory control.

14.9 Music and Executive Dysfunctions

Executive function deficit is found in many developmental disorders, with varying degrees and impacts. For example, although not explicitly involved in the diagnostic criteria, such disruption can be found in Attention Deficit and Hyperactivity Disorder (ADHD), Autistic Spectrum Disorder (ASD), Developmental coordination disorder (DCD), and others.

14.9.1 Attention Deficit and Hyperactivity Disorder (ADHD)

ADHD is characterized by inattention, hyperactivity, and Impulsivity. Executive functions are particularly disrupted, leading to poor concentration and sometimes also to difficult self-regulation. Affected children have difficulty controlling their impulses to automatic responses and delaying gratification.

Since ADHD has become more and more popular, it is often self-diagnosed by parents and children themselves, thus leading to some biases in the actual dimension of the disorder. Nevertheless, there has been a growing awareness of its implications. Music training and music therapy have both been effectively used in children with ADHD.

In a recent review, Jamey et al. found that in about 22 longitudinal studies involving more than 1700 children, "music training plays a privileged role compared to other activities (sports, visual arts, and drama) in improving children's executive functioning, with a particular effect on inhibition control." (Jamey et al. 2024)

The 22 studies included in this meta-analysis were carried out in 9 out of 11 so-called WEIRD countries (Western, Educated, Industrialized, Rich, and Democratic); only two studies were in countries outside the WEIRD definition, which is encouraging for the possibility of extending conclusions to different populations. Furthermore, the approaches used were variable, including multicomponent integrated music training, singing, body synchronization, rhythm-centered training, pitch-based training, violin Suzuki Method, and perceptual/motor music-based computer training. In this respect, it will be interesting to see more studies concentrating on methods and efficacy.

14.9.2 Social and Communication Skills

Jamey et al., in their conclusions, point out that besides a relative confirmation of the possibility that music could benefit inhibitory control, music should be included in curricula not because of any proven results in a given task but because of its intrinsic ability to "make people everywhere dance, dream, and connect with one another," as Sandra Trehub told one of the authors (Jamey et al. 2024).

And this underlines one of the most acknowledged benefits of music.

Since early infancy, music and singing have played a unique role in mother–child bonding. Sandra Trehub used to tell the story of her first steps in studying mother–child communication and infant-directed speech; when, as a young researcher, she was planning on recording the first speech exchanges in mother–child dyads, she was told that if mothers were left in a room with their babies, they would sooner sing rather than talk (personal communication). We are now aware of the power of such first interactions as a tool to draw and triangulate attention toward significant stimuli, calm and soothe during stressful events, and convey a rich spectrum of auditory information such as pitch, timbre, timing, and rhythm (Nguyen et al. 2023).

An interesting set of experiments has shown that kindergartners who participate in musical activities together tend to display prosocial behaviors when faced with social problems alongside their peers if they were involved in the same musical activity. However, if they had only been in the room or were doing other activities, their readiness to help was not as boosted, and the same applies to children and adults (Kirschner and Tomasello 2010).

14.9.3 Autistic Spectrum Disorder (ASD)

Colwyn Trevarthen (1980) described the first dyadic mother -infant interaction as "demonstrating that babies are born with the readiness to know another human." Yet some children lack some of these very first requisites of communication. Children with an ASD might experience, even at this stage, disruption of such physiological early means of communication, so infant-directed speech might be less efficient in conveying all the possible cues, and sometimes even singing is less effective to that end. Mothers can be at a loss when their children show early signs and are apparently nonresponsive to these cues. In these situations, it could be very helpful, for example, to engage in songwriting and, in general, singing together with a training music therapist to look for ways to engage infants, taking into account their peculiarities. Although a diagnosis is usually possible at around 36 months, these first signs can be detected, and their impact on the first exchanges can be alleviated.

Other children instead might show a typical development until 24–36 years and then present with a regression of their communication skills. The core symptoms crucial for ASD diagnosis are Social Communication Deficits (SCD) and Restricted and Repetitive Interests and Behaviors. However, more and more, the theoretical framework is being redefined to include the variability observed in the intellectual, language, and adaptive functioning and other symptoms that add to the clinical presentation (Rosen et al. 2021).

Music, and especially music therapy, has often been used as a helpful tool in children with ASD. Although the possibility of obtaining evidence-based results is still scarce, there are more and more attempts to systematize these interventions today. A recent multicentric international study has involved more than 300 children in nine countries. The objective was to evaluate the effect of improvisational music therapy (IMT), according to Nordoff Robbins, on the social affect score of Autism Diagnostic Observation Scale (ADOS) in 5 months. In the NIHR-Funded arm of the study that involved 103 children in the United Kingdom, the results did not give an apparent increase in social affect, although the proportion of those who did improve actually belonged to the subgroup randomized to IMT, and among them, those who received more sessions and had less intellectual disability showed more improvement (Crawford et al. 2017).

In a recent Cochrane Review (Geretsegger et al. 2022), the authors selected 26 studies for 1165 participants. The age of subjects varied from 2 to 12. The music therapy approach involved in 12 studies a highly structured intervention, sometimes addressing specific behaviors, with both receptive and active interventions, while the remaining studies were centered on relational music therapy, involving improvisation, songs, and structured games in a nondirective approach. Fifteen studies presented a control condition where no music was used, but in some studies, passive music listening was used as control; in 11 studies, standard care was the control condition. The authors found changes in social interaction and nonverbal communication. These changes were long-lasting even after the intervention. Notably, the most recent studies provided music therapy in group settings. The quality of evidence varied from moderate to very low. The authors suggest carefully indicating the type of intervention to make it comparable, thus rendering the results more generalizable and increasing external validity. More specific to the methods, there is still a lack of consensus on the most pertinent outcome measure. For example, a good solution might involve combining behavioral measures and physiological markers, as was done in one of the studies in the analysis.

In the search for interventions that parallel what we know of ASD, Lense and Camarata proposed the PRESS-Play framework, consisting of structured activities that use music and play to address some of the core features of ASD children and their caregivers: (1) Predictability; (2) Reinforcement; (3) Emotion Regulation; (4) Shared Attention; and (5) Social Play context. The authors stress that such activities should not be provided as standalone but as a meaningful and joyful addition to other interventions (Lense and Camarata 2020). In this way, we could ensure children enjoy pleasant experiences with their caregivers and peers while receiving multimodal stimulation such as music that carries possibilities for social interaction, communication, emotional connection, and sensory-motor integration.

14.10 Discussion and Perspectives

With regard to the multiplicity of variables that come into play in the course of a musical intervention, it is worth mentioning how, in the ReMus project, the self-esteem test (TMA) recorded improvements in both groups (average of the 48 children's perceived self-efficacy: before training 71, after training 91, average of the Scale 100, standard deviation of 15), probably also because the participants were guided in pleasant and creative group activities. The program was well-accepted by the children's parents, and was given for free thanks to the grant awarded by Fondazione Mariani (Grant R-11-85). The importance of these factors should not be overlooked when transferring the musical experience from a clinical research field to a more educational-laboratory field in which the additional variables that are introduced, if known and measured, can add invaluable content to the proposed activity in terms of formative spin-offs and its replicability in various settings.

Furthermore, as we have seen, certain traits are shared among various neurodevelopmental disorders, including inattention, impulsivity, and difficulties in different areas of learning. Additionally, gathering a large amount of data to ensure robust conclusions about the findings is increasingly crucial in all areas of research, particularly in neurodevelopmental disorders.

Siugzdaite and collaborators elegantly stated that "complex cognitive processes or deficits may have multiple different contributing factors. Conversely, the same local neural deficit could result in multiple cognitive symptoms across individuals" (Siugzdaite et al. 2020). In the authors' search for a solution to the problem often encountered in neurodevelopmental literature of ill-defined diagnostic labels and exclusion criteria, they analyzed data from over 400 children referred by their teachers, pediatricians, or Special Education Needs Coordinators (SENCO). They examined many cognitive and neuropsychological variables and imaging data through sophisticated machine-learning techniques. Their exciting results show that the children in their sample would not align or segregate based on their diagnosis but rather on their cognitive and neuropsychological profiles, irrespective of any label that had been given. The same applies to their brain imaging profile, particularly their cortical morphology as measured through diffusion tensor imaging (DTI) data. So, the actual differences seen among children could probably come from subtle differences in connectivity between structures ensuing during development. This line of reasoning brings back the windows of opportunity already hypothesized by Knudsen (2004), and it would be very plausible to think that music can be among the means to boost that kind of plasticity besides being pleasant, rewarding, and desirable from all points of view.

References

Anvari SH, Trainor LJ, Woodside J, Levy BA. Relations among musical skills, phonological processing, and early reading ability in preschool children. J Exp Child Psychol. 2002;83(2):111–30.

Bailey J, Penhune VB. A sensitive period for musical training: contributions of age of onset and cognitive abilities. Ann N Y Acad Sci. 2012;1252:163–70.

Barrett KC, Ashley R, Strait DL, Kraus N. Art and science: how musical training shapes the brain. Front Psychol. 2013;4(October):1e13. https://doi.org/10.3389/fpsyg.2013.00713.

Besson M, Chobert J, Marie C. Transfer of training between music and speech: common processing, attention, and memory. Front Psychol. 2011 May 12;2:94. https://doi.org/10.3389/fpsyg.2011.00094. PMID: 21738519; PMCID: PMC3125524.

Cancer A, Antonietti A. Music-based and auditory-based interventions for reading difficulties: a literature review. Heliyon. 2022 Apr 18;8(4):e09293. https://doi.org/10.1016/j.heliyon.2022.e09293. PMID: 35497042; PMCID: PMC9048091.

Chang HW, Trehub SE. Infants' perception of temporal grouping in auditory patterns. Child Dev. 1977 Dec;48(4):1666–70.

Chiappetta Cajola L, Rizzo AL. Didattica inclusiva e Musicoterapia: La prospettiva dell'ICF-CY e dell'Evidence based education. Roma: FrancoAngeli; 2016.

Crawford MJ, Gold C, Odell-Miller H, Thana L, Faber S, Assmus J, Bieleninik Ł, Geretsegger M, Grant C, Maratos A, Sandford S, Claringbold A, McConachie H, Maskey M, Mössler KA, Ramchandani P, Hassiotis A. International multicentre randomised controlled trial of improvisational music therapy for children with autism spectrum disorder: TIME-A study. Health Technol Assess. 2017 Oct;21(59):1–40. https://doi.org/10.3310/hta21590. PMID: 29061222; PMCID: PMC5672498.

Diamond A. Executive functions. Annu Rev Psychol. 2013;64:135–68. https://doi.org/10.1146/annurev-psych-113011-143750.

Flaugnacco E, Lopez L, Terribili C, Zoia S, Buda S, Tilli S, Monasta L, Montico M, Sila A, Ronfani L, Schön D. Rhythm perception and production predict reading abilities in developmental dyslexia. Front Hum Neurosci. 2014;8:392.

Flaugnacco E, Lopez L, Terribili C, Montico M, Zoia S, Schön D. Music training increases phonological awareness and reading skills in developmental dyslexia: a randomized control trial. PLoS One. 2015;10(9):e0138715.

Geretsegger M, Fusar-Poli L, Elefant C, Mössler KA, Vitale G, Gold C. Music therapy for autistic people. Cochrane Database Syst Rev. 2022 May 9;5(5):CD004381. https://doi.org/10.1002/14651858.CD004381.pub4. PMID: 35532041; PMCID: PMC9082683.

Gordon RL, Fehd HM, McCandliss BD. Does music training enhance literacy skills? A meta-analysis. Front Psychol. 2015;6:1777.

Goswami U. A temporal sampling framework for developmental dyslexia. Trends Cogn Sci. 2011;15(1):3–10.

Goswami U. Sensory theories of developmental dyslexia: three challenges for research. Nat Rev Neurosci. 2015;16:43–54.

Goswami U, Power AJ, Lallier M, Facoetti A. Oscillatory "temporal sampling" and developmental dyslexia: toward an over-arching theoretical framework. Front Hum Neurosci. 2014;8:904.

Habib M, Lardy C, Desiles T, Commeiras C, Chobert J, Besson M. Music and dyslexia: a new musical training method to improve reading and related disorders. Front Psychol. 2016 Jan 22;7:26. https://doi.org/10.3389/fpsyg.2016.00026. PMID: 26834689; PMCID: PMC4722115.

Hensch TK, Bilimoria PM. Re-opening windows: manipulating critical periods for brain development. Cerebrum. 2012;2012(August):11 PMID: 23447797; PMCID: PMC3574806.

Hepper PG. An examination of fetal learning before and after birth. Ir J Psychol. 1991;12:95–107. https://doi.org/10.1080/03033910.1991.10557830.

Ismail FY, Fatemi A, Johnston MV. Cerebral plasticity: windows of opportunity in the developing brain. Eur J Paediatr Neurol. 2017 Jan;21(1):23–48. https://doi.org/10.1016/j.ejpn.2016.07.007. Epub 2016 Aug 9.

Jamey K, Foster NEV, Hyde KL, Dalla Bella S. Does music training improve inhibition control in children? A systematic review and meta-analysis. Cognition. 2024 Nov;252:105913. https://doi.org/10.1016/j.cognition.2024.105913. Epub 2024 Aug 27. PMID: 39197250.

Kern P. Evidence-based practice in early childhood music therapy: a decision-making process. Music Ther Perspect. 2010;28(2):116–23.

Kirschner S, Tomasello M. Joint music making promotes prosocial behavior in 4-year-old children. Evol Hum Behav. 2010;31(5):354–64. https://doi.org/10.1016/j.evolhumbehav.2010.04.004.

Kisilevsky S, Hains SM, Jacquet AY, Granier-Deferre C, Lecanuet JP. Maturation of fetal responses to music. Dev Sci. 2004 Nov;7(5):550–9. https://doi.org/10.1111/j.1467-7687.2004.00379.x.

Knudsen EI. Sensitive periods in the development of the brain and behavior. J Cogn Neurosci. 2004 Oct;16(8):1412–25. https://doi.org/10.1162/0898929042304796.

Kraus N, Chandrasekaran B. Music training for the development of auditory skills. Nat Rev Neurosci. 2010;11:599–605. https://doi.org/10.1038/nrn2882.

Lense MD, Camarata S. PRESS-Play: Musical engagement as a motivating platform for social interaction and social play in young children with ASD. Music Sci (Lond). 2020 Jan-Dec;3:10.1177/2059204320933080. https://doi.org/10.1177/2059204320933080. Epub 2020 Jun 25. PMID: 32832103; PMCID: PMC7440205.

Loui P, Kroog K, Zuk J, Winner E, Schlaug G. Relating pitch awareness to phonemic awareness in children: implications for tone-deafness and dyslexia. Front Psychol. 2011;2:111. https://doi.org/10.3389/fpsyg.2011.00111. PMID: 21687467; PMCID: PMC3108552.

Macdonald K, Germine L, Anderson A, Christodoulou J, McGrath LM. Dispelling the myth: training in education or neuroscience decreases but does not eliminate beliefs in Neuromyths. Front Psychol. 2017 Aug 10;8:1314. https://doi.org/10.3389/fpsyg.2017.01314. PMID: 28848461; PMCID: PMC5554523.

Nguyen T, Flaten E, Trainor LJ, Novembre G. Early social communication through music: state of the art and future perspectives. Dev Cogn Neurosci. 2023 Oct;63:101279. https://doi.org/10.1016/j.dcn.2023.101279. Epub 2023 Jul 27. PMID: 37515832; PMCID: PMC10407289.

Overy K. Dyslexia and music: from timing deficits to musical intervention. Ann N Y Acad Sci. 2003;999:497–505.

Patel AD. Music, language, and the brain. New York: Oxford University Press; 2008.

Patel AD. Why would musical training benefit the neural encoding of speech? The OPERA hypothesis. Front Psychol. 2011 June 29;2:142. https://doi.org/10.3389/fpsyg.2011.00142. PMID: 21747773; PMCID: PMC3128244.

Patel AD. Can nonlinguistic musical training change the way the brain processes speech? The expanded OPERA hypothesis Hear Res. 2014 Feb;308:98–108. https://doi.org/10.1016/j.heares.2013.08.011. Epub 2013 Sep 20.

Pennington BF. Controversial therapies for dyslexia. Perspect Lang Literacy: Q. Publ. Int. Dyslexia Assoc. 2011:37.

Pennington BF, Santerre-Lemmon L, Rosenberg J, MacDonald B, Boada R, Friend A, Leopold DR, Samuelsson S, Byrne B, Willcutt EG, Olson RK. Individual prediction of dyslexia by single versus multiple deficit models. J Abnorm Psychol. 2012 Feb;121(1):212–24. https://doi.org/10.1037/a0025823.

Peterson RL, Pennington BF. Developmental dyslexia. Lancet 2012 May 26;379(9830):1997–2007. https://doi.org/10.1016/S0140-6736(12)60198-6. PMID: 22513218; PMCID: PMC3465717.

Pinker S. How the mind works. 2nd ed. New York, NY: W. W. Norton & Company; 2009.

Plantinga J, Trehub SE. Revisiting the innate preference for consonance. J Exp Psychol Hum Percept Perform. 2014 Feb;40(1):40–49. https://doi.org/10.1037/a0033471. Epub 2013 Jul 1.

Ramus F, Ahissar M. Developmental dyslexia: the difficulties of interpreting poor performance, and the importance of normal performance. Cogn Neuropsychol. 2012;29(1–2):104–22.

Ramus F, Rosen S, Dakin SC, Day BL, Castellote JM, White S, Frith U. Theories of developmental dyslexia: insights from a multiple case study of dyslexic adults. Brain. 2003;126:841–65.

Rauscher FH, Shaw GL, Ky KN. Music and spatial task performance. Nature. 1993 Oct 14;365(6447):611. https://doi.org/10.1038/365611a0.
Rosen NE, Lord C, Volkmar FR. The diagnosis of autism: from Kanner to DSM-III to DSM-5 and beyond. J Autism Dev Disord. 2021 Feb 24;51:4253. https://doi.org/10.1007/s10803-021-04904-1.
Schellenberg EG. Music lessons enhance IQ. Psychol Sci. 2004 Aug;15(8):511–4. https://doi.org/10.1111/j.0956-7976.2004.00711.x.
Schellenberg EG, Hallam S. Music listening and cognitive abilities in 10- and 11-year-olds: the blur effect. Ann N Y Acad Sci. 2005 Dec;1060:202–9. https://doi.org/10.1196/annals.1360.013.
Schellenberg EG, Lima CF. Music training and nonmusical abilities. Annu Rev Psychol. 2024 Jan 18;75:87–128. https://doi.org/10.1146/annurev-psych-032323-051354. Epub 2023 Sep 22.
Schellenberg EG, Trainor LJ. Sensory consonance and the perceptual similarity of complex-tone harmonic intervals: tests of adult and infant listeners. J Acoust Soc Am. 1996;100(5 Pt 1):3321–8. https://doi.org/10.1121/1.417355.
Siugzdaite R, Bathelt J, Holmes J, Astle DE. Transdiagnostic brain mapping in developmental disorders. Curr Biol. 2020 Apr 6;30(7):1245–1257.e4. https://doi.org/10.1016/j.cub.2020.01.078. Epub 2020 Feb 27. PMID: 32109389; PMCID: PMC7139199.
Stegemann T, Geretsegger M, Phan Quoc E, Riedl H, Smetana M. Music therapy and other music-based interventions in pediatric health care: an overview. Medicines (Basel). 2019 Feb 14;6(1):25. https://doi.org/10.3390/medicines6010025. PMID: 30769834; PMCID: PMC6473587.
Strait D, Kraus N. Playing music for a smarter ear: cognitive, perceptual and neurobiological evidence. Music Percept. 2011 Dec 1;29(2):133–146. https://doi.org/10.1525/MP.2011.29.2.133. PMID: 22993456; PMCID: PMC3444167.
Thompson EC, White-Schwoch T, Tierney A, Kraus N. Beat synchronization across the lifespan: intersection of development and musical experience. PLoS One. 2015;10(6):e0128839.
Thomson JM, Goswami U. Rhythmic processing in children with developmental dyslexia: auditory and motor rhythms link to reading and spelling. J Physiol Paris. 2008;102:120–9.
Tiernay A, Kraus N. The ability to move to a beat is linked to the consistency of neural responses to sound. J Neurosci. 2013;33(38):14981–8.
Trainor LJ. Are there critical periods for musical development? Dev Psychobiol. 2005 Apr;46(3):262–78. https://doi.org/10.1002/dev.20059.
Trainor LJ, Heinmiller BM. Infants prefer to listen to consonance over dissonance. Inf. Behav. Dev. 1998;21:77–88. https://doi.org/10.1016/S0163-6383(98)90055-8.
Trehub SE, Hannon EE. Infant music perception: domain-general or domain-specific mechanisms? Cognition. 2006;100(1):73–99. https://doi.org/10.1016/j.cognition.2005.11.006.
Trevarthen C. The foundations of intersubjectivity: development of interpersonal and cooperative understanding in infants. In: Olson D, editor. The social foundations of language and thought: essays in honor of Jerome S. Bruner. New York: Norton; 1980. p. 316–42.
Ullal-Gupta S, Vanden Bosch der Nederlanden CM, Tichko P, Lahav A, Hannon EE. Linking prenatal experience to the emerging musical mind. Front Syst Neurosci. 2013 Sep 3;7:48. https://doi.org/10.3389/fnsys.2013.00048. PMID: 24027502; PMCID: PMC3759965.
Winkler I, Háden GP, Ladinig O, Sziller I, Honing H. Newborn infants detect the beat in music. Proc Natl Acad Sci U S A. 2009 Feb 17;106(7):2468–2471. https://doi.org/10.1073/pnas.0809035106. Epub 2009 Jan 26. PMID: 19171894; PMCID: PMC2631079.

Music Therapy and Music-Based Interventions in Oncology and End-of-Life Care

15

Amy Clements-Cortés, Joyce Jing Yee Yip, and Sara Klinck

15.1 Introduction

Across the globe, cancer care (or oncology care) and end-of-life care (or palliative care) vary considerably in how they are actualized with adults and pediatric patients. In cancer care, factors that drive and influence the treatment and management of an individual with cancer includes the type of cancer, stage of the disease, disease trajectory, health practices and beliefs, and locations of cancer care (i.e., management by family physicians, specialized inpatient hospital units, specialized clinics and in the community, and the home). These management plans suggest a medical model of care with cancer patients, which can include pharmacological treatments to shrink or kill cancer cells, chemotherapy, radiotherapy, immunotherapy, targeted agents, and other novel treatments (Yazdanpanah et al. 2023). For end-of-life care, the medical model of care is specific to the terminal illness experienced by the patient such as cancer (Collins 2019; Heath and Lings 2012; Teut et al. 2014), malignant and non-malignant diseases (Bausewein et al. 2013), and dementia (Bradt and Dileo 2010; Garabedian and Kelly 2020; Uçaner Çifdalöz 2020). While pharmacological treatments are necessary, they do not provide a comprehensive whole person care beyond the concerns of the illness (such as the physical, psychological,

A. Clements-Cortés (✉)
Faculty of Music, University of Toronto, Toronto, ON, Canada
e-mail: a.clements.cortes@utoronto.ca

J. J. Y. Yip
Ontario Institute for Studies in Education, University of Toronto, Toronto, ON, Canada
e-mail: joycejingyee.yip@mail.utoronto.ca

S. Klinck
Faculty of Music, Wilfrid Laurier University, Waterloo, ON, Canada
e-mail: sklinck@wlu.ca

A. Raglio (ed.), *Music and Music Therapy Interventions in Clinical Practice*, Neurocultural Health and Wellbeing,
https://doi.org/10.1007/978-3-031-88578-5_15

spiritual, and social aspects of a person) (WHO 2020), necessitating an interdisciplinary approach to optimize quality of life by those with life-limiting conditions (Ferrell et al. 2018). Considerations of other factors affecting the patient are often not addressed, such as the impact of illness on the individuals' family or peers, home care network of practitioners, and economic concerns. This is where music therapy (MT) and music-based interventions (MBIs) can play an important role within cancer care and end-of-life.

This chapter considers MT and MBIs in cancer or oncology and end-of-life or palliative contexts, focusing broadly on the interventions commonly used to support these patients. MT and MBIs have increasingly been implemented to support presenting symptoms of a person's diagnosis (Bradt et al. 2021; Trigueros-Murillo et al. 2023), in addition to issues in multiple domains related to quality of life, not limited to physical, psychological, emotional, communication, and spiritual realms (Gao et al. 2019; Schmid et al. 2018; Toccafondi et al. 2018).

Raglio and Oasi (2015) explain that MBIs in cancer and end-of-life care are categorized as MT, music listening (music and medicine approaches), and generalized MBIs. MT differs from other MBIs, as it centralizes the therapeutic relationship between the practitioner and the patient requiring the service. According to Clements-Cortés (2016a), the development and efficacy of MT techniques used in end-of-life care have several emergent themes that address physical, psychosocial, and whole person care (Clements-Cortés 2016b). This finding suggests the intersections between these creative modalities for oncology and end-of-life patients. Applications of MT interventions in cancer and palliative care music therapy are: singing (Clements-Cortés and Yip 2024), instrument-play, improvisation (vocal and instrumental), songwriting, music-guided breathing exercises, verbal processing (Bradt et al. 2015), and the Bonny Method of Guided Imagery and Music (The Bonny Method) (Clements-Cortés 2019; Clements-Cortés and Yip 2021a). MT techniques are also flexible in oncology and end-of-life care, outlining receptive, improvisational/compositional and recreative interventions (Bruscia 2014; Klinck et al. 2021), implying the versatility of the practice. Receptive techniques have also been documented in these contexts, which involve interactive experiences like lyric analysis, somatic listening, relaxation, and music that the patient listens to passively to support physical, social, and cognitive development and spiritual domains (Grocke and Wigram 2007).

MBIs in cancer care are approaches classified under complementary and alternative medicine (Tsao et al. 2008) and can be administered by music therapists, musicians, and other health professionals such as medical students, trained volunteers to assist with hospitalized patients, and other persons interested in making music such as parents and guardians (Apps and Sunderland 2023; Bains et al. 2024; Blank et al. 2024; Bradt et al. 2021; Fancourt et al. 2016; Park and Lee 2022; Stegenga et al. 2024; Valero-Cantero et al. 2023). Similarly, in end-of-life care, MBIs have been utilized among inpatients and outpatients such as caregivers (Garabedian and Kelly 2020; Valero-Cantero et al. 2023), family members (Akard et al. 2021), hospice workers (Fiore 2021), music therapists (Mangiacotti et al. 2024), musicians and music educators (Potvin et al. 2023), and registered nurses (Robb et al. 2018), that considers environmental factors such as the living situation and social support from peers and the community (Foster et al. 2012). MBIs have been used for individuals with co-diagnoses or complex care (Akard et al. 2021), such as cancer patients facing end-of-life (Archie et al. 2013; Sampaio 2023); patients in neurologic palliative and hospice care (Potvin et al. 2023); patients admitted to the intensive care unit (Nazir 2023); dementia care (Dowlen et al. 2022; Johnston et al. 2022; Lepping et al. 2024; Mercadal-Brotons et al. 2021; van der Steen et al. 2018); neonatal care and neurorehabilitation (Chatterjee et al. 2021); and patients diagnosed with end-stage kidney disease (Burrai et al. 2018); aphasia (Zumbansen and Tremblay 2019); Parkinson's disease (Pohl et al. 2020) or early Alzheimer's disease (Leggieri et al. 2018); stroke and multiple sclerosis (Moumdjian et al. 2017); autism spectrum disorder, disability, epilepsy, and mental health (Stegemann et al. 2019).

15.2 Methodology

Narrative review allowed the authors of this chapter to offer a summary, critique, and interpretation (Greenhalg et al. 2018) of the range of research and descriptive literature in MBIs and MT in oncology and end-of-life care. Our results provide a synthesis of the foundational literature describing the current status of practice (Rumrill and Fitzgerald 2001). The discussion highlights the practical applications of MBIs and MT in cancer and end-of-life, sharing some areas for future research and development. To gather the relevant literature about MT and MBIs within oncology and end-of-life care, the following key terms were searched and combined to create appropriate search formulas: oncology, cancer, end-of-life, palliative care, MBIs, MT techniques, music medicine, MT, children, adolescents, and adults. For example, ["music therap*" AND "oncology" OR "cancer" OR "care" AND "adult"] were the terms used to search material related to MT utilized in cancer care for adults.[1] Several databases were used to support the search, including APA Psychinfo, Cochrane Library, Scopus, Medline, PubMed, CINHAL, and Google Scholar. Prior to generating the search, confounds were implemented: publications were to be written in English, published from the year 2000 onward, be peer reviewed, and available online or via institutional library access of the authors. Data saturation (Saunders et al. 2018) occurred in the collation of articles especially given literature often involved case studies and small sample sizes.

The types of literature that were reviewed in this chapter encompassed a wide range, such as individual research articles, descriptive articles, book chapters, scoping reviews, integrative, systematic, and meta reviews. Conference hearings and alternative reviews (i.e., book reviews, critiques in popular media such as

[1]An asterisk (*) is used to replace part of a word to find all variations of a root word. In this example, music therapy and music therapist could be in the return results. Quotations ("") are used to search for exact phrases and combinations of words in a specified order. The terms, AND and OR, are operators to refine and control the results by expanding or choosing particular search terms using Boolean search logic.

newspapers) were omitted. Once the search was generated, the authors screened each publication to seek relevance to the topic and duplicates. Folders were created per topic and were analyzed individually to explore the results and intersecting themes among the found literature.

15.3 Results

A total of two hundred thirty-nine (n=239) articles and reviews were found to be evaluated in this chapter. In the discussion section, tables of the key MT and MBIs used in oncology care and end-of-life care were created for adults and children to summarize the results.

15.3.1 Music Therapy for Adults with Cancer and at End-of-Life

Research has shown that MT has many benefits for persons in oncology settings, specifically for emotional processing and its efficacy in reducing anxiety, stress, and overall quality of life (Canadian Cancer Society 2021). By definition, oncology MT "… is the skilled and professionally informed use of MBIs within a therapeutic relationship to address biopsychosocial and/or spiritual concerns to alleviate discomfort, support coping, restore function, and improve life quality" (O'Callaghan and Magill 2017, p 11). Symptom management requires an interdisciplinary treatment approach, where art and MT can support psychological and social factors, adding to the quality of life of the individual(s) receiving the care (Yazdanpanah et al. 2022). Further, supportive therapies, such as MT, are critical throughout the cancer trajectory (Clements-Cortés and Yip 2024), especially when given support begins to decline within the first year of diagnosis (Manning-Walsh 2005). The summary of literature highlights MT applications pre-, during, and post-treatments of cancer and end-of-life illnesses.

15.3.2 Music Therapy During Treatment, Chemotherapy, and Radiation

MT has had a positive impact on various symptoms prevalent during chemotherapy and radiation treatment. Systematic review results (e.g., Kievisiene et al. 2020) indicate that MT was mostly researched for anxiety reduction and carried out during chemotherapy/radiotherapy or in preoperative, perioperative, or postoperative periods. Interventions that aimed to reduce anxiety included listening to recorded music following surgery and chemotherapy (Li et al. 2011), while waiting for chemotherapy time (Bulfone et al. 2009), and during radiation (Karadag et al. 2019). In particular, environmental music therapy (EMT) interventions combining live improvised and precomposed music significantly reduced perceived anxiety, distress, and wait-times in radiation oncology (Rossetti et al. 2023). Patient preferred live music has further been used to support reductions in negative affect, fatigue, and pain among post-transplant patients receiving chemotherapy and/or radiation (Fredenburg and Silverman 2014).

Management of chronic pain in advanced cancer was also investigated in Bradt et al.'s (2024) randomized controlled trial (RCT) comparing MT (music-based support) with social attention control (verbal-based support) sessions. The researchers found that MT interventions, such as joint music making, singing, playing instruments, instrumental or vocal improvisations, music-guided visualizations, music-guided deep breathing for relaxation, and music-based learning and skill acquisition, were mediated by self-efficacy and could be maximized by teaching music-based self-management strategies to patients (Bradt et al. 2024). Mondanaro et al. (2021) also found that live vocal and instrumental improvisation fostered feelings of resilience and increased emotional expression, while reducing depression and pain levels during chemotherapy infusion.

Köhler et al.'s (2020) systematic review and meta-analysis found mixed, but overall positive and significant evidence of MT's effects on psychological well-being, quality of life, and physical symptom distress in different phases of oncological treatment for adult cancer patients. MT techniques during curative treatment (chemotherapy and radiation) focused on relaxation and imagery, listening to music with a therapist, singing, improvisation, and songwriting, with the most promising effects on decreased anxiety, distress, depression, pain, and analgesic use. Reductions in anxiety and distress were beneficial outcomes when a multilevel combination of music listening, live music, and verbal processing with a therapist were applied in preparation for radiation (Rossetti et al. 2017). Similar techniques were fruitful in improving quality of life, facilitating emotional expression/regulation, and lowering levels of fatigue and depression during radiotherapy (Alcântara-Silva et al. 2018). Outcomes may also include improved physical parameters, such as heart rate, blood pressure, respiratory rate, and oxygen saturation alongside positive effects on pain, physical and respiratory comfort when receptive and active MT methods are implemented in this context (Clemens et al. 2023).

Compared to standard care alone, even as little as one 60-minute MT session reduced anxiety (self-reported and indicated through increased skin temperature) for patients receiving curative treatments (Lin et al. 2011). Other research points to similar positive effects on relaxation, comfort, happiness, and stress biomarkers, when compared with standard care alone for breast cancer patients receiving chemotherapy (Hanser et al. 2006).

Results of three RCTs compared music-based imagery with different control conditions: waitlist (Burns 2001), treatment as usual (Burns et al. 2007), and music listening (Burns et al. 2018), found guided music intervention improved mood states and quality of life to a greater degree than a waitlist control group (Burns 2001). Positive and negative affect, fatigue, and anxiety, all improved for both music imagery and treatment as usual groups (Burns et al. 2007), and music imagery led to higher responsiveness, emotionally focused, and treatment-specific outcomes, while preferred music listening improved distress (Burns et al. 2018). The third study (Burns et al. 2018) highlighted the complex ways that receptive music listening-based interventions can be experienced by cancer patients, potentially accessing both positive resources and emotional distress associated with diagnosis and treatment. Clinicians must be mindful of the psychological impact of supportive music and imagery, and monitor and adapt the unfolding clinical process in response to patients' needs. Supportive music and imagery has helped patients feel prepared for treatment and manage their treatment experience, and may be most beneficial as a brief intervention (i.e., 1–3 sessions) with goals to energize and replenish inner resources. Preferred music (genre) listening may also be beneficial when the goal is to contain emotional experience, or evoke a pleasant or narrower range of emotions (Burns et al. 2018).

To summarize, MT techniques focused on relaxation and imagery, listening to music with a therapist, improvisation, and songwriting were important and demonstrated the most beneficial effects for decreasing anxiety, distress, depression, and pain.

15.3.3 Music Therapy During Surgery and Transplantation

Evidence on the use of MT during surgery and transplantation is promising for supportive management of anxiety and pain. During surgery and transplantation, MT was beneficial for supportive management of anxiety and pain, and interventions focused on listening to the music therapist's live music, tailored recorded music, music listening and verbal reflection/conversation, and a variety of other techniques during the sessions (Köhler et al. 2020).

Music listening has been a key intervention in supporting multiple symptoms related to surgical procedures. Wang et al. (2015) found that listening to a music therapist play relaxing music, before and after surgery, resulted in lung cancer patients experiencing reduced anxiety, blood pressure, heart rate, and lower need for analgesics. Further, music listening with verbal reflection presurgery, followed by therapist-selected music during surgery, lessened recovery time, and reduced anxiety (Palmer et al. 2015). Yates and Silverman (2015) reported similar effects of receptive MT and therapeutic conversations on anxiety reduction and increased relaxation following surgery. Additionally, MT resulted in higher levels of hope (Verstegen 2016), improved mood (Dóro et al. 2017), reduced use of analgesics (Bates et al. 2017; Tuinmann et al. 2017), reduced pain perception and toxic side effects, and increased immunological parameters during stem cell transplantation (Cassileth et al. 2003).

Patient-preferred live music as a MT technique has been found to reduce fatigue and pain, and increase energy levels for adults hospitalized in a blood and marrow transplant unit (Fredenburg and Silverman 2014; Reimnitz and Silverman 2020; Reimnitz and Silverman 2020, 2021; Rosenow and Silverman 2014). This technique can further address hope (Verstegen and Silverman 2018), or reminiscence, emotional release, relaxation, and reflection (Reimnitz and Silverman 2021) within this context.

With respect to applications and outcomes of MT in the perioperative phase, Kievisiene et al.'s (2020) systematic review reported pain management was optimized with MT following surgery (Binns-Turner et al. 2011; Li et al. 2011), and when offered in-home for lasting effects on pain, intensity, fatigue (physical and emotional), and vigor (Hsieh et al. 2019). For breast cancer patients undergoing mastectomy, Lagattolla et al. (2023) found that individual receptive MT via music listening and guided relaxation further decreased anxiety levels. In comparison, integrated group MT consisting of improvisation, music and imagery, choral singing, verbal and reflective discussion resulted in higher perception of help received and interpersonal resources.

15.3.4 Music Therapy in End-of-Life

In end-of-life care, there are a variety of benefits that MT affords for all life-limiting issues when administered in individual and group MT sessions. Evidence for MT in end-of-life care was mixed and most studies offered tailored interventions or music-based relaxation, showing promising effects on quality of life, stress, pain, and spiritual well-being for those with terminal cancer (Köhler et al. 2020). For instance, O'Callaghan's (2024) systematic literature review of MT in palliative care found MT was effective for a reduction in pain and anxiety, improved mood, relaxation, spiritual well-being, and fostered relationship/connection with significant persons. Bowers and Wetsel (2014) reviewed 17 selected articles on adult palliative populations from various cultural backgrounds on the utilization and effectiveness of MT in adult palliative and/or hospice care. Results showed that anxiety and pain were the symptoms most commonly addressed and reduced by MT interventions, followed by depression and quality of life (Bowers and Wetsel 2014). Generally, receptive methods led to stronger improvements in psychological outcomes, as active methods may be more challenging for patients with cancer due to physical weakness or inhibition to express emotions (Köhler et al. 2020). The Bonny Method also demonstrated benefits in grief work, emotional expression, and processing (Clements-Cortés 2019). Specific techniques have demonstrated identified outcomes of the patient at end-of-life. This includes: song choice to promote social interaction (Clements-Cortés 2004; Gallagher et al. 2017; Kim and Dvorak 2018); lyric discussion and analysis to identify feelings and communicate messages (Black et al. 2020; Gallagher et al. 2017; Hilliard 2001); music for reminiscence to promote communication between family and friends (Clements-Cortés 2016c; Kim and Dvorak 2018); and musical life review which can assist in exploring remembering, and celebrating aspects of one's life (Klinck et al. 2021), with the prospect of songwriting (Black et al. 2020; Gallagher et al. 2017; Magill 2009a, 2011) and when patients have interest and energy to do so.

Pain management (Curtis 2011; Gallagher et al. 2006, 2018; Gutgsell et al. 2013; Krout 2001; McConnell et al. 2016; Vesel and Dave 2018) and emotional regulation (Gillespie et al. 2024) have generated the following outcomes: increased the patient's positive relationships with others (Kim and Dvorak 2018; Schmid et al.

2018); enhanced physical comfort, decreased anxiety (Gallagher et al. 2006, 2018); decreased agitation (Cadwalader et al. 2016); increased emotional well-being (McConnell and Porter 2017) and overall quality of life (Gallagher et al. 2017; Hilliard 2003b; Porter et al. 2018); death acceptance (Gallagher et al. 2017); and spiritual well-being (Burns et al. 2015; Liu et al. 2015; Magill 2009b; Salmon 2001; Warth et al. 2021).

Unique to end-of-life care is MT to support relationship completion (Clements-Cortés 2011; Clements-Cortés and Yip 2021b; Hsieh et al. 2024), legacy creation (O'Callaghan 2013; Mondanaro and Tsiris 2021; Potvin et al. 2018; Schreck et al. 2022) as well as physician-assisted suicide or medical assistance in dying (MAiD) (Black et al. 2020; Clements-Cortés and Yip 2020; Klinck and Clements-Cortés 2021), and bereavement (Gillespie et al. 2024; Klinck and Clements-Cortés 2021). MToffered for MAiD is helpful to engage in control, reflection, communication, and connection (Black et al. 2020). Songwriting, lyric discussion and analysis, life review, song dedications, and music improvisation (Clements-Cortés 2011; Klinck et al. 2021), song choice, and creation of playlists, The Bonny Method, entrainment, empathic improvisation, free associate singing, active vocal or instrumental improvisation, musical autobiographies, and legacy gifts (Klinck et al. 2021) are several techniques that are necessary for relationship completion.

End-of-life MT can also extend to informal carers or carer-patient dyads or shared MT experiences. Gillespie et al. (2024) conducted a systematic review of 34 studies that focused on the experience, characteristics, and effectiveness of MT interventions with informal carers pre- and post-bereavement loss. The majority of studies focused on informal carers of dementia and advanced cancer, with MT predominantly delivered in the pre-bereavement phase (Gillespie et al. 2024). In the studies, individual palliative care sessions, where the carer was present, patient-carer dyadic or family-based sessions at end-of-life, and bereavement group work were formats reflected in the studies. These interventions were delivered in-person, via telephone or virtual platform at home, in residential or daycare specialist facilities, public health or community facilities, hospices, or hospitals (Gillespie et al. 2024). Multiple receptive, improvisational, compositional, and recreative MT methods were targeted at improving health-related outcomes, such as quality of life, mental well-being, self-efficacy, communication, self-esteem, mood, relaxation, comfort, happiness, along with reduction in caregiver burden, depression, and anxiety (Gillespie et al. 2024). These results suggest a diverse range of improved pre- and post-bereavement core outcomes, measured via observation, clinician-administered instrument, or self-report (Gillespie et al. 2024).

15.3.4.1 Music Therapy in Adults with Terminal Cancer

With respect to terminal cancer there were more positive effects of MT with multiple techniques on quality of life (Hilliard 2003b), well-being, anxiety, depression, and overall symptom distress compared to standard care alone (Planas Domingo 2015). Hilliard (2003b) further noted that quality of life increased over time for patients with terminal cancer receiving one or more of the following MT interventions at home: song choice, music-prompted reminiscence, singing, lyric analysis, live music listening, instrument-playing, song parody, use of the iso-principle, planning of memorial services, music-assisted supportive counseling, and creation of song gifts.

Single-session MT has also demonstrated improvements in pain after one session of live music-facilitated relaxation compared to standard treatment (Gutgsell et al. 2013) and greater reduction in self-reported anxiety from palliative patients engaging in a single MT session (multiple techniques) as compared with volunteer visits (Horne-Thompson and Grocke 2008). Music therapists reported that singing client-preferred music and vocal work were frequently used for relaxation in both palliative and cancer care, as these interventions were effective and accessible (Clements-Cortés 2017). In end-of-life care, singing was found to improve mood, self-expression, and feelings of patient-caregiver/family togetherness (Clements-Cortés 2017).

Ramirez et al. (2018) found palliative patients showed increased emotional valence, arousal, and improved psychological well-being through participating in both active and receptive MT techniques in comparison to simply conversing about music (active control group). Similarly, Warth et al. (2015) found that guided music relaxation/mindfulness followed by receptive improvisation (listening to the therapist improvise vocally) improved relaxation and well-being while reducing fatigue in terminally ill patients.

Pre-loss MT interventions with advanced cancer patients could be shared with family caregivers, implemented by/with caregivers, and further impact caregivers' experiences of end-of-life and bereavement (Magill 2009a, b, c, 2011; O'Callaghan 2013; Potvin et al. 2018). Patient-carer dyads engaged in music listening and facilitated relaxation, breathing, visualization or mindfulness (Magill 2009a, b, c; Potvin et al. 2018), songwriting (Magill 2009a, 2011; O'Callaghan 2013), singing, song discussion and lyric analysis (Magill 2009a, b, c, 2011; Potvin et al. 2018), vocal/lyrical improvisation (Magill 2009a, c, 2011), and creation of recordings as legacy gifts (Magill 2009a, c; O'Callaghan 2013; Potvin et al. 2018). These MT interventions were aimed to promote empowerment, enhancing feelings of joy, connectedness, comfort, remembrance, hope, sense of meaning, and peace, while mitigating helplessness and distress. By engaging in MT sessions with loved ones, carers were provided with a range of opportunities for reducing patient symptoms, enhancing interpersonal communication, improving feelings of control, and affording anticipatory grief processes (Magill 2009a, b, c, 2011).

15.3.5 Music Therapy for Children and Adolescents

15.3.5.1 Cancer

MT is beneficial in providing holistic care for children and adolescents experiencing cancer. It is recognized as a non-pharmacological treatment used for stress and anxiety reduction for hospitalized children diagnosed with cancer (Fedhila et al. 2023). In pediatric settings, MT has demonstrated efficacy in reducing the impact of hospital treatments; building positive coping skills (Robb 2003; Robb et al. 2008); and assisting with adjustment, identity formation, positive transformation, and attachment (O'Callaghan 2013). Specifically, singing, songwriting, instrumental improvisation, music listening, and playing instruments led to enhanced feelings and mood for young hospitalized cancer patients (Barrera et al. 2002). Songwriting facilitated increased self-esteem, social interaction, and feelings of empowerment (Abad 2003), allowing expressions of messages, feelings, and stories (O'Callaghan 2005).

Cole et al.'s (2024) systematic review which included nine studies found MT resulted in increased quality of life with respect to relaxation, self-esteem, vitality, cognition, and community involving interpersonal relationships. The individual studies point to increased levels of mood (Barrera et al. 2002) and play engagement (Barrera et al. 2002; Wong et al. 2021); reduced pain, anxiety (Kemper and McLean 2008; Knoerl et al. 2022; Thrane 2013); fostered communication (Ferrari et al. 2015; Wong et al. 2021); increased attention, and memory (Wong et al. 2021); stress reduction (Kemper and McLean 2008; Knoerl et al. 2022; Wong et al. 2021); and enhanced quality of life (Cheung et al. 2021).

In Facchini and Ruini's (2021) systematic review of 19 MT studies with 596 participants in the treatment of childhood and adolescent cancer, reductions in psychological distress were found in nine studies, and an increase in well-being in eight studies, where receptive, active, and combined (active and receptive) MT were offered. Fedhila et al. (2023) shared that pain was significantly decreased, following MT in various scenarios after lumbar puncture (Nguyen et al. 2010) and when MT was performed during painful stimuli (Dobek et al. 2014). MT is also beneficial for lowering anxiety during anesthesia induction with songwriting (Robb and Ebberts 2003), and music listening during bone marrow transplant and lumbar puncture to facilitate distress reduction (Polat et al. 2015). Ghetti's (2012) examination of the literature showed that MT was beneficial during procedural support for medically invasive practices. Quality of life, pain, and anxiety reduction were the outcomes of MT for children undergoing cancer treatments, as reported similarly in da Silva Santa et al.'s (2021) systematic review and meta-analysis of music interventions in pediatric oncology.

A protocol has been developed called Active Music Engagement (AME) to alter the hospital environment through music enabling children to make choices and engage in a variety of age appropriate music interventions (Robb et al. 2008). In their RCT with 83 children aged 4–7, researchers found MT improved active engagement in social relationships, social interactivity, facial expression, and enhanced communication with family and medical staff (Robb et al. 2008).

Porter et al.'s (2017) study, with 251 children who were experiencing behavioral, emotional, and social difficulties, found that MT significantly decreased depressive symptoms and improvement in self-esteem and communication for the adolescents. In pediatric patients, the use of patient-created music during radiotherapy treatment resulted in enhanced communication and interaction (Barry et al. 2010). Further use of therapeutic music videos for adolescents and young adults, aged 11–24-years old undergoing hematopoietic stem cell transplant, resulted in significantly improved coping, and social integration 100 days post-transplant (Robb et al. 2014). Anxiety reduction was also an outcome of MT for adolescents with leukemia (Saghaei and Mostafazadeh 2019). Further, songwriting, song sharing, and discussion with adolescents and young adults were beneficial for reducing isolation and offering opportunities to express cancer experiences and connect with peers undergoing similar treatments (O'Callaghan and Barry 2009).

15.3.6 Music Therapy in End-of-Life Care

Kammin et al.'s (2024) systematic review and evidence synthesis shared that MT supported both the child and family's well-being pointing to: emotional and physical reprieve; normalized experiences; thriving (living) and enhancing family well-being alongside relaxation; coping; distraction from reality; normality; and quality of life. Quality of life was also a key outcome in end-of-life MT, as evidenced in Overå's (2023) scoping review of MT in pediatric palliative care.

Forrest (2021) outlined MT interventions implemented in these settings, which include singing, vocal or instrumental improvisations, story creation enabling symbolic representation, music listening, playlist creation, music relaxation, and song writing among others. Steinhardt et al. (2021) also described other interventions, such as songwriting, song lyric analysis, music listening, movement and music, guided music relaxation and imagery, and playing instruments. Songwriting has also been described by many researchers (e.g., Giordano et al. 2021, 2022); vibroacoustic therapy for pain and distress (Clark et al. 2017); and musical performance was mentioned by Scott et al. (2016), whereby empowerment and creativity can flourish in community hospice. Singing creates space for interactions between the family and child (Hilliard 2003a), while also establishing calm and strengthening independence, control, autonomy, reflection, and expression (Nall and Everitt 2005).

Through the focus on relationship connections, MT practice with terminally ill children and adolescents typically involves the family and can include both individual therapy sessions and sessions with family as a means of support and enhancing quality of life (Forrest 2021). Gallagher et al. (2017) found 82% of family members experienced improved mood, stress levels, and quality of life from participating in MT. Patient benefits included improved mood, pain control, and lower distress and depression. Emotional expression (Amadoru and McFerran 2007), communication (Amadoru and McFerran 2007; Lindenfelser et al. 2008; McFerran and Shanahan 2011), changed perceptions (Lindenfelser et al. 2008), happiness (Amadoru and McFerran 2007), and perspectives that MT is valued in family-centered care (Steinhardt et al. 2021) have also been documented.

Opportunities for play and fun (Hilliard 2003a), the need for normalcy (Daveson and Kennelly 2000), and song creation allows the child or adolescent to be considered as an individual beyond being a "patient" (Aasgaard 2001, 2005). Expression of emotions regarding illness (Daveson and Kennelly 2000), the reduction in pain perception (Duda 2013), and closure (Rigney 2011) are a few other patient-focused areas in end-of-life care for pediatric patients. A fairly newer practice in end-of-life care are Amplified Cardiopulmonary Recordings (ACPR). Known as heartbeat recordings (Schreck and Economos 2018), this is where heartbeat rhythms are synchronized into a favorite song (Walden et al. 2021) and are used for legacy work (Andrews et al. 2020). Research reflections from bereaved parents also showed its effectiveness in validating the child's life and finding meaning while offering support for grieving and coping through a legacy creation (Walden et al. 2021).

15.3.7 Music-Based Interventions and Oncology

There has been abundant literature surrounding the topics of oncology and MBIs, particularly for adults, adolescents, and children. MBIs have utilized interventions such as music sessions associated with percussion (Ploukou and Panagopoulou 2018); recorded (Bradt et al. 2021; Sun et al. 2023) or live music (Bro et al. 2019; Burns 2012; Toccafondi et al. 2017); music composition and improvisations (Colwell and Fiore 2020; Signoroni et al. 2019); group interventions (Chen et al. 2018) like singing (Fancourt et al. 2016; Warran et al. 2019) or other various musical instruments; music listening on a digital device selected by the patient (Bro et al. 2018; da Silva Santa et al. 2021; Henneghan et al. 2021; Kiernan et al. 2018; Merry and Silverman 2021; Valero-Cantero et al. 2023; Yang et al. 2024); music apps (Koehler et al. 2022); animation video (Turgut and Özgür 2021); rhythmic auditory cueing and real-time auditory feedback (Ghai and Ghai 2019); guided training from a music professional like orchestral performers (Cheung et al. 2019); passive listening interventions using headphones (Forbes et al. 2023; Sheikh-Wu et al. 2021); and music associated with other forms of art such as dances like the tango (Oei et al. 2023; Schad et al. 2023), music-guided movement (Blank et al. 2024), yoga (Malik et al. 2024), making art (Lawson et al. 2016), mindful awareness (Minasian 2023), acupressure (Peoples et al. 2019), and imagery (İriağaç et al. 2022). The emphasis on MBIs with culturally appropriate sensitivity during the music selection (Burns 2012; Sheikh-Wu et al. 2021) and flexibility in its modality are encouraged, including being offered in individual and groups (Chen 2020), hybrid, or fully in-person or remote (Blank et al. 2024; Minasian 2023) based in specific environments like the home (Hsieh et al. 2019).

15.3.7.1 Adults

For the majority of the resources, MBIs have been used to improve the well-being of patients directly (Gencer et al. 2019), but also to the practitioners in oncology care, such as nurses (Ploukou and Panagopoulou 2018), hospital staff, carers, and bereaved individuals who has been affected by cancer (Fancourt et al. 2016; Warran et al. 2019). Within adults, the types of patient use has been described in: postoperative oncology inpatients (Merry and Silverman 2021); adults on a medical oncology or hematology unit (Herbrand and Silverman 2021); patients with colon cancer (Tanriverdi et al. 2023); patients with active treatment of chemotherapy (Spilioti et al. 2017), screenings (colposcopy, mammography, and breast biopsy) (Burns 2012); adults with nero-oncological disorders (Vinciguerra et al. 2023); adult patients undergoing bone marrow procedures (Schandert et al. 2021); ovarian cancer patients (Malik et al. 2024); cancer patients receiving radiation therapy (Chen 2020); breast cancer survivors (Henneghan et al. 2021; Lima et al. 2020; Rodriguez-Wolfe et al. 2019; Schad et al. 2023); or patients with active breast cancer (Wang et al. 2018; Zeppegno et al. 2021). MBIs have been effective in decreasing levels of depression, anxiety (Forbes et al. 2023; Koca and Aylaz 2022; Nightingale et al. 2013; Schandert et al. 2021; Toccafondi et al. 2017), fatigue and energy levels (Herbrand and Silverman 2021; Hsieh et al. 2019; Oei et al. 2023; Qi et al. 2021; Schad et al. 2023), stress (Fancourt et al. 2016; Nguyen et al. 2023), psychosomatic symptoms (Ploukou and Panagopoulou 2018), nausea and vomiting (Kiernan et al. 2018; Wei et al. 2020), pain (Bro et al. 2018; Hsieh et al. 2019; Merry and Silverman 2021; Park and Lee 2022; Sun et al. 2023; Tola et al. 2022), and positive psychology through benefit-finding and positive thinking strategies (Sheikh-Wu et al. 2021) for enduring treatment and ongoing survival (O'Callaghan 2013). Beyond symptoms related to well-being, other aspects of the cancer patient have been addressed such as verbal fluency, immediate memory recall, perceived cognitive and impairment (Henneghan et al. 2021), systolic blood pressure (Spilioti et al. 2017; Wang et al. 2018), diastolic blood pressure and heart rate (Tanriverdi et al. 2023), building resilience (Warran et al. 2019; Zeppegno et al. 2021), financial concerns (Malik et al. 2024), spirituality and social bonding between family, staff (Toccafondi et al. 2018), or developing a sense of community (Blank et al. 2024) have also significantly improved within adult cancer patients when interacting with MBIs.

15.3.7.2 Children and Adolescents

Resources evaluating MBIs on adolescents and children in oncology care have been limited, but significant. Similar to adults, MBIs have profound impact on pediatric cancer patients with fewer depressive and anxiety-related symptoms (González-Martín-Moreno et al. 2021), higher levels of self-esteem, better quality of life (Cheung et al. 2019), mental health (Stegemann et al. 2019), and pain (da Silva Santa et al. 2021; Robb et al. 2023; Tsao et al. 2008), as well as improved symptoms outside of the cancer diagnosis such as gait and postural stability (Ghai and Ghai 2019), psychosocial support like their hopes, dreams, longing for romantic encounters, their urge to travel (Signoroni et al. 2019), heart rate, respiratory rate, and blood pressure (González-Martín-Moreno et al. 2021). The types of patients within pediatric oncology include pediatric brain tumor survivors (Cheung et al. 2019; Cheung et al. 2021), children with acute leukemia (Nie et al. 2024), and generalized pediatric and adolescent patients with cancer at any progress of the disease (i.e., diagnosis, treatment, and hospitalization) (González-Martín-Moreno et al. 2021).

15.3.8 Music-Based Interventions in End-of-Life Care

While MBIs are used within MT, they were eliminated in this results section to ensure the distinctive characteristics between MT and MBIs. There were also times where patients were part of both oncology and end-of-life care (Archie et al. 2013).

In these cases, these articles and reviews were included to ensure the intersections found in MBIs and palliative care.

The found articles and reviews in this area of research was limited, but explored the essential information related to MBIs and end-of-life care. The types of MBIs that have been used for patients in end-of-life care include preferred and passive music listening of new or familiar tunes (Garabedian and Kelly 2020; Leggieri et al. 2018); music playlist apps (Johnston et al. 2022; Richard-Lalonde 2023); gestures and improvisations (Dowlen et al. 2022; Moumdjian et al. 2017); music relaxation; multicomponent music interventions with other mediums (Moumdjian et al. 2017) such as music and dance (Shaffer 2022); aromatherapy and music (Akbaş Uysal et al. 2024); sedative music; music involving the voice, simple instruments such as percussion, and religious songs (Sampaio 2023); imagery with music; and group music activities (Robb et al. 2018). Symptoms that are targeted using MBIs can be threefold with the process of components, responses, and outcomes (Mercadal-Brotons et al. 2021). Components are aspects that can affect the patient experience, which range from esthetic engagement, engagement with themes of health, interaction with healthcare settings, evocation of emotion, involvement of the imagination, cognitive stimulation (Ramirez-Melendez 2023), social interaction, physical activity, and sensory activation (Mercadal-Brotons et al. 2021). Responses from patients and other parties can include psychological, physiological, social, and behavioral contexts (Mercadal-Brotons et al. 2021; Shaffer 2022). Finally, outcomes that arise from the components and responses can include prevention, promotion, management, and treatment, leading to an improved mental and physical health, as well as well-being of the individual (Mercadal-Brotons et al. 2021).

15.3.8.1 Adults

MBIs have been effective for patients in palliative care with neurological conditions, with attention to physical symptoms such as rehabilitation on upper limb function with fine motor skills, hand and arm capacity, and finger and hand velocity, mobility related to gait (Pohl et al. 2020; Zumbansen and Tremblay 2019), and cognition of verbal memory and focused attention span (Moumdjian et al. 2017). Specifically, familiar music was more activated than unfamiliar music due to the increased levels of connective tissue in the putamen, cerebellum, and frontal regions of the patient's brain, suggesting the benefits of MBIs on cognition (Leggieri et al. 2018). For patients with progressive neurologic disorders in hospice and palliative care, patient preferred music has been effective for everyday care, addressing situations like painful or invasive treatment (Potvin et al. 2023; Richard-Lalonde 2023), and improved symptoms such as positive mood, overall quality of life, motor functioning, self-efficacy, inclusion, promote life reflections, and foster feelings of connectedness with others; and decreased levels of emotional pain (Akbaş Uysal et al. 2024), depression, anxiety (Archie et al. 2013), and spiritual distress (Potvin et al. 2023). For persons with dementia as well as Parkinson's disease, MBIs have created lived experiences that showcase sharing life stories, building patient-family relationships and legacy for the future (Johnston et al. 2022), musical agency, and connections into everyday life (Dowlen et al. 2022).

15.3.8.2 Caregivers, Staff, and Other Members

Caregivers, staff, and managers of care have also benefitted from using MBIs, with most members calling the internalized experience as a haven, and in the moment with feelings and reflections (Dowlen et al. 2022; Johnston et al. 2022). These individuals have the ability to transport their reality into fulfilling their basic needs as a healthcare professional, such as "inclusion, comfort, identity, occupation, and attachment" (Garabedian and Kelly 2020) into patient–family relationships and supporting patients (Johnston et al. 2022). In particular, receptive and recreational music, such as drum circles, guitar lessons, and group singing, provides the aid and agency for caregivers, where they may feel powerless; for example, in dressing changes and repositioning of the patient (Potvin et al. 2023). The use of receptive music requires less musical training, making these interventions more accessible to the staff and facilitators that use them (Potvin et al. 2023).

15.3.8.3 Children and Adolescents

Similar to cancer care, the research surrounding the effectiveness of MBIs for children and adolescents have been sparse, but impactful. For children and adolescents with chronic diseases in palliative care, such as hemodialysis, bone marrow transplants and critically ill patients, MBIs were effective in addressing the patient's cognitive abilities and sociocultural issues and improved empathy (Sampaio 2023). MBIs have also helped children to identify and develop personal strengths that will help with coping with their terminal illness (Foster et al. 2012).

15.4 Discussion, Perspectives, and Future Directions

15.4.1 Music Therapy in Cancer Care and Palliative Care

As demonstrated by the extensive literature and multiple systematic reviews selected in this chapter, MT and MBIs offer valuable support in cancer and end-of-life care settings across the lifespan. However, there is considerably more research with adults than children and adolescents (Bradt et al. 2021) and the patients included in these studies do not represent the full scope of persons who would benefit from MT for cancer and end-of-life care such as the structurally vulnerable who cannot access MT. This can be due to a variety of issues, such as approval from research ethics, organizational limitations in providing music experiences, healthcare professional workload, inequitable healthcare, and funding. Specific to children and adolescents, more research is required at all stages, and in the various locations of care. More awareness is recommended to understand the mechanisms of music in the experience of pain, distress, quality of life, anxiety, and overall holistic symptom management. Wheeler et al. (2019) raised similar issues pertaining to the clinical value of quantitative versus qualitative studies in oncological MT and music medicine research. They argue that qualitative research could potentially produce a richer understanding of the patients' experiences and interventions' effects, potentially being more applicable for robust practice.

There are also several ongoing issues, not limited to the inadequate description of the MT technique or MBI used, misuse of terminology like MT, and incorrect words to describe who is providing the music experience. According to Kievisiene et al.'s (2020) systematic review, the challenge is the ability to translate the benefits of MT to patient symptoms into protocols or practice. Further complicating the issue, reviews such as Kievisiene et al. (2020) included studies that focused on listening to pre-recorded music, music intervention implemented with music therapist or clinical psychologist, other therapists singing to patients, and identifying patients singing to themselves as "music therapy." Similarly, Gillespie et al.'s (2024) review noted that MT interventions were either delivered by carers alone, carers trained by music therapists to implement techniques, facilitated by music therapists themselves, or in collaboration with other community or healthcare professionals. Determination of short- and long-term effects was also varied and point to the need for higher methodological quality and description of interventions in future studies. As such, the summarizing tables describe the various MT techniques and/or MBIs and what healthcare concerns they support are limited in naming specifics in a number of areas.

There is evidence to support that MT may be more beneficial and/or preferred by patients with cancer and those at end-of-life. Both MT and listening to playlists were beneficial for symptom management, elicited memories, facilitated connection with pre-illness self, and offered hope and inspiration (Bradt et al. 2015). Both were equally effective in improving anxiety, mood, relaxation, and pain. Whereas listening to prerecorded music afforded familiarity and predictability for those who felt insecure about making music, interactive music-making allowed for emotional expression and support from a music therapist. For instance, Bradt et al. (2015) found that the majority (74%) of cancer patients prefer MT over listening to a music playlist as there was more empathetic support provided by the music therapist and the opportunity to engage in joint music-making. This study suggests that patients who prefer music listening may be better served in the presence of a certified music therapist who can help them process their music-evoked responses and memories. Treatment benefits depended on the personality characteristics of the patient, along with their outlook on life and readiness to explore emotions. As such, the need for assessment to determine effective music interventions can address in-the-moment needs of the patients.

Bradt et al.'s (2021) Cochrane review assessed the effects of MT and music medicine interventions on physical and psychological outcomes with cancer patients, taken from 81 studies in 13 different countries, and compared with standard care. While MT interventions showed more consistent effects across trials than music medicine, Bradt et al. (2021) found that the overall music intervention may result in varied results, such as a large reduction in anxiety, small to moderate reduction in depression, moderate improvement in mood, large increase in hope, moderate to large improvement in pain, slight reduction in fatigue, and large improvement in quality of life. Further, comparative analyses suggested that MT interventions were more effective than music medicine interventions in improving quality of life and fatigue for adult cancer patients and they recommended more RCTs to determine the effectiveness of MT versus music medicine (Bradt et al. 2021).

Bradt et al. (2021) emphasized that more research is required to examine the following concerns: the relationship between the frequency and duration of music interventions, and treatment outcomes; studying effects other than anxiety reduction; evaluating the cost-benefit of MT and music medicine; and the use of MBIs in pediatric oncology. The primary focus should be on optimizing symptom management along the cancer trajectory (Bradt et al. 2015, 2021) and individual information of patients to determine who benefits from different MT interventions (Köhler et al. 2020). With respect to children, a clearer definition for pediatric palliative care is recommended to support inadequate research in this area (Overå 2023). With regards to music listening experiences, clinicians and researchers must carefully consider the potential negative impact of using headphones during procedures, as they may impede communication between the patient and medical personnel (Bradt et al. 2021; Kwekkeboom 2003).

Overall, music interventions can provide effective treatment options to adults with cancer, with MT interventions delivered by a trained MT leading to more consistent results. While the presentation of music differed between MT and music medicine studies, both produced similar beneficial outcomes on anxiety, pain, and depression with oncology patients, whereas quality of life, mood, and procedural support may be influenced differently since live MT interventions can be adapted moment-to-moment in response to patients' needs. The music therapist's role or implementation of MT interventions can be extended to training for patients, carers, or medical staff to deliver or continue strategies at home or when the music therapist was not present (Bradt et al. 2024; Gillespie et al. 2024; Kievisiene et al. 2020; Magill 2009c). Encouraging and preparing patients and carers to self-administer music interventions can promote empowerment (Magill 2009c), enhance self-efficacy for chronic pain management (Bradt et al. 2024), and foster patient-carer connection and relationship (Gillespie et al. 2024; Magill 2009c), and yet can often feel outside of the scope of MT practice. While patient-selected and self-administered music can present somewhat predictable musical contexts and reduce symptoms, Bradt et al. (2024) advocated for the presence of a music therapist, as music listening can evoke existential issues and strong emotional responses requiring psychotherapeutic support. Bowers and Wetsel (2014) further recommended that nurses and medical staff advocate for the unique approaches of music therapists and increase awareness of MT's efficacy in end-of-life through inclusion in palliative care treatment plans. Consideration of diverse MT models that bridge to music medicine in the contexts of oncology and palliative care is worthwhile, such as resource-oriented MT (Potvin et al. 2018), medical music psychotherapy (Loewy and Aldridge 2009), and integrative music therapy—a psychoneuroimmunological approach (Hanser 2016). Integration of MT and music medicine could result in a more comprehensive approach with cancer and palliative patients, with the role of music therapist as consultant potentially impacting the quality of music medicine research and accurately portraying best practices (Wheeler et al. 2019).

15.4.2 Music-Based Interventions in Oncology Care and End-of-Life Care

An overview of systematic reviews on the effect of MBIs in cancer care focuses on the benefits of MBIs in standard care (Trigueros-Murillo et al. 2023). As compared to the traditional care as a standalone, MBIs have decreased symptoms such as cancer-related distress, pain, and fatigue (Trigueros-Murillo et al. 2023). While the results were inconclusive for symptoms beyond cancer (such as anxiety, depression, mood, and quality of life), Bradt et al. (2021) noted the impact of MBIs on psychological and physical outcomes of persons with cancer in the following ways: reducing anxiety, a moderate impact on depression, and increasing feelings of hope in cancer patients (Bradt et al. 2021).

In both palliative and oncology care, studies that involve adult, adolescent, and children patients are specific to the sample selection as nonrandomized (Kiernan et al. 2018), particular to a demographic location (Chen et al. 2018; Toccafondi et al. 2018), and therefore cannot be generalized (Cheung et al. 2019; González-Martín-Moreno et al. 2021; Henneghan et al. 2021; Malik et al. 2024; Minasian 2023; Rodriguez-Wolfe et al. 2019), with the majority being quantitative studies (Koca and Aylaz 2022; Lima et al. 2020). Having patients select their music intervention according to Kiernan et al. 2018 "sacrifices control within the research design" (p 92), leading researchers to add studies within their literature reviews to be more logical and efficacious (Trigueros-Murillo et al. 2023) or having to change the music delivery for patients (Schandert et al. 2021). Certain environmental limitations of data collection, such as COVID-19 and cancer patients unable to use technology to respond (Koca and Aylaz 2022) and needing flexibility between work and life events (Rodriguez-Wolfe et al. 2019) may have also affected the final results. Complementary and integrative therapies of MBIs with other forms, such as mediation (Henneghan et al. 2021), can also make it difficult for researchers to evaluate the impact of MBIs within oncology patients (Henneghan et al. 2021), as the evidence is still limited and sometimes inconsistent and conflicting (Perkins et al. 2018; Zeppegno et al. 2021). Particularly for hospitalized children, no differences have been found in pain and fatigue scores (Nie et al. 2024; Robb et al. 2023), heart rate, respirations, narcotic, or non-narcotic medication usage as documented after the use of MBIs (Perkins et al. 2018). It is important for researchers to set a framework when treatment fidelity for MBIs to children and adolescents with cancer with the following recommendations: "study design, training providers, delivery of treatment, receipt of treatment, and [the] enactment of treatment skills" (MacLean et al. 2022, p 1).

Researchers (e.g., Blank et al. 2024) have also found that information about MBIs can be disseminated in various ways to the public, which can lead to increased access to patients, families, and community providers, but also misinformation based on the inadequate cultural and background approaches (Tola et al. 2022). There was also indication that MT had stronger evidence toward efficacy than MBIs in particular patients (Forbes et al. 2023; González-Martín-Moreno et al. 2021) such as cancer survivors (Sheikh-Wu et al. 2021), cancer patients receiving radiation therapy or that patients did not experience improvements in symptoms like depression and fatigue (Chen 2020). Further research between the relationship of MT and MBIs for cancer patients is recommended to pursue these perspectives forward. Specifically, investigation is needed to determine the response rate, the duration (Dallı et al. 2023) and effectiveness to MBIs for individual outcomes related to the symptoms of the cancer diagnosis (Archie et al. 2013; Nguyen et al. 2022). For example, it is unclear how the impact of music can be affected by the "tumor location, extent of disease, and impact of treatment with surgery, radiation and chemotherapy" (Vinciguerra et al. 2023, p 103). There has been mixed data on the efficacy of MBIs in cancers of the central nervous system versus MBIs on cancers that do not involve the brain (Vinciguerra et al. 2023). Despite these cases, there is growing and significant evidence that MBIs can improve the quality of life in cancer patients and other members impacted by cancer with promising research to the relationship of MBIs.

Similar to MBIs in cancer care, the effectiveness of MBIs is dependent on the patient and environmental factors, and are not always significant (Lepping et al. 2024) and generalized to all populations in palliative care (Dowlen et al. 2022). For example, prerecorded music has only worked for several participants, not all the found articles showcased the type of MBI being used (Lepping et al. 2024), and not every carer enjoyed the music experience (Garabedian and Kelly 2020). Environmental factors can include the physical room of colors and textures, the level of openness by management (Garabedian and Kelly 2020), and whether the patient hospital stays are long-lasting and repeated. Conversely, the patient factors can involve the length of the session based on the patient's responses, the stage of the disease (Dowlen et al. 2022), the preference to certain genres of music (Garabedian and Kelly 2020), inclination toward group sessions (Pohl et al. 2020), and their cultural and socioeconomic status (Sampaio 2023) in order to access the music experience (Shaffer 2022). Patients who are in hospice and palliative care will experience health declines over the course of their life that can be comorbid, not limited to reductions in strength and mobility, decreased ability to communicate and short-term memory call, and many more symptoms, ultimately affecting the readiness to musically engage and psychological safety (Potvin et al. 2023). These symptoms of patient decline can also affect the emotional and psychological wellness of caregivers and related members, affecting their capacity and motivation in the music experiences (Potvin et al. 2023). As communication may be difficult for these types of patients, facilitators who are administering MBIs are encouraged to use music as a way to cultivate new opportunities for communication, adapting to meet the needs of the patient and matching the patient's health journey (Potvin et al. 2023). MBIs that are recommended include using different instruments, selecting different repertoire, songwriting, or utilizing receptive music apps to support (Potvin et al. 2023).

15.4.3 Tables of Summary

Tables 15.1, 15.2, 15.3, and 15.4 outline a summary of the key MT and MBI applications in oncology and end-of-life care. The table is organized as follows:

- In the first row of the table, the population of interest (Adults or Children and Adolescents) is indicated.

Table 15.1 Key music therapy interventions for adults in cancer care and end-of-life care

Adults			
Cancer		End-of-life care	
Healthcare area/issue	**Key interventions (MT) indicated**	**Healthcare area/ issue**	**Key interventions (MT) indicated**
Pain	Patient preferred live music, recorded music, singing, humming, playing instruments, improvisation, guided imagery and music, music entrainment, music-guided deep breathing, X	Pain	Patient preferred live music, recorded music, singing, playing instruments, improvisation, music entrainment, music relaxation, X
Anxiety, distress, stress management	Patient preferred live music, recorded music and verbal processing, lyric analysis and discussion, improvisation, songwriting, guided imagery and music, music entrainment, music relaxation, music-guided deep breathing, X	Anxiety, distress, stress management	Music listening, lyric discussion and analysis, improvisation, songwriting, guided imagery and music, X
Relaxation comfort	Patient preferred live music, music entrainment, music-guided deep breathing, X	Relaxation comfort	Patient preferred live music, music listening and verbal processing, improvisation, guided imagery and music, music entrainment, music relaxation, music-guided deep breathing, X
Fatigue	Patient preferred live music, recorded music, music listening and verbal processing, X	Fatigue	Patient preferred live music, recorded music, music relaxation, X
Reduced anxiety, blood pressure, heart rate,	Music listening, singing, improvisation, guided imagery and music	Spiritual Well-being	Patient preferred live music, lyric discussion and analysis, improvisation, songwriting, music-assisted supportive counseling, X

(continued)

Table 15.1 (continued)

Adults			
Cancer		End-of-life care	
Quality of life	Music listening and verbal processing, the bonny method, music relaxation, Vibroacoustic therapy, X	Quality of life	Music listening, singing, song choice, lyric discussion and analysis, reminiscence, music-assisted supportive counseling, the bonny method, music entrainment, music relaxation, legacy gifts, Vibroacoustic therapy, X
Self-concept, connection to identity, self-esteem	Singing, lyric discussion and analysis, guided imagery and music, music relaxation, teaching music-based self-management strategies	Self-concept, connection to identity, self-esteem	Singing, lyric discussion and analysis, improvisation, music-assisted supportive counseling, guided imagery and music, music relaxation
Affect, depression, mood, Happiness	Patient preferred live music, music listening and verbal processing, singing, improvisation, songwriting, guided imagery and music, music relaxation, X	Affect, depression, mood	Music listening, improvisation, songwriting, music-assisted supportive counseling, guided imagery and music, X
Spiritual Well-being	Music listening and verbal processing, X	Social interaction, communication	Song choice, music for reminiscence
Psychological Well-being	X	Psychological Well-being	Music listening, improvisation, music-assisted supportive counseling, music relaxation, legacy work, X
Emotional expression and processing	Music listening and verbal processing, playing instruments, improvisation, guided imagery and music, X	Emotional processing, emotional reprieve	Free associative singing, lyric discussion and analysis, improvisation, songwriting, music-assisted supportive counseling, the bonny method, X
Treatment preparation and management	Music listening and verbal processing, guided imagery and imagery, music entrainment, ISO principle playlist	Celebrating one's life	Songwriting, musical life review, planning of funerals or memorial services, legacy gifts

(continued)

Table 15.1 (continued)

Adults			
Cancer		End-of-life care	
Decreased use of analgesics	Music listening, singing, improvisation, songwriting, guided imagery and music, music relaxation, X	Relationship and relationship completion	Free associative singing, singing, song choice, music playlists, improvisation, songwriting, the bonny method, improvisation, musical autobiographies, musical life review, legacy gifts
Reduced recovery time	Music listening with verbal processing	Legacy work, life review, grieving	Singing, lyric analysis and discussion, improvisation, songwriting, music-assisted supportive counseling, X
		Physician-assisted suicide, medical assistance in dying	Patient preferred live music, recorded music, X
		Death acceptance	Planning of funerals or memorial services, legacy gifts, X

- In the second row of the table, the type of patients and care is identified. In this case, it is cancer or end-of-life.
- In the third row of the table, two topics will be addressed.
  - Healthcare area/issue addresses the symptoms or concerns experienced by the patient.
  - Key interventions (MT/MBI) Indicated will describe the MT techniques or MBIs that address the healthcare area/issue.
- There will be symbols that will be used in this table.
  - An X indicates evidence for MT techniques indicated but not specified as documented in the RCT, literature, and systematic reviews as described above.

15.4.4 Conclusion

MT in adult cancer care has demonstrated its efficacy to support a variety of symptoms, including reduction in anxiety and pain related to surgery, overall physical symptom management during pre- and post-cancer treatment, enhancing psychological well-being, and quality of life. For adults at the end-of-life, a large variety of MT interventions have been utilized, many that are receptive in nature, but also

Table 15.2 Key music therapy interventions for children and adolescents in cancer care and end-of-life care

Children and Adolescents			
Cancer		End-of-life Care	
Healthcare area/issue	**Key interventions (MT) indicated**	**Healthcare area/issue**	**Key interventions (MT) indicated**
Pain	X	Pain	Vibroacoustic therapy, X
Anxiety	Music listening, songwriting, X	Anxiety, distress stress	Vibroacoustic therapy, X
Relaxation	X	Relaxation	Music listening, singing, guided music and imagery, music relaxation, X
Self-esteem/identity formation	Songwriting, X	Quality of life	Music listening, singing, playlist creation, playing instruments, improvisation, songwriting, story creation, music relaxation, X
Mood, depression	Music listening, singing, playlist creation, playing instruments, improvisation, songwriting, X	Mood, depression, happiness	X
Emotional expression	Song sharing and discussion, playing instruments, X	Emotional expression, emotional reprieve	Music listening, singing, playlist creation, improvisation, songwriting, story creation, music relaxation, X
Attachment	X	Attachment	Singing
Coping	Therapeutic music video, X	Coping	Music listening, singing, playlist creation, songwriting, music relaxation, X
Control/autonomy and choice-making	Singing, active music engagement, X	Control/autonomy	Singing, active music engagement, X
Psychological distress	Receptive techniques, active techniques, combined techniques, music listening, X	Normalized experiences	Music listening, singing, improvisation, songwriting, playlist creation, story creation, movement and music, music relaxation, X

(continued)

Table 15.2 (continued)

Children and Adolescents			
Cancer		End-of-life Care	
Attention, cognition, memory	X	Living	X
Adjustment/ transformation	X	Support and grieving	ACPR (heartbeat recordings), songwriting, X
Attachment, relationship	Singing, X	Attachment, relationship and relationship completion	Music listening, singing, playing instruments, songwriting, X
Social engagement and communication	Patient preferred music listening, song sharing, playing instruments, songwriting, active music engagement, therapeutic music video, X	Communication	Singing, X
Empowerment	Songwriting	Empowerment	Patient preferred music listening, musical performance, X
Increased Well-being	X	Legacy work	ACPR (heartbeat recordings), songwriting, X
Engagement	X	Finding meaning	ACPR (heartbeat recordings), songwriting, X
Reducing isolation	Song sharing, song discussion, songwriting, X	Family Well-being	Music listening, lyric discussion and analysis, playing instruments, songwriting
Procedural support, reducing impact of treatment	X	Distraction from reality	Music listening, singing, playlist creation, improvisation, songwriting, story creation, movement to music, music relaxation, X

Table 15.3 Key Music-based interventions for adults in cancer care or end-of-life care

Adults			
Cancer		End-of-life Care	
Healthcare area/ issue	**Key interventions (MBI) indicated**	**Healthcare area/ issue**	**Key interventions (MBI) indicated**
Pain	Music listening, individualized playlists, aromatherapy and music	Pain	Patient preferred music listening
Anxiety	Music listening; playlists	Anxiety	Patient preferred music listening, singing, improvisation, music and imagery, music and relaxation, X
Relaxation	Patient preferred music listening, music playlists	Well-being	Patient preferred music listening, music listening, playlist creation, music and dance, group music activities, aromatherapy and music, music and imagery, music relaxation
Fatigue and energy levels	Music listening, animation video and music, X	Physical activity	Patient preferred music listening
Distress	Music listening, group music listening and discussion, music lessons, music and art, aromatherapy and music, group guided physical relaxation, X	Quality of life	Patient preferred music listening
Mood, depression	Music listening, group music listening and discussion; singing, playlist creation, music and art, aromatherapy and music, group guided relaxation	Mood	Patient preferred music listening, singing
Self-efficacy and self-esteem	Group singing	Emotional expression	Patient preferred music listening; singing, playlist creation, improvisation, reminiscence, music and imagery, music and relaxation
Cognitive avoidance	Group music listening and discussion, group guided physical relaxation	Cognition, memory, attention span	Patient preferred music listening, singing

(continued)

Table 15.3 (continued)

Adults			
Cancer		End-of-life Care	
Communication and undergoing awake surgery	Music listening, singing, playing instruments	Communication and speech	Singing, song parodies
Reminiscence	Singing	Reminiscence	Singing
Social bonding and sense of community	Group singing, group instrumental ensembles	Social interaction and connection with others	Patient preferred music listening, music listening, songwriting
Quality of sleep	Music listening	Spiritual distress	Patient preferred music listening
Nausea and vomiting	Patient preferred music listening, music for relaxation	Procedural support	Patient preferred music listening
Loss of appetite	Music and art	Support for caregivers	Group singing, drum circles, guitar lessons

Table 15.4 Key music-based interventions for children and adolescents in cancer care or end-of-life care

Children and Adolescents			
Cancer		End-of-life care	
Healthcare area/issue	**Key interventions (MBI) indicated**	**Healthcare area/issue**	**Key interventions (MBI) indicated**
Pain	Music listening, X	Anxiety	Music listening
Anxiety	Music listening, X	Emotional expression	Music listening
Distress	Music and play	Cognition, memory	Playing instruments
Fatigue	X	Social interaction	Choosing and sharing instruments
Depression	X		
Psychological support and Well-being	Singing, songwriting, X		
Procedural pain	Recorded lullabies, live, music		

songwriting and legacy gift creation. Quality of life is, prevalent in the outcomes followed by efficacy for pain, anxiety, stress, mood, and spiritual well-being for those with life-limiting illnesses. In pediatric oncology, a focus and benefit of MT has been pain, anxiety, stress reduction, and procedural support. Similar to practice with adults, quality of life remained an overarching outcome. The role of MT for relationship completion, MAiD, and legacy creation is unique to end-of-life care with adults. For children, there was a focus on normalcy, thriving or "living," the presence of family in sessions, and implementation of Amplified Cardiopulmonary Recordings.

MBIs have been helpful for adults in reducing pain, anxiety, depression, nausea and vomiting, and stress management among other outcomes during cancer screening and active treatment. Further implications of the benefits of MBIs have been documented when caregivers and other members support the patient with cancer. Similarly, MBIs also enhanced standard care when applied in end-of-life treatments, but less evidence is showcased within children and adolescents.

Consistently, both MT and MBI in cancer care and end-of-life care would benefit from future research, examining the frequency, duration, and responses of patients, alongside with clearer descriptions of terminology, techniques, and service providers. Additional consideration and care needs to be a focus to ensure there is continual work toward equity-oriented cancer and end-of-life healthcare for all who would benefit. At present, studies and literature are limited in the diversity of patients who received services.

References

Aasgaard T. An ecology of love: aspects of music therapy in the pediatric oncology environment. J Palliat Care. 2001;17:177–82. https://doi.org/10.1177/082585970101700310.

Aasgaard T. Assisting children with malignant blood diseases to create and perform their own songs. In: Baker F, Wigwam T, editors. Songwriting: methods, techniques and clinical applications for music therapy clinicians, educators and students. London; 2005.

Abad V. A time of turmoil: music therapy interventions for adolescents in a paediatric oncology ward. Aust J Music Ther. 2003;14:20–37.

Akard TF, Dietrich MS, Friedman DL, Gerhardt CA, Given B, Hendricks-Ferguson V, Hinds PS, Ridner SH, Beckmann N, Gilmer MJ. Improved parent-child communication following a RCT evaluating a legacy intervention for children with advanced cancer. Prog Palliat Care. 2021;29:130–9. https://doi.org/10.1080/09699260.2020.1826778.

Akbaş Uysal D, Şenuzun Aykar F, Uyar M. The effects of aromatherapy and music on pain, anxiety, and stress levels in palliative care patients. Support Care Cancer. 2024;32:632. https://doi.org/10.1007/s00520-024-08837-0.

Alcântara-Silva TR, de Freitas-Junior R, Freitas NMA, de Paula JW, da Silva DJ, Machado GDP, Riberio MKA, Carneiro JP, Soares LR. Music therapy reduces radiotherapy-induced fatigue in patients with breast or gynecological cancer: a randomized trial. Integr Cancer Ther. 2018;17:628–35. https://doi.org/10.1177/1534735418757349.

Amadoru S, McFerran K. The role of music therapy in children's hospices. In: McFerran K, editor. Music therapy in pediatric palliative care: family-centered practice. Jessica Kingsley Publishers; 2007. p. 45–57.

Andrews E, Hayes A, Cerulli L, Miller EG, Slamon N. Legacy building in pediatric end-of- life care through innovative use of a digital stethoscope. Palliat Med Rep. 2020;1:149–55. https://doi.org/10.1089/pmr.2020.0028.

Apps K, Sunderland N. Live music in hospital oncology settings: environmental, interpersonal, and personal outcomes for staff, patients, and carers. Arts Health. 2023;15:1–17. https://doi.org/10.1080/17533015.2021.1946110.

Archie P, Bruera E, Cohen L. Music-based interventions in palliative cancer care: a review of quantitative studies and neurobiological literature. Support Care Cancer. 2013;21:2609–24. https://doi.org/10.1007/s00520-013-1841-4.

Bains KK, Jennings S, Bull C, Tilley L, Montgomery L, Lee AL. A systematic review of change in symptoms, well-being and quality of life with group singing in people with cancer and their caregivers. Support Care Cancer. 2024;32:246. https://doi.org/10.1007/s00520-024-08449-8.

Barrera ME, Rykov MH, Doyle SL. The effects of interactive music therapy on hospitalized children with cancer: a pilot study. Psycho-Oncology. 2002;11:379–88. https://doi.org/10.1002/pon.589.

Barry P, O'Callaghan C, Wheeler B, Grocke D. Music therapy CD creation for initial pediatric radiation therapy: a mixed methods analysis. J Music Ther. 2010;47:233–63. https://doi.org/10.1093/jmt/47.3.233.

Bates D, Bolwell B, Majhail NS, Rybicki L, Yurch M, Abounader D, Kohuth J, Jarancik S, Koniarczyk H, McLellan L, Dabney J, Lawrence C, Gallagher L, Kalaycio M, Sobecks R, Dean R, Hill B, Pohlman B, Hamilton BK, Gerds AT, Jagadeesh D, Liu HD. Music therapy for symptom management after autologous stem cell transplantation: results from a randomized study. Biol Blood Marrow Transplant. 2017;23:1567–72. https://doi.org/10.1016/j.bbmt.2017.05.015.

Bausewein C, Booth S, Gysels M, Higginson IJ. Non-pharmacological interventions for breathlessness in advanced stages of malignant and non-malignant diseases. Cochrane Database Syst Rev. 2013;2013:CD005623. https://doi.org/10.1002/14651858.CD005623.pub3.

Binns-Turner PG, Wilson LL, Pryor ER, Boyd GL, Prickett CA. Perioperative music and its effects on anxiety, hemodynamics, and pain in women undergoing mastectomy. AANA J. 2011;79(4 Suppl):S21–7. PMID: 22403963.

Black S, Bartel L, Rodin G. Exit music: the experience of music therapy within medical assistance in dying. Healthcare. 2020;8:331. https://doi.org/10.3390/healthcare8030331.

Blank CA, Biedka S, Montalmant A, Saft K, Lape M, Mao K, Bradt J, Liou KT. Scope, findability, and quality of information about music-based interventions in oncology: quantitative content analysis of public-facing websites at national cancer institute-designated cancer centers. JMIR Cancer. 2024;10 https://doi.org/10.2196/53440.

Bowers TA, Wetsel MA. Utilization of music therapy in palliative and hospice care: an integrative review. J Hosp Palliat Nurs. 2014;16:231–9. https://doi.org/10.1097/NJH.0000000000000060.

Bradt J, Dileo C. Music therapy for end-of-life care. Cochrane Database Syst Rev. 2010;20(1):CD007169. https://doi.org/10.1002/14651858.CD007169.pub2.

Bradt J, Potvin N, Kesslick A, Shim M, Radl D, Schriver E, Gracely EJ, Komarnicky-Kocher LT. The impact of music therapy versus music medicine on psychological outcomes and pain in cancer patients: a mixed methods study. Support Care Cancer. 2015;23:1261–71. https://doi.org/10.1007/s00520-014-2478-7.

Bradt J, Dileo C, Myers-Coffman K, Biondo J. Music interventions for improving psychological and physical outcomes in people with cancer. Cochrane Database Syst Rev. 2021;8:CD006911. https://doi.org/10.1002/14651858.CD006911.pub2.

Bradt J, Leader A, Worster B, Myers-Coffman K, Bryl K, Biondo J, Schneible B, Cottone C, Selvan P, Zhang F. Music therapy for pain management for people with advanced cancer: a randomized controlled trial. Psychooncology. 2024;33:e70005. https://doi.org/10.1002/pon.70005.

Bro ML, Jespersen KV, Hansen JB, Vuust P, Abildgaard N, Gram J, Johansen C. Kind of blue: a systematic review and meta-analysis of music interventions in cancer treatment. Psycho-Oncology. 2018;27:386–400. https://doi.org/10.1002/pon.4470.

Bro ML, Johansen C, Vuust P, Enggaard L, Himmelstrup B, Mourits-Anderson T, Brown P, d'Amore F, Andersen EAW, Abildgaard N, Gram J. Effects of live music during chemotherapy in lymphoma patients: a randomized, controlled, multi-center trial. Support Care Cancer. 2019;27:3887–96. https://doi.org/10.1007/s00520-019-04666-8.

Bruscia K. Defining music therapy. 3rd ed. Texas: Dallas; 2014.

Bulfone T, Quattrin R, Zanotti R, Regattin L, Brusaferro S. Effectiveness of music therapy for anxiety`reduction in women with breast cancer in chemotherapy treatment. Holist Nurs Pract. 2009;23(4):238–42. https://doi.org/10.1097/HNP.0b013e3181aeceee. PMID: 19574761.

Burns DS. The effect of the bonny method of guided imagery and music on the mood and life quality of cancer patients. J Music Ther. 2001;38:51–65. https://doi.org/10.1093/jmt/38.1.51.

Burns DS. Theoretical rationale for music selection in oncology intervention research: an integrative review. J Music Ther. 2012;49:7–22. https://doi.org/10.1093/jmt/49.1.7.

Burns DS, Azzouz F, Sledge R, Rutledge C, Hincher K, Monahan PO, Cripe LD. Music imagery for adults with acute leukemia in protective environments: a feasibility study. Support Care Cancer. 2007;16:507–13. https://doi.org/10.1007/s00520-007-0330-z.

Burns DS, Perkins SM, Tong Y, Hilliard RE, Cripe LD. Music therapy is associated with family perception of more spiritual support and decreased breathing problems in cancer patients receiving hospice care. J Pain Symptom Manag. 2015;50(2):225–31. https://doi.org/10.1016/j.jpainsymman.2015.02.022.

Burns DS, Meadows AN, Althouse S, Perkins SM, Cripe LD. Differences between supportive music and imagery and music listening during outpatient chemotherapy and potential moderators of treatment effects. J Music Ther. 2018;55(1):83–108. https://doi.org/10.1093/jmt/thy001.

Burrai F, Othman S, Brioni E, Silingardi M, Micheluzzi V, Luppi M, Apuzzo L, La Manna G. Virtual reality in dialysis: a new perspective on care. J Ren Care. 2018;44:195–6. https://doi.org/10.1111/jorc.12264.

Cadwalader A, Orellano S, Tanguay C, Roshan R. The effects of a single session of music therapy on the agitated behaviors of patients receiving hospice care. J Palliat Med. 2016;19(8):870–3. https://doi.org/10.1089/jpm.2015.0503. Epub 2016 Apr 26. PMID: 27115462.

Canadian Cancer Society. Complementary therapies/music therapy. 2021. https://www.cancer.ca/en/cancerinformation/diagnosis-and-treatment/complementary-therapies/music-therapy/?region=ab

Cassileth BR, Vickers AJ, Magill LA. Music therapy for mood disturbance during hospitalization for autologous stem cell transplantation: a randomized controlled trial. Cancer. 2003;98(12):2723–9. https://doi.org/10.1002/cncr.11842.

Chatterjee D, Hegde S, Thaut M, Thaut M. Neural plasticity: the substratum of music-based interventions in neurorehabilitation. NeuroRehabilitation. 2021;48:155–66. https://doi.org/10.3233/NRE-208011.

Chen HH. The effect of music intervention in cancer patients receiving radiation therapy: a systematic review and meta-analysis. Int J Radiat Oncol Biol Phys. 2020;108:e223.

Chen SC, Chou CC, Chang HJ, Lin MF. Comparison of group vs self-directed music interventions to reduce chemotherapy-related distress and cognitive appraisal: an exploratory study. Support Care Cancer. 2018;26:461–9. https://doi.org/10.1007/s00520-017-3850-1.

Cheung AT, Li WHC, Ho KY, Lam KKW, Ho LLK, Chiu SY, Chang GCF, Chung JOK. Efficacy of musical training on psychological outcomes and quality of life in Chinese pediatric brain tumor survivors. Psychooncology. 2019;28:174–80. https://doi.org/10.1002/pon.4929.

Cheung AT, Li WHC, Ho LLK, Xia W, Chan GCF, JOK C. Pediatric brain tumor survivors' lived experience of engaging in a musical training program which promoted their psychological Well-being: a qualitative study. Support Care Cancer. 2021;29:3145–54. https://doi.org/10.1007/s00520-020-05833-y.

Clark BA, Holsti L, Siden H. Pediatric palliative music therapy: pain, distress, and contentment in children with developmental delays associated with life-threatening severe neurological impairment. Can J Music Ther. 2017;23(1):22–39.

Clemens P, Szeverinski P, Tschann P, Dietl M, Gurk J, Kowatsch M, Tucek G, de Vries A. Physical and nonphysical effects of weekly music therapy intervention on the condition of radiooncology patients. Strahlenther Onkol. 2023;199:268–77. https://doi.org/10.1007/s00066-022-02033-x.

Clements-Cortés A. The use of music in facilitating emotional expression in the terminally ill. Am J Hosp Palliat Med. 2004;21:255–60. https://doi.org/10.1177/104990910402100406.

Clements-Cortés A. Portraits of music therapy in facilitating relationship completion at the end-of-life. Music Med. 2011;3:31–9. https://doi.org/10.1177/1943862110388181.

Clements-Cortés A. Development and efficacy of music therapy techniques within palliative care. Complement Ther Clin Pract. 2016a;23:125–9. https://doi.org/10.1016/j.ctcp.2015.04.004.

Clements-Cortés A. Music therapy in end-of-life care. In: Clements-Cortés A, Klink S, editors. Voices of the dying and bereaved: music therapy narratives. Barcelona Publishers; 2016b. p. 5–19.

Clements-Cortés A. Saying good-bye with song. In: Clements-Cortés A, Klinck S, editors. Voices of the dying and bereaved: music therapy narratives. Barcelona Publishers; 2016c. p. 48–62.

Clements-Cortés A. Singing and vocal interventions in palliative and cancer care: music therapists' perceptions of usage. J Music Ther. 2017;54:336–61. https://doi.org/10.1093/jmt/thx010.

Clements-Cortés A. Bereavement, grief, and loss at end-of-life. In: Grocke DE, editor. Guided imagery and music: the bonny method and beyond. 2nd ed. Barcelona Publishers; 2019. p. 245–58.

Clements-Cortés A, Yip J. Medical assistance in dying in Canada: implications and considerations for music therapists around the globe. Music Ther Perspect. 2020;39:11. https://doi.org/10.1093/mtp/miaa009.

Clements-Cortés A, Yip J. Chapter 6: the bonny method of guided imagery and music: evidence and potential for relationship completion. In: Clements-Cortés A, Yip J, editors. Relationship completion in palliative care music therapy. Barcelona Publishers; 2021a. p. 51–61.

Clements-Cortés A, Yip J, editors. Relationship completion in palliative care music therapy. Barcelona Publishers; 2021b.

Clements-Cortés A, Yip J. Benefits of community singing for cancer patients, survivors, and caregivers. In: Norton K, Morgan-Ellis E, editors. The Oxford handbook of singing. Oxford; 2024. p. 244–57. https://doi.org/10.1093/oxfordhb/9780197612460.001.0001.

Cole DM, Beane K, Engel M, Shaffer M, Tartabini S. The effect of music therapy as an adjunctive treatment in pediatric cancer patients receiving traditional therapies: a systematic review. J Adv Pract Oncol. 2024;15:265–76. https://doi.org/10.6004/jadpro.2024.15.4.4.

Collins A. 'it's very humbling': the effect experienced by those who facilitate a legacy project session within palliative care. Am J Hosp Palliat Med. 2019;36:65–71. https://doi.org/10.1177/1049909118787772.

Colwell CM, Fiore J. Feasibility of patient-created Orff chant as a music-based intervention in supportive cancer care. J Music Ther. 2020;57:E1–E31. https://doi.org/10.1093/jmt/thaa019.

Curtis SL. Music therapy and the symphony: a university-community collaborative project in palliative care. Music Med. 2011;3:20–6.

da Silva Santa IN, Schveitzer MC, Dos Santos MLBM, Ghelman R, Filho VO. Music interventions in pediatric oncology: systematic review and meta-analysis. Complement Ther Med. 2021;59:102725. https://doi.org/10.1016/j.ctim.2021.102725.

Dallı ÖE, Doğan DA, Pehlivan S, Yildrim Y, Evrensel T. The effect of two different types of music played to cancer patients during chemotherapy on anxiety, nausea, and satisfaction levels. Support Care Cancer. 2023;31:710. https://doi.org/10.1007/s00520-023-08165-9.

Daveson B, Kennelly J. Music therapy in palliative care for hospitalized children and adolescents. J Palliat Care. 2000;16(1):35–8.

Dobek CE, Beynon ME, Bosma RL, Stroman PW. Music modulation of pain perception and pain-related activity in the brain, brain stem, and spinal cord: a functional magnetic resonance imaging study. J Pain. 2014;15(10):1057–68. https://doi.org/10.1016/j.jpain.2014.07.006. Epub 2014 Jul 28. PMID: 25077425.

Dóro CA, Neto JZ, Cunha R, Dóro MP. Music therapy improves the mood of patients undergoing hematopoietic stem cells transplantation (controlled randomized study). Support Care Cancer. 2017;25:1013–8.

Dowlen R, Keady J, Milligan C, Swarbrick C, Ponsillo N, Geddes L, Riley B. In the moment with music: an exploration of the embodied and sensory experiences of people living with dementia during improvised music-making. Ageing Soc. 2022;42:2642–64. https://doi.org/10.1017/S0144686X21000210.

Duda LJ. Integrating music therapy into pediatric palliative care. Prog Palliat Care. 2013;21:65–77. https://doi.org/10.1179/1743291X13Y.0000000049.

Facchini M, Ruini C. The role of music therapy in the treatment of children with cancer: a systematic review of literature. Complement Ther Clin Pract. 2021;42:101289. https://doi.org/10.1016/j.ctcp.2020.101289.

Fancourt D, Williamon A, Carvalho LA, Steptoe A, Dow R, Lewis I. Singing modulates mood, stress, cortisol, cytokine and neuropeptide activity in cancer patients and carers. Ecancermedicalscience. 2016;10:631. https://doi.org/10.3332/ecancer.2016.631.

Fedhila F, Hannachi MW, Jbebli E, Selmi I, Rhayem S, Magouri I, Bellali H, Khemiri M. Impact of music therapy on quality of life in children with cancer. Children. 2023;10:1486. https://doi.org/10.3390/children10091486.

Ferrari A, Veneroni L, Clerici CA, Casanova M, Chiaravalli S, Magni C, Massimino M. Clouds of oxygen: adolescents with cancer tell their story in music. J Clin Oncol. 2015;33:218–21. https://doi.org/10.1200/JCO.2014.57.9888.

Ferrell BR, Twaddle ML, Melnick A, Meier DE. National consensus project clinical practice guidelines for quality palliative care guidelines, 4th edition. J Palliat Med. 2018;21:1684–9. https://doi.org/10.1089/jpm.2018.0431.

Fiore J. Randomized pilot study exploring an online pre-composed receptive music experience and a mindfulness-based intervention for hospice workers' stress and professional quality of life. Arts Psychother. 2021;74:101797. https://doi.org/10.1016/j.aip.2021.101797.

Forbes E, Baker AL, Britton B, Clover K, Skelton E, Moore L, Handley T, Oultram S, Oldmeadow C, Gibberd A, McCarter K. A systematic review of nonpharmacological interventions to reduce procedural anxiety among patients undergoing radiation therapy for cancer. Cancer Med. 2023;12:20396–422. https://doi.org/10.1002/cam4.6573.

Forrest L. Introducing relationship completion and key considerations in pediatric palliative care. In: Clements-Cortes A, Yip J, editors. Relationship completion in palliative care music therapy. Barcelona Publishers; 2021. p. 169–80.

Foster TL, Bell CJ, Gilmer MJ. Symptom management of spiritual suffering in pediatric palliative care. J Hosp Palliat Nurs. 2012;14:109–15. https://doi.org/10.1097/njh.0b013e3182491f4b.

Fredenburg HA, Silverman MJ. Effects of music therapy on positive and negative affect and pain with hospitalized patients recovering from a blood and marrow transplant: a randomized effectiveness study. Arts Psychother. 2014;41:174–80. https://doi.org/10.1016/j.aip.2014.01.007.

Gallagher LM, Lagman R, Walsh D, Davis MP, Legrand SB. The clinical effects of music therapy in palliative medicine. Support Care Cancer. 2006;14:859–66. https://doi.org/10.1007/s00520-005-0013-6.

Gallagher L, Lagman R, Bates D, Edsall M, Eden P, Janaitis J, Rybicki L. Perceptions of family members of palliative medicine and hospice patients who experienced music therapy. Support Care Cancer. 2017;25:1769–78. https://doi.org/10.1007/s00520-017-3578-y.

Gallagher LM, Lagman R, Rybicki L. Outcomes of music therapy interventions on symptom management in palliative medicine patients. Am J Hosp Palliat Care. 2018;35:250–7. https://doi.org/10.1177/1049909117696723.

Gao Y, Wei Y, Yang W, Jiang L, Li X, Ding J, Ding G. The effectiveness of music therapy for terminally ill patients: a meta-analysis and systematic review. J Pain Symptom Manag. 2019;57:319–29. https://doi.org/10.1016/j.jpainsymman.2018.10.504.

Garabedian CE, Kelly F. Haven: sharing receptive music listening to foster connections and well-being for people with dementia who are nearing the end-of-life, and those who care for them. Dementia. 2020;19:1657–71. https://doi.org/10.1177/1471301218804728.

Gencer D, Diel A, Klotzbach K, Christians K, Rauch M, Meissner R, Weiß C, Hofmann W-K, Hofheinz R-D. Cancer patients and music: (prospective) results from a survey to evaluate potential complementary treatment approaches. J Cancer Res Clin Oncol. 2019;145:2141–8. https://doi.org/10.1007/s00432-019-02959-3.

Ghai S, Ghai I. Role of sonification and rhythmic auditory cueing for enhancing gait associated deficits induced by neurotoxic cancer therapies: a perspective on auditory neuroprosthetics. Front Neurol. 2019;10:21. https://doi.org/10.3389/fneur.2019.00021.

Ghetti C. Music therapy as procedural support for invasive medical procedures: toward the development of music therapy theory. Nordic J Music Ther. 2012;21:3–25. https://doi.org/10.1080/08098131.2011.571278.

Gillespie K, McConnell T, Roulston A, Potvin N, Ghiglieri C, Gadde I, Anderson M, Kirkwood J, Thomas D, Roche L, O'Sullivan MO, McCullagh A, Graham-Wisener L. Music therapy for supporting informal carers of adults with life-threatening illness pre- and post-bereavement; a mixed-methods systematic review. BMC Palliat Care. 2024;23:55. https://doi.org/10.1186/s12904-024-01364-z.

Giordano F, Rutigliano C, Muggeo P, Fusaro T, Santoro N. Ettore's song: the hero who had the courage to fight Achilles. J Health Psychol. 2021;26:5–11. https://doi.org/10.1177/1359105320968144.

Giordano F, Rutigliano C, Baroni M, Grassi M, Muggeo P, Santoro N. Music therapy and pediatric palliative care: songwriting with children in the end-of-life. World J Pediatr. 2022;18:695–9. https://doi.org/10.1007/s12519-022-00578-6.

Greenhalgh T, Thorne S, Malterud K. Time to challenge the spurious hierarchy of systematic over narrative reviews? Eur J Clin Invest. 2018;48(6):e12931. https://doi.org/10.1111/eci.12931.

González-Martín-Moreno M, Garrido-Ardila EM, Jiménez-Palomares M, Gonzalez-Medina G, Oliva-Ruiz P, Rodriguez-Mansilla J. Music-based interventions in pediatric and adolescents oncology patients: a systematic review. Children. 2021;8:1–14. https://doi.org/10.3390/children8020073.

Grocke D, Wigram T. Receptive music therapy: techniques and clinical application for music therapy clinicians, educators, and students. London, UK: Jessica Kingsley; 2007.

Gutgsell KJ, Schluchter M, Margevicius S, DeGolia PA, McLaughlin B, Harris M, Mecklenburg J, Wiencek C. Music therapy reduces pain in palliative care patients: a randomized controlled trial. J Pain Symptom Manag. 2013;45:822–31. https://doi.org/10.1016/j.jpainsymman.2012.05.008.

Hanser SB. The journey from illness to wellness. In: Integrative health through music therapy. Palgrave Macmillan; 2016. p. 133–50. https://doi.org/10.1057/978-1-137-38477-5_9.

Hanser SB, Bauer-Wu S, Kubicek L, Healey M, Manola J, Hernandez M, et al. Effects of a music therapy intervention on quality of life and distress in women with metastatic breast cancer. J Soc Integr Oncol. 2006;4:116–24. https://doi.org/10.2310/7200.2006.014.

Heath B, Lings J. Creative songwriting in therapy at the end-of-life and in bereavement. Mortality. 2012;17:106–18. https://doi.org/10.1080/13576275.2012.673381.

Henneghan AM, Becker H, Phillips C, Kesler S. Sustained effects of mantra meditation compared to music listening on neurocognitive outcomes of breast cancer survivors: a brief report of a randomized control trial. J Psychosom Res. 2021;150:110628. https://doi.org/10.1016/j.jpsychores.2021.110628.

Herbrand MK, Silverman MJ. A randomized pilot study of patient-preferred live music addressing fatigue, energy, and pain in adults on a medical oncology/hematology unit. Psychol Music. 2021;49:1561–72. https://doi.org/10.1177/0305735620967723.

Hilliard R. The effects of music therapy-based bereavement groups on the mood and behavior of grieving children: a pilot study. J Music Ther. 2001;38:291–306. https://doi.org/10.1093/jmt/38.4.291.

Hilliard R. Music therapy in pediatric palliative care. Complementing the interdisciplinary approach. J Palliat Care. 2003a;19(2):127–32.

Hilliard RE. The effects of music therapy on the quality and length of life of people diagnosed with terminal cancer. J Music Ther. 2003b;40:113–37. https://doi.org/10.1093/jmt/40.2.113.

Horne-Thompson A, Grocke D. The effect of music therapy on anxiety in patients who are terminally ill. J Palliat Med. 2008;11:582–90. https://doi.org/10.1089/jpm.2007.0193.

Hsieh FC, Miao NF, Tseng IJ, Chiu H-L, Kao C-C, Liu D, Chen R, Tasi H-F, Chou K-R. Effect of home-based music intervention versus ambient music on breast cancer survivors in the community: a feasibility study in Taiwan. Eur J Cancer Care (Engl). 2019;28:e13064. https://doi.org/10.1111/ecc.13064.

Hsieh FN, Shoemark H, Magee WL. Music therapy to facilitate relationship completion at the end-of-life: a mixed-methods study. J Music Ther. 2024;61:102–31. https://doi.org/10.1093/jmt/thae005.

İriağaç Y, Çavdar E, Karaboyun K, Avci O, Tuna N, Selçuk E. The influence of visual objects and music on anxiety levels of breast cancer patients scheduled to experience chemotherapy for the first time: a prospective randomized clinical study. Support Care Cancer. 2022;30:4355–62. https://doi.org/10.1007/s00520-021-06778-6.

Johnston B, Bowman F, Carduff E, Donmez F, Lowndes A, McKeown A. 'Playlist for life' at the end-of-life: a mixed-methods feasibility study of a personalised music listening intervention in the hospice setting. Pilot Feasibility Stud. 2022;8:32. https://doi.org/10.1186/s40814-022-00983-8.

Kammin V, Fraser L, Flemming K, Hackett J. Experiences of music therapy in paediatric palliative care from multiple stakeholder perspectives: a systematic review and qualitative evidence synthesis. Palliat Med. 2024;38:364–78. https://doi.org/10.1177/02692163241230664.

Karadag E, Parlar Kilic S, Ugur O, Akyol MA. Attitudes of nurses in Turkey toward care of dying individual and the associated religious and cultural factors. J Relig Health. 2019;58:303–16. https://doi.org/10.1007/s10943-018-0657-4.

Kemper KJ, McLean TW. Parents' attitudes and expectations about music's impact on pediatric oncology patients. J Soc Integr Oncol. 2008;6:146–9.

Kiernan JM, Stark JC, Vallerand AH. Chemotherapy-induced nausea and vomiting mitigation with music interventions. Oncol Nurs Forum. 2018;45:88–95. https://doi.org/10.1188/18.ONF.88-95.

Kievisiene J, Jautakyte R, Rauckiene-Michaelsson A, Fatkulina N, Agostinis-Sobrinho C. The effect of art therapy and music therapy on breast cancer patients: what we know and what we need to find out – a systematic review. Evid Based Complement Alternat Med. 2020;2020(2):1–14. https://doi.org/10.1155/2020/7390321.

Kim B, Dvorak AL. Music therapy and intimacy behaviors of hospice family caregivers in South Korea: a randomized crossover clinical trial. Nord J Music Ther. 2018;27:218–34. https://doi.org/10.1080/08098131.2018.1427783.

Klinck S, Clements-Cortés A. Guidelines for using music for medical assistance in dying, funeral planning, and relationship completion and bereavement. In: Clements-Cortés A, Yip J, editors. Relationship completion in palliative care music therapy. Barcelona; 2021. p. 213–29.

Klinck S, Clements-Cortés A, Black SR. Music therapy techniques in end-of-life care. In: Clements-Cortés A, Yip J, editors. Relationship completion in palliative care music therapy. Barcelona; 2021. p. 33–42.

Knoerl R, Mazzola E, Woods H, Buchbinder E, Frazier L, LaCasce A, Li BT, Luskin MR, Phillips CS, Thornton K, Berry DL, Ligivel JA. Exploring the feasibility of a mindfulness-music therapy intervention to improve anxiety and stress in adolescents and young adults with cancer. J Pain Symptom Manag. 2022;63:e357–63. https://doi.org/10.1016/j.jpainsymman.2021.11.013.

Koca GY, Aylaz R. The effect of music on pain and anxiety in patients receiving chemotherapy during COVID-19. Eur J Cancer Care (Engl). 2022;31:e13715. https://doi.org/10.1111/ecc.13715.

Koehler AN, Rothman Y, Gomez Enriquez D, Kirschner M, Shatz R, Mahammedi A, Rebola CB, Sengupta S. The use of ARMCan app to improve the quality of life in breast cancer patients with chemobrain. J Clin Oncol. 2022;40:e13619. https://doi.org/10.1200/JCO.2022.40.16_suppl.e13619.

Köhler F, Martin ZS, Hertrampf RS, Gäbel C, Kessler J, Ditzen B, Warth M. Music therapy in the psychosocial treatment of adult cancer patients: a systematic review and meta-analysis. Front Psychol. 2020;11:651. https://doi.org/10.3389/fpsyg.2020.00651.

Krout RE. The effects of single-session music therapy interventions on the observed and self-reported levels of pain control, physical comfort, and relaxation of hospice patients. Am J Hosp Palliat Care. 2001;18:383–90. https://doi.org/10.1177/104990910101800607.

Kwekkeboom KL. Music versus distraction for procedural pain and anxiety in patients with cancer. Oncol Nurs Forum. 2003;30(3):433–40. https://doi.org/10.1188/03.onf.433-440.

Lagattolla F, Zanchi B, Pietro M, Cormio C, Lorusso V, Diotaiuti S, Fanizzi A, Massafra R, Costanzo S, Caporale F, Rieti E, Romito F. Receptive music therapy versus group music therapy with breast cancer patients hospitalized for surgery. Support Care Cancer. 2023;31:162. https://doi.org/10.1007/s00520-023-07624-7.

Lawson LM, Glennon C, Fiscus V, Harrell VS, Krause KA, Moore AB, Smith K. Effects of making art and listening to music on symptoms related to blood and marrow transplantation. Oncol Nurs Forum. 2016;43:E56–63. https://doi.org/10.1188/16.ONF.E56-E63.

Leggieri M, Fischer CE, Churchill NW, Fornazzari L, Barfett J, Munoz DG, Thaut MH, Vuong V, Schweizer TA. Repeated exposure to familiar music alters functional connectivity in Alzheimer's disease. Alzheimers Dement. 2018;14:P463. https://doi.org/10.1016/j.jalz.2018.06.422.

Lepping RJ, Hess BJ, Taylor JM, Hanson-Abrometi D, Williams KN. Inconsistent music-based intervention reporting in dementia studies: a systematic mapping review. J Alzheimers Dis. 2024;100:1145–59. https://doi.org/10.3233/JAD-240255.

Li XM, Yan H, Zhou KN, Dang SN, Wang DL, Zhang YP. Effects of music therapy on pain among female breast cancer patients after radical mastectomy: results from a randomized controlled trial. Breast Cancer Res Treat. 2011;128(2):411–9. https://doi.org/10.1007/s10549-011-1533-z.

Lima TU, Moura ECR, de Oliveira CMB, Leal RJDS, Neto JN, Pereira EC, Nascimento RVB, de Oliveira EJSG, Leal PAC. Impact of a music intervention on quality of life in breast cancer patients undergoing chemotherapy: a randomized clinical trial. Integr Cancer Ther. 2020;19:1534735420938430. https://doi.org/10.1177/1534735420938430.

Lin MF, Hsieh YJ, Hsu YY, Fetzer S, Hsu MC. A randomised controlled trial of the effect of music therapy and verbal relaxation on chemotherapy-induced anxiety. J Clin Nurs. 2011;20(7–8):988–99. https://doi.org/10.1111/j.1365-2702.2010.03525.x.

Lindenfelser KJ, Grocke D, McFerran K. Bereaved parents' experiences of music therapy with their terminally ill child. J Music Ther. 2008;45(3):330–48. https://doi.org/10.1093/jmt/45.3.330.

Liu X, Burns DS, Hilliard RE, Stump TE, Unroe KT. Music therapy clinical practice in hospice: differences between home and nursing home delivery. J Music Ther. 2015;52:376–93. https://doi.org/10.1093/jmt/thv012.

Loewy JV, Aldridge D. Music & medicine: debating evidence-based strategies and outcomes. Music Med. 2009;1:81–5. https://doi.org/10.1177/1943862109348968.

MacLean JA, Stegenga KA, Henley AK, Robb SL. Implementing NIH behavior change consortium treatment fidelity recommendations in a multi-site randomized controlled trial of an active music engagement intervention for young children with cancer and parents. Integr Cancer Ther. 2022;21:15347354221140491. https://doi.org/10.1177/15347354221140491.

Magill L. The meaning of the music: the role of music in palliative care music therapy as perceived by bereaved caregivers of advanced cancer patients. Am J Hosp Palliat Med. 2009a;26:33–9. https://doi.org/10.1177/1049909108327024.

Magill L. The spiritual meaning of pre-loss music therapy to bereaved caregivers of advanced cancer patients. Palliat Support Care. 2009b;7:97–108. https://doi.org/10.1017/S1478951509000121.

Magill L. Caregiver empowerment and music therapy: through the eyes of bereaved caregivers of advanced cancer patients. J Palliat Care. 2009c;25:68–75. https://doi.org/10.1177/082585970902500114.

Magill L. Bereaved family caregivers' reflections on the role of the music therapist. Music Med. 2011;3:56–63. https://doi.org/10.47513/mmd.v3i1.261.

Malik S, Sehrawat A, Chaturvedi J, Ranjeeta K, Suresh L, Sumit K, Sweety G. Impact of Nada yoga music therapy on anxiety and quality of life in ovarian cancer patients: a randomized controlled trial. Int J Yoga. 2024;17:138–45. https://doi.org/10.4103/ijoy.ijoy_69_24.

Mangiacotti AMA, Masotti A, Biasutti M. The impact of community music therapy intervention in older adults' care home communities: assessing community music therapists' views. Int J Community Music. 2024;17:37–60. https://doi.org/10.1386/ijcm_00096_1.

Manning-Walsh J. Social support as a mediator between symptom distress and quality of life in women with breast cancer. J Obstet Gynecol Neonatal Nurs. 2005;34:482–93. https://doi.org/10.1177/0884217505278310.

McConnell T, Porter S. Music therapy for palliative care: a realist review. Palliat Support Care. 2017;15:454–64. https://doi.org/10.1017/S1478951516000663.

McConnell T, Scott D, Porter S. Music therapy for end-of-life care: an updated systematic review. Palliat Med. 2016;30:877–83. https://doi.org/10.1177/0269216316635387.

McFerran K, Shanahan E. Music therapy practice in special education and children's hospice: a systematic comparison of two music therapists' strategies with three preadolescent boys'. Music Ther Persp. 2011;29:103–11. https://doi.org/10.1093/mtp/29.2.103.

Mercadal-Brotons M, Tomaino CM, Alcântara Silva TR, Vianna Moreira S. Music therapy & music based interventions in the context of dementia: recommendations for clinical guidelines – part II. Music Med. 2021;13:169–73. https://doi.org/10.47513/mmd.v13i3.822.

Merry M, Silverman MJ. Effects of patient-preferred live music on positive and negative affect and pain with adults on a post-surgical oncology unit: a randomized study. Arts Psychother. 2021;72:101739. https://doi.org/10.1016/j.aip.2020.101739.

Minasian S. Mindful awareness of music: a modality for symptom management. Clin J Oncol Nurs. 2023;27:233–6. https://doi.org/10.1188/23.CJON.233-236.

Mondanaro J, Tsiris G. Music therapy and relationship completion in palliative care: themes and orientations for contemporary education. In: Clements-Cortés A, Yip J, editors. Relationship completion in palliative care music therapy. Barcelona; 2021. p. 71–95.

Mondanaro JF, Sara GA, Thachil R, Pranjić M, Rossetti A, Sim GEH, Canga B, Harrison IB, Loewy JV. The effects of clinical music therapy on resiliency in adults undergoing infusion: a randomized, controlled trial. J Pain Symptom Manag. 2021;61:1099–108. https://doi.org/10.1016/j.jpainsymman.2020.10.032.

Moumdjian L, Sarkamo T, Leone C, Leman M, Feys P. Effectiveness of music-based interventions on motricity or cognitive functioning in neurological populations: a systematic review. Eur J Phys Rehabil Med. 2017;53:466–82. https://doi.org/10.23736/S1973-9087.16.04429-4.

Nall K, Everitt E. From hospice to home: music therapy outreach. In: Pavlicevic M, editor. Music therapy in children's hospices: Jessie's fund in action. London: Jessica Kingsley; 2005. p. 147–58.

Nazir A. The effect of listening to the holy qur'an recitation therapy on physiological parameters and neuropsychological functions in intensive care unit patients: a narrative review from physical and rehabilitation medicine point of view. Iranian Rehab J. 2023;21:215–22. https://doi.org/10.32598/irj.21.2.1540.7.

Nguyen TN, Nilsson S, Hellström AL, Bengtson A. Music therapy to reduce pain and anxiety in children with cancer undergoing lumbar puncture: a randomized clinical trial. J Pediatr Oncol Nurs. 2010;27:146–55. https://doi.org/10.1177/1043454209356830.

Nguyen KT, Xiao J, Chan DNS, Zhang M, Chan CWH. Effects of music intervention on anxiety, depression, and quality of life of cancer patients receiving chemotherapy: a systematic review and meta-analysis. Support Care Cancer. 2022;30:5615–26. https://doi.org/10.1007/s00520-022-06881-2.

Nguyen KT, Vu NTH, Tran MTT, Chan CWH. A qualitative study on stress, coping strategies and feasibility of music intervention among women with cancer receiving chemotherapy during COVID-19 pandemic in Vietnam. Sci Rep. 2023;13:542. https://doi.org/10.1038/s41598-023-27654-9.

Nie Y, Tian Y, Han X. Music nursing as complementary therapy improves anxiety, fatigue, and quality of life in children with acute leukaemia: a retrospective study. Noise Health. 2024;26:25–9. https://doi.org/10.4103/nah.nah_33_24.

Nightingale CL, Rodriguez C, Carnaby G. The impact of music interventions on anxiety for adult cancer patients: a meta-analysis and systematic review. Integr Cancer Ther. 2013;12:393–403. https://doi.org/10.1177/1534735413485817.

O'Callaghan C. Song writing in threatened lives. In: Dileo C, Lowy J, editors. Music therapy at the end-of-life. Cherryl Hill; 2005. p. 117–27.

O'Callaghan C. Music therapy preloss care through legacy creation. Prog Palliat Care. 2013;21:78–82. https://doi.org/10.1179/1743291X12Y.0000000044.

O'Callaghan C. Research on hospice music therapy. In: Dileo C, Baroni M, editors. Music therapy at the end-of-life. 2nd ed. Cherryl Hill; 2024.

O'Callaghan C, Barry P. Music therapists practice-based research in cancer and palliative care: creative methods and situated findings. Voices A World Forum Music Ther. 2009;9(3) https://voices.no/index.php/voices/article/view/1803.

O'Callaghan C, Magill L. Music therapy with adults diagnosed with cancer and their families. In: Edwards J, editor. The Oxford handbook of music therapy. Oxford University Press; 2017. p. 112–34.

Oei SL, Thronicke A, Groß J, Rieser T, Becker S, Grabowski P, Grieb G, Matthes H, Schad F. Does the Argentine tango sustainably improve cancer-associated fatigue and quality of life in breast cancer survivors? Cancers (Basel). 2023;15(23):5678. https://doi.org/10.3390/cancers15235678.

Overå M. Music therapy in paediatric palliative care: a scoping review. Br J Music Ther. 2023;37:58–70. https://doi.org/10.1177/13594575231196406.

Palmer JB, Lane D, Mayo D, Schluchter M, Leeming R. Effects of music therapy on anesthesia requirements and anxiety in women undergoing ambulatory breast surgery for cancer diagnosis and treatment: a randomized controlled trial. J Clin Oncol. 2015;33:3162–8. https://doi.org/10.1200/JCO.2014.59.6049.

Park YJ, Lee MK. Effects of nurse-led nonpharmacological pain interventions for patients with cancer: a systematic review and meta-analysis. J Nurs Scholarsh. 2022;54:422–33. https://doi.org/10.1111/jnu.12750.

Peoples AR, Culakova E, Heckler CE, Shayne M, O'Connor TL, Kirshner JJ, Bushunow PW, Morrow GR, Roscoe JA. Positive effects of acupressure bands combined with relaxation music/instructions on patients most at risk for chemotherapy-induced nausea. Support Care Cancer. 2019;27:4597–605. https://doi.org/10.1007/s00520-019-04736-x.

Perkins RS, Boyce M, Byrtek MC, Ellis RC, Hill C, Fitzpatrick PS, Demirel S. Roadmap to wellness: exploring live customized music at the bedside for hospitalized children. Front Oncol. 2018;8:21. https://doi.org/10.3389/fonc.2018.00021.

Planas Domingo J. Effectiveness of music therapy in advanced cancer patients admitted to a palliative care unit: a non-randomized controlled, clinical trial. Music Med. 2015;7(1):23–31.

Ploukou S, Panagopoulou E. Playing music improves Well-being of oncology nurses. Appl Nurs Res. 2018;39:77–80. https://doi.org/10.1016/j.apnr.2017.11.007.

Pohl P, Wressle E, Lundin F, Enthoven P, Dizdar N. Group-based music intervention in Parkinson's disease—findings from a mixed-methods study. Clin Rehabil. 2020;34:533–44. https://doi.org/10.1177/0269215520907669.

Polat S, Gürol A, Çelebioğlu A, Yildirim ZK. The effect of therapeutic music on anxiety in children with acute lymphoblastic leukaemia. Indian J Tradit Knowl. 2015;1:5.

Porter S, McConnell T, McLaughlin K, Lynn F, Cardwell C, Braiden J-J, Boylan J, Holmes V, Music in Mind Study Group. Music therapy for children and adolescents with behavioural and emotional problems: a randomised controlled trial. J Child Psychol Psychiatry. 2017;58:586–94. https://doi.org/10.1111/jcpp.12656.

Porter S, McConnell T, Graham-Wisener L, Regan J, McKeown M, Kirkwood J, Clarke M, Gardner E, Dorman S, McGrillen K, Reid J. A randomised controlled pilot and feasibility study of music therapy for improving the quality of life of hospice inpatients. BMC Palliat Care. 2018;17:125. https://doi.org/10.1186/s12904-018-0378-1.

Potvin N, Bradt J, Ghetti C. A theoretical model of resource-oriented music therapy with informal hospice caregivers during pre-bereavement. J Music Ther. 2018;55(1):27–61. https://doi.org/10.1093/jmt/thx019.

Potvin N, Morrow M, Pegg C. Chapter 9: music therapy and music-based interventions for neurologic palliative care. In: Devlin K, Kang K, Pantelyat A, editors. Music therapy and music-based interventions in neurology. Springer Nature; 2023. p. 109–22.

Qi Y, Lin L, Dong B, Xu E, Bao Z, Qi J, Chen X, Tian L. Music interventions can alleviate cancer-related fatigue: a meta-analysis. Support Care Cancer. 2021;29:5965–76. https://doi.org/10.1007/s00520-021-05986-4.

Raglio A, Oasi O. Music and health: what interventions for what results? Front Psychol. 2015;6:230. https://doi.org/10.3389/fpsyg.2015.00230.

Ramirez R, Planas J, Escude N, Mercade J, Farriols C. EEG-based analysis of the emotional effect of music therapy on palliative care cancer patients. Front Psychol. 2018;9:254. https://doi.org/10.3389/fpsyg.2018.00254.

Ramirez-Melendez R. Neurocognitive music therapy: intersecting music, medicine, and technology for health and Well-being. Springer; 2023.

Reimnitz L, Silverman MJ. A randomized pilot study of music therapy in the form of patient-preferred live music on fatigue, energy, and pain in hospitalized adult oncology patients on a blood and marrow transplant unit. Arts Health. 2020;12:154–68. https://doi.org/10.1080/17533015.2018.1534251.

Reimnitz L, Silverman M. Perceived mechanisms targeting cancer-related fatigue, song choice rationale, and song function: an interpretivist study of patient-preferred live music with adult oncology patients on a blood and marrow transplant unit. Psychol Music. 2021;49(5):1401–14. https://doi.org/10.1177/0305735620942299.

Richard-Lalonde M. Development and crossover pilot randomized controlled trial of a patient-oriented music intervention to reduce pain in the adult intensive care unit. J Pain Symptom Manag. 2023;66:978–86. https://escholarship.mcgill.ca/concern/theses/tt44pt24f.

Rigney M. Using reflexive tools for coping and bringing closure in pediatric palliative care: a music therapist's story of working with a terminally ill child. Voices: A World Forum Music Ther. 2011;11 https://doi.org/10.15845/voices.v11i3.287.

Robb SL. Designing music therapy interventions for hospitalized children and adolescents using a contextual support model of music therapy. Music Ther Perspect. 2003;21:27–39. https://doi.org/10.1093/mtp/21.1.27.

Robb SL, Ebberts AG. Songwriting and digital video production interventions for pediatric patients undergoing bone marrow transplantation. Part I: an analysis of depression and anxiety levels according to phase of treatment. J Pediatr Oncol Nurs. 2003;20:2–15. https://doi.org/10.1053/jpon.2003.3.

Robb SL, Clair AA, Watanabe M, Monahan PO, Azzouz F, Stouffer JW, Ebberts A, Darsie E, Whitmer C, Walker J, Nelson K, Hanson-Abromeit D, Lane D, Hannan A. Randomized controlled trial of the active music engagement (AME) intervention on children with cancer. Psycho-Oncology. 2008;17:699–708. https://doi.org/10.1002/pon.1301.

Robb SL, Burns DS, Stegenga KA, Haut PR, Monahan PO, Meza J, Stump TE, Cherven BO, Docherty SL, Hendricks-Ferguson VL, Kintner EK, Haight AE, Wall DA, Haase JE. Randomized clinical trial of therapeutic music video intervention for resilience outcomes in adolescents/young adults undergoing hematopoietic stem cell transplant: a report from the children's oncology group. Cancer. 2014;120:909–17. https://doi.org/10.1002/cncr.28355.

Robb SL, Hanson-Abromeit D, May L, Hernandez-Ruiz E, Allison M, Beloat A, Daugherty S, Kurtz R, Ott A, Oyedele OO, Polasik S, Rager A, Rifkin J, Wolf E. Reporting quality of music intervention research in healthcare: a systematic review. Complement Ther Med. 2018;38:24–41. https://doi.org/10.1016/j.ctim.2018.02.008.

Robb SL, Stegenga K, Perkins SM, Stump TE, Moody KM, Henley AK, MacLean J, Jacob SA, Delgado D, Haut PR. Mediators and moderators of active music engagement to reduce traumatic stress symptoms and improve Well-being in parents of young children with cancer. Integr Cancer Ther. 2023;22:15347354231218266. https://doi.org/10.1177/15347354231218266.

Rodriguez-Wolfe M, Anglade D, Gattamorta KA, Hurwitz WB, Pirl WF. Individualized piano instruction for improving cognition in breast cancer survivors. Oncol Nurs Forum. 2019;46:605–15. https://doi.org/10.1188/19.ONF.605-615.

Rosenow SC, Silverman MJ. Effects of single session music therapy on hospitalized patients recovering from a bone marrow transplant: two studies. Arts Psychother. 2014;41:65–70. https://doi.org/10.1016/j.aip.2013.11.003.

Rossetti A, Chadha M, Torres BN, Lee JK, Hylton D, Loewy JV, Harrison LB. The impact of music therapy on anxiety in cancer patients undergoing simulation for radiation therapy. Int J Radiat Oncol Biol Phys. 2017;99:103–10. https://doi.org/10.1016/j.ijrobp.2017.05.003.

Rossetti A, Loewy J, Fischer Z, Deshpande S, Chadha M. A clinical pilot study on the effects of environmental music therapy on anxiety and waiting in radiation oncology: a randomized control trial. Music Med. 2023;15:1–8. https://doi.org/10.47513/mmd.v15i1.911.

Rumrill P, Fitzgerald S. Using narrative literature reviews to build a scientific knowledge base. Work. 2001;16:165–70. https://doi.org/10.3233/WOR-2001-00173.

Saghaei S, Mostafazadeh A. The effectiveness of music therapy on anxiety sensitivity and self-efficacy in adolescents with leukemia in Tehran. Iran Int J Body Mind Cult. 2019;6:112–7. https://doi.org/10.22122/ijbmc.v6i2.163.

Salmon D. Music therapy as psychospiritual process in palliative care. J Palliat Care. 2001;17(3):142–6. https://doi.org/10.1177/082585970101700304.
Sampaio ADSC. Music-based interventions in rehabilitation of children and adolescents with chronic diseases: sharing an experience from a Brazilian public hospital. Front Rehabil Sci. 2023;4:1116914. https://doi.org/10.3389/fresc.2023.1116914.
Saunders B, Sim J, Kingstone T, Baker S, Waterfield J, Bartlam B, Burroughs H, Hinks C. Saturation in qualitative research: exploring its conceptualization and operationalization. Qual Quant. 2018;52:1893–907. https://doi.org/10.1007/s11135-017-0574-8.
Schad F, Rieser T, Becker S, Groß J, Matthes H, Oei SL, Thronicke A. Efficacy of tango argentino for cancer-associated fatigue and quality of life in breast cancer survivors: a randomized controlled trial. Cancers (Basel). 2023;15:2920. https://doi.org/10.3390/cancers15112920.
Schandert LC, Lou AM, Prince MS, Schneider SM. Music intervention nonpharmacologic method to reduce pain and anxiety in adult patients undergoing bone marrow procedures. Clin J Oncol Nurs. 2021;25:314–20. https://doi.org/10.1188/21.CJON.314-320.
Schmid W, Rosland JH, Von Hofacker S, Hunskår I, Bruvik F. Patient's and health care provider's perspectives on music therapy in palliative care – an integrative review. BMC Palliat Care. 2018;17:32. https://doi.org/10.1186/s12904-018-0286-4.
Schreck B, Economos A. Heartbeat recording and composing in perinatal palliative care and hospice music therapy. Music Med. 2018;10:22–5.
Schreck B, Loewy J, Larocca RV, Harman E, Archer-Nanda E. Amplified cardiopulmonary recordings: music therapy legacy intervention with adult oncology patients and their families – a preliminary program evaluation. J Palliat Med. 2022;25:1409–12. https://doi.org/10.1089/jpm.2022.0017.
Scott R, Sheridan M, Blair A, Stewart L. Creativity and empowerment in a children's hospice community. Eur J Palliat Care. 2016;23:28–31.
Shaffer J. Enhancing neuroplasticity is urgent: music and dance for the UN/WHO decade of action for healthy ageing for all. J Ageing Longev. 2022;2:178–92. https://doi.org/10.3390/jal2030015.
Sheikh-Wu SF, Kauffman MA, Anglade D, Shamsaldeen F, Ahn S, Downs C. Effectiveness of different music interventions on managing symptoms in cancer survivors: a meta-analysis. Eur J Oncol Nurs. 2021;52:101968. https://doi.org/10.1016/j.ejon.2021.101968.
Signoroni S, Veneroni L, Bagliacca EP, Gaggiotti P, Silva M, Casanova M, Chairavalli S, Clerici CA, Massimino M, Ferrari A. "Summer is you": Adolescents and young adults with cancer sing about their desire for summer. Pediatr Blood Cancer. 2019;66:e27630. https://doi.org/10.1002/pbc.27630.
Spilioti ED, Galanis PA, Konstantakopoulou OK, Kalokairinou AG. The effects of music on cancer patients submitted to chemotherapy treatment. Int J Caring Sci. 2017;10:1465–77.
Stegemann T, Geretsegger M, Phan Quoc E, Riedl H, Smetana M. Music therapy and other music-based interventions in pediatric health care: an overview. Medicines. 2019;6:25. https://doi.org/10.3390/medicines6010025.
Stegenga K, Henley AK, Harman E, Robb SL. Shifting perspectives and transformative change: parent perspectives of an active music engagement intervention for themselves and their child with cancer. Pediatr Blood Cancer. 2024;71:e30913. https://doi.org/10.1002/pbc.30913.
Steinhardt TL, Mortvedt S, Trondalen G. Music therapy in the hospital-at-home: a practice for children in palliative care. Br J Music Ther. 2021;35:53–62. https://doi.org/10.1177/13594575211029109.
Sun X, Yang T, Zhang X, Ma C, Yu H, Lu C, Zhang W, Wang Y, Miao X, Li Y, Wang L, Liu Z. Music listening improves patients' satisfaction with colonoscopic interventions: a single-center randomized clinical trial. Eurasian J Med Oncol. 2023;7:345–9. https://doi.org/10.14744/ejmo.2023.46885.
Tanriverdi O, Karaoglu T, Aydemir FN. Can music and medicine be effective on anxiety, depression and chemotherapy? Related nausea and vomiting? (PEGASUS study). Indian J Cancer. 2023;60:282–91. https://doi.org/10.4103/ijc.IJC_387_20.

Teut M, Dietrich C, Deutz B, Mittring N, Witt CM. Perceived outcomes of music therapy with body tambura in end-of-life care – a qualitative pilot study. BMC Palliat Care. 2014;13(1):18. https://doi.org/10.1186/1472-684X-13-18.

Thrane S. Effectiveness of integrative modalities for pain and anxiety in children and adolescents with cancer: a systematic review. J Pediatr Oncol Nurs. 2013;30:320–32. https://doi.org/10.1177/1043454213511538.

Toccafondi A, Bonacchi A, Mambrini A, Miccinesi G, Prosseda CM. Live concerts reduce cancer inpatients' anxiety. Eur J Cancer Care (Engl). 2017;26 https://doi.org/10.1111/ecc.12590.

Toccafondi A, Bonacchi A, Mambrini A, Miccinesi G, Prosseda CM. Live music intervention for cancer inpatients: the music givers format. Palliat Support Care. 2018;16:777–84. https://doi.org/10.1017/S1478951517000165.

Tola YO, Iloba NG, Chow KM. Perception of music and its cultural elements on acute post-mastectomy pain management among Nigerian women: an exploratory qualitative study. Support Care Cancer. 2022;30:2527–35. https://doi.org/10.1007/s00520-021-06426-z.

Trigueros-Murillo A, Martinez-Calderon J, Casuso-Holgado MJ, González-García P, Heredia-Rizo AM. Effects of music-based interventions on cancer-related pain, fatigue, and distress: an overview of systematic reviews. Support Care Cancer. 2023;31:488. https://doi.org/10.1007/s00520-023-07938-6.

Tsao JCI, Evans S, Meldrum M, Altman T, Zeltzer LK. A review of CAM for procedural pain in infancy: Part II. Other interventions. J Evid Based Complement Altern Med. 2008;5:399–407. https://doi.org/10.1093/ecam/nem089.

Tuinmann G, Preissler P, Böhmer H, Suling A, Bokemeyer C. The effects of music therapy in patients with high-dose chemotherapy and stem cell support: a randomized pilot study. Psychooncology. 2017;26:377–84. https://doi.org/10.1002/pon.4142.

Turgut H, Özgür GK. The effect of an animation video and music on anxiety and pain scores before TRUS-guided biopsy. Bull Urooncol. 2021;20:7–10. https://doi.org/10.4274/uob.galenos.2020.1791.

Uçaner Çifdalöz B. Special feature | music therapy in dementia and end-of-life care: Mediterranean perspectives music therapy in Turkey: historical background and current perspectives on dementia and end-of-life care. Interdiscip J Music Ther. 2020;12

Valero-Cantero I, Casals C, Espinar-Toledo M, Barón-López FJ, Martínez-Valero FJ, Soler NG-A, Vázquez-Sánchez MA. Effect of self-chosen music in alleviating the burden on family caregivers of patients with advanced cancer: a randomised controlled trial. Int J Environ Res Public Health. 2023;20(5):4662. https://doi.org/10.3390/ijerph20054662.

van der Steen JT, Smaling HJ, van der Wouden JC, Bruinsma MS, Scholten RJ, Vink AC, van der Steen JT. Music-based therapeutic interventions for people with dementia. Cochrane Database Syst Rev. 2018;2018:CD003477. https://doi.org/10.1002/14651858.CD003477.pub4.

Verstegen A. Effects of hope-based music therapy on hope and pain in hospitalized patients on blood and marrow transplant unit: a convergent parallel mixed-methods pilot study (Master's thesis). University of Minnesota, Minneapolis 2016. Retrieved from: http://hdl.handle.net/11299/183312.

Verstegen AL, Silverman MJ. Effects of music therapy on mood and pain with patients hospitalized for bone marrow transplantation: a randomized effectiveness pilot study. J Creat Ment Health. 2018;13(4):418–28. https://doi.org/10.1080/15401383.2018.1486257.

Vesel T, Dave S. Music therapy and palliative care: systematic review. J Pain Symptom Manag. 2018;56:e74. https://doi.org/10.1016/j.jpainsymman.2018.10.276.

Vinciguerra C, Nardone V, Holdhoff M. Chapter 8: music for neuro-oncological disorders. In: Devlin K, Kang K, Pantelyat A, editors. Music therapy and music-based interventions in neurology. Springer Nature; 2023. p. 97–108.

Walden M, Charley Elliott E, Ghrayeb A, Lovenstein A, Ramick A, Adams G, Fairchild B, Schreck B. And the beat goes on: heartbeat recordings through music therapy for parents of children with progressive neurodegenerative illnesses. J Palliat Med. 2021;24:1023–9. https://doi.org/10.1089/jpm.2020.0447.

Wang Y, Tang H, Guo Q, Liu J, Liu X, Luo J, Yang W. Effects of intravenous patient-controlled sufentanil analgesia and music therapy on pain and hemodynamics after surgery for lung cancer: a randomized parallel study. J Altern Complement Med. 2015;21:667–72. https://doi.org/10.1089/acm.2014.0310.

Wang X, Zhang Y, Fan Y, Tan X-S, Lei X. Effects of music intervention on the physical and mental status of patients with breast cancer: a systematic review and meta-analysis. Breast Care. 2018;13:183–91. https://doi.org/10.1159/000487073.

Warran K, Fancourt D, Wiseman T. How does the process of group singing impact on people affected by cancer? A grounded theory study. BMJ Open. 2019;9 https://doi.org/10.1136/bmjopen-2018-023261.

Warth M, Keßler J, Hillecke TK, Bardenheuer HJ. Music therapy in palliative care. Dtsch Ärztebl Int. 2015;112(46):788–94. https://doi.org/10.3238/arztebl.2015.0788.

Warth M, Koehler F, Brehmen M, Weber M, Bardenheuer HJ, Ditzen B, Kessler J. "Song of life": results of a multicenter randomized trial on the effects of biographical music therapy in palliative care. Palliat Med. 2021;35(6):1126–36. https://doi.org/10.1177/02692163211010394.

Wei TT, Tian X, Zhang F-Y, Qiang W-M, Bai A-L. Music interventions for chemotherapy-induced nausea and vomiting: a systematic review and meta-analysis. Support Care Cancer. 2020;28:4031. https://doi.org/10.1007/s00520-020-05409-w.

Wheeler BL, Lesiuk TL, Burns DS, Hanser SB, Rossetti A, Cassity MD. Music therapy and music medicine studies in oncology: part I: a comparison. Music Med. 2019;11:145. https://doi.org/10.47513/mmd.v11i3.671.

Wong KC, Tan BWZ, Tong JWK, Chan MY. The role of music therapy for children undergoing cancer treatment in Singapore. Healthcare (Basel, Switzerland). 2021;9(12):1761. https://doi.org/10.3390/healthcare9121761.

World Health Organization. Palliative care. 2020. https://www.who.int/news-room/fact-sheets/detail/palliative-care#:~:text=Each%20year%2C%20an%20estimated%2040,palliative%20care%20currently%20receive%20it

Yang HF, Chang WW, Chou YH, Huang J-Y, Liao Y-S, Liao T-E, Tseng H-C, Chang S-T, Chen HL, Ke Y-F, Tsai P-F, Chan H-M, Chang B-J, Hwang Y-T, Tsai H-Y, Lee Y-C. Impact of background music listening on anxiety in cancer patients undergoing initial radiation therapy: a randomized clinical trial. Radiat Oncol. 2024;19:73. https://doi.org/10.1186/s13014-024-02460-3.

Yates GJ, Silverman MJ. Immediate effects of single-session music therapy on affective state in patients on a post-surgical oncology unit: a randomized effectiveness study. Arts Psychother. 2015;44:57–61. https://doi.org/10.1016/j.aip.2014.11.002.

Yazdanpanah N, Mojtabavi H, Ziaei H, Pirkoohi ZR, Rayzan E, Rezaei N. The clinical benefits of art therapy: definition, history, and outcomes with a focus on music therapy. In: Multidisciplinarity and Interdisciplinarity in Health. Springer; 2022. p. 457–82. https://doi.org/10.1007/978-3-030-96814-4_20.

Yazdanpanah N, Dochy F, Darmstadt GL, Peters GJ, Tsitlakidis A, Aifantis EC, Cerda A, Comini E, Brand S, Gupta M, Cheson BD, Thomas S, Tanzer M, Weiskirchen R, Bella F, Fereshtehnejad SM, Nikita K, Ali I, Kato K, Poggi A, Jon ECK, Rao IM, Tao X, He JH, Rao LJM, Leemans A, Pomponio A, Hernandez AM, Ahmadieh H, Sahraian MA, Kelishadi R, Thongboonkerd V, Bahinipati S, Toi M, Herrath MV, Sellke F, Sherwood S, Perry G, Nieto JJ, Gupta S, Dorigo T, Mobasher B, Ochs HD, Rezaei N. Cancer: a complex problem requiring interdisciplinary research. In: Rezaei N, editor. Cancer treatment: an interdisciplinary approach. Interdisciplinary cancer research, vol. 2. Cham: Springer; 2023. https://doi.org/10.1007/16833_2022_116.

Zeppegno P, Krengli M, Ferrante D, Bagnati M, Burgio V, Farruggio S, Rolla R, Gramaglia C, Grossini E. Psychotherapy with music intervention improves anxiety, depression and the redox status in breast cancer patients undergoing radiotherapy: a randomized controlled clinical trial. Cancers (Basel). 2021;13(8):1752. https://doi.org/10.3390/cancers13081752.

Zumbansen A, Tremblay P. Music-based interventions for aphasia could act through a motor-speech mechanism: a systematic review and case–control analysis of published individual participant data. Aphasiology. 2019;33:466–97. https://doi.org/10.1080/02687038.2018.1506089.

Music Therapy and Music-Based Interventions in Pain Medicine

16

Sandra M. Saade-Lemus, Danna P. Garcia-Guaqueta, and Juan Sebastian Martin-Saavedra

Key Points

- Music-based interventions have a moderate analgesic effect when compared to no intervention.
- Music-induced analgesia ranges from 1 to 2 points in a 0–10 visual analogue scale or numeric rating scale.
- Standardizing music properties improves statistical heterogeneity.
- The only strong predictor of music-induced analgesia effect size is duration, with 30 minutes being the minimum required to achieve a minimal effect.
- Instrumental, slow-tempo (60–80 beats per minute), non-percussive music is a reliable analgesic intervention and should be the starting point when choosing an intervention in the clinical context.
- Patient-preferred music is slightly superior to non-preferred music.

S. M. Saade-Lemus
Sleep Medicine and Neurology Departments, Boston Medical Center, Boston, MA, USA

Grupo de Investigacion en Neurociencias (NeURos), Universidad del Rosario, Bogotá D.C., Colombia

D. P. Garcia-Guaqueta
Grupo de Investigacion en Neurociencias (NeURos), Universidad del Rosario, Bogotá D.C., Colombia

Pediatric Neurology, Oregon Health & Science University, Portland, OR, USA

J. S. Martin-Saavedra (✉)
Pediatric Neurology, Massachusetts General Hospital – Harvard Medical School, Boston, MA, USA

Grupo de Investigacion Clinica, Universidad del Rosario, Bogotá D.C., Colombia
e-mail: jmartinsaavedra@mgh.harvard.edu; juans.martin@urosario.edu.co

A. Raglio (ed.), *Music and Music Therapy Interventions in Clinical Practice*, Neurocultural Health and Wellbeing,
https://doi.org/10.1007/978-3-031-88578-5_16

16.1 Introduction

Our body is wise. It can tell us when there is a risk of physical and mental harm. We call this pain and it is a subjective and sensorial experience. It is personal, it is affected by our environment and life experiences, and it can be expressed verbally and through other behaviors (Raja et al. 2020).

In the Caribbean region of Colombia, the Wayuu women get together and cry in a high-pitched lament, while in the Cuna from Darien region of Colombia and Panama, the Inatuledi (medical figure) chants during delivery (Música indígena colombiana 1987). Similarly, David, in the Abrahamic sacred books, played the harp to King Saul to ease his spirit (Babikian et al. 2013). These are just a few examples of how music, which has been present since the dawn of society (Killin 2018; Nikolsky 2020), has always found its way into healing rituals and very consistently to alleviate pain.

Music and language cannot be separated when studying their evolution. Some believe that at some point there was a communicative musical language that evolved in two different forms: music and language (Nikolsky 2020). However, there is archeological evidence of possible proto-music behaviors hundreds of thousands of years ago and definite instruments such as paleolithic flutes from 40,000 years ago (Nikolsky 2020), which is prior to the oldest evidence of written language. This raises the question: did music lead to the development of language or were these two parallel and coincidental evolutionary processes? Then, what is the evolutionary need of music persisting and continuing to evolve with humans if language is a better communicative tool?

For example, the prosodic component of language, which shares features with music, develops and remains contralateral to language centers (Perani et al. 2011). This function is usually located in the right hemisphere, where multiple authors have found music processing also takes place (Peretz 1990; Peretz et al. 1994; Angulo-Perkins et al. 2014; Rosslau et al. 2016). Furthermore, fetuses recognize rhythm and prosody early during development which will evolve to phoneme recognition, but not words, at birth (Vandormael et al. 2019). Therefore, there might be a link between music and language development. Nonetheless, this does not explain why we continue to appreciate, enjoy, and seek music. Additionally, people with hearing impairments at birth, or with music-related disorders (e.g., amusia or arrhythmia) can develop language.

Without diving into the philosophical aspect of this question, we might assume that there is an evolutionary benefit from remaining musical beings beyond complementing language and communication. Medical literature has grown demonstrating these benefits in the form of therapeutic effects of music. One of the most investigated is pain relief.

Now we have a strong body of evidence supporting that music does alleviate pain in different clinical settings (Martin-Saavedra et al. 2018a, b). However, there are still a lot of questions that remain unanswered and that require a lot of research (Martin-Saavedra et al. 2018b). In this chapter, we will review the context of music-induced analgesia, the types of music interventions, the current level of evidence, and provide evidence-based guidelines for clinical practice and research.

16.2 Music Theory

To better understand the analgesic effects of music, we must start with the therapeutic tool: how we define and create music. Music is highly complex and subjective. Like any form of art, perception and appreciation is an essential part of living music. Therefore, having a common, objective language to discuss music helps limit the subjectivity and variability of music. From a healthcare perspective, this is an imperative need if we want the field of music therapy to continue advancing and strengthen its evidence-based practice. In this setting, occidental or other forms of music theory provide objective rules to write, describe, and discuss musical pieces (Martin-Saavedra and Saade-Lemus 2019).

Music is defined by occidental theorists as the art of organizing sounds (Williams 1984). This organization can be done in terms of timing (rhythm) or sound quality (melody, harmony, and instrumentation). The temporal organization is traditionally determined by the note duration and hits. Note duration is classified and described in fractions of the "whole note" or semibreve. For example, the most known note is the crotchet or "quarter note" that lasts one-quarter of a whole note. Then, the two main components of rhythm in a musical piece are the time signature (e.g., 4/4) and the tempo (e.g., 60 beats of crotchet per minute) (Nikolsky 2020).

The quality of the sound depends on its physical properties (volume, pitch, timbre, and waveform). Twelve different waveforms are repeated throughout the spectrum of sound frequency (pitch). These "waveforms" are the musical notes (A or La, B or Si, C or Do, D or Re, E or Mi, F or Fa, and G or Sol) (Williams 1984). The distance between each of these notes is the same and is known as intervals, except for the distance between B and C, and between E and F which is half of a regular interval. Therefore, the other five notes are produced by modifying one of the notes by half an interval; this is called an accidental (Williams 1984).

If notes are played (organized) in singular progressions it is known as melody, and if produced in plural (played at the same time) it is known as harmony. Chords are specific harmonic organization of notes and are described in terms of these 12 notes. Music theory uses scales or modes to describe in an objective manner the quality of the sounds to play.

Finally, there are also the physical properties of sound that provide timbre or voice, pitch (frequency), and volume or intensity (described in decibels). All these are dependent on the tools (instruments) used for playing music. The voice is that unique quality of the instrument, the pitch (measured in Hz) is described in terms of high or low, and volume determines how the instrument is played or amplified.

In summary, A (La) can be played at 420 Hz (middle pitch) on a piano, violin, or guitar, and it will sound similar but not the same. Using these terms, tempo, time-signature, mode or scale, specify the instrument (voice), pitch, and intensity; music-based interventions could be replicated and will allow to standardize interventions, and improve heterogeneity of studies. This is in accordance with recommendations by Robb et al. (Robb et al. 2011, 2018) and is encouraged by the authors of this chapter (Martin-Saavedra and Saade-Lemus 2019).

16.3 Materials and Methods

A systematic review methodology following the PRISMA (Page et al. 2021) guidelines was performed. Search, study screening by title, abstract, and full text was done independently by JSMS and DG. Selected studies were compared after independent selection and any discrepancies in selected or excluded studies were resolved by consensus of all three authors. Data extraction was done by DG and JSMS and reviewed by JSMS and SSL afterward.

16.3.1 Search Strategy

JSMS published a systematic review with meta-analysis (Martin-Saavedra et al. 2018b) and an umbrella review (Martin-Saavedra et al. 2018a). The objective will be to expand the results from these studies with a slightly modified search. Search was done in four databases: Pubmed, ScienceDirect (includes gray literature), Cochrane Library, and Google Scholar (includes gray literature).

Given this prior experience, we modified that search slightly and instead of doing search entries individually for each combination of terms, we decided to combine all terms in an advanced search modality. We also deleted the following terms: "instrumental music," "slow music," "rapid music," "unpleasant music," "music tempo," "music tonality," "pitch range music," "music structural features," and "pleasant music" that yielded no additional results during the search of those studies.

Final search entry for each search engine was: ("music" OR "music-supported therapy" OR "music therapy" OR "music medicine") AND ("pain" OR "pain relief") AND ("systematic review" OR "meta-analysis" OR "trial"). We expanded to all types of languages and authors aimed to find translators for languages different from French (spoken by JSMS), English (spoken by all authors), German (spoken by SSL), and Spanish (spoken by all) for this search. No limitations on the publication date were set.

16.3.2 Study Selection

Studies were screened by title, then by abstract, and finally during full text read. Clinical or controlled trials exploring the effects of music medicine or music therapy to manage pain were included. Studies in which music was added to other forms of therapy and those in which music is part of another type of therapy (e.g., dance therapy) were excluded. Studies using non-validated measurements of pain intensity were also excluded. Given initial results yielded a very large amount of papers we decided to also exclude abstracts, trial registries, and reviews from results and analysis.

16.3.3 Data Validation

In order to validate our data extraction process, we randomly reviewed studies before 2017 and used the first 22 studies that met inclusion criteria. Data was then extracted from these studies and compared to the meta-analysis published by the senior author of this chapter (Martin-Saavedra et al. 2018b). After validating the data extraction process, we moved forward to review studies published between 2018 and now. Two of the 22 random studies before 2017 were included in the meta-analysis from 2018 and a total of 75 variables were shared between the two studies with agreement in 67 (89%).

16.3.4 Variable Definition

16.3.4.1 Clinical Context and Demographic Variables

We explored the effects of age, sex, pain etiology, and pain chronicity for subgroup analysis. Age categories were predefined as adults (>18 years of age), children (12 months to 18 years of age), infants (2 months to 12 months of age), term newborns (0–60 days of age born at 37 weeks or later), and preterm newborns (0–60 days of age born <37 weeks of gestation). Sex was categorized as male-only (studies including only male population), female-only (studies including only female population), or both (studies including both sexes).

Pain etiology was classified as: surgical (pain caused by surgical procedure understood as any procedure with breaking of skin and subcutaneous layers, except dental); nonsurgical procedures (pain caused by procedures that do not fit the surgical definition, except for dental procedures); experimental (pain caused in experimental settings and not by intervention or medical cause); dental procedure (any surgical or nonsurgical procedure of the teeth and related structures); and no procedure (any pain not caused by a procedure according to the prior definitions).

Type of pain was classified as: acute (pain lasting <6 months); chronic (pain lasting >6 months); and acute on chronic (pain lasting <6 months caused by a new medical condition or procedure in a patient with known chronic pain condition).

16.3.4.2 Music Intervention Characteristics

Music intervention was categorized by type as: music therapy (direct involvement of certified music therapist) and music medicine; receptive (passive listening of music) and active (participant was actively involved during music session either by doing mindfulness exercises, physical activity, music production, or other). We further categorized active music interventions in type, but due to a small number of studies it was not used for meta-analysis.

Additionally, we extracted if predesigned composition was used (music was composed prior to study with the objective of alleviating pain). Music preference was evaluated by categorizing if patients and researchers participated in music selection. We also assessed timing of music intervention in procedural pain in three separate subgroups (before, during, and after) in four categories (presence, absence, not described, and no procedure). Duration of music was tested via meta-regression only.

16.3.4.3 Music Properties

Music properties were categorized similarly to what was published previously by one of our authors (Martin-Saavedra et al. 2018b). Tempo was categorized in <60 bpm (very slow), 60–80 bpm (slow), or >80 (moderate to rapid). Time signature (new to this chapter) was categorized in odd (e.g. ¾) or even (e.g. 4/4). Melodic progression was classified as sustained (harmonic or melodic structure is sustained throughout 2 or more music bars after changing chord) or unsustained (most melodic/harmonic changes occur in < than 2 time bars).

Melodic/harmonic structure was categorized by the mode (music scale) of the composition in major modes or minor modes, or if Persian/Turkish Maqam were used. Quality of melody/harmony was categorized in high consonance (smooth music by interval progression in Western music, for example, 1st > 5th interval progression) and low consonance (nonsmooth music, usually limited to experimental music and atonal music not following usual interval progressions).

Instrumentation was categorized based on the presence of lyrical content as: present (if lyrical singing was present in the composition) and not present (no lyrical singing, excluding nonlyrical vocalizations such as humming). We also analyzed the presence of percussive instruments as present or not in the composition.

Certain predesigned music for pain has been available for a while, and thus, we extracted two main ones (u-sequence compositions) and binaural music (music composed using binaural beats). Binaural beats are defined as the use of pure tones (sinusoidal tones) at different frequency in each ear that creates a delta frequency which helps define the type of beat (for example, 10 hz Binaural beats). We analyzed based on the presence or not of binaural beats. We excluded studies using U-sequence (which uses a specific progression of mode, instrumentation, tempo, and other features) and used them in a separate analysis.

Volume control was categorized in low (<60 dB), moderate (60–85 dB), high (>85 dB), controlled with unspecified dB, and controlled by patient. We also look into the amount of songs used as single (one music used for all patients) and multiple (if more than one song was used). Summary of subgroup analysis is shown in Fig. 16.6. Given U-sequence is a type of predesigned intervention characterized by changing music properties, we excluded them from the subgroup meta-analysis as we did a separate model for it.

16.3.5 Data Analysis

Given the broad aim of this chapter, a multilevel meta-analysis by subgroups was performed. Primary outcome was pain relief. To assess efficacy, we calculated post-intervention pain standardized mean differences between patients receiving music interventions compared to controls (usual care).

We only used random effects methods due to the known heterogeneity between studies (Martin-Saavedra et al. 2018b). For all models, pooled effect was estimated using Hedges 'G' corrected standardized mean difference with inverse variance methods. Heterogeneity is described in terms of I-square statistics using a restricted maximum-likelihood estimator and Q-profile method for tau-square and its confidence interval, respectively.

Given there is no reliable method for pre-post measurement meta-analysis, we tried to estimate adjusted means from reported post-intervention means in studies also reporting baseline pain scores. We used studies reporting means and standard deviation, as this assumes normality of the distribution of those means. We applied a log function to transform means given different pain scores were used.

We then ran a linear regression and Pearson's R to evaluate correlation of pre-post which was significant (Adjusted $R2 = 68\%$, $F = 167.6$ on DF 1 to 79, $p < 0.0001$, Pearson's $R = 0.82$ for music values; Adjusted $R2 = 68\%$, $F = 172.6$ on DF 1 to 79, $p < 0.0001$, Pearson's $R = 0.83$). Linearity was assessed with residual and fitted estimates q-q plots. Of note, studies reporting pre-values of 0 were removed as those cannot be computed on regression or meta-analysis. We then used the intercept, estimates, and their standard errors to calculate adjusted means and their standard deviation.

We used the packages "meta" and "metafor" in R for the analysis. For graphs we used "metafor" and "ggplot2" packages. For maps we used the "tidyverse" package and the "maps" coordinates within that package. For statistical results, we will use N to refer to number of patients and K to refer to number of studies. Effect size was determined based on Cohen's convention according to the absolute value of SMD. SMD of 0.2–0.49 was considered small effect, 0.5–0.8 was considered moderate, and >0.8 was considered large. We used metaregression to assess the effect on residual heterogeneity and size of the effect (test of moderators) per variable.

16.4 Results

16.4.1 General

Figure 16.1 summarizes search results and Fig. 16.2 shows where music-related research is being published. The following is the article ID and its respective reference included in this study: 1 (Voss et al. 2004), 2 (Hsieh et al. 2014), 3 (Graversen and Sommer 2013), 4 (Bergomi et al. 2014), 5 (Dabu-Bondoc et al. 2010), 6 (Fowler-Kerry and Lander 1987), 7 (Mitchell and MacDonald 2006), 8 (Clark et al. 2006), 10 (Shabani et al. 2016), 11 (Arruda et al. 2016), 12 (Tuinmann et al. 2017), 14 (Hsu et al. 2016), 15 (Alam et al. 2016), 16 (Bradt et al. 2016),17 (Cho and Choi 2016), 18 (Rapolienė et al. 2016), 19 (Karalar et al. 2016), 20 (Soo et al. 2016), 21 (Madson and Silverman 2010), 22 (Téllez et al. 2016), 23 (Yinger 2016), 24 (Huang et al. 2016), 25 (Düzgün and Karadakovan 2024), 26 (Ünal Toprak et al. 2024), 27 (Daihimfar et al. 2024), 28 (Mounier et al. 2024), 29 (Harper et al. 2023), 30 (Barlas et al. 2023), 31 (Giordano et al. 2023), 32 (Obersnel et al. 2023), 34 (Demirci et al.

2023), 37 (Gürkan and Kaya 2023), 38 (Chen et al. 2023), 39 (Paoin et al. 2023), 42 (Billar et al. 2023), 43 (Demir and Konuk 2023), 44 (Tse et al. 2023), 45 (Anbalagan et al. 2023), 46 (Öztaş et al. 2023), 47 (Kakar et al. 2023), 48 (Orak et al. 2023), 49 (Werner et al. 2023), 50 (Goktas and Avci 2023), 51 (Colebaugh et al. 2023), 52 (Küçük Alemdar et al. 2023), 54 (Sadeghi et al. 2023), 55 (Kakde et al. 2023), 56 (Dallı et al. 2023), 57 (Durgun and Yaman 2023), 59 (Choi et al. 2023), 60 (Öztürk et al. 2023), 61 (Golino et al. 2023), 62 (Sorribes De Ramón et al. 2023), 63 (Yılmaz and Ölçücü 2023), 64 (Us et al. 2023), 65 (Tripyla et al. 2023), 66 (Hedayati et al. 2023), 67 (Prasad et al. 2023), 68 (Aly et al. 2023), 69 (Raglio et al. 2023), 70 (Esteban Pellicer et al. 2023), 71 (Rabinowitch et al. 2023), 72 (Hohneck et al. 2023), 73 (Dong et al. 2023), 74 (Dur et al. 2023), 75 (Cici et al. 2023), 76 (Nelson et al. 2023), 77 (Sun et al. 2022), 78 (Karakuş Selçuk and Baysal 2022), 80 (Du et al. 2022), 81 (Koca and Aylaz 2022), 82 (Bozkurt et al. 2022), 84 (Schell et al. 2022), 85 (Brosh et al. 2022), 87 (Merliot-Gailhoustet et al. 2022), 88 (Inayama et al. 2022), 89 (Bueno-Serrano et al. 2022), 90 (Terzi 2022), 92 (Loong et al. 2022), 93 (Howlin et al. 2022), 94 (Ganesan et al. 2022), 95 (Özdemir et al. 2019), 96 (Zohaib et al. 2022), 97 (Nandeibam et al. 2022), 98 (Brix and Pedersen 2022), 99 (Bertacco et al. 2022), 100 (Ghasemi et al. 2022), 101 (Lunde et al. 2022), 104 (Sharara-Chami et al. 2022), 105 (Jacquier et al. 2022), 107 (Chen et al. 2022), 109 (Deng et al. 2022), 110 (Rodgers-Melnick et al. 2022), 111 (Wood et al. 2021), 112 (Jacq et al. 2018), 113 (Tang et al. 2021), 115 (Miladinia et al. 2021), 116 (de Melo et al. 2021), 117 (Kim and Jeong 2021), 119 (McClintock et al. 2021), 120 (Sorensen et al. 2021), 121 (Guerrier et al. 2021), 122 (Yiğit et al. 2021), 123 (Casarin et al. 2021), 124 (Lee et al. 2021), 125 (Antonacci et al. 2021), 126 (Reynaud et al. 2021), 127 (Bicego et al. 2021), 128 (Eid et al. 2021), 129 (Browne et al. 2021), 130 (Mumm et al. 2021), 131 (Muzzi et al. 2021), 133 (Azeem et al. 2021), 134 (Toker et al. 2021), 135 (Contreras-Molina et al. 2021), 136 (Anglin et al. 2021), 137 (Mondanaro et al. 2021), 138 (Etienne et al. 2021), 139 (Konar et al. 2021), 140 (Akın 2021), 141 (Bay et al. 2021), 142 (Ferraz et al. 2021), 143 (Law et al. 2021), 144 (Laframboise-Otto et al. 2021), 145 (Merry and Silverman 2021),146 (Mateu et al. 2018), 147 (Ölçücü et al. 2021), 148 (Bulut et al. 2020), 149 (Uggla et al. 2018), 150 (Gezginci et al. 2018), 151 (Verstegen and Silverman 2018), 152 (Çetinkaya et al. 2018), 153 (Hilal et al. 2018), 154 (Mackintosh et al. 2018), 155 (Rossi et al. 2018), 156 (Citlik-Saritas et al. 2018), 157 (Innes et al. 2018), 158 (Choi et al. 2018a), 159 (Cheung et al. 2018), 160 (Packiam et al. 2018), 161 (Corrigan et al. 2020), 162 (Torres et al. 2018), 163 (Rodgers-Melnick et al. 2018), 164 (Choi et al. 2018b), 165 (Warth et al. 2018), 166 (Yarahmadi et al. 2018), 167 (Shukla et al. 2018), 168 (Tang et al. 2018), 169 (Doğan Bakı et al. 2018), 170 (Tolunay et al. 2018), 171 (van der Heijden et al. 2018), 172 (Drzymalski et al. 2020), 173 (Blichfeldt-Ærø et al. 2020), 174 (Gür and Apay 2020), 175 (Dhokia et al. 2020), 176 (Ebrahimi et al. 2020), 177 (Amanak 2020), 178 (Lin et al. 2020a), 179 (Chan et al. 2020), 180 (Orak et al. 2020), 181 (Tan et al. 2020), 182 (Viana et al. 2020), 183 (Martin-Saavedra and Ruiz-Sternberg 2020), 185

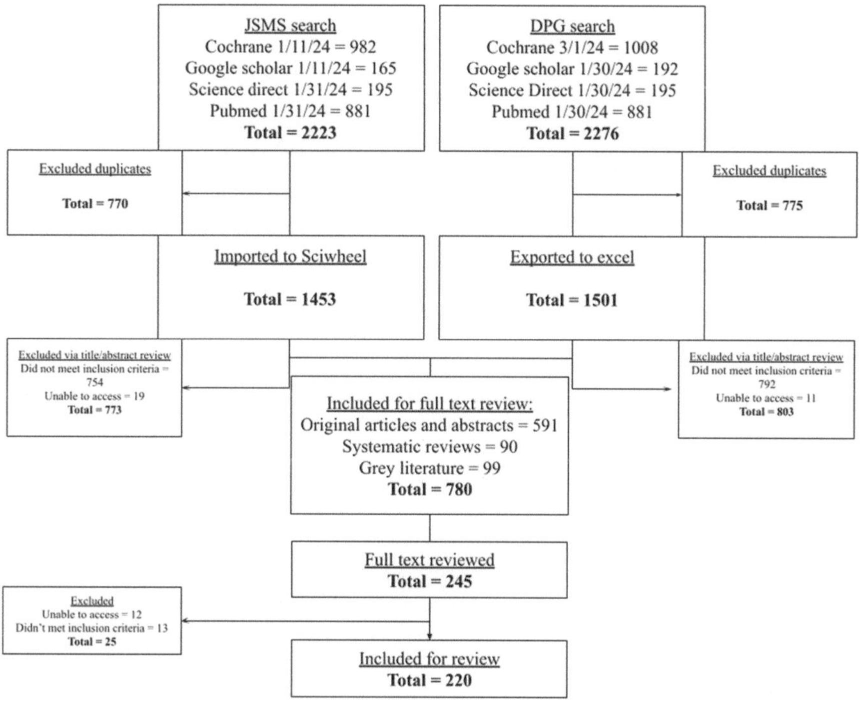

Fig. 16.1 Study selection flow chart

(Zhang et al. 2020), 186 (Chai et al. 2020), 187 (Doro et al. 2020), 188 (Belloeil et al. 2020), 189 (Cimen et al. 2020), 191 (Tran et al. 2020), 192 (Buglione et al. 2020), 193 (Li et al. 2020a), 194 (Kavak Akelma et al. 2020), 195 (Howard et al. 2020), 197 (Çelebi et al. 2020), 198 (Low et al. 2020), 199 (Çift and Benlioglu 2020), 200 (Roshani et al. 2020), 201 (Barandouzi et al. 2020), 202 (El-Khoury et al. 2020), 203 (Kiani et al. 2019), 204 (Delimar et al. 2019), 206 (van der Heijden et al. 2019), 207 (Jethani 2019), 208 (Ortega et al. 2019), 209 (Luis et al. 2019), 210 (Wren et al. 2019), 211 (Mateu-Capell et al. 2019), 212 (Diri et al. 2019), 213 (Hsieh et al. 2019), 214 (Kavakli et al. 2019), 215 (Ko et al. 2019), 216 (Yaman Aktaş and Karabulut 2019), 217 (Young et al. 2021), 218 (Leonard 2019), 219 (Li et al. 2019), 220 (Tekgündüz et al. 2019), 221 (Aktaş and Karabulut 2019), 223 (Sánchez-Jáuregui et al. 2019), 224 (Öztürk et al. 2019), 225 (Burrai et al. 2019), 226 (Haqiqi et al. 2023), 227 (Mousaviasl et al. 2023), 228 (Soyeux and Marchand 2022), 229 (Halder et al. 2022), 230 (Giordano et al. 2022), 231 (Soliva et al. 2022) 232 (Shoghi et al. 2022), 234 (Johnson and Elkins 2020), 235 (Gökçek and Kaydu 2020), 236 (Gochenour et al. 2020), 237 (Ramezani et al. 2020), 238 (Pongan et al. 2020), 239 (Fernando et al. 2019), 240 (Gupta et al. 2019), 241 (Quigley et al. 2019),

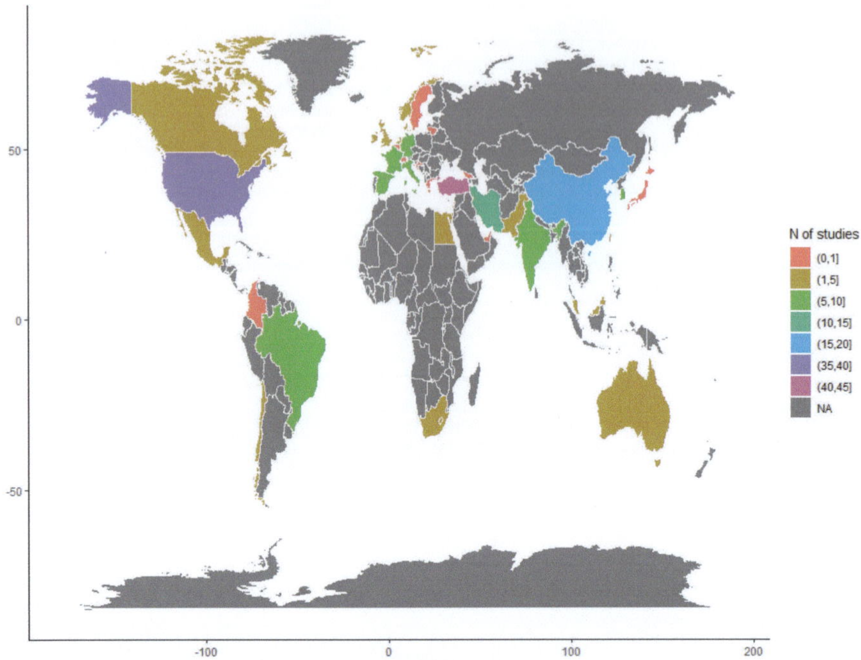

Fig. 16.2 Geographic frequency of publications

242 (Gallagher et al. 2018), 243 (James and Drummond 2018), 244 (Bashiri et al. 2018), 245 (Fen et al. 2018), 246 (Duimaz 2020), and 247 (Victoria et al. 2018).

16.4.2 Immediate Music-Induced Analgesia

Most studies compared pain scores right after the intervention against control. We included pooled meta-analysis studies that reported mean and standard deviation within the next 24 hours of the last music intervention. In case of multiple measures within 24 hours, we chose the one measured closest to 30 minutes after the intervention. Twelve studies did not report mean or standard deviations (or other distribution statistics) so they were excluded from meta-analysis.

A final sample of 120 studies was included in this meta-analysis with 9660 individuals exposed to a total of 17,524.5 minutes of music (162 minutes per week on average per study). Funnel plot showed some studies scattered outside standard deviation (see Fig. 16.3) suggestive of large heterogeneity that was confirmed in the pooled meta-analysis (SMD = −0.63, CI 95% −0.78 to −0.48; I2 = 95%, $\tau 2 = 0.7477$).

In order to assess effects by publication bias from the funnel plot, we did sensitivity analysis by removing possible outliers. Specifically, we identified five studies with very large effects (Shabani et al. 2016; Yinger 2016; Mounier et al. 2024;

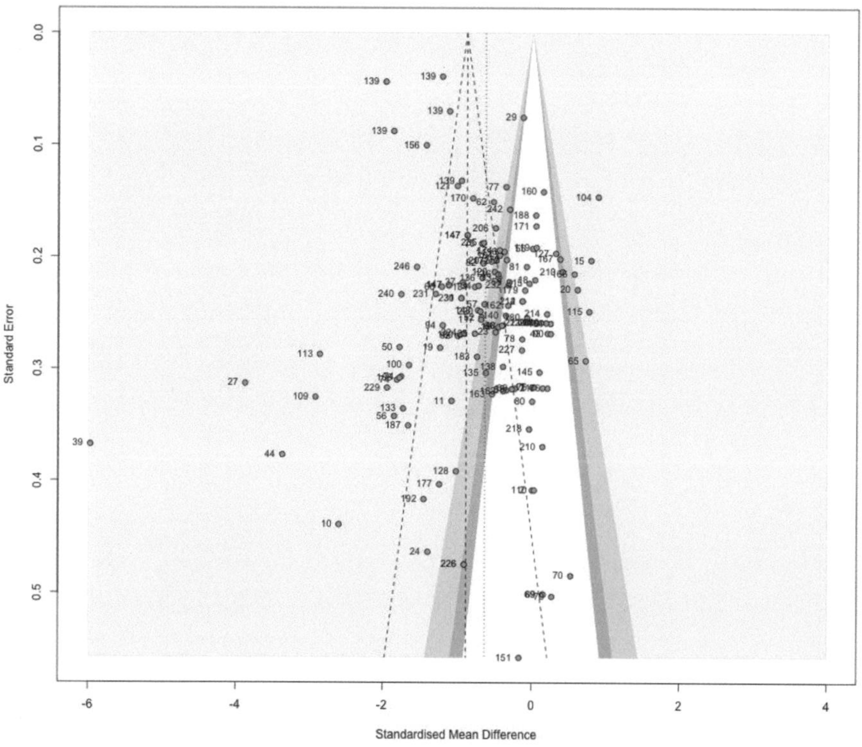

Fig. 16.3 Funnel plot including all studies

Chen et al. 2022; Jacq et al. 2018). Pooled meta-analysis' heterogeneity (I2) remained at 94–95% after removing individual studies (Shabani et al. 2016; Yinger 2016; Mounier et al. 2024; Chen et al. 2022; Jacq et al. 2018), and all at the same time. Therefore, none of these studies were removed from further analysis.

Twenty studies reported median with interquartile range (three studies had more than 1 music group). Shi method of approximation of SD was used for the model and the found effect was slightly larger ($K = 24$, N music = 1098, N control = 1138, MD −0.88, CI 95% −1.43 to −0.33, I2 = 92%) to pooled meta-analysis from normally distributed data.

16.4.3 Clinical Effect of Music-Induced Analgesia

Figure 16.4 shows the forest plot for logarithmic adjusted means by pre-intervention values. We also identified 14 studies reporting mean differences, but three had missing means or their standard deviation so were excluded. Given all of the studies used the same scale (0–10 VAS or NRS), we did weighted mean differences (WMD, Fig. 16.5) instead of SMD (Fig. 16.4).

Study	Experimental Total	Experimental Mean	Experimental SD	Control Total	Control Mean	Control SD	SMD	95%-CI	Weight (common)	Weight (random)
1	19	3.39	1.8773	21	3.67	1.3639	-0.17	[-0.79; 0.45]	0.7%	1.1%
2	12	3.65	1.5699	12	3.94	1.0963	-0.21	[-1.01; 0.60]	0.4%	0.9%
10	20	-1.84	-0.0641	20	-0.13	-0.3338			0.0%	0.0%
11	22	0.31	0.7926	21	1.49	0.3607	-1.86	[-2.59; -1.14]	0.5%	1.0%
14	35	0.60	1.1456	35	0.88	0.5877	-0.30	[-0.77; 0.17]	1.1%	1.4%
17	20	1.58	1.2365	20	1.80	0.7542	-0.22	[-0.84; 0.41]	0.7%	1.1%
18	35	0.69	1.1915	50	0.87	0.7483	-0.18	[-0.62; 0.25]	1.4%	1.4%
20	40	0.56	1.2016	40	0.62	0.6090	-0.06	[-0.50; 0.37]	1.3%	1.4%
25	30	1.17	1.3273	30	1.70	0.7672	-0.48	[-0.99; 0.03]	1.0%	1.3%
29	376	0.53	3.6336	332	0.87	1.7148	-0.12	[-0.27; 0.03]	11.7%	1.8%
39	84	0.64	1.8009	81	1.88	0.9156	-0.86	[-1.18; -0.54]	2.5%	1.6%
44	41	0.49	1.1768	30	1.18	0.4989	-0.72	[-1.20; -0.23]	1.1%	1.4%
48	30	0.97	1.2334	30	1.38	0.6887	-0.40	[-0.91; 0.11]	1.0%	1.3%
52	33	-1.57	0.0495	33	-0.46	-0.3184			0.0%	0.0%
55	55	-0.52	0.7246	53	-0.36	0.1390	-0.30	[-0.68; 0.08]	1.8%	1.5%
56	25	1.03	1.1515	25	1.70	0.6500	-0.70	[-1.28; -0.13]	0.8%	1.2%
57	36	0.41	1.0651	36	0.95	0.5151	-0.63	[-1.11; -0.16]	1.1%	1.4%
59	41	0.78	1.3362	41	1.05	0.7166	-0.25	[-0.68; 0.19]	1.3%	1.4%
65	25	1.65	1.4141	25	1.63	0.8697	0.02	[-0.53; 0.57]	0.8%	1.2%
66	30	1.22	1.3475	30	1.63	0.7841	-0.37	[-0.88; 0.15]	1.0%	1.3%
68	20	3.13	1.8304	20	3.55	1.2510	-0.26	[-0.88; 0.37]	0.7%	1.1%
68	20	3.09	1.8133	20	3.55	1.2367	-0.29	[-0.91; 0.34]	0.7%	1.1%
69	8	1.41	0.7422	8	1.57	0.4437	-0.25	[-1.23; 0.74]	0.3%	0.7%
69	8	1.43	0.7476	8	1.57	0.4482	-0.21	[-1.20; 0.77]	0.3%	0.7%
73	43	1.64	1.8481	43	2.00	1.1352	-0.24	[-0.66; 0.19]	1.4%	1.4%
74	30	1.23	1.3540	30	2.00	0.7895	-0.69	[-1.21; -0.16]	0.9%	1.3%
74	30	1.19	1.3353	30	2.00	0.7739	-0.73	[-1.26; -0.21]	0.9%	1.3%
75	60	1.37	2.0034	60	1.75	1.1906	-0.23	[-0.59; 0.13]	2.0%	1.5%
76	20	2.04	1.4142	20	2.28	0.9028	-0.20	[-0.82; 0.43]	0.7%	1.2%
76	20	2.08	1.4270	20	2.28	0.9136	-0.17	[-0.79; 0.46]	0.7%	1.2%
78	25	1.59	1.3870	29	1.86	0.9123	-0.23	[-0.77; 0.30]	0.9%	1.3%
80	19	1.75	1.2706	18	1.98	0.7688	-0.21	[-0.86; 0.43]	0.6%	1.1%
81	45	1.15	1.6128	47	1.42	0.9493	-0.20	[-0.61; 0.21]	1.5%	1.5%
94	35	1.01	1.3491	35	1.57	0.7580	-0.51	[-0.99; -0.04]	1.1%	1.4%
109	40	1.17	1.5327	40	1.88	0.8859	-0.56	[-1.01; -0.11]	1.3%	1.4%
110	12	1.44	0.9172	12	1.64	0.5502	-0.26	[-1.07; 0.54]	0.4%	0.9%
113	50	0.74	1.4517	50	1.65	0.7714	-0.78	[-1.19; -0.37]	1.5%	1.5%
121	119	-1.20	0.4390	124	0.07	-0.3226			0.0%	0.0%
122	30	-0.72	0.4447	30	-0.56	0.0289	-0.49	[-1.00; 0.03]	1.0%	1.3%
127	59	1.62	2.1543	47	1.77	1.1790	-0.08	[-0.47; 0.30]	1.7%	1.5%
128	15	0.01	0.5563	15	0.51	0.2227	-1.14	[-1.92; -0.37]	0.4%	0.9%
133	25	0.21	0.7999	25	1.31	0.3559	-1.75	[-2.41; -1.09]	0.6%	1.1%
134	42	1.53	1.7681	42	2.00	1.0731	-0.32	[-0.75; 0.11]	1.4%	1.4%
134	42	1.51	1.7535	42	2.00	1.0609	-0.34	[-0.77; 0.09]	1.4%	1.4%
135	21	0.78	0.9563	25	1.43	0.5596	-0.83	[-1.44; -0.22]	0.7%	1.2%
136	53	0.61	1.4162	38	1.40	0.6169	-0.68	[-1.10; -0.25]	1.4%	1.4%
136	53	0.78	1.5216	38	1.40	0.6916	-0.49	[-0.91; -0.07]	1.4%	1.4%
138	23	1.53	1.3064	23	1.92	0.7924	-0.36	[-0.94; 0.22]	0.7%	1.2%
143	54	1.39	1.9176	53	1.85	1.1332	-0.28	[-0.67; 0.10]	1.8%	1.5%
145	24	1.03	1.1282	20	1.17	0.5814	-0.15	[-0.74; 0.44]	0.7%	1.2%
148	35	0.53	1.1086	35	1.06	0.5568	-0.60	[-1.08; -0.12]	1.1%	1.4%
151	6	0.43	0.4385	7	0.78	0.2304	-0.95	[-2.13; 0.22]	0.2%	0.6%
156	250	0.74	3.2515	250	1.50	1.7295	-0.29	[-0.46; -0.11]	8.2%	1.8%
162	40	0.79	1.3260	30	1.12	0.6175	-0.30	[-0.78; 0.18]	1.1%	1.4%
163	20	1.49	1.2049	20	1.85	0.7277	-0.36	[-0.98; 0.27]	0.7%	1.1%
163	20	1.42	1.1792	20	1.85	0.7063	-0.43	[-1.06; 0.20]	0.6%	1.1%
166	45	0.14	1.0331	45	-0.16	0.4440	0.37	[-0.05; 0.78]	1.5%	1.5%
168	30	2.29	1.8463	30	2.71	1.2013	-0.27	[-0.78; 0.24]	1.0%	1.3%
171	71	2.36	2.8957	64	2.60	1.7986	-0.10	[-0.43; 0.24]	2.2%	1.6%
174	55	1.58	2.0505	54	1.92	1.2392	-0.20	[-0.58; 0.18]	1.8%	1.5%
177	15	3.43	1.6814	15	3.91	1.1639	-0.33	[-1.05; 0.39]	0.5%	1.0%
183	29	1.02	1.2362	23	1.66	0.6205	-0.62	[-1.18; -0.06]	0.8%	1.2%
187	24	0.35	0.8441	21	1.58	0.3734	-1.80	[-2.50; -1.10]	0.5%	1.0%
188	74	0.94	1.9140	77	1.11	1.0836	-0.11	[-0.43; 0.21]	2.5%	1.6%
200	30	-0.28	0.6477	30	-0.44	0.1987	0.32	[-0.19; 0.83]	1.0%	1.3%
201	30	1.18	1.3308	30	1.34	0.7701	-0.14	[-0.65; 0.37]	1.0%	1.3%
206	75	0.76	1.7927	62	1.48	0.8703	-0.50	[-0.84; -0.16]	2.2%	1.6%
207	50	-0.49	0.7114	50	0.28	0.1522	-1.48	[-1.92; -1.03]	1.3%	1.4%
210	46	0.22	1.0936	44	-0.06	0.4792	0.33	[-0.09; 0.75]	1.5%	1.5%
210	12	0.91	0.7611	19	1.02	0.5281	-0.17	[-0.89; 0.56]	0.5%	1.0%
217	21	3.53	2.0298	19	3.79	1.3420	-0.15	[-0.77; 0.47]	0.7%	1.1%
218	16	1.55	1.0974	16	1.80	0.6674	-0.26	[-0.96; 0.43]	0.5%	1.0%
220	35	1.74	1.7188	34	2.16	1.0518	-0.29	[-0.76; 0.18]	1.1%	1.4%
221	30	0.54	1.0312	30	0.76	0.5195	-0.27	[-0.78; 0.24]	1.0%	1.3%
226	10	1.40	0.8283	10	1.89	0.4948	-0.69	[-1.59; 0.22]	0.3%	0.8%
226	10	1.40	0.8283	10	1.89	0.4948	-0.69	[-1.59; 0.22]	0.3%	0.8%
227	25	1.29	1.2616	25	1.54	0.7421	-0.23	[-0.79; 0.32]	0.8%	1.2%
231	47	2.81	2.6166	43	3.98	1.6828	-0.52	[-0.94; -0.10]	1.4%	1.5%
232	40	1.11	1.4969	40	1.56	0.8560	-0.37	[-0.81; 0.07]	1.3%	1.4%
242	84	0.91	2.0137	79	1.33	1.0768	-0.26	[-0.56; 0.05]	2.7%	1.6%
246	60	-0.41	0.8319	60	1.45	0.2107	-3.05	[-3.58; -2.52]	0.9%	1.3%
Common effect model	**3389**			**3269**			**-0.36**	**[-0.41; -0.31]**	**100.0%**	.
Random effects model							**-0.43**	**[-0.54; -0.32]**	.	**100.0%**

Heterogeneity: $I^2 = 71\%$, $\tau^2 = 0.1616$, $p < 0.01$

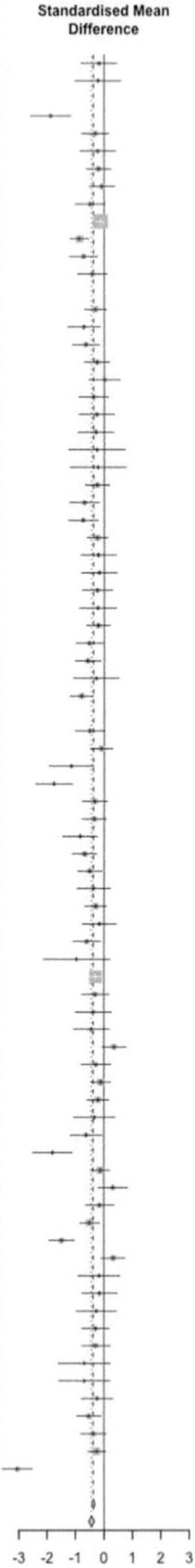

Fig. 16.4 Pooled forest using estimated post-intervention mean scores adjusted by pre-intervention pain scores

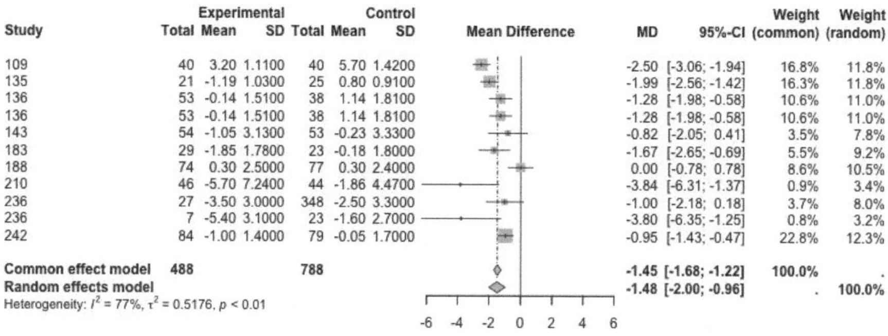

Fig. 16.5 Forest plot comparing pre-post mean differences between music and usual care (control)

Comparing 488 individuals exposed to music and 788 to control (usual care), music improves pain by 1.48 (CI 95% −2.0 to −0.96) units on a 0–10 VAS/NRS ($I2$ = 77%, $t2$ = 0.5176, $p < 0.01$) (see Fig. 16.5). When compared to SMD and WMD (Figs. 16.4 and 16.5) both showed a small to moderate effect size with similar heterogeneity.

16.4.4 Study Design and Clinical Context

Subgroup analysis showed that there was a between-groups difference in sex of patients (Chi2 = 11.04, p = 0.004) and with blinding (Chi2 = 6.48, p = 0.04), see Fig. 16.6. Given the subgroup country had so many categories, only meta regression was done for location of study (country, not included in Fig. 16.6).

Meta-regressions showed that none of the categories within each subgroup impacted effect size significantly ($p > 0.05$) except for the subgroup country. Publications coming from China (K = 10), India (K = 9), Thailand (K = 1), Georgia (K = 1), and Pakistan (K = 1) were associated with larger effect sizes. A trend of age was observed in meta-regression (QM(df = 3) = 6.86, p = 0.07), with ages 12 months to 18 years predicting larger pain reduction ($p < 0.0001$). No subgroup was accountable for the heterogeneity of the results ($p < 0.0001$).

16.4.5 Music Intervention Characteristics

Subgroup meta-analysis results are summarized in Fig. 16.7. Music presentation (Chi2 = 12.61, p = 0.006) and all three subgroups for moment of music intervention (Chi2 = 18.62, 17.62, and 19.09, for pre, intra, and post-procedure analysis; $p < 0.001$) demonstrated between group differences. Meta-regression showed that none of the specific categories had a significant impact on effect size or heterogeneity. Differences were mostly coming from studies that did not provide details on the music intervention.

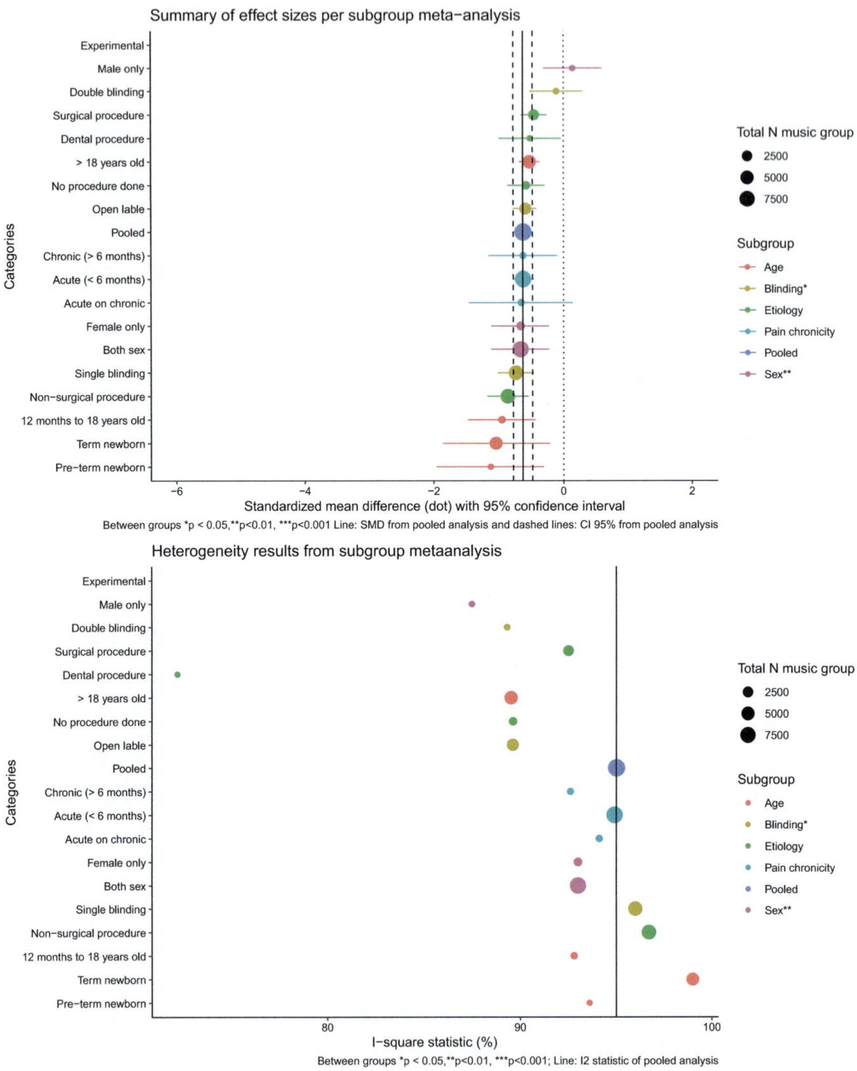

Fig. 16.6 Variation of pooled effect sizes and heterogeneity per clinical and demographic categories

Duration of music intervention was a significant predictor of effect size but did not explain the heterogeneity. Longer duration in minutes was associated with −0.006 SMD increase in difference for every minute added to music-based intervention (QM(df 1) = 17.001, $p < 0.0001$). This was not observed for the number of interventions per day, days per week of intervention, or weeks of intervention ($p > 0.05$).

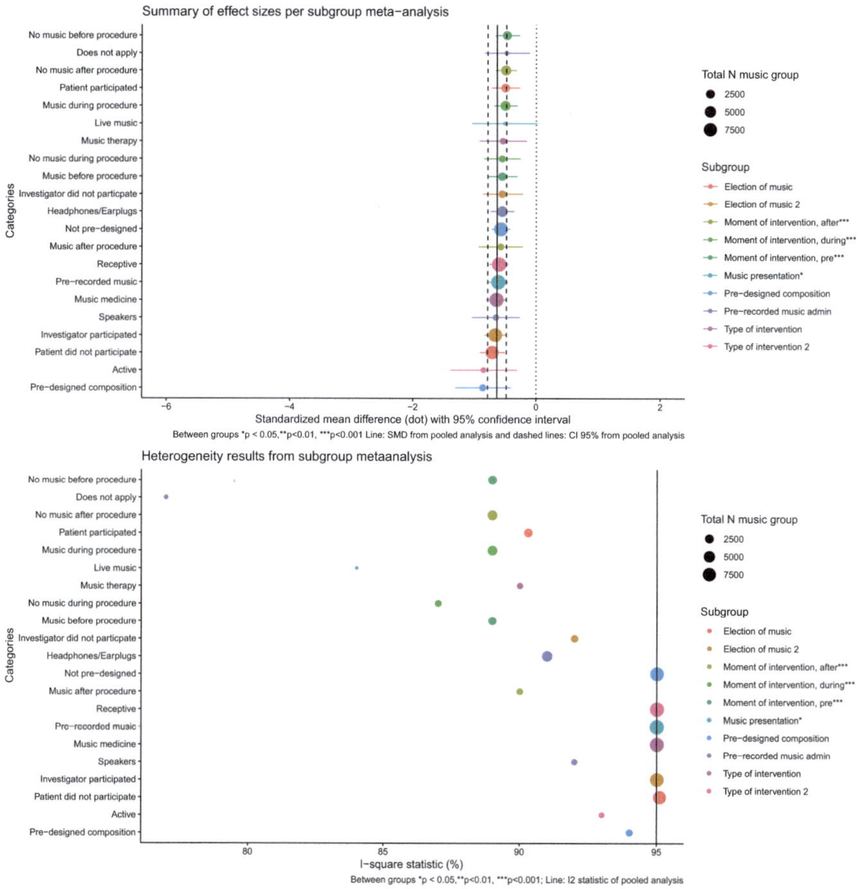

Fig. 16.7 Variation of pooled effect sizes and heterogeneity based on characteristics of music intervention

The total music exposure time, estimated by multiplying duration of intervention in minutes by number of interventions per day, days of interventions per week, and weeks of intervention yielded no significant effects either ($p = 0.81$). No subgroup or variable (including duration) explained a significant part of the heterogeneity.

Ten studies had two music groups, one for music selected by patient (preferred, entered as control) and music chosen by investigator alone (non-preferred, entered as experimental). Preferred music was minimally superior to non-preferred one (*N* non-preferred = 445, *N* preferred = 442, SMD = 0.15, CI 95% −0.01 to 0.31; I2 = 13%).

16.4.6 Music Properties

Subgroup analysis for music properties is shown in Fig. 16.8. When melodic/harmonic consonance was described (or song given), all were of high consonance so it was excluded from Fig. 16.8. A trend for between group differences was observed for sustained melody/harmony (Chi2 = 4.76, p = 0.09), music mode (Chi2 = 6.4, p = 0.09), and volume of music (Chi2 = 8.36, p = 0.08). However, metaregression did not show a significant category to predict a larger effect size or its heterogeneity.

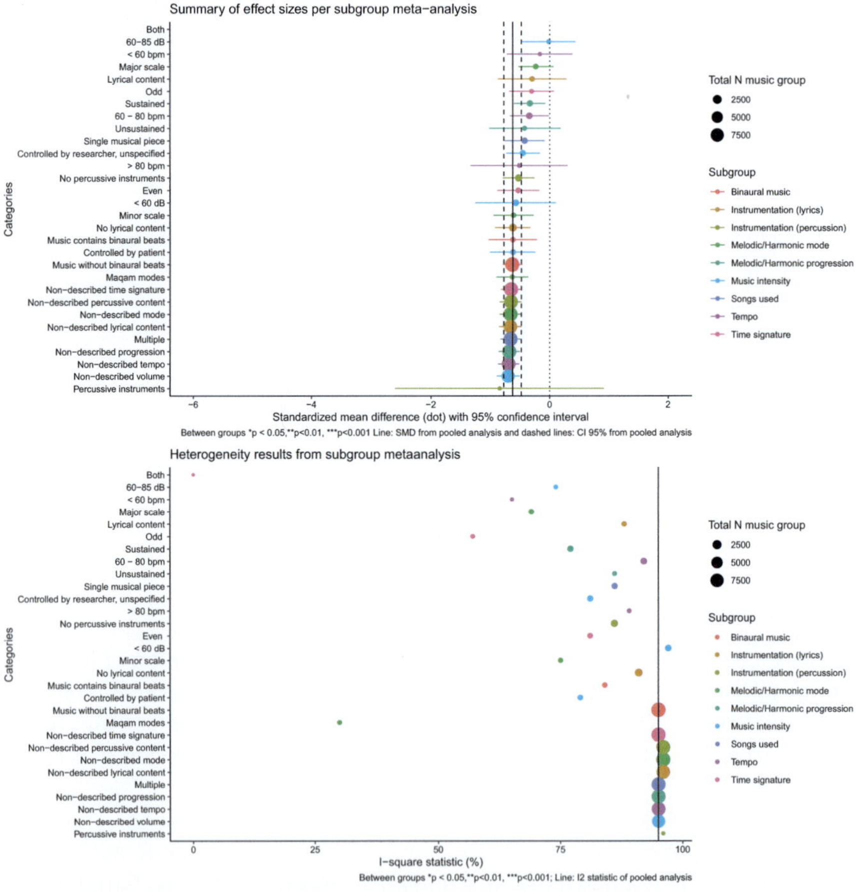

Fig. 16.8 Variation of pooled effect sizes and heterogeneity based on music properties of songs

16.4.7 Ideal Clinical Context

Based on results from subgroup analysis of clinical context and demographics, studies on adults, including both sex, and studying acute surgical pain seem to have the best effect sizes and heterogeneity. We selected all studies meeting this criteria for analysis. Heterogeneity did not improve and effect size was small (I2 = 92%, SMD −0.38, CI 95% −0.62 to −0.15).

16.4.8 Ideal Music Properties

Results from subgroup analysis do not allow for strong conclusions on ideal subgroups of music qualities. We chose as inclusion criteria the following characteristics: music without percussion, without lyrics, without binaural beats, and of tempo 60–80 bpm. This selection was done based on sample size, stability of SMD and its CI 95%, and I2 from subgroup meta-analysis. Also, these are common qualities reported in the literature to be "relaxing" and there is prior evidence showing effectiveness (Martin-Saavedra et al. 2018b). Significant moderate effect was identified with minimally improved heterogeneity (I2 = 84%, SMD = −0.49, CI 95% −0.94 to −0.03; Fig. 16.9.

16.4.9 Predesigned Interventions

Four studies evaluated binaural and non-binaural music as intervention groups (studies 5, 67, 68, and 76). We used non-binaural music as controls and ran a meta-analysis that showed a minimal significant effect favoring non-binaural music (N = 135 both groups, SMD = 0.29, CI 95% 0.01 to 0.57, I2 = 0%). Three studies used U-sequence (Music Care) interventions. One of these had two groups exposed to music. When compared to controls, U-sequence had a minimal to moderate pain-reducing effect with high heterogeneity (I2 = 88, SMD = −0.48, CI 95% −0.97 to 0.01).

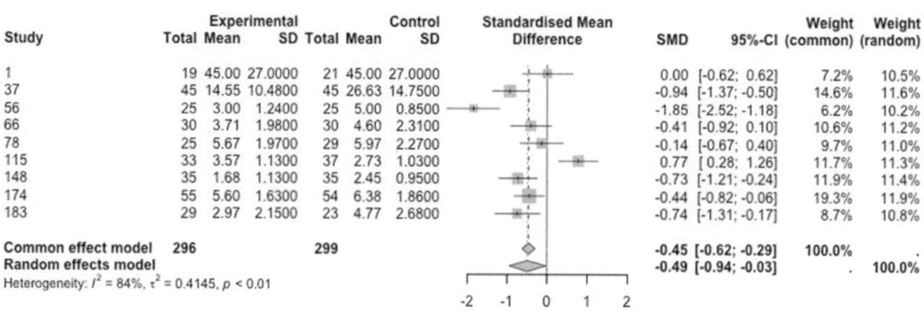

Fig. 16.9 Subgroup meta-analysis of studies using music of 60–80 bpm with no lyrics or percussion

16.4.10 Length of Music-Induced Analgesia

To evaluate the length of music-induced analgesia, we evaluated studies with multiple measurements after a single music intervention. Figure 16.10 summarizes the results by subgroup analysis based on the timing of pain measurement after a single

Study	Music Total	Music Mean	Music SD	Control Total	Control Mean	Control SD	SMD	95%-CI	Weight (common)	Weight (random)
Timing = < 30 min after										
5	20	4.50	2.4000	20	4.30	2.2000	0.09	[-0.53; 0.71]	1.3%	2.1%
5	20	3.60	2.8000	20	4.30	2.2000	-0.27	[-0.90; 0.35]	1.3%	2.1%
24	12	33.16	14.7400	12	53.83	13.8600	-1.39	[-2.30; -0.49]	0.6%	1.7%
25	30	3.53	1.9700	30	5.00	1.8000	-0.77	[-1.29; -0.24]	1.8%	2.3%
59	41	2.24	0.5300	41	2.41	0.5400	-0.31	[-0.75; 0.12]	2.6%	2.4%
65	25	6.00	1.9000	25	4.40	2.3000	0.75	[0.17; 1.32]	1.5%	2.2%
68	20	33.70	21.5000	20	39.20	24.4000	-0.23	[-0.86; 0.39]	1.3%	2.1%
68	20	32.00	26.9000	20	39.20	24.4000	-0.27	[-0.90; 0.35]	1.3%	2.1%
121	119	0.23	0.4000	124	0.81	0.7000	-1.01	[-1.28; -0.74]	7.0%	2.6%
127	59	5.91	1.4500	47	5.42	1.6600	0.31	[-0.07; 0.70]	3.4%	2.5%
133	25	1.16	1.2300	25	3.23	1.1200	-1.73	[-2.39; -1.07]	1.2%	2.1%
134	42	5.33	1.7500	42	7.00	2.4800	-0.77	[-1.21; -0.33]	2.5%	2.4%
134	42	5.17	2.5300	42	7.00	2.4800	-0.72	[-1.17; -0.28]	2.6%	2.4%
138	23	3.80	2.0000	23	4.00	2.2200	-0.09	[-0.67; 0.49]	1.5%	2.2%
177	15	47.14	9.0100	15	59.12	9.7800	-1.24	[-2.03; -0.45]	0.8%	1.9%
183	29	2.97	2.1500	23	4.77	2.6800	-0.74	[-1.31; -0.17]	1.6%	2.2%
188	74	4.00	2.9000	77	3.60	2.5000	0.15	[-0.17; 0.47]	4.9%	2.6%
210	12	2.60	1.8400	19	2.33	1.8800	0.14	[-0.58; 0.86]	1.0%	2.0%
229	30	0.01	0.0100	30	0.40	0.5000	-1.09	[-1.63; -0.54]	1.7%	2.3%
242	84	2.60	2.3000	79	3.30	2.2000	-0.31	[-0.62; -0.00]	5.2%	2.6%
246	60	0.57	0.9300	60	3.80	2.7700	-1.55	[-1.96; -1.14]	3.0%	2.5%
Common effect model	802			794			-0.50	[-0.61; -0.40]	48.0%	.
Random effects model							-0.52	[-0.79; -0.24]	.	47.4%
Heterogeneity: $I^2 = 85\%$, $\tau^2 = 0.3369$, $p < 0.01$										
Timing = 30-120 min after										
5	20	3.40	1.4000	20	4.10	2.4000	-0.35	[-0.97; 0.28]	1.3%	2.1%
5	20	3.50	2.0000	20	4.10	2.4000	-0.27	[-0.89; 0.36]	1.3%	2.1%
56	25	3.00	1.2400	25	5.00	0.8500	-1.85	[-2.52; -1.18]	1.1%	2.1%
65	25	3.50	1.8000	25	3.60	1.7000	-0.06	[-0.61; 0.50]	1.6%	2.2%
73	43	6.02	2.1000	43	7.01	2.2200	-0.45	[-0.88; -0.03]	2.7%	2.4%
138	23	5.30	2.6000	23	6.40	2.9000	-0.39	[-0.98; 0.19]	1.5%	2.2%
242	84	1.17	0.3800	79	1.38	0.5000	-0.47	[-0.78; -0.16]	5.2%	2.6%
Common effect model	240			235			-0.49	[-0.68; -0.31]	14.7%	.
Random effects model							-0.53	[-0.92; -0.14]	.	15.8%
Heterogeneity: $I^2 = 68\%$, $\tau^2 = 0.2019$, $p < 0.01$										
Timing = 3 - 24 h after										
59	41	2.24	0.5300	41	2.41	0.5400	-0.31	[-0.75; 0.12]	2.6%	2.4%
109	40	3.53	0.7200	40	6.13	1.0200	-2.92	[-3.55; -2.28]	1.2%	2.1%
133	25	5.33	1.6700	25	6.72	1.6500	-0.82	[-1.40; -0.24]	1.5%	2.2%
183	29	2.37	2.3100	23	3.63	2.8300	-0.49	[-1.04; 0.07]	1.6%	2.2%
188	74	2.70	2.4000	77	2.60	2.4000	0.04	[-0.28; 0.36]	4.9%	2.6%
Common effect model	209			206			-0.52	[-0.73; -0.32]	11.9%	.
Random effects model							-0.88	[-1.89; 0.13]	.	11.6%
Heterogeneity: $I^2 = 94\%$, $\tau^2 = 1.2611$, $p < 0.01$										
Timing = 24-48 h after										
5	20	3.90	1.7000	20	5.00	2.0000	-0.58	[-1.21; 0.05]	1.2%	2.1%
5	20	3.50	1.5000	20	5.00	2.0000	-0.83	[-1.48; -0.18]	1.2%	2.1%
25	30	5.37	1.9200	30	4.70	1.4800	0.39	[-0.13; 0.90]	1.9%	2.3%
56	25	3.83	0.8300	25	4.66	1.0700	-0.85	[-1.43; -0.27]	1.5%	2.2%
59	41	1.46	0.6700	41	1.59	0.5900	-0.20	[-0.64; 0.23]	2.7%	2.4%
133	25	6.23	1.4300	25	7.89	1.2200	-1.23	[-1.84; -0.62]	1.4%	2.2%
144	24	5.05	.	23	5.67	.			0.0%	0.0%
Common effect model	185			184			-0.45	[-0.68; -0.23]	9.8%	.
Random effects model							-0.53	[-1.00; -0.06]	.	13.3%
Heterogeneity: $I^2 = 76\%$, $\tau^2 = 0.2556$, $p < 0.01$										
Timing = 2 day or more after										
59	41	1.07	0.2600	41	1.34	0.4800	-0.69	[-1.14; -0.25]	2.5%	2.4%
73	43	2.03	1.2600	43	3.85	1.2400	-1.44	[-1.92; -0.97]	2.2%	2.4%
121	119	0.10	0.3000	124	0.20	0.4000	-0.28	[-0.53; -0.03]	7.8%	2.6%
133	25	1.78	1.8800	25	2.34	1.4300	-0.33	[-0.89; 0.23]	1.6%	2.2%
138	23	3.40	2.9000	23	3.20	2.9000	0.07	[-0.51; 0.65]	1.5%	2.2%
Common effect model	251			256			-0.48	[-0.66; -0.30]	15.6%	.
Random effects model							-0.54	[-1.03; -0.05]	.	11.9%
Heterogeneity: $I^2 = 82\%$, $\tau^2 = 0.2593$, $p < 0.01$										
Common effect model	**1687**			**1675**			**-0.50**	**[-0.57; -0.43]**	**100.0%**	**.**
Random effects model							**-0.56**	**[-0.76; -0.37]**	**.**	**100.0%**

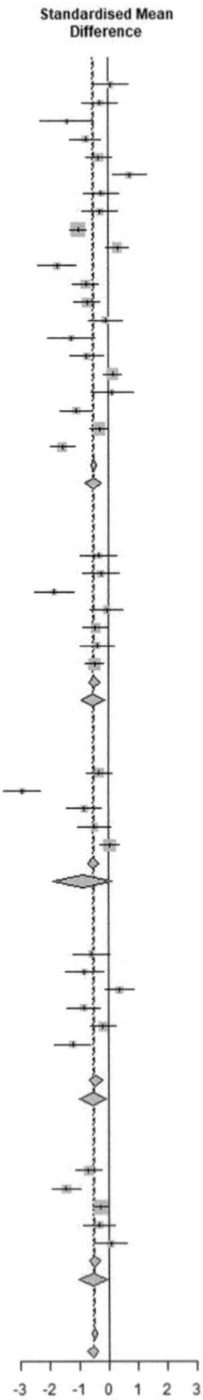

Heterogeneity: $I^2 = 84\%$, $\tau^2 = 0.3553$, $p < 0.01$
Test for subgroup differences (common effect): $\chi^2_4 = 0.27$, df = 4 ($p = 0.99$)
Test for subgroup differences (random effects): $\chi^2_4 = 0.47$, df = 4 ($p = 0.98$)

Fig. 16.10 Subgroup analysis by timing of pain measurement

music intervention. The average effect size remained similar, but the precision of the effect decreased with time.

16.5 Discussion

Music-based interventions are effective but highly heterogeneous in reducing pain when compared to usual care. The overall difference is moderate. Pain scores are on average 0.6 standard deviations lower (ranging from 0.5 to 1.0) than usual care independent of the scoring tool. This effect was clinically significant when adjusting by pre-pain scores or when assessing pre-post mean differences. On average, music-induced pain reduction by 1.5/11 (ranging 1–2, based on NRS/VAS of 0–10) units on average when compared to controls, which is considered a small analgesic effect (Jensen et al. 2003; Lee et al. 2003; Martin et al. 2013). The heterogeneity of the results is explained in small part by pain reporting methods and by musical properties of used songs, and much less by demographics, clinical context, or intervention design.

The strongest predictor of music-induced analgesia was duration of intervention. Based on our results from meta-regression, music interventions should last around 33 minutes to achieve a minimally significant small effect size (SMD −0.2). Interestingly, duration did not explain the large heterogeneity observed, likely due to other hidden variables. For example, music duration effect might depend on the duration of the pain stimuli. A brief pain, like in short procedures, might not require the same amount of music exposure as a longer surgical procedure. Also the severity of the pain; it is possible that more severe pain might require longer musical analgesic interventions, but current data is not enough to assess this hypotheses.

Our subgroup results for different variables related to the clinical setting and population show that currently there is no specific context in which music-induced analgesia will work best or worse. This finding is consistent with the available literature. The effect size of our meta-analysis is similar to those reported in broad meta-analysis in all types of pain (Martin-Saavedra et al. 2018b; Lee 2016), acute surgical pain (Hole et al. 2015; Li et al. 2024; Fu et al. 2021; Hung et al. 2018; Kühlmann et al. 2018; van der Heijden et al. 2015; Lee et al. 2023), cancer and chronic pain (Bradt et al. 2021; Bro et al. 2018; Yangöz and Özer 2019; Garza-Villarreal et al. 2017; Tsai et al. 2014; Li et al. 2020b; da Silva Santa et al. 2021), palliative care (Gao et al. 2019), and pain in pediatric patients (Ting et al. 2022).

This moderate analgesic effect of music remains constant even throughout different conditions such as hemodialysis (Yangöz and Özer 2022; Wu et al. 2021), cardiac procedures (Chandrababu et al. 2021; Kakar et al. 2021; Wang et al. 2020a), abdominal surgery (Dale 2021), patients with burns (Monsalve-Duarte et al. 2022; Li et al. 2022; Fardin et al. 2020), post-cesarean delivery (Khaity et al. 2023; Weingarten et al. 2021), endoscopic procedures (Wang et al. 2014; Sorkpor et al. 2021; García-Perdomo et al. 2018; Abd-ElGawad et al. 2023), orthopedic surgery (Lin et al. 2020b; Patiyal et al. 2021), dental procedures (Tan et al. 2023), biopsy procedures (Wu et al. 2021; Song et al. 2018; Ashour et al. 2022), venipuncture

(Yamada et al. 2023), urologic procedures (Kyriakides et al. 2018), and fibromyalgia (Wang et al. 2020b).

Larger effect sizes have only been reported in labor-related pain (Maleki and Youseflu 2023; Chuang et al. 2019; Santiváñez-Acosta et al. 2020; Wu et al. 2020; Hakimi et al. 2021), reproductive assistive therapies (Mahmoud et al. 2022), burn-care-related procedures (Li et al. 2017). Nonsignificant effects or lower pooled effects were described in meta-analysis in colonoscopy (Bechtold et al. 2009; Shanmuganandan et al. 2017), one meta-analysis in advanced cancer (Huda et al. 2023), plastic surgery (Zapata-Copete et al. 2019), and one in orthopedic surgery (Yu et al. 2020). Therefore, music can be used in any type of pain and clinical condition and a moderate but variable effect should be expected.

The following special situations should be taken into account when deciding if music-based interventions could be used. Pain in male-only conditions might not respond to music as it does in conditions affecting female only or both sexes. Adult patients seem to experience less music-induced analgesia than children and infants. Music-induced analgesia also seems to be more consistent in adults than in pediatric populations. The analgesic effect of music might also be larger in nonsurgical procedural pain. Dental procedures seem to respond to music more homogeneously but with less consistency compared to other procedures.

As expected, quality of the studies does affect reported results. This was clear from subgroup analysis showing that blinding impacted the effect size. Given music is an intervention in which the patient will rarely be blinded, single blinding is the minimum degree of concealment that music research should continue to achieve. Interestingly, tests of moderators in metaregression did not show that blinding had a significant effect on the size of music-induced analgesia. Therefore, the current result and available evidence, despite being open label in many cases, is reliable.

Double blinding might be possible with certain designs, such as factorial crossover trials with multiple groups, music given during procedures under general anesthesia, or not disclosing to patients music is known to have analgesic properties (given the benign nature of the intervention). Our study suggested a trend for double blinding to be associated with a nonsignificant range of music-induced analgesia. This was likely due to underpowering (low number of studies and patients), so we encourage authors to develop mixed-methods studies to achieve double or triple blinding in the future.

Another evidence of quality (or risk of bias) affecting results is that the lack of intervention details described yielded larger effects in most subgroup meta-analyses. This was mostly evident in subgroup analysis of musical properties of used songs and characteristics of the intervention itself. Subgroup meta-analysis showed that the effect size tended to be larger in studies not providing details. This was particularly evident in analysis of the timing of the intervention (pre-, intra-, or post-procedural). Meta-regression showed that studies not describing these details predicted larger effects.

Preferred music is consistently more effective than non-preferred music. However, the effect size is minimal (SMD < 0.2). This was similar to our subgroup meta-analysis in which there was no significant difference based on participation of researcher or patient in the selection of music. However, a trend favoring research selection without patient involvement was observed. Therefore, we strongly recommend using music based on the patient's preference in clinical practice, whereas in research, music should be controlled solely by the investigator. Researcher-controlled music will allow control of music properties, intervention design, and clinical context in order to advance music-based research.

Although nonsignificant differences were noted, active music interventions and predesigned songs yielded a moderate to large effect size, with slightly better heterogeneity. Music, pre-, intra-, and postoperatively, was effective in reducing pain with no significant differences when comparing effect sizes. This is something that has been reported in prior meta-analysis on surgical pain (Hole et al. 2015; Dale 2021; Fu et al. 2020). This is even true in music played during general anesthesia (Fu et al. 2021). Live music was the only modality of administration of music that might be not effective in certain situations; however, this is likely due to underpowered results.

Regarding music properties, results have improved compared to meta-analysis from 2018. Description of music in terms of music theory or specifying song used (allowing for musically analyzing the intervention) have increased. That is reflected in our subgroup meta-analysis that was feasible and yielded results for most studied variables which was not achievable back in 2018.

In this sense, the main conclusion, similar to meta-analysis from 2018, is that music with no lyrics, no percussion, and slow (60–80 bpm) tempo provides a reliable but heterogeneous analgesic effect. We recommend using these properties as a starting point to choose a specific song for interventions in clinical practice if Western music is being used. Turkish/Persian folk music modes were the only musical modality that was associated with a homogeneous moderate size of analgesia and is strongly recommended to be used in clinical practice. Individual maqams were not able to be tested but the most commonly used in studies were Acemaşiran and Rehavi. Given the superiority of these qualities of Western and Middle Eastern music has not been assessed or proven, we recommend starting to use these as "music analgesic controls" for future research.

Trends from subgroup analysis suggest that certain music properties should be avoided. Fast or very slow tempo (<60 bpm or >80 bpm), percussive content, too high (65–80 dB) or too low (<60 dB) volume, lyrical content, and major modes may be ineffective in certain cases. Particularly percussive content and high intensity (65–80 dB) should be avoided in clinical practice but may be used in research as control (or placebo). We strongly recommend avoiding binaural beats, despite being effective too (see subgroup analysis), music without binaural beats has a small but significantly larger analgesic effect.

Predesigned interventions tended to have larger effects with smaller heterogeneity. Using single musical pieces yielded a smaller effect but improved heterogeneity. Given that single songs and predesigned interventions seem to be equivalent to multiple and non-predesigned interventions; we recommend using single and predesigned interventions for future research. We specially encourage researchers to do this to directly compare specific music properties.

Binaural music and U-sequence (Music Care) interventions were used by different researchers. As mentioned above, despite being effective, binaural music is less effective than non-binaural music and should be avoided if pain is the therapeutic target. U-sequence is effective but there are not enough studies comparing non-U-sequenced songs to assess superiority, equivalence, or inferiority. Occasio adolore is a predesigned composition that was created exclusively for a study, so it is not known by common public (controls familiarity) and has been effective in its original study and a second study in Turkey. We invite researchers to use these predesigned interventions as readily available interventions for clinical practice, as guides to compose new interventions, and particularly as controls for research.

Heterogeneity improved by >10 points by the method in which pain was compared or reported. Pain is a personal experience (Raja et al. 2020). In other words, 3/10 is never the same pain for two different individuals. In fact, pain intensity perception can change with time (Raja et al. 2020). Therefore, pain changes (pre-post mean differences) and post-intervention scores adjusted by pre-interventions scores is the recommended way of studying analgesia.

Given the lack of good pre-post test meta-analysis methods (Cuijpers et al. 2017), we decided to estimate adjusted means from the available data. The resulting data is a "prediction" from a fitted model and therefore does not reflect a true effect. Therefore, we expected that our adjusted-means meta-analysis would fall into sampling and calculation biases leading to overestimation of effect size. Surprisingly a separate meta-analysis with pre-post mean differences yielded similar effect sizes and heterogeneity (71% and 77%). In consequence, we strongly recommend reporting pre or basal pain scores or the mean changes between study timepoints.

Another problem with music-induced analgesia research is the lack of robust trials. Considering pain is the most prevalent complaint or symptom, the number of included individuals per studies is low. Low number of patients will make studies underpowered and ultimately increase heterogeneity. Research in this field should start moving into larger trials to provide stronger conclusions based on stronger statistics.

16.6 Conclusion and Summary of Recommendations

16.6.1 Music Selection/Preparation for Clinical Practice

We recommend using music or preparing music of moderate to slow tempo between 60 and 80 beats per minute and with no lyrics or percussion. For Middle Eastern music, we recommend songs composed under Persian/Turkish Acemaşiran and Rehavi maqams. For Western music, we recommend favoring compositions in minor scales. Using binaural beats or music is not recommended as they are less effective. Volume should be controlled by the patient or researcher within 60–65 dB. We strongly recommend using these characteristics to choose songs based on a patient's preferences, or to provide patients with a list of songs of these characteristics for them to choose.

16.6.2 Type of Music Intervention

Music therapists or music experts should be involved in hospital and clinical care as given active music interventions may induce larger analgesia, and choosing songs based on music properties might require musical expertise. Using predesigned compositions is also recommended for groups or institutions that cannot involve music therapists, or for large clinical populations in which individual therapist involvement cannot be achieved. We strongly recommend music interventions of 30 minutes or more to achieve a clinically relevant effect. Music interventions can be given every other day as the effects may last for over 24 hours.

16.6.3 Clinical Context

Music provides a small to moderate clinical analgesia that is consistent among different populations and clinical context. Pediatric patients seem to respond better to music-induced analgesia than adults but it is recommended for all ages. Analgesia might be challenging to achieve with music in conditions affecting only males. Music should be offered peri-operatively to patients undergoing any type of surgical, nonsurgical, or dental procedure.

16.6.4 Music-Induced Analgesia Research

Music research should move to large (population-based sample calculation), single or double blinded, randomized clinical trials using two control groups: usual care and an analgesic music control. We recommend using as analgesic music control a predesigned/composed single song intervention of 60–80 bpm, without lyrics or percussion, in minor scales (Western music) or Acemaşiran/Rehavi maqams (Middle Eastern music). Participation of patients in music selection for research should be avoided to improve controlled settings and intervention. Analgesic music control should be compared to predesigned/compose single song interventions with the desired property to be tested. For example, comparing specific instrumentation or proving inferiority of slow tempo (< 60 bpm). Results of music-induced analgesia should be reported in terms of pre-post differences, or include basal (pre-intervention scores) when able. When not able to report basal pain scores, provide explanation.

References

Abd-ElGawad M, Abdelsattar NK, Kamel MA, Sabri YA, Fathy EM, El-Moez NA, et al. The effect of music intervention in decreasing pain and anxiety during outpatient hysteroscopy procedure: a systematic review and meta-analysis of randomized control trials. BMC Womens Health. 2023;23(1):360.

Akın ME. Effect of music on anxiety and pain during ultrasound-guided core needle breast biopsy: a randomized controlled trial. Diagn Interv Radiol. 2021;27(3):360–5.

Aktaş YY, Karabulut N. The use of cold therapy, music therapy and lidocaine spray for reducing pain and anxiety following chest tube removal. Complement Ther Clin Pract. 2019;34:179–84.

Alam M, Roongpisuthipong W, Kim NA, Goyal A, Swary JH, Brindise RT, et al. Utility of recorded guided imagery and relaxing music in reducing patient pain and anxiety, and surgeon anxiety, during cutaneous surgical procedures: a single-blinded randomized controlled trial. J Am Acad Dermatol. 2016;75(3):585–9.

Aly AE, Hansa I, Ferguson DJ, Vaid NR. The effect of alpha binaural beat music on orthodontic pain after initial archwire placement: a randomized controlled trial. Dental Press J Orthod. 2023;27(6):e2221150.

Amanak K. The effect of the sound of the ney (reed flute) on women in labour in Bursa, Turkey. J Pak Med Assoc. 2020;70(11):1934–7.

Anbalagan S, Velasquez JH, Staufert Gutierrez D, Devagiri S, Nieto D, Ankola P. Music for pain relief of minor procedures in term neonates. Pediatr Res. 2023;95:679.

Anglin C, Knoll P, Mudd B, Ziegler C, Choi K. Music's effect on pain relief during outpatient urological procedures: a single center, randomized control trial focusing on gender differences. Transl Androl Urol. 2021;10(6):2332–9.

Angulo-Perkins A, Aubé W, Peretz I, Barrios FA, Armony JL, Concha L. Music listening engages specific cortical regions within the temporal lobes: differences between musicians and non-musicians. Cortex. 2014;59:126–37.

Antonacci K, Steele N, Wheatley J, Weyant DM, Brozanski B, Stone B, et al. Effects of guitar accompaniment patterns on hospitalized infants: a randomized controlled trial. Music Ther Perspect. 2021;39(2):172–83.

Arruda MALB, Garcia MA, Garcia JBS. Evaluation of the effects of music and poetry in oncologic pain relief: a randomized clinical trial. J Palliat Med. 2016;19(9):943–8.

Ashour ASA, Abd-ElGawad M, Yohanna M, El-Nagar M, Fadl AN, Goda GM, et al. Is music intervention effective in reducing anxiety and pain during breast biopsy procedure? A systematic review and meta-analysis of randomized controlled trials. Support Care Cancer. 2022;30(12):10379–89.

Azeem M, Ejaz Z, Ashraf A, Bukhari F, Ali MM, Rashid A. Music for pain control following orthodontic initial archwire placement. PJMHS. 2021;15(6):1347–8.

Babikian T, Zeltzer L, Tachdjian V, Henry L, Javanfard E, Tucci L, et al. Music as medicine: a review and historical perspective. Alternative and Complementary Therapies. 2013;19(5):251–4.

Barandouzi ZA, Keshavarz M, Montazeri A, Ashayeri H, Rajaei Z. Comparison of the analgesic effect of oral sucrose and/or music in preterm neonates: a double-blind randomized clinical trial. Complement Ther Med. 2020;48:102271.

Barlas T, Sodan HN, Avci S, Cerit ET, Yalcin MM. The impact of classical music on anxiety and pain perception during a thyroid fine needle aspiration biopsy. Hormones (Athens). 2023;22(4):581–5.

Bashiri M, Akçalı D, Coşkun D, Cindoruk M, Dikmen A, Çifdalöz BU. Evaluation of pain and patient satisfaction by music therapy in patients with endoscopy/colonoscopy. Turk J Gastroenterol. 2018;29(5):574–9.

Bay C, Henriquez R, Villarroel L, Gana JC. Effect of music on pediatric endoscopic examinations: a randomized controlled trial. Endosc Int Open. 2021;9(4):E599–605.

Bechtold ML, Puli SR, Othman MO, Bartalos CR, Marshall JB, Roy PK. Effect of music on patients undergoing colonoscopy: a meta-analysis of randomized controlled trials. Dig Dis Sci. 2009;54(1):19–24.

Belloeil V, Tessier Cazeneuve C, Leclercq A, Mercier MB, Legendre G, Corroenne R. Impact of music therapy before first-trimester instrumental termination of pregnancy: a randomised controlled trial. BJOG. 2020;127(6):738–45.

Bergomi P, Chieppi M, Maini A, Mugnos T, Spotti D, Tzialla C, et al. Nonpharmacological techniques to reduce pain in preterm infants who receive heel-lance procedure: a randomized controlled trial. Res Theory Nurs Pract. 2014;28(4):335–48.

Bertacco M, Soyeux O, Durand R, Boudrias P, Wiseman L, Rompré P, et al. Effect of personalized musical intervention on burden of care in dental implant surgery: a pilot randomized controlled trial. J Dent. 2022;120:104091.

Bicego A, Monseur J, Collinet A, Donneau A-F, Fontaine R, Libbrecht D, et al. Complementary treatment comparison for chronic pain management: a randomized longitudinal study. PLoS One. 2021;16(8):e0256001.

Billar R, Kappen P, Mohammadian S, van den Berg C, de Rijke Y, van den Akker E, et al. The effect of recorded music on pain endurance (CRESCENDo) – a randomized controlled trial. Complement Ther Med. 2023;77:102969.

Blichfeldt-Ærø SC, Knutsen TM, Hagen HM, Diep LM, Trondalen G, Halvorsen S. Music therapy as an adjunct in cardiac device lead extraction procedures: a randomized controlled trial. Appl Nurs Res. 2020;56:151376.

Bozkurt M, Erkoc M, Danis E, Can O, Kandemir E, Canat HL. The effect of listening to music on reducing anxiety and pain during extracorporeal shock wave lithotripsy; a randomized controlled study. Med Bull Haseki. 2022;60(5):406–10.

Bradt J, Norris M, Shim M, Gracely EJ, Gerrity P. Vocal music therapy for chronic pain Management in Inner-City African Americans: a mixed methods feasibility study. J Music Ther. 2016;53(2):178–206.

Bradt J, Dileo C, Myers-Coffman K, Biondo J. Music interventions for improving psychological and physical outcomes in people with cancer. Cochrane Database Syst Rev. 2021;10(10):CD006911.

Brix LD, Pedersen ASB. Effect of music intervention in colonoscopy-naïve adults: a randomised controlled trial. Br J Nurs. 2022;31(10):526–32.

Bro ML, Jespersen KV, Hansen JB, Vuust P, Abildgaard N, Gram J, et al. Kind of blue: a systematic review and meta-analysis of music interventions in cancer treatment. Psychooncology. 2018;27(2):386–400.

Brosh K, Roditi E, Wasser LM, Aryan A, Hanhart J, Potter MJ. Effect of music selection on anxiety level during Intravitreal injections for individuals of varying cultures. Ophthalmic Epidemiol. 2022;29(5):582–7.

Browne C, Redmond E, Kelly T, Rogers E, O'Malley P, Nusrat N, et al. Strategies to maximise patient comfort during extracorporeal shockwave lithotripsy – a randomised controlled trial. Surgeon. 2021;19(4):207–11.

Bueno-Serrano G, Alcoba-García MP, Tabares-Jiménez J, González-López R, Llanos-Jiménez L, Mahillo-Fernández I, et al. Value of music and nitrous oxide for pain control during Extracorporeal Shock Wave Lithotripsy (ESWL). Arch Esp Urol. 2022;75(7):624–9.

Buglione A, Saccone G, Mas M, Raffone A, Di Meglio L, di Meglio L, et al. Effect of music on labor and delivery in nulliparous singleton pregnancies: a randomized clinical trial. Arch Gynecol Obstet. 2020;301(3):693–8.

Bulut M, Küçük Alemdar D, Bulut A, Şalcı G. The effect of music therapy, hand massage, and kaleidoscope usage on postoperative nausea and vomiting, pain, fear, and stress in children: a randomized controlled trial. J Perianesth Nurs. 2020;35(6):649–57.

Burrai F, Lupi R, Luppi M, Micheluzzi V, Donati G, Lamanna G, et al. Effects of listening to live singing in patients undergoing hemodialysis: a randomized controlled crossover study. Biol Res Nurs. 2019;21(1):30–8.

Casarin J, Cromi A, Sgobbi B, Di Siena A, Serati M, Bolis ME, et al. Music therapy for preoperative anxiety reduction in women undergoing total laparoscopic hysterectomy: a randomized controlled trial. J Minim Invasive Gynecol. 2021;28(9):1618–1624.e1.

Çelebi D, Yılmaz E, Şahin ST, Baydur H. The effect of music therapy during colonoscopy on pain, anxiety and patient comfort: a randomized controlled trial. Complement Ther Clin Pract. 2020;38:101084.

Çetinkaya F, Aşiret GD, Yilmaz CK, İnci S. Effect of listening to music on anxiety and physiological parameters during coronary angiography: a randomized clinical trial. Eur J Integr Med. 2018;23:37–42.

Chai PR, Schwartz E, Hasdianda MA, Azizoddin DR, Kikut A, Jambaulikar GD, et al. A brief music app to address pain in the emergency department: prospective study. J Med Internet Res. 2020;22(5):e18537.

Chan JC-H, Chan LP, Yeung CP, Tang TW, Yip Mang O, Lam WC. Effect of music on patient experience during Intravitreal injection. J Ophthalmol. 2020;2020:9120235.

Chandrababu R, Ramesh J, Sanatombi Devi E, Nayak BS, George A. Effectiveness of music on anxiety and pain among cardiac surgery patients: a quantitative systematic review and meta-analysis of randomized controlled trials. Int J Nurs Pract. 2021;27(4):e12928.

Chen G-Y, Guo L-Y, Chuang I-C, Kuo H-C, Tsai Y-C, Liu S-F. Effect of music intervention on lung expansion exercises after cardiothoracic surgery. J Clin Med. 2022;11(6):1589.

Chen R, Duan S, Wang Y, He F, Ren L, Peng W. Effects of music therapy on pain relief during fundus screening in infants: randomized controlled clinical trial. Medicine (Baltimore). 2023;102(44):e35878.

Cheung CWC, Yee AWW, Chan PS, Saravelos SH, Chung JPW, Cheung LP, et al. The impact of music therapy on pain and stress reduction during oocyte retrieval – a randomized controlled trial. Reprod Biomed Online. 2018;37(2):145–52.

Cho SW, Choi HJ. Effect of music on reducing anxiety for patients undergoing Transrectal ultrasound-guided prostate biopsies: randomized prospective trial. Urol J. 2016;13(2):2612–4.

Choi S, Park S-G, Lee H-H. The analgesic effect of music on cold pressor pain responses: the influence of anxiety and attitude toward pain. PLoS One. 2018a;13(8):e0201897.

Choi S, Park S-G, Bellan L, Lee H-H, Chung SK. Crossover clinical trial of pain relief in cataract surgery. Int Ophthalmol. 2018b;38(3):1027–33.

Choi EK, Baek J, Lee D, Kim DY. Effect on music therapy on quality of recovery and postoperative pain after gynecological laparoscopy. Medicine (Baltimore). 2023;102(9):e33071.

Chuang C-H, Chen P-C, Lee CS, Chen C-H, Tu Y-K, Wu S-C. Music intervention for pain and anxiety management of the primiparous women during labour: a systematic review and meta-analysis. J Adv Nurs. 2019;75(4):723–33.

Cici R, Bulbuloglu S, Kapikiran G. Effect of meditation music and comedy movie interventions on postoperative kinesiophobia and pain in patients undergoing total knee arthroplasty. ANZ J Surg. 2023;93(1–2):302–9.

Çift A, Benlioglu C. Effect of different musical types on patient's relaxation, anxiety and pain perception during shock wave lithotripsy: a randomized controlled study. Urol J. 2020;17(1):19–23.

Cimen SG, Oğuz E, Gundogmus AG, Cimen S, Sandikci F, Ayli MD. Listening to music during arteriovenous fistula surgery alleviates anxiety: a randomized single-blind clinical trial. World J Transplant. 2020;10(4):79–89.

Citlik-Saritas S, Saritas S, Cevik-Akyil R, Isik K. The effects of Turkish classical music on physiological parameters, pain and analgesic use in patients with myocardial infarction: a non-randomized controlled study. Eur J Integr Med. 2018;22:50–3.

Clark M, Isaacks-Downton G, Wells N, Redlin-Frazier S, Eck C, Hepworth JT, et al. Use of preferred music to reduce emotional distress and symptom activity during radiation therapy. J Music Ther. 2006;43(3):247–65.

Colebaugh CA, Wilson JM, Flowers KM, Overstreet D, Wang D, Edwards RR, et al. The impact of varied music applications on pain perception and situational pain catastrophizing. J Pain. 2023;24(7):1181–92.

Contreras-Molina M, Rueda-Núñez A, Pérez-Collado ML, García-Maestro A. Effect of music therapy on anxiety and pain in the critical polytraumatised patient. Enferm Intensiva (Engl Ed). 2021;32(2):79–87.

Corrigan MJ, Keeler JR, Miller HD, Ben Khallouq BA, Fowler SB. Music therapy and retinopathy of prematurity screening: using recorded maternal singing and heartbeat for post exam recovery. J Perinatol. 2020;40(12):1780–8.

Cuijpers P, Weitz E, Cristea IA, Twisk J. Pre-post effect sizes should be avoided in meta-analyses. Epidemiol Psychiatr Sci. 2017;26(4):364–8.

da Silva Santa IN, Schveitzer MC, Dos Santos MLBM, Ghelman R, Filho VO. MUSIC INTERVENTIONS IN PEDIATRIC ONCOLOGY: systematic review and meta-analysis. Complement Ther Med. 2021;59:102725.

Dabu-Bondoc S, Vadivelu N, Benson J, Perret D, Kain ZN. Hemispheric synchronized sounds and perioperative analgesic requirements. Anesth Analg. 2010;110(1):208–10.

Daihimfar F, Babamohamadi H, Ghorbani R. A comparison of the effects of acupressure and music on venipuncture pain intensity in children: a randomized controlled clinical trial. Pain Res Manag. 2024;2024:2504732.

Dale VH. The impact of perioperative music on abdominal surgery patients' experience of postoperative pain: a systematic review and meta-analysis. J Perioper Pract. 2021;31(1–2):31–43.

Dallı ÖE, Yıldırım Y, Aykar FŞ, Kahveci F. The effect of music on delirium, pain, sedation and anxiety in patients receiving mechanical ventilation in the intensive care unit. Intensive Crit Care Nurs. 2023;75:103348.

de Melo GM, Cardoso MVLML, de Almeida PC, Rodrigues EC. Effect of music combined with swaddling on pain in full-term newborns: randomized clinical trial. Rev Bras Enferm. 2021;75(3):e20210017.

Delimar V, Miloš O, Hančević M, Bilić H, Krbot Skorić M, Milivojević I, et al. Factors contributing to the reduction of pain during electromyography and nerve conduction studies. Psychiatr Danub. 2019;31(Suppl 5):774–80.

Demir K, Konuk Şener D. The effect of auditory stimuli on the pain and physiological parameters of children on mechanical ventilation during aspiration procedure: a randomized controlled trial. J Spec Pediatr Nurs. 2023;28(4):e12416.

Demirci H, van der Storm SL, Huizing NJ, Fräser M, Stufkens SAS, Krips R, et al. Watching a movie or listening to music is effective in managing perioperative anxiety and pain: a randomised controlled trial. Knee Surg Sports Traumatol Arthrosc. 2023;31(12):6069–79.

Deng C, Xie Y, Liu Y, Li Y, Xiao Y. Aromatherapy plus music therapy improve pain intensity and anxiety scores in patients with breast cancer during perioperative periods: a randomized controlled trial. Clin Breast Cancer. 2022;22(2):115–20.

Dhokia M, Elander J, Clements K, Gilbert P. A randomized-controlled pilot trial of an online compassionate mind training intervention to help people with chronic pain avoid analgesic misuse. Psychol Addict Behav. 2020;34(7):726–33.

Diri MA, Çetinkaya F, Gül M. The effects of listening to music on anxiety, pain, and satisfaction during urodynamic study: a randomized controlled trial. Urol Int. 2019;103(4):444–9.

Doğan Bakı E, Ulu Ş, Yüksek A, Arıcan H, Sıvacı R. Does listening to music during tonsillectomy affect Sevoflurane consumption? Med Princ Pract. 2018;27(4):343–9.

Dong Y, Zhang L, Chen L-W, Luo Z-R. Music therapy for pain and anxiety in patients after cardiac valve replacement: a randomized controlled clinical trial. BMC Cardiovasc Disord. 2023;23(1):32.

Doro CA, Neto JZ, Kowalski S. Music therapy reduced nauseas and pain of the patients undergoing hematopoietic stem cells transplantation autologous (randomized clinical trial). 2020.

Drzymalski DM, Lumbreras-Marquez MI, Tsen LC, Camann WR, Farber MK. The effect of patient-selected or preselected music on anxiety during cesarean delivery: a randomized controlled trial. J Matern Fetal Neonatal Med. 2020;33(24):4062–8.

Du J, Shi P, Fang F, Yu H. Effect of music intervention on subjective scores, heart rate variability, and prefrontal hemodynamics in patients with chronic pain. Front Hum Neurosci. 2022;16:1057290.

Duymaz T. The effects of music therapy on gross motor function, pain, and level of functional independence in children with cerebral palsy. Ann Clin Anal Med. 2020:11(2):115–19. https://doi.org/10.4328/ACAM.6171.

Dur Ş, Çevik SG, Ustabaş Yıldız N. The effect of white noise and classical music on pain and physiologic parameters in preterm infants during retinopathy of prematurity examinations: a randomized controlled trial. Early Child Dev Care. 2023;193(1):60–71.

Durgun H, Yaman Aktaş Y. A randomized controlled trial on the effect of music listening on procedural pain, anxiety and comfort levels during cystoscopy. Psychol Health Med. 2023;28(4):1004–12.

Düzgün G, Karadakovan A. Effect of music on pain in cancer patients in palliative care service: a randomized controlled study. Omega (Westport). 2024;88(3):1085–100.

Ebrahimi R, Shroyer AL, Dennis P, Currier J, Lendvai Wischik D. Music can reduce the need for pharmacologic conscious sedation during invasive coronary angiography. J Invasive Cardiol. 2020;32(11):440–4.

Eid MM, Abdelbasset WK, Abdelaty FM, Ali ZA. Effect of physical therapy rehabilitation program combined with music on children with lower limb burns: a twelve-week randomized controlled study. Burns. 2021;47(5):1146–52.

El-Khoury HJ, Brookes JDL, Tan B, Shahbaz S, McCahy PJ. Impact of modern media on analgesic requirements during extracorporeal shockwave lithotripsy. ANZ J Surg. 2020;90(1–2):53–6.

Esteban Pellicer LÁ, Conde Villar AJ, Martínez Rubio JL, Casañas E, Estévez Luaña R. Can music decrease anxiety and pain during dental implant surgery? A randomized clinical trial. J Oral Maxillofac Surg. 2023;81(2):194–200.

Etienne R, Laurent M, Henry A, Bioy A, Salleron J, Schohn CH, et al. Interest of a standardized hypnotic message for the reduction of pain and anxiety in cancer patients treated by capsaicin patch for neuropathic pain: a randomized controlled trial. BMC Complement Med Ther. 2021;21(1):154.

Fardin A, Rezaei SA, Maslakpak MH. Non-pharmacological interventions for anxiety in burn patients: a systematic review and meta-analysis of randomized controlled trials. Complement Ther Med. 2020;49:102341.

Fen BW, Hashim MN, Ju TW, Latiff ZA. Music listening intervention vs local Anaesthetic cream for pain management in infants undergoing Venepuncture: a collaborative trans-disciplinary research. J Pediatr Res. 2018;5(1):1–10.

Fernando GVMC, Wanigabadu LU, Vidanagama B, Samaranayaka TSP, Jeewandara JMKC. "Adjunctive effects of a short session of music on pain, Low-mood and anxiety modulation among cancer patients" – a randomized crossover clinical trial. Indian J Palliat Care. 2019;25(3):367–73.

Ferraz MCL, Santana-Santos E, Pinto JS, Nunes Ribeiro CJ, Santana JFNB, Alves JAB, et al. Analgesic effect of music during wound care among patients with diaphyseal tibial fractures: randomized controlled trial. Eur J Pain. 2021;25(3):541–9.

Fowler-Kerry S, Lander JR. Management of injection pain in children. Pain. 1987;30(2):169–75.

Fu VX, Oomens P, Klimek M, Verhofstad MHJ, Jeekel J. The effect of perioperative music on medication requirement and hospital length of stay: a meta-analysis. Ann Surg. 2020;272(6):961–72.

Fu VX, Sleurink KJ, Janssen JC, Wijnhoven BPL, Jeekel J, Klimek M. Perception of auditory stimuli during general anesthesia and its effects on patient outcomes: a systematic review and meta-analysis. Can J Anaesth. 2021;68(8):1231–53.

Gallagher LM, Gardner V, Bates D, Mason S, Nemecek J, DiFiore JB, et al. Impact of music therapy on hospitalized patients post-elective Orthopaedic surgery: a randomized controlled trial. Orthop Nurs. 2018;37(2):124–33.

Ganesan P, Manjini KJ, Bathala Vedagiri SC. Effect of music on pain, anxiety and physiological parameters among postoperative sternotomy patients: a randomized controlled trial. J Caring Sci. 2022;11(3):139–47.

Gao Y, Wei Y, Yang W, Jiang L, Li X, Ding J, et al. The effectiveness of music therapy for terminally ill patients: a meta-analysis and systematic review. J Pain Symptom Manag. 2019;57(2):319–29.

García-Perdomo HA, Montealegre Cardona LM, Cordoba-Wagner MJ, Zapata-Copete JA. Music to reduce pain and anxiety in cystoscopy: a systematic review and meta-analysis. J Complement Integr Med. 2018;16(3) https://doi.org/10.1515/jcim-2018-0095.

Garza-Villarreal EA, Pando V, Vuust P, Parsons C. Music-induced analgesia in chronic pain conditions: a systematic review and meta-analysis. Pain Physician. 2017;20(7):597–610.

Gezginci E, Iyigun E, Kibar Y, Bedir S. Three distraction methods for pain reduction during cystoscopy: a randomized controlled trial evaluating the effects on pain, anxiety, and satisfaction. J Endourol. 2018;32(11):1078–84.

Ghasemi M, Hoseinialiabadi P, Yazdanpanah F, Mahani MA, Malekyan L, Najafi K, et al. Comparison of music and vapocoolant spray in reducing the pain of venous cannulation in children age 6-12: a randomized clinical trial. BMC Pediatr. 2022;22(1):237.

Giordano F, Mitrotti A, Losurdo A, Pesino A, Cortese C, Rossini M, et al. Effect of receptive music therapy on pain, anxiety and heart rate variability during percutaneous renal biopsy: a randomized controlled trial. Signa vitae. 2022;16:2721.

Giordano F, Mitrotti A, Losurdo A, Esposito F, Granata A, Pesino A, et al. Effect of music therapy intervention on anxiety and pain during percutaneous renal biopsy: a randomized controlled trial. Clin Kidney J. 2023;16(12):2721–7.

Gochenour KS, Ellis RS, Meredith SL, Vesely KC, Kang P, Haefner S. Music and medicine come together over pain in the air medical transport environment. Air Med J. 2020;39(6):484–8.

Gökçek E, Kaydu A. The effects of music therapy in patients undergoing septorhinoplasty surgery under general anesthesia. Braz J Otorhinolaryngol. 2020;86(4):419–26.

Goktas N, Avci D. The effect of visual and/or auditory distraction techniques on children's pain, anxiety and medical fear in invasive procedures: a randomized controlled trial. J Pediatr Nurs. 2023;73:e27–35.

Golino AJ, Leone R, Gollenberg A, Gillam A, Toone K, Samahon Y, et al. Receptive music therapy for patients receiving mechanical ventilation in the intensive care unit. Am J Crit Care. 2023;32(2):109–15.

Graversen M, Sommer T. Perioperative music may reduce pain and fatigue in patients undergoing laparoscopic cholecystectomy. Acta Anaesthesiol Scand. 2013;57(8):1010–6.

Guerrier G, Bernabei F, Lehmann M, Pellegrini M, Giannaccare G, Rothschild P-R. Efficacy of preoperative music intervention on pain and anxiety in patients undergoing cataract surgery. Front Pharmacol. 2021;12:748296.

Gupta S, Das SK, Jana D, Pal DK. Distraction during cystoscopy to reduce pain and increase satisfaction: randomized control study between real-time visualization versus listening to music versus combined music and real-time visualization. Urol Ann. 2019;11(1):33–8.

Gür EY, Apay SE. The effect of cognitive behavioral techniques using virtual reality on birth pain: a randomized controlled trial. Midwifery. 2020;91:102856.

Gürkan O, Kaya MF. Effect of music on anxiety and pain levels of patients undergoing thyroid fine needle aspiration biopsy: a randomized controlled study. Acad Radiol. 2023;31:538.

Hakimi S, Hajizadeh K, Hasanzade R, Ranjbar M. A systematic review and meta-analysis of the effects of music therapy on postpartum anxiety and pain levels. J Caring Sci. 2021;10(4):230–7.

Halder A, Kumar A, Hariharan U, Manjhi B. Effect of perioperative music therapy/medicine on postoperative pain in women undergoing elective lower segment caesarean section delivery under spinal Anaesthesia: a case-control study. JCDR. 2022;16:UC10–5.

Haqiqi M, Hashem-Dabaghian F, Ghandhari A, Amini-Behbahani F, Akhtari E. Comparing the therapeutic effects of two Iranian musical modes with standard treatment in acute sciatica pain: a pilot study. J Popul Ther Clin Pharmacol. 2023;30(15):94–102.

Harper FWK, Heath AS, Moore TF, Kim S, Heath EI. Using music as a tool for distress reduction during cancer chemotherapy treatment. JCO Oncol Pract. 2023;19(12):1133–42.

Hedayati J, Bagheri-Nesami M, Elyasi F, Hosseinnataj A. The effect of music therapy on the pain and anxiety levels of patients experiencing wound healing by suturing in the emergency wards. Anesth Pain Med. 2023;13(1):e132943.

Hilal Z, Alici F, Tempfer CB, Rath K, Nar K, Rezniczek GA. Mozart for reducing patient anxiety during colposcopy: a randomized controlled trial. Obstet Gynecol. 2018;132(4):1047–55.

Hohneck A, Meissner R, Reyser C, Heinemann L, Christians K, Merx K, et al. Effects of a sound intervention on physical and emotional Well-being in patients with cancer: a prospective randomized trial. Oncol Res Treat. 2023;46(1–2):1–10.

Hole J, Hirsch M, Ball E, Meads C. Music as an aid for postoperative recovery in adults: a systematic review and meta-analysis. Lancet. 2015;386(10004):1659–71.

Howard C, Powell AS, Pavlidis E, Pavel A, Finn D, Allen A, et al. No effect of a musical intervention on stress response to venepuncture in a neonatal population. Acta Paediatr. 2020;109(3):511–7.

Howlin C, Stapleton A, Rooney B. Tune out pain: agency and active engagement predict decreases in pain intensity after music listening. PLoS One. 2022;17(8):e0271329.

Hsieh C, Kong J, Kirsch I, Edwards RR, Jensen KB, Kaptchuk TJ, et al. Well-loved music robustly relieves pain: a randomized, controlled trial. PLoS One. 2014;9(9):e107390.

Hsieh F-C, Miao N-F, Tseng I-J, Chiu H-L, Kao C-C, Liu D, et al. Effect of home-based music intervention versus ambient music on breast cancer survivors in the community: a feasibility study in Taiwan. Eur J Cancer Care (Engl). 2019;28(4):e13064.

Hsu K-C, Chen LF, Hsiep PH. Effect of music intervention on burn patients' pain and anxiety during dressing changes. Burns. 2016;42(8):1789–96.

Huang R, Wang J, Wu D, Long H, Yang X, Liu H, et al. The effects of customised brainwave music on orofacial pain induced by orthodontic tooth movement. Oral Dis. 2016;22(8):766–74.

Huda N, Banda KJ, Liu A-I, Huang T-W. Effects of music therapy on spiritual Well-being among patients with advanced cancer in palliative care: a meta-analysis of randomized controlled trials. Semin Oncol Nurs. 2023;39(6):151481.

Hung T-T, Liu Y-C, Tsai P-C, Lin M-F. The pain-relief efficacy of passive music-based interventions in cancer patients undergoing diagnostic biopsies and surgery: a systematic review and meta-analysis. Hu Li Za Zhi. 2018;65(1):70–82.

Inayama E, Yamada Y, Kishida M, Kitamura M, Nishino T, Ota K, et al. Effect of music in reducing pain during hemodialysis access cannulation: a crossover randomized controlled trial. Clin J Am Soc Nephrol. 2022;17(9):1337–45.

Innes KE, Selfe TK, Kandati S, Wen S, Huysmans Z. Effects of mantra meditation versus music listening on knee pain, function, and related outcomes in older adults with knee osteoarthritis: an exploratory Randomized Clinical Trial (RCT). Evid Based Complement Alternat Med. 2018;2018:7683897.

Jacq G, Melot K, Bezou M, Foucault L, Courau-Courtois J, Cavelot S, et al. Music for pain relief during bed bathing of mechanically ventilated patients: a pilot study. PLoS One. 2018;13(11):e0207174.

Jacquier S, Nay M-A, Muller G, Muller L, Mathonnet A, Lefèvre-Benzekri D, et al. Effect of a musical intervention during the implantation of a central venous catheter or a dialysis catheter in the intensive care unit: a prospective randomized pilot study. Anesth Analg. 2022;134(4):781–90.

James K, Drummond PD. RAPID INDUCTION ANALGESIA FOR CAPSAICIN-INDUCED PAIN IN UNIVERSITY STUDENTS: a randomized, controlled trial. Int J Clin Exp Hypn. 2018;66(4):428–50.

Jensen MP, Chen C, Brugger AM. Interpretation of visual analog scale ratings and change scores: a reanalysis of two clinical trials of postoperative pain. J Pain. 2003;4(7):407–14.

Jethani B. Influence of music therapy on anxiety, pain perception, heart rate and blood pressure of patients undergoing endodontic treatment—a randomized control trial. IJSR. 2019:1–5.

Johnson AJ, Elkins GR. Effects of music and relaxation suggestions on experimental pain. Int J Clin Exp Hypn. 2020;68(2):225–45.

Kakar E, Billar RJ, van Rosmalen J, Klimek M, Takkenberg JJM, Jeekel J. Music intervention to relieve anxiety and pain in adults undergoing cardiac surgery: a systematic review and meta-analysis. Open Heart. 2021;8(1):e001474.

Kakar E, Ottens T, Stads S, Wesselius S, Gommers DAMPJ, Jeekel J, et al. Effect of a music intervention on anxiety in adult critically ill patients: a multicenter randomized clinical trial. J Intensive Care. 2023;11(1):36.

Kakde A, Lim MJ, Shen H, Tan HS, Tan CW, Sultana R, et al. Effect of music listening on perioperative anxiety, acute pain and pain catastrophizing in women undergoing elective cesarean delivery: a randomized controlled trial. BMC Anesthesiol. 2023;23(1):109.

Karakuş Selçuk A, Baysal E. The effect of dark chocolate and music on pain and anxiety in young women with primary dysmenorrhea: randomized controlled trial. Eur J Integr Med. 2022;56:102192.

Karalar M, Keles I, Doğantekin E, Kahveci OK, Sarici H. Reduced pain and anxiety with music and noise-canceling headphones during shockwave lithotripsy. J Endourol. 2016;30(6):674–7.

Kavak Akelma F, Altınsoy S, Arslan MT, Ergil J. Effect of favorite music on postoperative anxiety and pain. Anaesthesist. 2020;69(3):198–204.

Kavakli AS, Kavrut Ozturk N, Yavuzel Adas H, Kudsioglu ST, Ayoglu RU, Özmen S, et al. The effects of music on anxiety and pain in patients during carotid endarterectomy under regional anesthesia: a randomized controlled trial. Complement Ther Med. 2019;44:94–101.

Khaity A, Tarek M, Alabdallat Y, Albakri K, Gabra MD, Ghaith Hazem S. The effect of music intervention on anxiety and pain during cesarean delivery: a meta-analysis of 1513 patients. Int J Med Students. 2023;10:S227.

Kiani MA, Heydarian F, Feyzabadi Z, Saeidi M, Jafari SA, Hebrani P. Effect of music and toys on reducing pain during colonoscopy and acceptance of colonoscopy by children: a randomized clinical trial. Electron Physician. 2019;11(4):7652–9.

Killin A. The origins of music. Music Sci. 2018;1:205920431775197.

Kim S, Jeong H. Effects of patient-selected music listening on the pain and anxiety of patients undergoing hemodialysis: a randomized controlled trial. Healthcare (Basel). 2021;9(11):1437.

Ko SY, Leung DY, Wong EM. Effects of easy listening music intervention on satisfaction, anxiety, and pain in patients undergoing colonoscopy: a pilot randomized controlled trial. Clin Interv Aging. 2019;14:977–86.

Koca GY, Aylaz R. The effect of music on pain and anxiety in patients receiving chemotherapy during COVID-19. Eur J Cancer Care (Engl). 2022;31(6):e13715.

Konar MC, Islam K, Sil A, Nayek K, Barik K. Effect of music on outcomes of birth asphyxia: a randomized controlled trial. J Trop Pediatr. 2021;67(2):fmab009.

Küçük Alemdar D, Bulut A, Yilmaz G. Impact of music therapy and hand massage in the pediatric intensive care unit on pain, fear and stress: randomized controlled trial. J Pediatr Nurs. 2023;71:95–103.

Kühlmann AYR, de Rooij A, Kroese LF, van Dijk M, Hunink MGM, Jeekel J. Meta-analysis evaluating music interventions for anxiety and pain in surgery. Br J Surg. 2018;105(7):773–83.

Kyriakides R, Jones P, Geraghty R, Skolarikos A, Liatsikos E, Traxer O, et al. Effect of music on outpatient urological procedures: a systematic review and meta-analysis from the European Association of Urology section of Uro-technology. J Urol. 2018;199(5):1319–27.

Laframboise-Otto JM, Horodyski M, Parvataneni HK, Horgas AL. A randomized controlled trial of music for pain relief after arthroplasty surgery. Pain Manag Nurs. 2021;22(1):86–93.

Law HY, Ng DYT, Chung CD. Use of music in reducing pain during outpatient hysteroscopy: prospective randomized trial. J Obstet Gynaecol Res. 2021;47(3):904–12.

Lee JH. The effects of music on pain: a meta-analysis. J Music Ther. 2016;53(4):430–77.

Lee JS, Hobden E, Stiell IG, Wells GA. Clinically important change in the visual analog scale after adequate pain control. Acad Emerg Med. 2003;10(10):1128–30.

Lee BC, Kim HO, Chung HS, Heo SH, Jeong YY, Kim MS, et al. Does music from noise-canceling headphones have a beneficial effect on men undergoing transrectal ultrasound-guided prostate biopsy? Prostate Int. 2021;9(3):145–50.

Lee HY, Nam ES, Chai GJ, Kim DM. Benefits of music intervention on anxiety, pain, and physiologic response in adults undergoing surgery: a systematic review and meta-analysis. Asian Nurs Res (Korean Soc Nurs Sci). 2023;17(3):138–49.

Leonard H. Live music therapy during rehabilitation after total knee arthroplasty: a randomized controlled trial. J Music Ther. 2019;56(1):61–89.

Li J, Zhou L, Wang Y. The effects of music intervention on burn patients during treatment procedures: a systematic review and meta-analysis of randomized controlled trials. BMC Complement Altern Med. 2017;17(1):158.

Li L, Shu W, Li Z, Liu Q, Wang H, Feng B, et al. Using yoga nidra recordings for pain management in patients undergoing colonoscopy. Pain Manag Nurs. 2019;20(1):39–46.

Li W, Bryan RG, Kheterpal A, Simeone FJ, Chang CY, Torriani M, et al. The effect of music on pain and subjective experience in image-guided musculoskeletal corticosteroid injections: a randomized controlled trial. Skeletal Radiol. 2020a;49(3):435–41.

Li Y, Xing X, Shi X, Yan P, Chen Y, Li M, et al. The effectiveness of music therapy for patients with cancer: a systematic review and meta-analysis. J Adv Nurs. 2020b;76(5):1111–23.

Li Y, Liu FL, Yuan J, Li ZW, Liu NX, Guan N. Meta-analysis of the interventional effects of music therapy on pain and anxiety of burn patients in wound dressing change. Zhonghua Shao Shang Za Zhi. 2022;38(11):1079–84.
Li G, Yu L, Yang Y, Deng J, Shao L, Zeng C. Effects of perioperative music therapy on patients with postoperative pain and anxiety: a systematic review and meta-analysis. J Integr Complement Med. 2024;30(1):37–46.
Lin Z-W, Huang S-T, Xu N, Cao H, Chen L-W, Chen Q. Effect of music therapy on the chronic pain and midterm quality of life of patients after mechanical valve replacement. Ann Thorac Cardiovasc Surg. 2020a;26(4):196–201.
Lin C-L, Hwang S-L, Jiang P, Hsiung N-H. Effect of music therapy on pain after orthopedic surgery-a systematic review and meta-analysis. Pain Pract. 2020b;20(4):422–36.
Loong LJ, Ling KK, Tai ELM, Kueh YC, Kuan G, Hussein A. The effect of binaural beat audio on operative pain and anxiety in cataract surgery under topical anaesthesia: a randomized controlled trial. Int J Environ Res Public Health. 2022;19(16):10194.
Low MY, Lacson C, Zhang F, Kesslick A, Bradt J. Vocal music therapy for chronic pain: a mixed methods feasibility study. J Altern Complement Med. 2020;26(2):113–22.
Luis M, Doss R, Zayed B, Yacoub M. Effect of live oud music on physiological and psychological parameters in patients undergoing cardiac surgery. Glob Cardiol Sci Pract. 2019;2019(2):e201917.
Lunde SJ, Vuust P, Garza-Villarreal EA, Kirsch I, Møller A, Vase L. Music-induced analgesia in healthy participants is associated with expected pain levels but not opioid or dopamine-dependent mechanisms. Front Pain Res (Lausanne). 2022;3:734999.
Mackintosh J, Cone G, Harland K, Sriram KB. Music reduces state anxiety scores in patients undergoing pleural procedures: a randomised controlled trial. Intern Med J. 2018;48(9):1041–8.
Madson AT, Silverman MJ. The effect of music therapy on relaxation, anxiety, pain perception, and nausea in adult solid organ transplant patients. J Music Ther. 2010;47(3):220–32.
Mahmoud MY, Labib K, Sileem SA, Mustafa FA, Hamed WM, Abd Elhamid A, et al. The impact of music therapy on anxiety and pregnancy rate among infertile women undergoing assisted reproductive technologies: a systematic review and meta-analysis. J Psychosom Obstet Gynaecol. 2022;43(2):205–13.
Maleki A, Youseflu S. The effect of music-based interventions on short-term postpartum episiotomy pain: a systematic review and meta-analysis. Heliyon. 2023;9(4):e14785.
Martin WJJM, Ashton-James CE, Skorpil NE, Heymans MW, Forouzanfar T. What constitutes a clinically important pain reduction in patients after third molar surgery? Pain Res Manag. 2013;18(6):319–22.
Martin-Saavedra JS, Ruiz-Sternberg AM. The effects of music listening on the management of pain in primary dysmenorrhea: a randomized controlled clinical trial. Nord J Music Ther. 2020;29:1–18.
Martin-Saavedra JS, Saade-Lemus S. Music's objective classification improves quality of music-induced analgesia studies. Pain. 2019;160(6):1482–3.
Martin-Saavedra JS, Vergara-Mendez LD, Talero-Gutiérrez C. Music is an effective intervention for the management of pain: an umbrella review. Complement Ther Clin Pract. 2018a;32:103–14.
Martin-Saavedra JS, Vergara-Mendez LD, Pradilla I, Vélez-van-Meerbeke A, Talero-Gutiérrez C. Standardizing music characteristics for the management of pain: a systematic review and meta-analysis of clinical trials. Complement Ther Med. 2018b;41:81–9.
Mateu M, Alda O, Inda M-D-M, Margarit C, Ajo R, Morales D, et al. Randomized, controlled, crossover study of self-administered Jacobson relaxation in chronic, nonspecific, low-back pain. Altern Ther Health Med. 2018;24(6):22–30.
Mateu-Capell M, Arnau A, Juvinyà D, Montesinos J, Fernandez R. Sound isolation and music on the comfort of mechanically ventilated critical patients. Nurs Crit Care. 2019;24(5):290–8.
McClintock G, Wong E, Mancuso P, Lalak N, Gassner P, Haghighi K, et al. Music during flexible cystoscopy for pain and anxiety – a patient-blinded randomised control trial. BJU Int. 2021;128(Suppl 1):27–32.
Merliot-Gailhoustet L, Raimbert C, Garnier O, Carr J, De Jong A, Molinari N, et al. Discomfort improvement for critically ill patients using electronic relaxation devices: results of the cross-

over randomized controlled trial E-CHOISIR (electronic-CHOIce of a system for intensive care relaxation). Crit Care. 2022;26(1):263.
Merry M, Silverman MJ. Effects of patient-preferred live music on positive and negative affect and pain with adults on a post-surgical oncology unit: a randomized study. Arts Psychother. 2021;72:101739.
Miladinia M, Voss JG, Molavynejad S, Malehi AS, Zarea K, Nouri EM, et al. Slow-stroke Back massage compared with music therapy for leukemia-related pain and fatigue: a randomized controlled trial. JCO Oncol Pract. 2021;17(11):e1614–21.
Mitchell LA, MacDonald RAR. An experimental investigation of the effects of preferred and relaxing music listening on pain perception. J Music Ther. 2006;43(4):295–316.
Mondanaro JF, Sara GA, Thachil R, Pranjić M, Rossetti A, EunHye Sim G, et al. The effects of clinical music therapy on resiliency in adults undergoing infusion: a randomized, controlled trial. J Pain Symptom Manag. 2021;61(6):1099–108.
Monsalve-Duarte S, Betancourt-Zapata W, Suarez-Cañon N, Maya R, Salgado-Vasco A, Prieto-Garces S, et al. Music therapy and music medicine interventions with adult burn patients: a systematic review and meta-analysis. Burns. 2022;48(3):510–21.
Mounier S, Cambonie G, Baleine J, Le Roux M, Bringuier S, Milési C. Music therapy during basic daily care in critically ill children: a randomized crossover clinical trial. J Pediatr. 2024;264:113736.
Mousaviasl S, Naeimi S, Maghsoudi F, Darekati SN, Mosaviasl SZ. The effect of distraction techniques on pain intensity and acetaminophen received after tonsillectomy in children aged 5-12 years old. J Evid Based Care. 2023;13:52–60.
Mumm J-N, Eismann L, Rodler S, Vilsmaier T, Zehni AZ, Apfelbeck M, et al. Listening to music during outpatient cystoscopy reduces pain and anxiety and increases satisfaction: results from a prospective randomized study. Urol Int. 2021;105(9–10):792–8.
Música indígena colombiana. Maguaré 1987;5.
Muzzi E, Ronfani L, Bossini B, Lezcano C, Orzan E, Barbi E. Effects of intraoperative auditory stimulation on pain and agitation on awakening after pediatric adenotonsillectomy: a randomized clinical trial. JAMA Otolaryngol Head Neck Surg. 2021;147(7):638–45.
Nandeibam Y, Joseph T, Antonisamy B, Kamath MS, Kunjummen AT. Effectiveness of music therapy as an adjuvant to conscious sedation in women undergoing transvaginal oocyte retrieval: a randomized controlled trial. J Obstet Gynaecol Res. 2022;48(6):1409–17.
Nelson D, Berry R, Szczepura K, Mercer CE. Assessing the impact of binaural and non-binaural auditory beat intervention to pain and compression in mammography. Radiography (Lond). 2023;29(1):101–8.
Nikolsky A. The pastoral origin of semiotically functional tonal organization of music. Front Psychol. 2020;11:1358.
Obersnel M, Nardin B, Canepari E, Torelli L, Rizzitelli P, Buchini S, et al. Active production of music as distraction for venipuncture in children and adolescents: a randomized clinical trial. Eur J Pediatr. 2023;182(12):5455–63.
Ölçücü MT, Yılmaz K, Karamık K, Okuducu Y, Özsoy Ç, Aktaş Y, et al. Effects of listening to binaural beats on anxiety levels and pain scores in male patients undergoing cystoscopy and ureteral stent removal: a randomized placebo-controlled trial. J Endourol. 2021;35(1):54–61.
Orak Y, Bakacak SM, Yaylali A, Tolun FI, Kiran H, Boran OF, et al. Effects of music therapy on pain and oxidative stress in oocyte pick-up: a randomized clinical trial. Braz J Anesthesiol. 2020;70(5):491–9.
Orak Y, Tolun FI, Tok A, Turgut C, Bakacak M, Yaylali A, et al. Effect of music therapy on glutathione peroxidase, malondialdehyde and pain in patients undergoing oocyte retrieval: a randomized controlled trial. Eur J Integr Med. 2023;61:102266.
Ortega A, Gauna F, Munoz D, Oberreuter G, Breinbauer HA, Carrasco L. Music therapy for pain and anxiety management in nasal bone fracture reduction: randomized controlled clinical trial. Otolaryngol Head Neck Surg. 2019;161(4):613–9.

Özdemir Ü, Taşcı S, Yıldızhan E, Aslan S, Eser B. The effect of classical turkish music on pain severity and anxiety levels in patients undergoing bone marrow aspiration and biopsy. Pain Manag Nurs. 2019;20(1):82–7.

Öztaş HG, Gökbulut N, İbici Akça E. The effects of sacral massage and music therapy applied to primaparous women in labor on labor pain, postpartum comfort, and posttraumatic growth: a randomized controlled trial. Int J Tradit Complement Med Res. 2023;4(2):38–49.

Öztürk E, Hamidi N, Yikilmaz TN, Özcan C, Başar H. Effect of listening to music on patient anxiety and pain perception during urodynamic study: randomized controlled trial. Low Urin Tract Symptoms. 2019;11(1):39–42.

Öztürk FU, Turnaoğlu H, Uslu N. Preferred music lowers anxiety levels and pain perception while promoting patient satisfaction in women undergoing ultrasound-guided breast biopsy: randomized controlled study. Acta Radiol. 2023;64(3):993–8.

Packiam VT, Nottingham CU, Cohen AJ, Eggener SE, Gerber GS. No effect of music on anxiety and pain during transrectal prostate biopsies: a randomized trial. Urology. 2018;117:31–5.

Page M, McKenzie J, Bossuyt P, Boutron I, Hoffmann T, Mulrow CD, et al. The PRISMA 2020 statement: an updated guideline for reporting systematic reviews. BMJ. 2021;372:n71.

Paoin P, Prasongvej P, Chanthasenanont A, Niumpradit T, Pongrojpaw D, Suwannarurk K. Efficacy of music therapy and Zingiber officinale roscoe aromatherapy for reducing pain during the first stage of labor: a randomized controlled trial. SMJ. 2023;75(10):707–12.

Patiyal N, Kalyani V, Mishra R, Kataria N, Sharma S, Parashar A, et al. Effect of music therapy on pain, anxiety, and use of opioids among patients underwent orthopedic surgery: a systematic review and meta-analysis. Cureus. 2021;13(9):e18377.

Perani D, Saccuman MC, Scifo P, Anwander A, Spada D, Baldoli C, et al. Neural language networks at birth. Proc Natl Acad Sci USA. 2011;108(38):16056–61.

Peretz I. Processing of local and global musical information by unilateral brain-damaged patients. Brain. 1990;113(Pt 4):1185–205.

Peretz I, Kolinsky R, Tramo M, Labrecque R, Hublet C, Demeurisse G, et al. Functional dissociations following bilateral lesions of auditory cortex. Brain. 1994;117(Pt 6):1283–301.

Pongan E, Delphin-Combe F, Krolak-Salmon P, Leveque Y, Tillmann B, Bachelet R, et al. Immediate benefit of art on pain and well-being in community-dwelling patients with mild Alzheimer's. Am J Alzheimers Dis Other Dement. 2020;35:1533317519859202.

Prasad M, Sethi P, Kumari K, Sharma A, Kaur M, Dixit PK, et al. Comparison of binaural tone music vs patient choice music vs midazolam on perioperative anxiety in patients posted for surgery under spinal anaesthesia: a randomized control trial. Cureus. 2023;15(2):e35091.

Quigley C, Ellard R, Arreyedh HA, Droney T, Harney F, Townley D. Classical music for analgesia in laser Panretinal photocoagulation for treatment of diabetic retinopathy. Ir Med J. 2019;112:941.

Rabinowitch T-C, Dassa A, Sadot AS, Trincher A. Outcomes and experiences of an online balance-space music therapy intervention for cancer patients: a mixed methods study. Arts Psychother. 2023;82:101998.

Raglio A, Bettaglio R, Manera MR, Aiello EN, Gontero G, Imbriani C, et al. Feasibility of therapeutic music listening in fibromyalgia: a randomised controlled pilot study. Neurol Sci. 2023;44(2):723–7.

Raja SN, Carr DB, Cohen M, Finnerup NB, Flor H, Gibson S, et al. The revised International Association for the Study of Pain definition of pain: concepts, challenges, and compromises. Pain. 2020;161(9):1976–82.

Ramezani Z, Pasha YZ, Amiri SJ, Hajiahmadi M, Pirnia B. Comparison of the effectiveness of warm compress and music on the pain caused by heel blood sampling in neonates: a single-blind, prospective, randomized controlled trial. Crescent J Med Biol Sci. 2020;7:138–9.

Rapolienė L, Razbadauskas A, Sąlyga J, Martinkėnas A. Stress and fatigue management using Balneotherapy in a short-time randomized controlled trial. Evid Based Complement Alternat Med. 2016;2016:9631684.

Reynaud D, Bouscaren N, Lenclume V, Boukerrou M. Comparing the effects of self-selected MUsic versus predetermined music on patient ANXiety prior to gynaecological surgery: the MUANX randomized controlled trial. Trials. 2021;22(1):535.

Robb SL, Burns DS, Carpenter JS. Reporting guidelines for music-based interventions. J Health Psychol. 2011;16(2):342–52.

Robb SL, Hanson-Abromeit D, May L, Hernandez-Ruiz E, Allison M, Beloat A, et al. Reporting quality of music intervention research in healthcare: a systematic review. Complement Ther Med. 2018;38:24–41.

Rodgers-Melnick SN, Matthie N, Jenerette C, Griest Pell TJ, Lane D, Fu P, et al. The effects of a single electronic music improvisation session on the pain of adults with sickle cell disease: a mixed methods pilot study. J Music Ther. 2018;55(2):156–85.

Rodgers-Melnick SN, Lin L, Gam K, Souza de Santana Carvalho E, Jenerette C, Rowland DY, et al. Effects of Music Therapy on Quality of Life in Adults with Sickle Cell Disease (MUSIQOLS): a mixed methods feasibility study. J Pain Res. 2022;15:71–91.

Roshani B, Rezaei M, Azadi P, Jalilian A. The effect of binaural beat music on reducing anxiety and pain and increasing satisfaction of ophthalmic patients. J Kermanshah Univ Med Sci. 2020;23(4):e99914.

Rossi A, Molinaro A, Savi E, Micheletti S, Galli J, Chirico G, et al. Music reduces pain perception in healthy newborns: a comparison between different music tracks and recoded heartbeat. Early Hum Dev. 2018;124:7–10.

Rosslau K, Herholz SC, Knief A, Ortmann M, Deuster D, Schmidt C-M, et al. Song perception by professional singers and actors: an MEG study. PLoS One. 2016;11(2):e0147986.

Sadeghi M, Sarlak H, Nakhostin A, Almasi-Hashiani A. Which audio distraction technique is more effective for reduction the pain and anxiety of pediatric dental patients; "music" or "kids-story"? A randomized split-mouth crossover clinical trial. J Psychosom Res. 2023;168:111218.

Sánchez-Jáuregui T, Téllez A, Juárez-García D, García CH, García FE. Clinical hypnosis and music in breast biopsy: a randomized clinical trial. Am J Clin Hypn. 2019;61(3):244–57.

Santiváñez-Acosta R, de Las Nieves Tapia-López E, Santero M. Music therapy in pain and anxiety management during labor: a systematic review and meta-analysis. Medicina (Kaunas). 2020;56(10):526.

Schell A, Wassmer F, Zaubitzer L, Kramer B, Sadick H, Rotter N, et al. The effect of complementary music intervention on the patients' quality of life after septoplasty and rhinoplasty. BMC Complement Med Ther. 2022;22(1):282.

Shabani F, Nayeri ND, Karimi R, Zarei K, Chehrazi M. Effects of music therapy on pain responses induced by blood sampling in premature infants: a randomized cross-over trial. Iran J Nurs Midwifery Res. 2016;21(4):391–6.

Shanmuganandan AP, Siddiqui MRS, Farkas N, Sran K, Thomas R, Mohamed S, et al. Does music reduce anxiety and discomfort during flexible sigmoidoscopy? A systematic review and meta-analysis. World J Gastrointest Endosc. 2017;9(5):228–37.

Sharara-Chami R, El-Hout Y, Lakissian Z, Hafez B, Abi-Gerges C, Fayad J, et al. Music as an adjunct to combination analgesia for neonatal circumcision: a randomized controlled trial. J Pediatr Urol. 2022;18(2):184.e1–6.

Shoghi M, Aghtaii MZ, Kheradmand M. The effect of the active and passive distraction techniques on the burn children's pain intensity and anxiety during dressing changes. J Nurs Midwifery Sci. 2022;9:167.

Shukla VV, Bansal S, Nimbalkar A, Chapla A, Phatak A, Patel D, et al. Pain control interventions in preterm neonates: a randomized controlled trial. Indian Pediatr. 2018;55(4):292–6.

Soliva MS, Salvador IR, Testal AG, López CC, Ramón RO, Coca JV, et al. Intervention study to verify the effect of live classic music during hemodialysis on the quality of life of patients with chronic kidney disease. Nefrologia. 2022;42(5):559–67.

Song M, Li N, Zhang X, Shang Y, Yan L, Chu J, et al. Music for reducing the anxiety and pain of patients undergoing a biopsy: a meta-analysis. J Adv Nurs. 2018;74(5):1016–29.

Soo MS, Jarosz JA, Wren AA, Soo AE, Mowery YM, Johnson KS, et al. Imaging-guided Core-needle breast biopsy: impact of meditation and music interventions on patient anxiety, pain, and fatigue. J Am Coll Radiol. 2016;13(5):526–34.

Sorensen EP, Gu H, Tabacchi M, Council ML. Music reduces pain and anxiety associated with local anesthesia for dermatologic procedures: a randomized controlled trial. J Am Acad Dermatol. 2021;85(4):989–91.

Sorkpor SK, Johnson CM, Santa Maria DM, Miao H, Moore C, Ahn H. The effect of music listening on pain in adults undergoing colonoscopy: a systematic review and meta-analysis. J Perianesth Nurs. 2021;36(5):573–580.e1.

Sorribes De Ramón LA, Ferrández Martínez AF, García Carricondo AR, Espín Gálvez F, Alarcón Rodríguez R. Effect of virtual reality and music therapy on anxiety and perioperative pain in surgical extraction of impacted third molars. J Am Dent Assoc. 2023;154(3):206–14.

Soyeux O, Marchand S. A web app-based music intervention reduces experimental thermal pain: a randomized trial on preferred versus least-liked music style. Front Pain Res (Lausanne). 2022;3:1055259.

Sun D-J, You Y-X, He X-J, Li H-T, Zeng X-P, Li D-Z, et al. Effects of light music played by piano intervention on satisfaction, anxiety, and pain in patients undergoing colonoscopy: a randomized controlled trial. Medicine (Baltimore). 2022;101(52):e32339.

Tan P, Lester LH, Lin AM. Music therapy treatments in an inpatient setting—a randomized pilot study. Arts Psychother. 2020;69:101660.

Tan K, Liu H, Huang S, Li C. Efficacy of music intervention for dental anxiety disorders: a systematic review and meta-analysis. Medicina (Kaunas). 2023;59(2):209.

Tang L, Wang H, Liu Q, Wang F, Wang M, Sun J, et al. Effect of music intervention on pain responses in premature infants undergoing placement procedures of peripherally inserted central venous catheter: a randomized controlled trial. Eur J Integr Med. 2018;19:105–9.

Tang H, Chen L, Wang Y, Zhang Y, Yang N, Yang N. The efficacy of music therapy to relieve pain, anxiety, and promote sleep quality, in patients with small cell lung cancer receiving platinum-based chemotherapy. Support Care Cancer. 2021;29(12):7299–306.

Tekgündüz KŞ, Polat S, Gürol A, Apay SE. Oral glucose and listening to lullaby to decrease pain in preterm infants supported with NCPAP: a randomized controlled trial. Pain Manag Nurs. 2019;20(1):54–61.

Téllez A, Sánchez-Jáuregui T, Juárez-García DM, García-Solís M. Breast biopsy: the effects of hypnosis and music. Int J Clin Exp Hypn. 2016;64(4):456–69.

Terzi E. The effect of listening to the music of the patient's own or others' choice during cesarean sections on pain, and its contribution to anesthesia technicians. J Exp Clin Med. 2022;39(3):786–92.

Ting B, Tsai C-L, Hsu W-T, Shen M-L, Tseng P-T, Chen DT-L, et al. Music intervention for pain control in the pediatric population: a systematic review and meta-analysis. J Clin Med. 2022;11(4):991.

Toker E, Demirel G, Doganer A, Karakucuk S. Effects of turkish classical music on postpartum pain and anxiety in cesarean deliveries: a randomized controlled trial. Altern Ther Health Med. 2021;27(S1):120–7.

Tolunay T, Bicici V, Tolunay H, Akkurt MO, Arslan AK, Aydogdu A, et al. Rhythm and orthopedics: the effect of music therapy in cast room procedures, a prospective clinical trial. Injury. 2018;49(3):593–8.

Torres E, Pedersen IN, Pérez-Fernández JI. Randomized trial of a Group Music and Imagery Method (GrpMI) for women with fibromyalgia. J Music Ther. 2018;55(2):186–220.

Tran BW, Nowrouz MY, Dhillon SK, Xie KK, Breslin KM, Golladay GJ. The impact of music and noise-cancellation on sedation requirements during Total knee replacement: a randomized controlled trial. Geriatr Orthop Surg Rehabil. 2020;11:2151459320910844.

Tripyla N, Katsas K, Karagkouni K, Liosis I, Ntelis S, Linos D. Evaluation of the effect of Mozart music on pain and respiratory rate after thyroidectomy. Hormones (Athens). 2023;22(1):113–9.

Tsai HF, Chen YR, Chung MH, Liao YM, Chi MJ, Chang CC, et al. Effectiveness of music intervention in ameliorating cancer patients' anxiety, depression, pain, and fatigue: a meta-analysis. Cancer Nurs. 2014;37(6):E35–50.

Tse MMY, Yan E, Tang ASK, Cheung D, Ng S. A music-with-movement exercise programme for community-dwelling older adults suffering from chronic pain: a pilot randomized controlled trial. Nurs Open. 2023;10(9):6566–74.

Tuinmann G, Preissler P, Böhmer H, Suling A, Bokemeyer C. The effects of music therapy in patients with high-dose chemotherapy and stem cell support: a randomized pilot study. Psychooncology. 2017;26(3):377–84.

Uggla L, Bonde LO, Hammar U, Wrangsjö B, Gustafsson B. Music therapy supported the health-related quality of life for children undergoing haematopoietic stem cell transplants. Acta Paediatr. 2018;107(11):1986–94.

Ünal Toprak F, Uysal N, Göksel F, Soylu Y. The effect of music on anxiety, pain levels, and physiological parameters in women undergoing brachytherapy: a randomized controlled trial. Semin Oncol Nurs. 2024;40:151575.

Us MC, Saran MG, Cebeci B, Akkuş E, Şeker E, Aybar ŞSŞ. A randomized comparative effectiveness study of reflexology, sucrose, and other treatments for needle procedures in newborns. Pediatr Neurol. 2023;140:78–85.

van der Heijden MJE, Oliai Araghi S, van Dijk M, Jeekel J, Hunink MGM. The effects of perioperative music interventions in pediatric surgery: a systematic review and meta-analysis of randomized controlled trials. PLoS One. 2015;10(8):e0133608.

van der Heijden MJE, Jeekel J, Rode H, Cox S, van Rosmalen J, Hunink MGM, et al. Can live music therapy reduce distress and pain in children with burns after wound care procedures? A randomized controlled trial. Burns. 2018;44(4):823–33.

van der Heijden MJE, Mevius H, van der Heijde N, van Rosmalen J, van As S, van Dijk M. Children listening to music or watching cartoons during ER procedures: a RCT. J Pediatr Psychol. 2019;44(10):1151–62.

Vandormael C, Schoenhals L, Hüppi PS, Filippa M, Borradori Tolsa C. Language in preterm born children: atypical development and effects of early interventions on neuroplasticity. Neural Plast. 2019;2019:6873270.

Verstegen AL, Silverman MJ. Effects of music therapy on mood and pain with patients hospitalized for bone marrow transplantation: a randomized effectiveness pilot study. J Creat Ment Health. 2018;13(4):418–28.

Viana TRFV, de Melo GM, Cardoso MVLML, de Almeida PC, de Oliveira LM, de Santos DAS. Pain in full term newborns submitted to music and swaddling during venipunctures. Rev Rene. 2020;21:e43904.

Victoria G, Eliane G, Claude K, Philippe FJ. The effects of standardized musical intervention (Music Care© type) during painful cares on vigils patients in intensive care unit. Ann Intensive Care. 2018;8(1):F-60.

Voss JA, Good M, Yates B, Baun MM, Thompson A, Hertzog M. Sedative music reduces anxiety and pain during chair rest after open-heart surgery. Pain. 2004;112(1–2):197–203.

Wang MC, Zhang LY, Zhang YL, Zhang YW, Xu XD, Zhang YC. Effect of music in endoscopy procedures: systematic review and meta-analysis of randomized controlled trials. Pain Med. 2014;15(10):1786–94.

Wang Y, Wei J, Guan X, Zhang Y, Zhang Y, Zhang N, et al. Music intervention in pain relief of cardiovascular patients in cardiac procedures: a systematic review and meta-analysis. Pain Med. 2020a;21(11):3055–65.

Wang M, Yi G, Gao H, Wu B, Zhou Y. Music-based interventions to improve fibromyalgia syndrome: a meta-analysis. Explore (NY). 2020b;16(6):357–62.

Warth M, Kessler J, van Kampen J, Ditzen B, Bardenheuer HJ. "Song of life": music therapy in terminally ill patients with cancer. BMJ Support Palliat Care. 2018;8(2):167–70.

Weingarten SJ, Levy AT, Berghella V. The effect of music on anxiety in women undergoing cesarean delivery: a systematic review and meta-analysis. Am J Obstet Gynecol MFM. 2021;3(5):100435.

Werner LM, Skouras S, Bechtold L, Pallesen S, Koelsch S. Sensorimotor synchronization to music reduces pain. PLoS One. 2023;18(7):e0289302.

Williams A. De la música. In: La Quena, editor. Teoría de la música. Buenos Aires; 1984. p. 5.

Wood C, Cutshall SM, Lawson DK, Ochtrup HM, Henning NB, Larsen BE, et al. Music therapy for anxiety and pain after spinal cord injury: a pilot study. Glob Adv Health Med. 2021;10:21649561211058696.

Wren AA, Shelby RA, Soo MS, Huysmans Z, Jarosz JA, Keefe FJ. Preliminary efficacy of a lovingkindness meditation intervention for patients undergoing biopsy and breast cancer surgery: a randomized controlled pilot study. Support Care Cancer. 2019;27(9):3583–92.

Wu Q, Liu Z, Pang X, Cheng L. Efficacy of five-element music interventions in perinatal mental health and labor pain: a meta-analysis. Complement Ther Clin Pract. 2020;40:101217.

Wu XL, Ji B, Yao SD, Wang LL, Jiang ZY. Effect of music intervention during hemodialysis: a comprehensive meta-analysis. Eur Rev Med Pharmacol Sci. 2021;25(10):3822–34.

Yamada Y, Kitamura M, Inayama E, Kishida M, Kataoka Y, Ikenoue T. Acoustic stimulation for relieving pain during venipuncture: a systematic review and network meta-analysis. BMJ Open. 2023;13(12):e077343.

Yaman Aktaş Y, Karabulut N. Relief of procedural pain in critically ill patients by music therapy: a randomized controlled trial. Complement Med Res. 2019;26(3):156–65.

Yangöz ŞT, Özer Z. The effect of music intervention on patients with cancer-related pain: a systematic review and meta-analysis of randomized controlled trials. J Adv Nurs. 2019;75(12):3362–73.

Yangöz ŞT, Özer Z. Effects of music intervention on physical and psychological problems in adults receiving haemodialysis treatment: a systematic review and meta-analysis. J Clin Nurs. 2022;31(23–24):3305–26.

Yarahmadi S, Mohammadi N, Ardalan A, Najafizadeh H, Gholami M. The combined effects of cold therapy and music therapy on pain following chest tube removal among patients with cardiac bypass surgery. Complement Ther Clin Pract. 2018;31:71–5.

Yiğit Ü, İlçe A, Karagöz İ. The effect of music therapy on pain, anxiety and vital signs in patients undergoing spinal anaesthesia: a randomized controlled trial. TFSD. 2021;2:35–44.

Yılmaz K, Ölçücü MT. The effects of listening to music embedded binaural beats on anxiety levels and pain scores in male patients undergoing prostate biopsy: a randomized placebo-controlled study. J Urol Surg. 2023;10(1):62–6.

Yinger OS. Music therapy as procedural support for young children undergoing immunizations: a randomized controlled study. J Music Ther. 2016;53(4):336–63.

Young H-J, Mehta T, Herman C, Baidwan NK, Lai B, Rimmer JH. The effects of a movement-to-music (M2M) intervention on physical and psychosocial outcomes in people Poststroke: a randomized controlled trial. Arch Rehabil Res Clin Transl. 2021;3(4):100160.

Yu R, Zhuo Y, Feng E, Wang W, Lin W, Lin F, et al. The effect of musical interventions in improving short-term pain outcomes following total knee replacement: a meta-analysis and systematic review. J Orthop Surg Res. 2020;15(1):465.

Zapata-Copete JA, Cordoba-Wagner MJ, García-Perdomo HA. Role of music in a plastic surgery setting: a systematic review and meta-analysis. Indian J Plast Surg. 2019;52(2):160–5.

Zhang X-H, Gao X-X, Wu W-W, Yu J-A. Impact of orally administered tramadol combined with self-selected music on adult outpatients with burns undergoing dressing change: a randomized controlled trial. Burns. 2020;46(4):850–9.

Zohaib A, Siddiq A, Khalid SE, Hassan W, Saleem M, Fareed W. Music harmonizes extracorporeal shockwave lithotripsy experience by reducing anxiety and pain—a randomized control trial. PJMHS. 2022;16(6):161–3.

A Systematic Review of Music Therapy and Music-Based Interventions in Healthcare Applications: Surgery, NICU, and Dementia Care in Acute Settings and Transition

17

Amy Clements-Cortés and Joyce Jing Yee Yip

17.1 Introduction

According to Raglio and Oasi (2015), applications of music in healthcare contexts can be organized as music therapy (MT), music listening (including music and medicine approaches) and general music-based interventions (MBIs). Music therapy has been used as a treatment in a variety of healthcare contexts such as hospitals, clinics, long-term homes, hospices, correctional centers, schools, community centers, private practice (CAMT 2024) at home, via telehealth (Clements-Cortés et al. 2023), and many more applications. Music-based interventions have also increasingly been used in these contexts (Foster et al. 2021). Raglio and Oasi (2015) also explain that MT interventions are distinguished from MBIs, as there is a relational component. MBIs can involve musical activity that is based on an objective to improve aspects of well-being such as socialization, cognitive stimulations, and mood elevation (Raglio and Oasi 2015). Alternatively, applications of music listening, an example of a MBI, can either be individualized music experience (Gerdner 2012; Särkämö et al. 2008) or can be considered a music medicine approach, as they are targeted toward a specific symptom or disease (Haas and Brandes 2009).

Part 1 of this systematic review provides an analysis of evidence-based literature in areas of MT and MBIs in the following healthcare applications: surgery, neonatal intensive care unit (NICU), and dementia care in acute settings and transition. While the topics covered in these chapters are not an exhaustive list of the MBIs and MT

A. Clements-Cortés (✉)
Faculty of Music, University of Toronto, Toronto, ON, Canada
e-mail: a.clements.cortes@utoronto.ca

J. J. Y. Yip
Ontario Institute for Studies in Education, University of Toronto, Toronto, ON, Canada
e-mail: joycejingyee.yip@mail.utoronto.ca

A. Raglio (ed.), *Music and Music Therapy Interventions in Clinical Practice*, Neurocultural Health and Wellbeing,
https://doi.org/10.1007/978-3-031-88578-5_17

applications within these healthcare contexts and concerns, it is a reflection of the research that has taken place to develop foundational knowledge through these areas. The authors of these chapters have accomplished this overview through a narrative synthesis systematic review aimed to assess the efficacy and benefits of MT, MBIs, or a combination of both practices in the existing research and literature within the respective healthcare context.

17.2 Methodology

The use of systematic review allowed the authors to account for the vast and various types of resources found, including experimental studies, systematic reviews, scoping reviews, narrative reviews, book chapters, or meta-analyses. Further, an additional approach utilizing narrative synthesis has enabled the results to be presented that considers a wide range of questions and not solely focused on one specific intervention (Popay et al. 2006), allowing the authors to consider all MT and MBIs discussed.

This systematic review includes the research and scholarly literature published in English within the last two decades (2004–2024), assessing MT and MBIs in the following healthcare contexts and/or concerns: Part 1 involves surgery, neonatal intensive care unit (NICU), and dementia care in acute settings and transition; Part 2 describes eating disorders, work-related stress, homelessness, artists in residence, and concerts/music and medicine. To identify relevant articles, the authors used data indexes that were found at the University of Toronto Libraries Databases, and included the following: CINAHL, MEDLINE, Music Index, Music Periodicals Database, PubMed, PsychInfo, and Scopus. Outside of these indexes, Google Scholar was also used as part of the search. At this stage, papers were removed before screening due to several reasons: duplication; articles that were published outside of the 2004–2024 timeline; and articles that were not peer-reviewed.

An exception to including the source into this systematic review is in specific instances when there was a dearth of literature on a topic. Individual experimental studies, book chapters, and narrative reviews were considered on a case-by-case basis. The keywords that were used in the search formula combined various terms based on the topic of inquiry, and included the following for Part 1: music, music therapy, music-based interventions, music medicine, music in medicine, music and medicine, music and health, music listening, dementia, acute care, transition, hospital, surgery, and NICU. For instance, if the authors were interested in searching results of MBIs and MT with surgery, the search term can be formulated as: ["music therapy" OR "music-based intervention*" AND "surgery"].[1]

[1] The asterisk (*) broadens the search term by finding words that start with the word and retrieve variations of the term. In the case of the music-based intervention, this can involve the term being in plural (i.e., music-based interventions) as the extension to the search word.

Figure 17.1 shares a summary of the identification, screening, and retrieval process (Page et al. 2021).

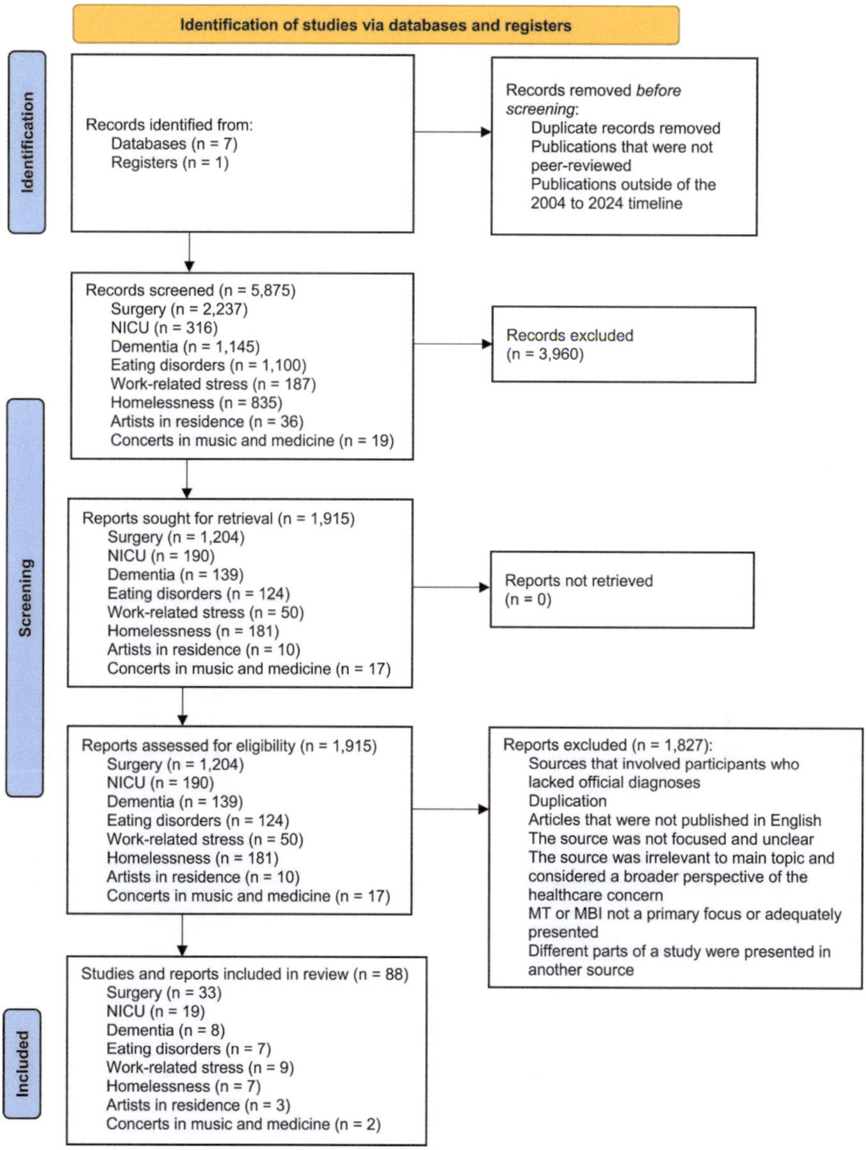

Fig. 17.1 PRISMA Chart of searched results for Part 1 and Part 2 (Page et al. 2021)

17.3 Results

After searched results on databases ($n = 7$) and registers ($n = 1$), 5875 articles were screened and 1915 reports were sought for retrieval and assessed for eligibility. The exclusion criteria during this stage of screening included sources where participants lacked official diagnosis; duplication; articles that were not published in English; lack of study clarity; results being irrelevant to the main topic and considered a broader perspective of the health concern; MT and MBIs that were not a primary focus or adequately presented; and different parts of the article were presented in another source.

A total of 88 resources ($n = 88$) were used in these chapters. Within each healthcare context, the number of papers screened, sought for retrieval, and assessed for eligibility after the initial review is noted. An overview of the healthcare setting is also provided, based on empirical-based research. The authors also recognized that it was difficult to separate out MBIs from MT independently. Many articles evaluated all music-based experiences and at times, the terminology (MT and MBIs) were not consistent. This was often evident if the source and perspectives were from an allied healthcare perspective. Therefore, there is some overlap in how MT and MBIs are presented in the found sources.

The authors documented elements of each study included in the review source into a summary of MT, MBIs, or MT and MBI combinations (Table 17.1). The table is prepared with the following headings and descriptions:

- *Healthcare Area/Issue*: Healthcare context or issue.
- *Author, Title & Year*: An abbreviated reference to the article of interest. The full reference of each source is available in the reference list.
- *Type of Source*: Systematic reviews, scoping reviews, narrative reviews, meta-analysis, book chapters, or experimental studies.
- *Main Applications*: Whether the found resource showcased MT, MBIs, or a combination of both MT and MBIs. An "X" symbol was used to indicate if MT or MBI was reported, but no further description or specifics were given. The combination category indicated the music interventions that were not categorized as MT or MBIs or they were used in both applications by varied health care professionals and others.
- *Benefits*: Outlined benefits of the main applications.
- *Considerations*: Future implications or issues to note.

17.3.1 Surgery

The authors of this chapter found an abundance of research and literature, focusing on MBIs and MT in surgery. A total of 1204 reports ($n = 1204$) were sought for retrieval. Thirty-three sources ($n = 33$) were analyzed in further detail, which ranged from 18 experimental studies ($n = 18$), seven systematic reviews ($n = 7$), six systematic review/meta-analysis ($n = 6$), and two scoping reviews ($n = 2$).

Table 17.1 A systematic review of music therapy and music based interventions in healthcare applications: Surgery, NICU, and dementia care in acute settings and transition

Healthcare area/issue	Authors, title & year	Type of source	Main applications			Benefits	Considerations
			Music therapy (MT)	Music-based Interventions (MBIs)	Combination		
Surgery	Azi et al. (2021). Benefits of intraoperative music on orthopedic surgeries under spinal anesthesia: a randomized clinical trial.	Experimental			Music group (patients listening to instrumental music through headset during procedure)	Reduced anxiety and sedative requirements	
Surgery	Chandrababu et al. (2021). Effectiveness of music on anxiety and pain among cardiac surgery patients: a quantitative systematic review and meta-analysis of randomized controlled trials.	Systematic review and meta-review		X		Significant reduction in anxiety and pain among patients who received musical intervention	
Surgery	Cici and Özkan (2022). Effects on anxiety and vital signs of the emotional freedom technique and music before surgery for lumbar disc hernia.	Experimental			X	Music reduced blood pressure	Emotional freedom technique was more effective than music

(continued)

Table 17.1 (continued)

Healthcare area/issue	Authors, title & year	Type of source	Main applications			Benefits	Considerations
			Music therapy (MT)	Music-based Interventions (MBIs)	Combination		
Surgery	Criss et al. (2023). The healthcare experience of autistic patients in orthopaedic surgery and closely related fields: a scoping review.	Scoping review			Animal-assisted therapy, aquatic environment therapy, music therapy, movement-based therapy, equine-assisted therapy, therapy in an aquatic setting, exercise and social play, sensory management and accommodations, caregiver/parent training, and technology		No clear methods that are most effective. More understanding on the impact of music participation (i.e., singing)
Surgery	Dahshan et al. (2021). A role for music in cataract surgery: a systematic review.	Systematic review			Music listening through earphones: non-specified music, Korean traditional music, binaural beat embedded music, and no music	Reduced perceived pain, anxiety, and improved vitals by reducing heart rate and blood pressure with binaural beat-embedded music	

Surgery	Dale (2021). The impact of perioperative music on abdominal surgery patients' experience of postoperative pain: a systematic review and meta-analysis.	Systematic review and meta-analysis		Pre-selected: soothing music, music without lyrics, relaxing, orchestral classical, song collection	Listening to music	Significantly positive impact on postoperative pain	Minimal difference between intra- and postoperative interventions, or between patient- and researcher-selected music
Surgery	Demir et al. (2021). Effect of music on fatigue, comfort, and vital signs in patients after liver transplant surgery: a randomized controlled trial.	Experimental	MT intervention involved curated listening playlists of nature sounds at maximum 60 dB			Fatigue scores and vital signs decreased after music, higher comfort levels	
Surgery	El Boghdady and Ewalds-Kvist (2020). The influence of music on the surgical task performance: a systematic review.	Systematic review		X		Classical music at a low to medium volume improves surgery task performance by increasing both accuracy and speed	Volume of music during operations

(continued)

Table 17.1 (continued)

Healthcare area/issue	Authors, title & year	Type of source	Main applications			Benefits	Considerations
			Music therapy (MT)	Music-based Interventions (MBIs)	Combination		
Surgery	Fenko and Loock (2014). The influence of ambient scent and music on patients' anxiety in a waiting room of a plastic surgeon.	Experimental			Ambient scents and music in a waiting room	Music and scent significantly reduced patient's anxiety when used separately	Scent and music together should be used with caution
Surgery	Fu et al. (2021). The perception and attitude toward noise and music in the operating room: a systematic review.	Systematic review		X		Significant reduction of complications in surgical patients when noise levels were lower	Higher volume and noise levels
Surgery	Gallagher et al. (2018). Impact of music therapy on hospitalized patients post-elective orthopaedic surgery: a randomized controlled trial.	Experimental	X			Improvements of pain, emotional status, and nausea with MT sessions	Effects on narcotic and antiemetic usage, as well as length of stay, were not observed

Surgery	Grafton-Clarke et al. (2019). Music therapy following cardiac surgery—is it an effective method to reduce pain and anxiety?	Systematic review	Postoperative music therapy with music protocol Music protocols: short session on day 1 postoperatively to multiple sessions per day over a 72-h period Music type: relaxing music, typically between 50 and 60 dB			Helps with pain and reduction in analgesia; improvements in anxiety	
Surgery	Guerrier et al. (2021). Efficacy of a web app–based music intervention during cataract surgery: a randomized clinical trial.	Experimental		Web-based music invention during cataract surgery		Less incidence of hypertension, lower anxiety, and less use of sedative drug injections in the music arm	

(continued)

Table 17.1 (continued)

Healthcare area/issue	Authors, title & year	Type of source	Main applications			Benefits	Considerations
			Music therapy (MT)	Music-based Interventions (MBIs)	Combination		
Surgery	Hole et al. (2015). Music as an aid for postoperative recovery in adults: a systematic review and meta-analysis.	Systematic review and meta-analysis			Patient's own, easy listening, relaxation, slow and soft, soft piano, music, sedative, instrumental, various, Baroque, Spanish guitar, flute, prescriptive, Turkish classical	Music reduced postoperative pain, anxiety, and analgesia use, and increased patient satisfaction	No differences in the length of stay, choice of music, and timing of delivery
Surgery	Kakar et al. (2022). Implementation of music in colorectal perioperative standard care—barriers and facilitators among patients and healthcare professionals.	Experimental	Perioperatively applied music interventions			Reduced pain and anxiety in patients, reduced use of sedatives and opioids for surgery	Benefits only applied to one location and small number of participants
Surgery	Kühlmann et al. (2018). Meta-analysis evaluating music interventions for anxiety and pain in surgery.	Systematic review		X		Music interventions significantly decreased anxiety and pain during general anesthesia	No significant effects of music interventions and age, sex, choice and timing of music, and type of anesthesia

Surgery	Kühlmann et al. (2020). Music interventions in pediatric surgery (the music under surgery in children study): a randomized clinical trial.	Experimental		Preoperative music intervention; pre- and intraoperative music intervention		Significant reduced heart rate after preoperative music intervention.	Music interventions do not benefit all young infants in surgery. Weak evidence between music exposure and behaviors.
Surgery	Lagattolla et al. (2023). Receptive music therapy versus group music therapy with breast cancer patients hospitalized for surgery.	Experimental	Individual/ receptive vs. group/ active-recepted integrated music therapy to patients undergoing breast surgery			Both types of MT interventions reduced stress, depression, anger, and anxiety	
Surgery	Lattimore (2017). Assessing healthcare providers perspective: music intervention for open heart surgery patients.	Experimental		X		Majority endorsed music interventions due to significant influence on patient outcomes	Unfamiliarity of the modality, music in care. Participants were neutral to very likely to implement music intervention, if available.

(continued)

Table 17.1 (continued)

Healthcare area/issue	Authors, title & year	Type of source	Main applications			Benefits	Considerations
			Music therapy (MT)	Music-based Interventions (MBIs)	Combination		
Surgery	Lin et al. (2020). Effect of music therapy on pain after orthopedic surgery—a systematic review and meta-analysis.	Systematic review and meta-analysis			MT and MBIs on postoperative pain (patient selected)	Relieves pain and anxiety	Length of stay showed little differences
Surgery	Miyata et al. (2016). Music before dental surgery suppresses sympathetic activity.	Experimental			Music listening from the time of arriving at the outpatient client before entering the operating room at low/high frequency	Reduced anxiety before dental procedures	Only affects the sympathetic nervous system, not parasympathetic
Surgery	Narayanan et al. (2022). The effect of background music on stress in the operating surgeon: a scoping review.	Scoping review				Reduced anxiety and mental workload; significant physiological improvement; positive perception among surgeons and professionals involved in managing stress	
Surgery	Oomens et al. (2019). The effect of music on simulated surgical performance: a systematic review.	Systematic review		X		Efficient surgical task completion	Insufficient evidence of music having beneficial effects on surgical performance

Surgery	Rivera et al. (2024). Music during cataract surgery: impact on anxiety.	Experimental			Music group (selecting own music)	Lower self-reported anxiety, feeling less frightened, nervous, and confused during surgery	No difference between groups on types of sedatives given
Surgery	Sadideen et al. (2012). Is there a role for music in reducing anxiety in plastic surgery minor operations?	Experimental	Music playlists developed by a music therapist			Popular music genres in pre-operation were Disney songs, classical music, and the Piano Guys. In post-operation: classical music, Disney songs, and the Beatles. Decreased anxiety and depression	
Surgery	Tan et al. (2020). The effect of perioperative music listening on patient satisfaction, anxiety, and depression: a quasi-experimental study.	Experimental	Music playlists of selected music and noise-cancelling earphones			Significant reduction in anxiety and depression, improved patient satisfaction	Implications of perioperative music listening to patient care
Surgery	van der Heijden et al. (2015). The effects of perioperative music interventions in pediatric surgery: a systematic review and meta-analysis of randomized controlled trials.	Systematic review and meta-analysis			Live MT or recorded music	Overall positive effects on postoperative pain, anxiety, and distress	

(continued)

Table 17.1 (continued)

Healthcare area/issue	Authors, title & year	Type of source	Main applications			Benefits	Considerations
			Music therapy (MT)	Music-based Interventions (MBIs)	Combination		
Surgery	Weldon et al. (2015). Music and communication in the operating theatre.	Experimental			Music in the operating room	Playing music added anxiety in the operation	Interfere with team communication
Surgery	Williams and Hine (2018). An investigation into the use of recorded music as a surgical intervention: a systematic, critical review of methodologies used in recent adult controlled trials.	Systematic review			Recorded music, selection and composition of music for future interventions	Patients are frequently allowed to select music during surgery; improves psychological states and physiological arousal	Music for distraction, relaxation, emotional shift, entrainment, and endogenous analgesia has been rarely assessed Patient music history is rarely assessed; lack of scientific rigor and theoretical frameworks
Surgery	Wu et al. (2017). Effects of music listening on anxiety and physiological responses in patients undergoing awake craniotomy.	Experimental		Patients selecting music to listen to in a waiting room		Significant decrease in anxiety and heartbeat rate and blood pressure over time	

Surgery	Xu et al. (2021). The impact of music on patient satisfaction, anxiety, and depression in patients undergoing gynecologic surgery.	Experimental	Music played in the operating theater			Music reduced intraoperative anxiety	Easy listening music and chart classics are suitable
Surgery	Yang et al. (2022). Effect of genre and amplitude of music during laparoscopic surgery.	Experimental		Music listening: soft rock by the Beatles and hard rock by AC/DC		Soft rock: patients were faster in peg transfer and intracorporeal knot. Hard rock was good for precision cutting	Depends on music genre and amplitude for surgery
Surgery	Yeoh and Spence (2023). Background music's impact on patients waiting in surgery and radiology clinics.	Experimental		Music listening in a waiting room (Western classical, lo-fi) or no music at a surgical and radiology clinic		No music resulted in less anxiety and higher patient's perceptions of the hospital	Choice of background music that matches the day; negative perceptions of background music; the cultural product of music; specific curated playlists are necessary

(continued)

Table 17.1 (continued)

Healthcare area/issue	Authors, title & year	Type of source	Main applications			Benefits	Considerations
			Music therapy (MT)	Music-based Interventions (MBIs)	Combination		
NICU	Jayamala et al. (2015). Impact of music therapy on breast milk secretion in mothers of premature newborns.	Experimental	X			Reduced stress and cortisol; increase in breast milk expression in mothers	
NICU	Burrows (2020). Developmental care in the NICU: best practices for preterm infants, expectations of healthcare providers, and impact on parents and families.	Experimental	X			Parent-infant attachment is beneficial in kangaroo care	Music therapists are part of a healthcare team Development care may not be as effective
NICU	Caparros-Gonzalez et al. (2018). Listening to relaxing music improves physiological responses in premature infants: a randomized controlled trial.	Experimental	X			After each session, the respiratory rate decreased. Across the sessions, the heart rate increased in the control	

NICU	Costa et al. (2022). Clinical benefits of music-based interventions on preterm infants' health: a systematic review of randomised trials.	Systematic review			MBIs were divided into music medicine and music therapy	MBIs were associated with pain relief; MT for: improvements in cardiac and respiratory function, weight gain, eating behavior, and quiet alert and sleep states	
NICU	Ettenberger (2017a). Music therapy during end-of-life care in the neonatal intensive care unit (NICU)–Reflections from early clinical practice in Colombia.	Experimental	X			Three case vignettes of ideas and experiences among music therapists and other healthcare professionals concerned with end-of-life care in the NICU.	Cultural differences, family-centered care principles, sensitive language for communication
NICU	Ettenberger (2017b). Music therapy in the neonatal intensive care unit: putting the families at the centre of care.	Scoping review	Family-centered music therapy			Early relational and communicative experiences between parents and their babies	Needs to be a balance between babies, parents, and emerging relationships

(continued)

Table 17.1 (continued)

Healthcare area/issue	Authors, title & year	Type of source	Main applications			Benefits	Considerations
			Music therapy (MT)	Music-based Interventions (MBIs)	Combination		
NICU	Ettenberger et al. (2016). Family-centred music therapy with preterm infants and their parents in the neonatal intensive care unit (NICU) in Colombia – a mixed-methods study.	Experimental	Kangaroo care with preterm infants			Significant improvements in maternal state-anxiety and weight gain per day; parents improved bonding and anxiety scores	
NICU	Filippa et al. (2020). Early vocal contact and music in the NICU: new insights into preventive interventions.	Literature review	Early vocal contact and music on the preterm infant's brain development and early development			Maternal, direct, and recorded voice and music were beneficial in the NICU	Long-term effects of music and early vocal contact on preterm infants' neurodevelopment needs be further investigated
NICU	Haslbeck and Bassler (2020). Clinical practice protocol of creative music therapy for preterm infants and their parents in the neonatal intensive care unit.	Experimental	Creative MT; humming or singing; improvised and sung lullaby style; parent involvement through kangaroo care and parental voice bonding			Relaxing, stimulating, and coregulating premature infants; advantageous for intuitive parenting by the traumatic experience of preterm birth	Creative MT is only effective for infants who are clinically stable. Parents who are available and receptive make it easier for creative MT to be integrated

NICU	Kim (2022). The experience of music therapists working with the parents of premature infants in the neonatal intensive care unit (NICU).	Experimental	X			Music therapists are responsible for: witnessing parents' difficulties and providing support; music therapy advocacy; serving as a bridge between parents and their babies; utilizing various interventions; mediating between parents and medical staff; and setting boundaries	Recognize the roles and challenges of music therapists in the NICU
NICU	Loewy (2015). NICU music therapy: song of kin as critical lullaby in research and practice.	Experimental	Live music; the *song of kin* intervention: parent selects songs and compares to well-known theme			Parents in music psychotherapy sessions before working with their infants exhibit support from instances of fear or anxiety related to premature birth and movement	Culturally based, parent-selected, personalized musical tunes

(continued)

Table 17.1 (continued)

Healthcare area/issue	Authors, title & year	Type of source	Main applications			Benefits	Considerations
			Music therapy (MT)	Music-based Interventions (MBIs)	Combination		
NICU	Menke et al. (2021). Family-centered music therapy—empowering premature infants and their primary caregivers through music: results of a pilot study.	Experimental	X			Shortening of caffeine therapy, nasogastric/orogastric tube feed and hospitalization. Parents showed a significant reduction in stress factors	No difference between MT treatment and control of having no MT
NICU	Pineda et al. (2019). Health care professionals' perceptions about sensory-based interventions in the NICU.	Experimental		Infant holding, recorded music/singing, occupational and physical therapy, infant swings		69% of respondents used recorded music and singing in the NICU for 30–32 weeks Conditions of sensory-based interventions like music were based on personnel that provided them and varied across settings	No standard protocol in place for type, timing, and frequency of interventions Sensory-based interventions used less and tactile interventions being used most often; interventions were initiated early after preterm birth and timed with development

NICU	Pinto (2023). Prematurity: can music have a role in neonatal intensive care unit?.	Experimental			MT or musical stimulation (MS)	Complementary therapy at NICU, such as vital signs, sleep quality, neurodevelopment and growth, and parent-infant bonding. Good for an individualized approach	Investigate the effects of MT and MS interventions on NICU based on their characteristics, situation, and recommendations
NICU	Rabold (2013). The effects of music therapy in the NICU on behavior, weight, and length of stay: a systematic review.	Systematic review	X			Infants and their families decreased stress, had more comfort, and a shorter stay Families are more agreeable to calming music and nurses being less attentive	Nurses address which patients can benefit most from music
NICU	Roa and Ettenberger (2018). Music therapy self-care group for parents of preterm infants in the neonatal intensive care unit: a clinical pilot intervention.	Experimental	Music guided relaxations, breathing techniques, and self-expression			Improvements in anxiety, stress, mood, restfulness, and motivation by parents; ability to relax, distract from worries, and having time for themselves	

(continued)

Table 17.1 (continued)

Healthcare area/issue	Authors, title & year	Type of source	Main applications			Benefits	Considerations
			Music therapy (MT)	Music-based Interventions (MBIs)	Combination		
NICU	Stegemann et al. (2019). Music therapy and other music-based interventions in pediatric health care: an overview.	Systematic review			Live music: minimal change in rhythm, harmony, dynamics, and volume; minimal range in melody and pitch range. Both are required to sound like a lullaby Recording of mother's voice MT and MBIs in pediatric healthcare	Beneficial effects of MT, music medicine, and other MBIs for children and adolescents; alleviate symptoms and improve quality of life.	More research is required
NICU	Ullsten (2019). Singing, sharing, soothing: family-centred music therapy during painful procedures in neonatal care.	Experimental	Live music, family-centered music therapy, biopsychosocial parental infant-directed singing			Pain relief and attachment formation during painful procedures for parents	Neonatal music therapy is still young in the Nordic countries. Further development of NICU MT as a family-centered approach

NICU	van der Heijden et al. (2016). Do hospitalized premature infants benefit from music interventions? A systematic review of randomized controlled trials.	Systematic review		X		Live music interventions improved sleep and heart rate; recorded music improved heart rate; better feeding and sucking outcomes good for live and recorded music	Variation in quality of the studies, age, outcome, and timing of the interventions across studies makes it difficult to draw strong conclusions
Dementia care in acute settings and transition	Abraha et al. (2017). Systematic review of systematic reviews of nonpharmacological interventions to treat behavioural disturbances in older patients with dementia.	Systematic review	Music therapy utilizing music listening vs. more active music therapy more effective			Reducing BPSD	
Dementia care in acute settings and transition	Hack et al. (2021). The effectiveness of music as an intervention for dementia patients in acute settings.	Systematic review			X	Improvement in mood and well-being, reducing BPSD	
Dementia care in acute settings and transition	Lam et al. (2020). Effects of music therapy on patients with dementia—a systematic review.	Systematic review	X			Improvement in verbal fluency, BPSD-anxiety, depression, apathy	Lack of standardization of MT

(continued)

Table 17.1 (continued)

Healthcare area/issue	Authors, title & year	Type of source	Main applications			Benefits	Considerations
			Music therapy (MT)	Music-based Interventions (MBIs)	Combination		
Dementia care in acute settings and transition	Leggieri et al. (2019). Music intervention approaches for Alzheimer's disease: a review of the literature.	Narrative review Systematic review	Active music therapy		Personalized MBIs	Socialization, relaxation, improve behavior and cognition	
Dementia care in acute settings and transition	Moreno-Morales et al. (2020). Music therapy in the treatment of dementia: a systematic review and meta-analysis.	Systematic review and meta-analysis	Listening to music and singing			Improvement in cognitive function, quality of life, and long-term depression	Standardization of protocols is needed or stage of dementia
Dementia care in acute settings and transition	Soufineyestani et al. (2021). Impacts of music intervention on dementia: a review using meta-narrative method and agenda for future research.	Narrative review	Active and receptive MT—live and recorded	Active and receptive MBIs—live and recorded		Safe, cost effective non-pharmacological approach Overall benefits—balance blood pressure, heart rate, reduce mood fluctuations Improvement in cognition, boost communication skills, memory, self-esteem, emotional and BPSD, quality of life	Lack of definitions between MT and MBIs, lack of protocols and standardized definitions of MBIs, small sample sizes

Dementia care in acute settings and transition	Tsoi et al. (2018). Receptive music therapy is more effective than interactive music therapy to relieve behavioral and psychological symptoms of dementia: a systematic review and meta-analysis.	Systematic review and meta-analysis	Music therapy utilizing music listening			Reducing BPSD	Studies in the analysis demonstrated considerable contradictions
Dementia care in acute settings and transition	van der Steen et al. (2018). Music-based therapeutic interventions for people with dementia.	Systematic review	X			Depression and reduction of BPSD	

An "X" symbol was used to indicate if MBI or MT was reported, but no further description or specifics were given

In general, music has been an effective medium for patients undergoing surgery and health professionals performing surgery, including healthcare applications not limited to: pediatric surgery (Kühlmann et al. 2020; van der Heijden et al. 2015); cataract surgery (Dahshan et al. 2021; Guerrier et al. 2021; Rivera et al. 2024); orthopedic surgery (Azi et al. 2021; Lin et al. 2020); abdominal and laparoscopic surgery (Dale 2021; Yang et al. 2022); cardiology (Grafton-Clarke et al. 2019); limb surgeries (Cici and Özkan 2022); dental surgery (Miyata et al. 2016); cancer-related treatments (Lagattolla et al. 2023); liver transplants (Demir et al. 2021); and waiting rooms of surgeries (Yeoh and Spence 2023). Within these settings, various MT and MBI practices have been used with patients, whether administered by healthcare professionals or music therapists. This can involve the following: preoperative music (music listening or receptive music) in the operating theater (Kakar et al. 2022; Tan et al. 2020; Weldon et al. 2015; Xu et al. 2021) or the waiting room (Wu et al. 2017); playlists developed by a music therapist (Sadideen et al. 2012; Tan et al. 2020); music and movement (Criss et al. 2023); and weekly sessions of MT (Gallagher et al. 2018). Patients experienced a variety of benefits as a result of music engagement, including reduced anxiety, pain, and stress (Chandrababu et al. 2021; Fenko and Loock 2014; Hole et al. 2015; Kühlmann et al. 2018; Miyata et al. 2016; Rivera et al. 2024; van der Heijden et al. 2015; Weldon et al. 2015; Wu et al. 2017; Xu et al. 2021); reduced use of sedatives and opioids (Azi et al. 2021; Kakar et al. 2022); lowered blood pressure and trauma (Cici and Özkan 2022; Dahshan et al. 2021); decreased levels of depression (Tan et al. 2020) and anger (Lagattolla et al. 2023); less incidence of hypertension (Guerrier et al. 2021); and higher comfort levels (Demir et al. 2021). There were also preferences in the type of music used in the pre-, during, and post-surgery procedures, including popular music and classical music (Sadideen et al. 2012); and relaxing music between 50 and 60 decibels (Grafton-Clarke et al. 2019).

For healthcare professionals, preoperative music has been used to perform surgical tasks at particular volumes (Kakar et al. 2022; Fu et al. 2021; Oomens et al. 2019); with preferences to classical music (El Boghdady and Ewalds-Kvist 2020); easy listening genres (Xu et al. 2021) like soft rock (Yang et al. 2022); and nature sounds, which have been recommended as repeated requests to be played in the background (Weldon et al. 2015). By increasing both accuracy, speed of surgical tasks (El Boghdady and Ewalds-Kvist 2020; Oomens et al. 2019) and reduced complications of patients (Fu et al. 2021), symptoms of healthcare professionals of using music in surgery were similar to patients. This included evidence of reduced anxiety and workload among surgeons and operating theater staff (Narayanan et al. 2022).

17.3.2 Neonatal Intensive Care Unit (NICU)

MT and MBIs in the NICU involves the administration of music for the healthcare of preterm infants (Caparros-Gonzalez et al. 2018) and related populations into intervention, which can comprise of parents of the patients (Ettenberger et al. 2016;

Jayamala et al. 2015; Loewy 2015; Menke et al. 2021; Roa and Ettenberger 2018; Ullsten 2019), healthcare personnel (Pineda et al. 2019), or facilitators like music therapists (Burrows 2020; Kim 2022). Music practitioners, such as performing musicians, classify as music makers who administer MBI in NICU conditions (Koivisto 2021). Their work is inspired by music performance, such as simple, smooth, and tranquil sedative music or silence, that can be showcased to patients in the NICU without the intention of health benefits (Koivisto 2021). These music performances can involve a lullaby or modifications of traditional music, which are performed using string instruments or humming in low tones (Koivisto 2021).

The research and literature surrounding MBIs in the NICU have not been documented as readily as MT. However, the relationship between MT and NICU has been profound, and the extensive amount of research and literature cannot be covered in this overview. The authors sought out 190 reports ($n = 190$) which resulted in the 19 sources ($n = 19$) included. These are categorized into 13 experimental designs ($n = 13$), four systematic reviews ($n = 4$), one literature review ($n = 1$), and one scoping review ($n = 1$), whereby case vignettes (Ettenberger 2017a, b; Costa et al. 2022) were most popular to researchers.

Researchers like Costa et al. (2022) attempted to differentiate between MT and MBIs and their benefits in the NICU. There are two categories of music care in the NICU: music medicine and music therapy. Music medicine involves the use of music to address pain relief, while music therapy optimizes the improvements of the patient which can include improvements in the following areas: weight gain, eating habits, cardiac and respiratory function, sleep states, and cardiac and respiratory function (Costa et al. 2022).

Studies documented significant benefits of MT to a variety of populations in the NICU, not limited to prenatal children with the following diagnoses: disability, neurorehabilitation, autism spectrum disorder, and epilepsy (Stegemann et al. 2019). Within MT, live music (Loewy 2015; Ullsten 2019), recorded music (Stegemann et al. 2019), and silence with only hospital sounds (Caparros-Gonzalez et al. 2018) have been used most readily in pediatric healthcare. Vocal contact (Filippa et al. 2020) such as utilizing the mother's voice into music recordings or early vocal contact with infant holding and infant swings (Pineda et al. 2019) has also been incorporated into the music experience for NICU patients (Filippa et al. 2020). These musical practices form the foundation of family-centered music therapy (Ettenberger 2017b; Roa and Ettenberger 2018) and creative music therapy (Haslbeck and Bassler 2020) in the NICU, acknowledging the significance of music therapists as part of a healthcare team (Burrows 2020). Patients have expressed various positive symptoms as a result of MT exposure, including significant improvements in anxiety and weight gain (Ettenberger 2017a); stress levels and mood (Roa and Ettenberger 2018); neurodevelopment growth and parent-infant bonding (Pinto 2023); heart rate and sucking outcomes (van der Heijden et al. 2016); respiratory rate (Caparros-Gonzalez et al. 2018); and earlier discharge from the hospital (Menke et al. 2021). For parents, MT and MBI showed a significant reduction in stress and cortisol (Jayamala et al. 2015), and preferences to calming music with nurses being less attentive to the music experience (Rabold 2013).

17.3.3 Dementia Care in Acute Settings and Transition

Dementia care is a large topic that requires its own full analysis that is beyond this chapter. In this section, a general overview is discussed on the efficacy of music in supporting persons with dementia in hospital for acute or crisis support, and those in hospital transitioning home following rehabilitation, other hospitalization, or waiting for long-term care. In these settings, the behavioral and psychological symptoms of dementia (BPSD) can be intensified, given the inadequate familiarity of the environment. These include aggression, agitation, apathy, and depression (Cloak et al. 2024). MBIs, specifically individuals listening to music, offer benefits in dementia care as a realistic and feasible option, as well as active MT, which was discussed in other parts of this book.

In this section, the authors have assessed 139 articles (n = 139) and included eight articles (n = 8) in this review. Four articles are classified as systematic reviews (n = 4), two are narrative and systematic reviews (n = 2), one narrative review (n = 1), and one systematic review and meta-analysis (n = 1).

Studies like Kobets (2011) acknowledge that music should be used in dementia care in medical settings and further integration of MBIs especially MT as a core treatment is needed. One commonly reported issue noted in the systematic reviews below is a lack of protocol standardization of MBIs and MT interventions. Systematic reviews on music interventions and dementia found music applications were the best for reducing BPSD among non-pharmacological interventions (Abraha et al. 2017), and specifically MT, which included listening versus more active MT approaches were more beneficial in reducing BPSD (Tsoi et al. 2018) and MT assisted with BPSD and depression (van der Steen et al. 2018).

Hack et al.'s (2021) systematic review of ten studies involving music interventions for persons with dementia in acute settings found impact for the use of MBIs for mood and well-being as well as the BPSD symptoms of dementia. The challenge in these settings is assessing long-term effects and recruiting participants given the short stay environment. However, further research is needed given individuals with dementia in acute care settings are likely to experience other critical health issues impacting the use of MBIs.

In Leggieri et al.'s (2019) systematic review on the cognitive and behavioral outcomes of music listening versus MT interventions from 2009 to 2019, as well as individualized versus non-individualized music for Alzheimer's disease (AD) researchers found personalized individual music regardless of intervention provided optimal benefits for the person with AD. While a large pool of papers were initially identified, only six papers were included in their analysis' criteria. Results highlighted that active MT provided socialization and acute benefits, and music listening offered relaxation and a longer term impact. Similarly in Moreno-Morales et al.'s (2020) systematic review and meta-analysis of MT in dementia care, authors concluded that MT interventions, such as listening to music and singing, demonstrated improvement in quality of life, cognitive function, and long-term depression.

Further, Lam et al.'s (2020) systematic review of MT in dementia care included 82 studies (43 clinical trials and 39 systematic review and meta-analyses). Lam et al. (2020) found that there were significant reductions in common BPSD symptoms, such as anxiety, depression, and apathy, as well as improvements in verbal fluency following MT. In contrast to Moreno-Morales et al. (2020), Lam et al. (2020) were unable to determine MT's efficacy in quality of life or agitation.

In Soufineyestani et al.'s (2021) meta-narrative study, researchers investigated the evidence for active versus receptive music interventions, as well as either recorded or live music. Some issues were the lack of standardized music protocols, descriptions of the music-based interventions (MBIs), inadequate definition between MT and music-based interventions, the selection of appropriate music, and the role of music therapists in providing the MT or MBI. Researchers called for "... a comprehensive non-pharmacological music treatment approach to be designed for each stage of dementia to be employed alongside pharmacological treatments" (Soufineyestani et al. 2021, p. 1). Benefits of MBIs and MT included improvement in cognition, memory, self-esteem, emotional and BPSD symptoms of dementia, and quality of life.

17.4 Discussion

While this chapter aims to report the best practices for MT, MBIs, or a combination of both practices, many articles do not separate the interventions, making it difficult to write about them independently. What is an ongoing challenge is the lack of description of the MT and MBI interventions included in the individual studies, which comprise systematic reviews and other reviews. This inadequate description makes it difficult for clinicians to replicate and implement the MBIs in the care that they provide. Further, insufficient protocols and small sample sizes of studies included in the large reviews are also an issue. These are not easy issues to resolve, given that MT and MBIs require tailoring to some degree (personalization) in order to be effective. Below are specific points of discussion that were found in the resources of this chapter. They are discussed in each healthcare context.

17.4.1 Surgery

The majority of sources informing this section do not separate the type of music used in surgical environments (Lattimore 2017). This finding proposes challenges for the field of MT, as researchers categorize MBIs such as listening to music playlists, (Demir et al. 2021; Sadideen et al. 2012), the patient, or a healthcare team (Tan et al. 2020; Yeoh and Spence 2023) creates as music therapy.

The experimental articles included in this review offered quantitative results of a patient or the healthcare professional's symptoms based on the completion of self-reported scales, implying the possibilities of bias and inaccuracy of completion. Quantitative research is often found in the field of surgery, as it is a practice that is empirical and clinical by nature. Some studies (e.g., Lattimore 2017) offered a qualitative understanding of healthcare providers in their concerns about music by asking healthcare professionals about the use of music in these environments and the likelihood of utilizing music interventions in procedures. However, results of this study were analyzed quantitatively via percentages to understand the proportion of healthcare professionals using music interventions and the endorsement of music in surgery (Lattimore 2017) as opposed to responses to interviews of each participant, eliminating the possible qualitative data collection that can be performed in music and surgery.

As there are numerous benefits in the use of MT and MBIs in surgery for both patients and healthcare professionals, there are recommendations for future directions in this area. Music can be a potential distraction of work influenced by the volume levels (El Boghdady and Ewalds-Kvist 2020; Weldon et al. 2015); thus, impairing communication between operating staff and surgeons (Fu et al. 2021; Weldon et al. 2015), and hinder work climate and culture (Kakar et al. 2022). As well, an evaluation of patient music history is required (Williams and Hine 2018), as there is limited research and literature surrounding the nature of active music making by patients within the surgery environment (Criss et al. 2023). In addition, consideration in the music for patients and the healthcare team should include the following: music that matches the day of surgery; the genre (Yang et al. 2022) and cultural association of the music (Yeoh and Spence 2023); the volume of the music during operating treatment (El Boghdady and Ewalds-Kvist 2020); and the age of the patient in which music exposure can be administered in surgery (Kühlmann et al. 2020).

17.4.2 Neonatal Intensive Care Unit (NICU)

Case studies and case vignettes have highlighted the nature of MT and MBIs among patients, music therapists, other healthcare professionals in the NICU (Ettenberger 2017a), and parents of the patients (Kim 2022). While preterm infants do not have the capabilities of forming decisions, existing research suggests that there are preferences for these patients. For instance, Loewy (2015) mentioned that parents were asked to select culturally based and personalized music for infants in the NICU as a non-invasive intervention for enhanced quality of care. It was also recommended for parents to consider alternatives before engaging in music therapy, such as psychotherapy, to support the fear and anxiety associated with premature birth (Loewy 2015). Similarly, Pinto (2023) suggested that the effects of MBI and MT should consider the particular situations of the patients and their characteristics, implying the individualized approach to these services. These considerations may cause variations in the quality of MT and MBI, making it difficult to draw strong conclusions (van der Heijden et al. 2016).

Several studies recommended a balance between the participants involved in MBI and MT is essential to visualize the benefits. This can include babies in the NICU, parents, family members, and emerging relationships developed in the ward with other healthcare professionals (Ettenberger 2017b). For some music therapists, there were some difficulties in providing the necessary support of MT to their prenatal patients in the NICU, suggesting challenges of boundaries and inadequate knowledge to administer practice without a certified healthcare professional on site (Kim 2022).

17.4.3 Dementia Care in Acute Settings and Transition

In the case of MBIs for persons with dementia in acute settings, Hack et al.'s (2021) systematic review of ten studies summarized the impact of MBIs, addressing its implications for mood, well-being, and behavioral and psychological symptoms of dementia (BPSD). The challenge in these settings is assessing long-term effects and recruiting participants given the short stay environment. Further research is needed, given individuals with dementia in acute care settings are likely to experience other critical health issues impacting the use of MBIs. Lam et al. (2020) were unable to determine MT's efficacy in quality of life or agitation compared to the study by Moreno-Morales et al. (2020), who found improvements in cognitive function, quality of life, and long-term depression. As such, standardization of MT protocols is recommended to meet the needs of populations with dementia.

MT and MBIs are being used at an increasing rate in dementia care, but are not typically applied in the acute settings and transition. The National Institute of Health is calling for rigorously structured, well-powered clinical trials of MBIs (Edwards et al. 2023). Given that music is assessed to be the most beneficial non-pharmacological treatment for persons with dementia (Abraha et al. 2017), MT and MBIs should be implemented systematically in acute care settings as a tool to transition to the next care setting. Specifically, studies should be conducted to determine how MBIs and MT could support the BPSD of dementia during transition and integration into the next or new setting. As personalized music is central to the success of many MBIs, it is essential to ensure personalized music profiles are prepared to support the creation and implementation of MT and MBIs for each individual.

17.5 Conclusion

Table 17.2 outlines a summary of the key Music Therapy and Music Based Interventions applications effective for each healthcare area or issue.

Table 17.2 Key interventions in each healthcare area/issue

Healthcare area/issue	Key interventions (MBIs and MT) indicated
Surgery	Perioperatively applied MT and MBIs, music listening before surgery, music listening in the waiting room, music in the operating room, music playlists developed by a music therapist and with noise-cancelling earphones, web app music intervention, music with lower volume, instrumental music, music groups, individual/receptive MT, group/active-receptive integrated MT
Neonatal intensive care unit (NICU)	Live music sounding like a lullaby, sedative music, recorded music using the mother's voice, music guided relaxations, early vocal contact, medical MT, humming or improvised singing, family-centered MT, live music
Dementia	Music listening, active and receptive MT, singing, live and recorded music

17.6 Future Directions

This systematic review has presented an overview of MT and MBIs in several healthcare contexts including surgery, NICU, and dementia care in acute settings and transition. Further assessment is required on the efficacy and selection of music with a specific focus on defining and describing the music interventions utilized. Without this specification, there is difficulty to realize the benefits of MT and MBIs that may or may not be reported and their empirical significance to the results. Researchers are still documenting the benefits and considerations for each healthcare issue or context with a broad encompassing of music interventions, ranging from passive to active applications and in combination with other arts-based methods. Consistently, the assessment on the preferences for music is required, particularly to be culturally responsive. Future research should focus on not only the considerations listed in this chapter, but on developing necessary protocols where applicable, piloting these protocols in all global regions, and the inclusion of equity deserving groups and the voices of marginalized individuals. The service user voice is often absent in research study design. To resolve this concern, researchers can engage in more participatory action studies to advance the use of MT and MBIs in inclusion and the service user voice.

Acknowledgments Thank you, Elienna Wang, for assisting in the format of the references.

References

Abraha I, Rimland JM, Trotta FM, Dell'Aquila G, Cruz-Jentoft A, Petrovic M, Gudmundsson A, Soiza R, O'Mahony D, Guaita A, Cherubini A. Systematic review of systematic reviews of nonpharmacological interventions to treat behavioural disturbances in older patients with dementia. BMJ Open. 2017;7:e012759. https://doi.org/10.1136/bmjopen-2016-012759.

Azi LMTA, Azi ML, Viana MM, Panont ALP, Oliveira RMF, Sadigursky D, Alencar DF. Benefits of intraoperative music on orthopedic surgeries under spinal anesthesia: a randomized clinical trial. Complement Ther Med. 2021;63:102777. https://doi.org/10.1016/j.ctim.2021.102777.

Burrows A. Developmental care in the NICU: best practices for preterm infants, expectations of healthcare providers, and impact on parents and families. Assumption University; 2020. https://digitalcommons.assumption.edu/honorstheses/74

Canadian Association of Music Therapists. About music therapy. 2024. https://www.musictherapy.ca/about-camt-music-therapy/about-music-therapy/. Accessed 26 May 2024.

Caparros-Gonzalez RA, de la Torre-Luque A, Diaz-Piedra C, Vico FJ, Buela-Casal G. Listening to relaxing music improves physiological responses in premature infants: a randomized controlled trial. Adv Neonatal Care. 2018;18(1):58–69. https://doi.org/10.1097/ANC.0000000000000448.

Chandrababu R, Ramesh J, Sanatombi Devi E, Nayak BS, George A. Effectiveness of music on anxiety and pain among cardiac surgery patients: a quantitative systematic review and meta-analysis of randomized controlled trials. Int J Nurs Pract. 2021;27(4):e12928. https://doi.org/10.1111/ijn.12928.

Cici R, Özkan M. Effects on anxiety and vital signs of the emotional freedom technique and music before surgery for lumbar disc hernia. Altern Ther Health Med. 2022;28(5):20–7.

Clements-Cortés A, Pranjić M, Knott D, Mercadal-Brotons M, Fuller A, Kelly L, Selvarajah I, Vaudreuil R. International music therapists' perceptions and experiences in telehealth music therapy provision. Int J Environ Res Public Health. 2023;20(8):5580. https://doi.org/10.3390/ijerph20085580.

Cloak N, Schoo C, Khalili YA. Behavioral and psychological symptoms in dementia. StatPerals; 2024.

Costa VS, Bündchen DC, Sousa H, Pires LB, Felipetti FA. Clinical benefits of music-based interventions on preterm infants' health: a systematic review of randomised trials. Acta Paediatr. 2022;111(3):478–89. https://doi.org/10.1111/apa.16222.

Criss SD, Kakulamarri S, Xu RF, Fajardo M, Keeney T, Tolchin DW, May CJ. The healthcare experience of autistic patients in orthopaedic surgery and closely related fields: a scoping review. Children (Basel). 2023;10(5):906. https://doi.org/10.3390/children10050906.

Dahshan D, Kuzbel J, Verma V. A role for music in cataract surgery: a systematic review. Int Ophthalmol. 2021;41(12):4209–15. https://doi.org/10.1007/s10792-021-01986-9.

Dale VH. The impact of perioperative music on abdominal surgery patients' experience of postoperative pain: a systematic review and meta-analysis. J Perioper Pract. 2021;31(1–2):31–43. https://doi.org/10.1177/1750458920943375.

Demir B, Kapıkıran G, Özkan M. Effect of music on fatigue, comfort, and vital signs in patients after liver transplant surgery: a randomized controlled trial. Holist Nurs Pract. 2021;35(3):150–7. https://doi.org/10.1097/HNP.0000000000000444.

Edwards E, St Hillaire-Clarke C, Frankowski DW, Finkelstein R, Cheever T, Chen WG, Onken L, Poremba A, Riddle R, Schloesser D, Burgdorf CE, Wells N, Fleming R, Collins FS. NIH music-based intervention toolkit: music-based interventions for brain disorders of aging. Neurology. 2023;100(18):868–78. https://doi.org/10.1212/WNL.0000000000206797.

El Boghdady M, Ewalds-Kvist BM. The influence of music on the surgical task performance: a systematic review. Int J Surg. 2020;73:101–12. https://doi.org/10.1016/j.ijsu.2019.11.012.

Ettenberger M. Music therapy during end-of-life care in the neonatal intensive care unit (NICU) – reflections from early clinical practice in Colombia. Voices. 2017a;17(2):1–19. https://doi.org/10.15845/voices.v17i2.921.

Ettenberger M. Music therapy in the neonatal intensive care unit: putting the families at the centre of care. Br J Music Ther. 2017b;31(1):12–7. https://doi.org/10.1177/1359457516685881.

Ettenberger M, Rojas Cárdenas C, Parker M, Odell-Miller H. Family-centred music therapy with preterm infants and their parents in the neonatal intensive care unit (NICU) in Colombia – a mixed-methods study. Nord J Music Ther. 2016;26(3):207–34. https://doi.org/10.1080/08098131.2016.1205650.

Fenko A, Loock C. The influence of ambient scent and music on patients' anxiety in a waiting room of a plastic surgeon. HERD. 2014;7(3):38–59. https://doi.org/10.1177/193758671400700304.

Filippa M, Lordier L, De Almeida JS, Monaci MG, Adam-Darque A, Grandjean D, Kuhn P, Hüppi PS. Early vocal contact and music in the NICU: new insights into preventive interventions. Pediatr Res. 2020;87(2):249–64. https://doi.org/10.1038/s41390-019-0490-9.

Foster B, Pearson S, Berends A, Mackinnon C. The expanding scope, inclusivity, and integration of music in healthcare: recent developments, research illustration, and future direction. Healthcare (Basel). 2021;9(1):99. https://doi.org/10.3390/healthcare9010099.

Fu VX, Oomens P, Merkus N, Jeekel J. The perception and attitude toward noise and music in the operating room: a systematic review. J Surg Res. 2021;263:193–206. https://doi.org/10.1016/j.jss.2021.01.038.

Gallagher LM, Gardner V, Bates D, Mason S, Nemecek J, Difiore JB, Bena J, Li M, Bethoux F. Impact of music therapy on hospitalized patients post-elective orthopaedic surgery: a randomized controlled trial. Orthop Nurs. 2018;37(2):124–33. https://doi.org/10.1097/NOR.0000000000000432.

Gerdner LA. Individualized music for de entia: evolution and application of evidence-based protocol. World J Psychiatry. 2012;2(2):26–32. https://doi.org/10.5498/wjp.v2.i2.26.

Grafton-Clarke C, Grace L, Harky A. Music therapy following cardiac surgery—is it an effective method to reduce pain and anxiety? Interact Cardiovasc Thorac Surg. 2019;28(5):722–7. https://doi.org/10.1093/icvts/ivy311.

Guerrier G, Abdoul H, Jilet L, Rothschild P-R, Baillard C. Efficacy of a web app–based music intervention during cataract surgery: a randomized clinical trial. Arch Ophthalmol. 2021;139(9):1007–13. https://doi.org/10.1001/jamaophthalmol.2021.2767.

Haas R, Brandes V, editors. Music that works: contributions of biology, neurophysiology, psychology, sociology, medicine and musicology. Vienna: Springer; 2009. https://doi.org/10.1007/978-3-211-75121-3.

Hack K, Martin K, Atkinson C. The effectiveness of music as an intervention for dementia patients in acute settings: a literature review. Music Med. 2021;13(4):229–42. https://doi.org/10.47513/mmd.v13i4.787.

Haslbeck FB, Bassler D. Clinical practice protocol of creative music therapy for preterm infants and their parents in the neonatal intensive care unit. J Vis Exp. 2020;(155):e60412. https://doi.org/10.3791/60412.

Hole J, Hirsch M, Ball E, Meads C. Music as an aid for postoperative recovery in adults: a systematic review and meta-analysis. Lancet. 2015;386(10004):1659–71. https://doi.org/10.1016/S0140-6736(15)60169-6.

Jayamala AK, Lakshmanagowda PB, Pradeep GCM, Goturu J. Impact of music therapy on breast milk secretion in mothers of premature newborns. J Clin Diagn Res. 2015;9(4):CC04–6. https://doi.org/10.7860/JCDR/2015/11642.5776.

Kakar E, Ruler O, Straten B, Hoogteijling B, Graaf EJR, Ista E, Lange JF, Jeekel J, Klimek M. Implementation of music in colorectal perioperative standard care—barriers and facilitators among patients and healthcare professionals. Color Dis. 2022;24(7):868–75. https://doi.org/10.1111/codi.16102.

Kim H. The experience of music therapists working with the parents of premature infants in the neonatal intensive care unit (NICU). Dissertation, Molloy College. 2022

Kobets AJ. Harmonic medicine: the influence of music over mind and medical practice. Yale J Biol Med. 2011;84(2):161–7.

Koivisto T-A. Making our way through the deep waters of life: music practitioners' professional work in neonatal intensive care units. In: Westerlund H, Gaunt H, editors. Expanding professionalism in music and higher music education, vol. 1. 1st ed. Routledge; 2021. p. 115–28. https://doi.org/10.4324/9781003108337-10.

Kühlmann AYR, de Rooij A, Kroese LF, van Dijk M, Hunink MGM, Jeekel J. Meta-analysis evaluating music interventions for anxiety and pain in surgery. Br J Surg. 2018;105(7):773–83. https://doi.org/10.1002/bjs.10853.

Kühlmann AYR, van Rosmalen J, Staals LM, Keyzer-Dekker CMG, Dogger J, de Leeuw TG, van der Toorn F, Jeekel J, Wijnen RMH, van Dijk M. Music interventions in pediatric surgery (the music under surgery in children study): a randomized clinical trial. Anesth Analg. 2020;130(4):991–1001. https://doi.org/10.1213/ANE.0000000000003983.

Lagattolla F, Zanchi B, Pietro M, Cormio C, Lorusso V, Diotaiuti S, Fanizzi A, Massafra R, Costanzo S, Caporale F, Rieti E, Romito F. Receptive music therapy versus group music therapy with breast cancer patients hospitalized for surgery. Support Care Cancer. 2023;31(3):162. https://doi.org/10.1007/s00520-023-07624-7.

Lam HL, Li WTV, Laher I, Wong RY. Effects of music therapy on patients with dementia – a systematic review. Geriatrics (Basel). 2020;5(4):62. https://doi.org/10.3390/GERIATRICS5040062.

Lattimore K. Assessing healthcare providers perspective: music intervention for open heart surgery patients. St. John Fisher University; 2017. https://fisherpub.sjf.edu/cgi/viewcontent.cgi?article=1055&context=nursing_etd_masters

Leggieri M, Thaut MH, Fornazzari L, Schweizer TA, Barfett J, Munoz DG, Fischer CE. Music intervention approaches for Alzheimer's disease: a review of the literature. Front Neurosci. 2019;13:132. https://doi.org/10.3389/fnins.2019.00132.

Lin C, Hwang S, Jiang P, Hsiung N. Effect of music therapy on pain after orthopedic surgery—a systematic review and meta-analysis. Pain Pract. 2020;20(4):422–36. https://doi.org/10.1111/papr.12864.

Loewy J. NICU music therapy: song of kin as critical lullaby in research and practice. Ann N Y Acad Sci. 2015;1337(1):178–85. https://doi.org/10.1111/nyas.12648.

Menke BM, Hass J, Diener C, Pöschl J. Family-centered music therapy – empowering premature infants and their primary caregivers through music: results of a pilot study. PLoS One. 2021;16:e0250071. https://doi.org/10.1371/journal.pone.0250071.

Miyata K, Odanaka H, Nitta Y, Shimoji S, Kanehira T, Kawanami M, Fujisawa T. Music before dental surgery suppresses sympathetic activity derived from preoperative anxiety: a randomized controlled trial. JDR Clin Trans Res. 2016;1(2):153–62. https://doi.org/10.1177/2380084416650613.

Moreno-Morales C, Calero R, Moreno-Morales P, Pintado C. Music therapy in the treatment of dementia: a systematic review and meta-analysis. Front Med. 2020;7:160. https://doi.org/10.3389/fmed.2020.00160.

Narayanan A, Pearson L, Fisher JP, Khashram M. The effect of background music on stress in the operating surgeon: scoping review. BJS Open. 2022;6(5):zrac112. https://doi.org/10.1093/bjsopen/zrac112.

Oomens P, Fu VX, Kleinrensink GJ, Jeekel J. The effect of music on simulated surgical performance: a systematic review. Surg Endosc. 2019;33(9):2774–84. https://doi.org/10.1007/s00464-019-06868-x.

Page MJ, McKenzie JE, Bossuyt PM, Boutron I, Hoffmann TC, Mulrow CD, Shamseer L, Tetzlaff JM, Akl EA, Brennan SE, Chou R, Glanville J, Gimshaw JM, Hróbjartsson A, Lalu MM, Li T, Loder EW, Mayo-Wilson E, McDonald S, McGuinness LA, Stewart LA, Thomas J, Tricco AC, Welch VA, Whiting P, Moher D. The PRISMA 2020 statement: an updated guideline for reporting systematic reviews. BMJ. 2021;372:n71. https://doi.org/10.1136/bmj.n71.

Pineda R, Roussin J, Heiny E, Smith J. Health care professionals' perceptions about sensory-based interventions in the NICU. Am J Perinatol. 2019;36(12):1229–36. https://doi.org/10.1055/s-0038-1676536.

Pinto DPS. Prematurity: can music have a role in neonatal intensive care unit? Centro Hospitalar e Universitário de Coimbra – Hospital Pediátrico; 2023. https://estudogeral.uc.pt/handle/10316/111563

Popay J, Roberts H, Sowden A, Petticrew M, Arai L, Rodgers M, Britten N, Roen K, Duffy S. Guidance on the conduct of narrative synthesis in systematic reviews. A product from the ESRC methods programme. Version 1. Lancaster University; 2006. https://www.lancaster.ac.uk/media/lancaster-university/content-assets/documents/fhm/dhr/chir/NSsynthesisguidanceVersion1-April2006.pdf. Accessed 1 June 2024.

Rabold S. The effects of music therapy in the NICU on behavior, weight, and length of stay: a systematic review. San Marcos: California State University; 2013. https://scholarworks.calstate.edu/concern/theses/td96k303s#

Raglio A, Oasi O. Music and health: what interventions for what results? Front Psychol. 2015;6:230. https://doi.org/10.3389/fpsyg.2015.00230.

Rivera PA, Linderman WL, Miguez S, Chow J, DeBroff B, Diaz V. Music during cataract surgery: impact on anxiety. J Cataract Refract Surg. 2024;50:688. https://doi.org/10.1097/j.jcrs.0000000000001444.

Roa E, Ettenberger M. Music therapy self-care group for parents of preterm infants in the neonatal intensive care unit: a clinical pilot intervention. Medicines (Basel). 2018;5(4):134. https://doi.org/10.3390/medicines5040134.

Sadideen H, Parikh A, Dobbs T, Pay A, Critchley PS. Is there a role for music in reducing anxiety in plastic surgery minor operations? Ann R Coll Surg Engl. 2012;94:1–3. https://doi.org/10.1308/003588412X13171221501861.

Särkämö T, Tervaniemi M, Laitinen S, Forsblom A, Soinila S, Mikkonen M, Autti T, Silvennoinen HM, Erkkilä J, Laine M, Peretz I, Hietanen M. Music listening enhances cognitive recovery and mood after middle cerebral artery stroke. Brain. 2008;131(3):866–76. https://doi.org/10.1093/brain/awn013.

Soufineyestani M, Khan A, Sufineyestani M. Impacts of music intervention on dementia: a review using meta-narrative method and agenda for future research. Neurol Int. 2021;13(1):1–17. https://doi.org/10.3390/neurolint13010001.

Stegemann T, Geretsegger M, Phan Quoc E, Riedl H, Smetana M. Music therapy and other music-based interventions in pediatric health care: an overview. Medicines (Basel). 2019;6(1):25. https://doi.org/10.3390/medicines6010025.

Tan DJA, Polascik BA, Kee HM, Hui Lee AC, Sultana R, Kwan M, Raghunathan K, Belden CM, Sng BL. The effect of perioperative music listening on patient satisfaction, anxiety, and depression: a quasiexperimental study. Anesthesiol Res Pract. 2020;2020(1):3761398. https://doi.org/10.1155/2020/3761398.

Tsoi KKF, Chan JYC, Ng Y-M, Lee MMY, Kwok TCY, Wong SYS. Receptive music therapy is more effective than interactive music therapy to relieve behavioral and psychological symptoms of dementia: a systematic review and meta-analysis. J Am Med Dir Assoc. 2018;19(7):568–76. https://doi.org/10.1016/j.jamda.2017.12.009.

Ullsten A. Singing, sharing, soothing: family-centred music therapy during painful procedures in neonatal care. Dissertation, Örebro University. 2019.

van der Heijden MJE, Oliai Araghi S, van Dijk M, Jeekel J, Hunink MGM. The effects of perioperative music interventions in pediatric surgery: a systematic review and meta-analysis of randomized controlled trials. PLoS One. 2015;10(18):e0133608. https://doi.org/10.1371/journal.pone.0133608.

van der Heijden MJE, Oliai Araghi S, Jeekel J, Reiss IKM, Hunink MGM, van Dijk M. Do hospitalized premature infants benefit from music interventions? A systematic review of randomized controlled trials. PLoS One. 2016;11(9):e0161848. https://doi.org/10.1371/journal.pone.0161848.

van der Steen JT, Smaling HJA, van der Wouden JC, Bruinsma MS, Scholten RJPM, Vink AC. Music-based therapeutic interventions for people with dementia. Cochrane Database Syst Rev. 2018;(7):CD003477. https://doi.org/10.1002/14651858.CD003477.pub4.

Weldon S-M, Korkiakangas T, Bezemer J, Kneebone R. Music and communication in the operating theatre. J Adv Nurs. 2015;71(12):2763–74. https://doi.org/10.1111/jan.12744.

Williams C, Hine T. An investigation into the use of recorded music as a surgical intervention: a systematic, critical review of methodologies used in recent adult controlled trials. Complement Ther Med. 2018;37:110–26. https://doi.org/10.1016/j.ctim.2018.02.002.

Wu P-Y, Huang M-L, Lee W-P, Wang C, Shih W-M. Effects of music listening on anxiety and physiological responses in patients undergoing awake craniotomy. Complement Ther Med. 2017;32:56–60. https://doi.org/10.1016/j.ctim.2017.03.007.

Xu X, Sun BL, Huang F, Chia HLA, Sultana R, Teo A, Tuner BS. The impact of music on patient satisfaction, anxiety, and depression in patients undergoing gynecologic surgery. J Perianesth Nurs. 2021;36(2):122–7. https://doi.org/10.1016/j.jopan.2020.08.014.

Yang C, Möttig F, Weitz J, Reissfelder C, Mees ST. Effect of genre and amplitude of music during laparoscopic surgery. Langenbeck's Arch Surg. 2022;407(5):2115–21. https://doi.org/10.1007/s00423-022-02490-z.

Yeoh JPS, Spence C. Background music's impact on patients waiting in surgery and radiology clinics. HERD. 2023;16(3):278–90. https://doi.org/10.1177/19375867231161094.

A Systematic Review of Music Therapy and Music-Based Interventions in Healthcare Applications: Eating Disorders, Work-Related Stress, Homelessness, Artists and Concerts in Music and Medicine

18

Amy Clements-Cortés and Joyce Jing Yee Yip

18.1 Introduction

A full introduction, including details on the methodology, is presented in Part 1 (Chap. 17), alongside the assessment on surgery, NICU, and dementia care in acute settings and transition. In this chapter, the authors will report Part 2 of this systematic review. The results will describe eating disorders (EDs), work-related stress, homelessness, artists in residence, and concerts/music and medicine and is presented below. This narrative synthesis systematic review was aimed to assess the effectiveness and utility of MT, MBIs, or a combination of both practices in the existing research and literature within the respective healthcare context. With the last two areas (artists in residence and concerts/music and medicine), the analysis is focused on MBIs, some of which are informed by music therapy practices and foundations.

18.2 Methodology

Part 2 of this systematic review includes the research and scholarly literature published in English within the last two decades (2004–2024), assessing MT and MBIs in the following healthcare contexts and/or concerns: eating disorders, work-related

A. Clements-Cortés (✉)
Faculty of Music, University of Toronto, Toronto, ON, Canada
e-mail: a.clements.cortes@utoronto.ca

J. J. Y. Yip
Ontario Institute for Studies in Education, University of Toronto, Toronto, ON, Canada
e-mail: joycejingyee.yip@mail.utoronto.ca

A. Raglio (ed.), *Music and Music Therapy Interventions in Clinical Practice*, Neurocultural Health and Wellbeing,
https://doi.org/10.1007/978-3-031-88578-5_18

stress, homelessness, artists in residence, and concerts/music and medicine. The keywords that were used in the search formula combined various terms based on the topic of inquiry, and included these terms: music, music therapy, music-based interventions, music medicine, music in medicine, music and medicine, music and health, music listening, eating disorders, workplace, stress, artists in residence, concerts in music and medicine, homelessness, and unhoused individuals. Please refer to Fig. 18.1 for the PRISMA chart, which provides a summary of the identification, screening, and retrieval process (Page et al. 2021).

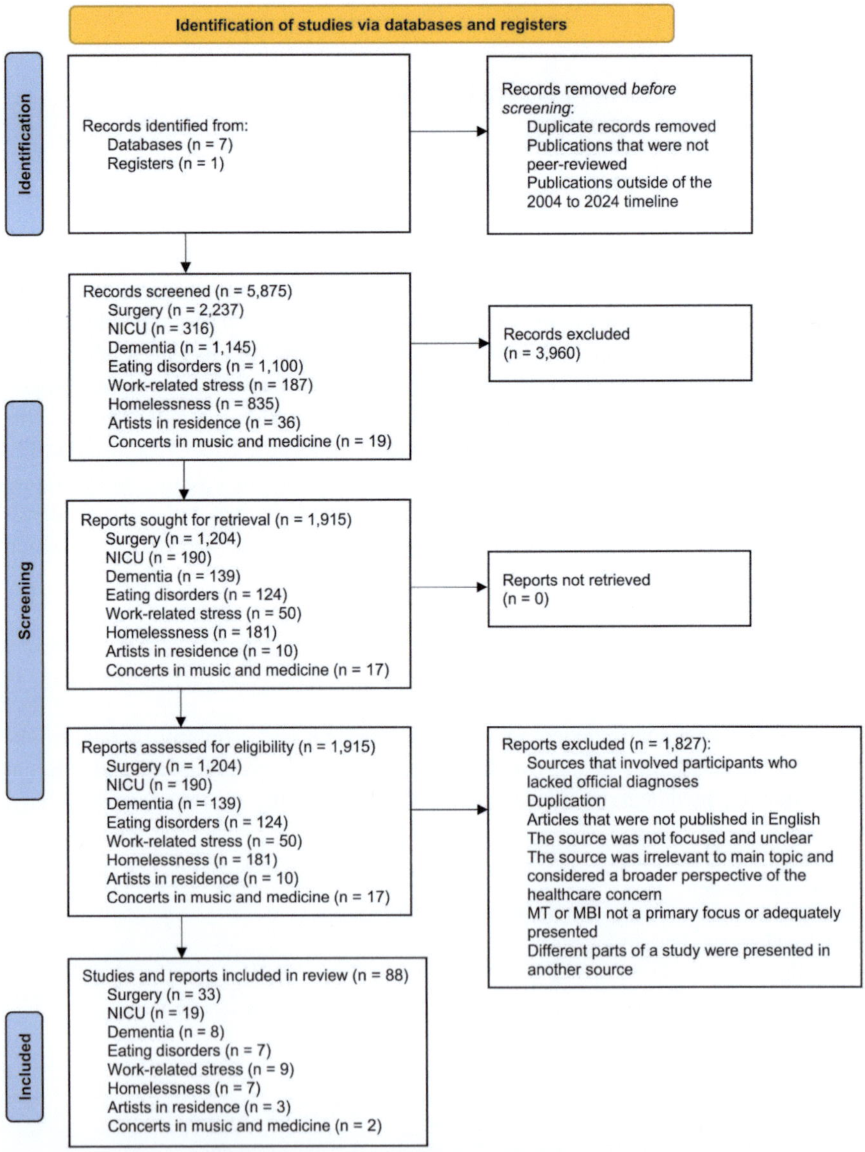

Fig. 18.1 PRISMA Chart of searched results for Part 1 and Part 2 (Page et al. 2021)

18.3 Results

Eighty-eight resources ($n = 88$) were used in Chap. 17 and this chapter. The number of papers after the initial review is noted for each healthcare context and an overview of the healthcare setting is also provided. A total of 5875 articles were identified and screened from databases ($n = 7$) and register ($n = 1$). A total of 1915 reports were sought for retrieval and assessed for eligibility. The exclusion criteria at this stage was as follows: sources lacking official diagnoses; duplicate records; sources not published in English; inadequate study clarity; irrelevancy to the main topic or presented a broader perspective of the health concern; MT and MBIs that were not clearly described or not the focus; or parts of the article were presented in another report.

The authors recognized the difficulty to separate out MBIs from MT independently as individual categories, as descriptors provided by researchers were unclear and have perspectives from allied healthcare professions. Many articles evaluated all music-based experiences and at times, the terminology (MT and MBIs) were not consistent. Hence, some overlap is presented within the resources found.

Please see Table 18.1 to observe the details of each source included in the review with the following categories: Healthcare area/issue; Author, title & year; Type of source; and Main applications, Benefits, and Considerations.

18.3.1 Eating Disorders (EDs)

One hundred and twenty-four articles ($n = 124$) have been initially reviewed with seven sources ($n = 7$) being included in this review. The breakdown of these sources resulted in: two narrative reviews ($n = 2$); two mixed methods ($n = 2$); two classified as both meta-analysis and systematic review ($n = 2$) and one systematic review ($n = 1$). Only five articles (Chang et al. 2023; Dvorak 2023; Pasiali et al. 2020; Shah et al. 2023; Testa et al. 2020) were documented in Table 18.1, as these resources best resonate with the focus of music as the primary intervention.

A key takeaway from work in the area of MT and MBIs in ED was that the outcomes and efficacy of MT and MBIs depended on context, age, theoretical framework, and cultural factors. This has been attested in the selected sources. Testa et al.'s (2020) systematic literature review analyzed the use of music for persons with eating disorders. In the review, 16 studies found that group singing reduced post-prandial anxiety in individuals with anorexia nervosa (AN), and songwriting was seen as valuable when paired with processing of related image perception topics (Testa et al. 2020). Further, individuals with AN benefitted from listening to classical music to increase or assist with food consumption while individuals with bulimia nervosa (BN) found benefit in vodcasts with visual or autobiographical stimuli with respect to body image (Testa et al. 2020). Testa et al. (2020) found that music videos reinforced body dissatisfaction for persons with ED, suggesting the transition into social media and other digital sources as a place for information and influence.

Table 18.1 A systematic review of music therapy and music-based interventions in healthcare applications: Eating disorders, work-related stress, homelessness, artists and concerts in music and medicine

			Main applications				
Healthcare area/issue	Authors, title & year	Type of source	Music therapy (MT)	Music-based Interventions (MBIs)	Combination	Benefits	Considerations
Eating disorders	Chang et al. (2023). Music-based intervention impacts for people with eating disorders: a narrative synthesis systematic review.	Systematic review			X	Improved mood regulation, emotional well-being, and management of meal-related distress. Video podcasts (Vodcast) were also used for healthy eating for non-inpatients	Suboptimal description of MBIs and quality reporting of complex MBIs make it challenging to see how MT can help people with EDs to live healthier lives
Eating disorders	Dvorak (2023). Explanatory sequential descriptive analysis of music therapists' clinical practice for individuals with eating disorders.	Experimental	Improvisation, composition, receptive and recreative interventions			Self-expression, coping skills, improvement for depression, identify, and express feelings	

Eating disorders	Pasiali et al. (2020). Music therapy programming for persons with eating disorders: a review with clinical examples.	Narrative review	Improvisation, song autobiography, song discussion, song writing, music assisted relaxation and imagery, Bonny method of guided imagery and music			Pathway to explore sense of self and identity Search for meaning and emotional healing feelings, anxiety, body image, self-esteem exploration	
Eating disorders	Shah et al. (2023). The impact of group music therapy for individuals with eating disorders.	Experimental	Improvisation, singing, drumming, listening to recorded improvisation, creating art, mindfulness-based exercise			Express emotions, foster social connections, reduced negative affect	
Eating disorders	Testa et al. (2020). A systematic review of scientific studies on the effects of music in people with or at risk for eating disorders.	Systematic review	Music listening, songwriting, singing, vodcasts			Reduced anxiety, increased food consumption, processing of body image perception	

(continued)

Table 18.1 (continued)

			Main applications				
Healthcare area/issue	Authors, title & year	Type of source	Music therapy (MT)	Music-based Interventions (MBIs)	Combination	Benefits	Considerations
Work-related stress	Beck et al. (2015). Coping with work-related stress through guided imagery and music (GIM): randomized controlled trial.	Experimental	Guided imagery music (GIM) and MT			Improved well-being, mood, physical distress, and managed cortisol levels. Job return was quicker when participants started GIM closer to sick leave	
Work-related stress	de Witte et al. (2020). Effects of music interventions on stress-related outcomes: a systematic review and two meta-analyses.	Systematic review and meta analyses	X	Music as medicine, music listening		Stress reduction in physiological (heart rate, blood pressure, hormones) and psychological (anxiety, restlessness) outcomes	
Work-related stress	de Witte et al. (2022). Development of a music therapy micro-intervention for stress reduction.	Scoping review	Active and passive protocols			Stress reduction replicability by other therapists, short-term intervention, transferability to daily life	

Work-related stress	Matoso et al. (2022). The effect of organizational music therapy on reducing the stress level of health care professionals in a public hospital.	Experimental	Receptive MT			Reduces stress and improves work-life quality of hospital professionals	
Work-related stress	McFerran et al. (2018). Intentional music use to reduce psychological distress in adolescents accessing primary mental health care.	Experimental	X			Improvements in distress and social engagement among peers	
Work-related stress	O'Brien et al. (2021). Evolving and thriving—keeping music therapy alive in a pandemic world: the royal Melbourne hospital music therapy response in 2020.	Scoping review	X			Challenges, new ways of working, and celebrates live music in public hospitals	Cultural and gender limitations; adapting physical restrictions during COVID; developing long COVID clinic with MT as part of recovery program; evolution of MT

(continued)

Table 18.1 (continued)

Healthcare area/issue	Authors, title & year	Type of source	Main applications			Benefits	Considerations
			Music therapy (MT)	Music-based Interventions (MBIs)	Combination		
Work-related stress	Son et al. (2019). Effects of aromatherapy combined with music therapy on anxiety, stress, and fundamental nursing skills in nursing students: a randomized controlled trial.	Experimental	X		MT and aromatherapy	Aroma and MT had a significant effect on reducing anxiety & stress, and nursing performance	
Work-related stress	Wang et al. (2022). Light acupuncture and five-element music therapy for nurses' mental health and well-being during and post-COVID-19: protocol for a randomised cross-over feasibility study.	Experimental	Before and after light acupuncture treatment and 5-element music therapy			Improved nurses' mental well-being in hospitals after using light acupuncture and MT	

Work-related stress	Yıldırım and Çiriş Yıldız (2022). The effect of mindfulness-based breathing and music therapy practice on nurses' stress, work-related strain, and psychological well-being during the COVID-19 pandemic.	Experimental	Mindfulness-based breathing and music therapy			Decreased stress and work-related strain, increased psychological well-being	
Homelessness	Bailey and Davidson (2005). Effects of group singing and performance for marginalized and middle-class singers.	Experimental	Songwriting, improvisation, instrument playing and composition	Choral singing		Social engagement, mental stimulation, increased adaptive skills, reduced substance misuse and emotional and physical stress as well as the ability to make progress toward goals	
Homelessness	Cournoyer Lemaire et al. (2020). A critical scoping review about the impact of music in the lives of young adults who use drugs.	Scoping review	Improvisation, songwriting, and lyric analysis			Coping mechanism from stressors, emotional regulation, self-expression and connection to individuals with addiction	

(continued)

Table 18.1 (continued)

Healthcare area/issue	Authors, title & year	Type of source	Main applications			Benefits	Considerations
			Music therapy (MT)	Music-based Interventions (MBIs)	Combination		
Homelessness	Gregory et al. (2024). Music therapy in shelters for people who are unhoused: a scoping review.	Scoping review	Songwriting, song sharing, singing, musical games, lyric analysis, improvisation, progressive muscles relaxation, drumming, and performance			Promoted empowerment and well-being	Challenge of attendance, lack of studies with families Inability to generalize the results given variability in issues of homelessness Protocols needed to advance this area of practice
Homelessness	Rio (2005). Adults in recovery: a year in members of the choirhouse.	Experimental	Songwriting, improvisation, instrument playing and composition	Choral singing		Participants achieved greater insights of personal issues of homelessness, substance abuse, interpersonal relationships, music, creativity, and spirituality	Church provided shelter for the homeless, but very little provided in the way of mental health support; benefits for a day treatment approach to recovery

Artists in residence	Beard (2023). Artists in residence: music therapy students in intergenerational relationships with older adults residing in an assisted living facility.	Experimental		.	Group singing to highly familiar music	Developed music therapy student education and curriculums; growth of leadership, musical, and clinical skills for students	Improvements in all dependent measures for older adults; significant. Intergenerational relationships
Artists in residence	Danila et al. (2018). A performing arts intervention improves cognitive dysfunction in 50 hospitalized older adults.	Experimental		Storytelling and poetry intervention		High satisfaction between the patient and the artist with lower delirium scores at discharge	
Artists in residence	Sonke et al. (2017). Nurse perceptions of artists as collaborators in interprofessional care teams.	Experimental		X		Artists are valued as part of the interprofessional care team, focusing on patient-centered care by providing holistic dimensions, cognitive and social engagement, and meaningful interactions	Cost-effective for creativity and collaboration

(continued)

Table 18.1 (continued)

			Main applications				
Healthcare area/issue	Authors, title & year	Type of source	Music therapy (MT)	Music-based Interventions (MBIs)	Combination	Benefits	Considerations
Concerts in music and medicine	da Rocha et al. (2022). Effects of concert music on cognitive, physiological, and psychological parameters in the elderly with dementia: a quasi-experimental study.	Experimental		Music listening sessions, once a week, versus a control group		Statistically significant reduction in apathy	Music preferences are required for behavior changes
Concerts in music and medicine	Shibazaki and Marshall (2017). Exploring the impact of music concerts in promoting well-being in dementia care.	Experimental		Concerts of professional musicians		Increased cooperation, interaction, conversation, care and opportunities for assessment and well-being; decreased levels of agitation and anti-social behavior	Musical preferences were present

An "X" symbol was used to indicate if MBI or MT was reported, but no further description or specifics were given

With respect to MT, Pasiali et al.'s (2020) narrative literature review examined six clinical interventions: songwriting, song discussion, song autobiography, improvisation, music-assisted relaxation and imagery, and the Bonny method of guided imagery and music. The results in this review found that music served as a container to explore feelings, anxiety, body image, self-esteem, and identity (Pasiali et al. 2020). Similarly, Shah et al. (2023) examined improvisation, singing, drumming, listening to recorded improvisation, creating art and using mindfulness-based exercise in MT groups for persons with ED. Findings augment the role of playing, creating music, assisting participants to discover various aspects of self in their recovery process and provide the avenue to stay with those emotions, share them, and foster social connections (Shah et al. 2023). There were lower levels of negative affect reported post sessions, even when considering anxiety was high prior to sessions (Shah et al. 2023). From the perspective of music therapists practicing from a variety of theoretical frameworks of MT (including cognitive behavior therapy, humanistic, psychoanalytic, and neurologic MT), Dvorak (2023) reported participants used receptive, recreative, improvisation, and composition methods to achieve outcomes of identification and expression of feelings, managing depression, enhancing self-expression, and coping skills.

Chang et al. (2023) published a systematic review of 16 studies, examining MT ($n = 5$), MBIs ($n = 4$), and "other MBIs" ($n = 7$) for persons with ED. Other MBIs were defined as interventions of music delivered by a practitioner other than a music therapist, such as a healthcare worker or musician (Chang et al. 2023). They noted the efficacy of singing, songwriting, and guided imagery and music in group settings supported emotional wellness and psychosocial development (Chang et al. 2023). Dance or movement therapy interventions, which include music into the creative arts, were also found to increase mood, self-awareness, and relationship building, but the use of music or its functionality and efficacy were not explored (Padrao and Coimbra 2011; Savidaki et al. 2020).

18.3.2 Work-Related Stress

In this systematic review, 50 results ($n = 50$) were sought for retrieval and only nine articles ($n = 9$) were evaluated. Six articles ($n = 6$) were classified as experimental studies, one was a systematic review and meta-analysis ($n = 1$), and two were scoping reviews ($n = 2$). None of the sources ($n = 0$) addressed the impact of MBIs on this topic. Hence, this section will focus on the impact of MT on work-related stress.

To begin, O'Brien et al. (2021) offered a definition of work-related stress and the impact of MT through a systematic review. Work-related stress involves situations where there are significant changes to the physiological and psychological health of a person in either clinical, medical, work, or study-related studies (O'Brien et al. 2021). MT in work-related stress entails a personalized approach of music therapists, which can include the creation of active and passive micro music intervention protocols via improvisation, client song choice, and adjustments of tempo and dynamics (de Witte et al. 2022); as well as the use of modified-guided imagery and music interventions that utilize MT philosophies (Beck et al. 2015).

Researchers focused on the quantitative nature of MT in work-related stress through administering receptive music therapy and visualizing stress levels after a period of time (Matoso et al. 2022); intervention of treatment groups (e.g., mindfulness and breathing in MT) versus control of no MT (Yıldırım and Çiriş Yıldız 2022); facilitating MT alone in a guided imagery and music modified intervention (Beck et al. 2015); and MT with another treatment such as light acupuncture treatment (Wang et al. 2022) or aromatherapy (Son et al. 2019). Results showed that MT reduced stress and work-related strain (in measures like anxiety and job performance) to improve the well-being of various populations like nurses in hospitals (Son et al. 2019; Wang et al. 2022; Yıldırım and Çiriş Yıldız 2022); other hospital healthcare professionals (Matoso et al. 2022); young individuals in mental healthcare (McFerran et al. 2018); and individuals looking to return to work after sick leave (Beck et al. 2015). These studies emphasized the impact of holistic approaches in congruence with MT to address aspects of well-being (Wang et al. 2022) like changes of physiological outcomes (e.g., heart rate, blood pressure, and hormones), psychological outcomes (e.g., measures of anxiety and restlessness) (de Witte et al. 2020; O'Brien et al. 2021), and other bio-social measures such as improved levels of mood disturbance and cortisol concentrations (Beck et al. 2015).

18.3.3 Homelessness

The authors retrieved 181 articles (n = 181) and retained seven articles (n = 7) to include in this review. Two papers are classified as qualitative experimental investigations (n = 2) and two focused on scoping reviews (n = 2). The three remaining articles (n = 3) included one systematic review of singing for mental health which references group singing among individuals experiencing homelessness (n = 1), one scoping review of housing interventions for adults experiencing homelessness which included music-based studies (n = 1), and one systematic narrative review of arts-based methods with young persons having complex psychosocial needs, which references one paper on homelessness (n = 1). However, the last three articles (Nathan et al. 2023; Semborski et al. 2021; Williams et al. 2018) are not indexed in Table 18.1, as they were not solely focused on the use of music with unhoused individuals.

In the research, MBIs and MT have an impact on individuals experiencing homelessness, with more emphasis on MT than MBIs. Many issues and factors result in persons being unhoused. For instance, being aged out of foster care (Yoshioka-Maxwell 2022); discharge from the military (Tsai and Kelton 2022) or criminal justice system (Almquist and Walker 2022); family violence (Clark et al. 2019); discrimination (Gutman et al. 2022); substance abuse and addiction (Cournoyer Lemaire et al. 2020; Rio 2005); and extreme poverty (Hepburn et al. 2022) were situations where one could become homeless. MT has been observed as an accessible and beneficial resource for addressing complex needs of these individuals. A variety of interventions were administered such as songwriting (Nathan et al. 2023); lyric analysis (Cournoyer Lemaire et al. 2020); composition, song sharing, singing, musical games, improvisation progressive muscle relaxation, drumming, and performance (Gregory et al. 2024); and choral singing (Bailey and Davidson 2005; Rio 2005). Benefits of MT were significant to the homeless population, including improvements in social engagement, mental stimulation, increased adaptive skills, reduced substance misuse and emotional and physical stress, and the ability to make progress toward goals (Bailey and Davidson 2005; Rio 2005). It is also important to consider implications beyond the use of music in these environments, which included coping mechanisms, emotional regulation, and self expression (Cournoyer Lemaire et al. 2020); spirituality, substance abuse, and relationships (Rio 2005); housing interventions and mental health (Semborski et al. 2021; Williams et al. 2018); and co-created knowledge with others using other arts-based methods (Nathan et al. 2023).

18.3.4 Artists in Residence

Artists in residence in healthcare can be defined as a visiting professional artist or group of artists that are brought into an environment of care to share their creative knowledge and practice to everyday lives of patients, family, visitors, and staff (Sonke 2015). In this systematic literature search, no scoping reviews or other reviews ($n = 0$) were found about this topic. Ten reports ($n = 10$) were sought for retrieval. The three resources ($n = 3$) documented in this review described the work of artists in residence in healthcare environments, whereby all were experimental designs. The creative endeavors of artists in residence in these articles were present in a medical center or unit (Danila et al. 2018; Sonke et al. 2017) and assisted living facility (Beard 2023). These endeavors contained facilitating storytelling and poetry (Danila et al. 2018); group singing to highly familiar music (Beard 2023); and performing in concerts as a professional musician (Shibazaki and Marshall 2017). For patients, positive effects were highlighted through the work of artists in residence, including high levels of satisfaction and lower delirium scores of elders in acute care (Danila et al. 2018); improvements in quality of life and well-being, lower self-reported depression and anxiety levels of older adults, and increased awareness of intergenerational relationships with music (Beard 2023).

18.3.5 Concerts in Music and Medicine

Broadly, music and medicine can be understood as the encouragement and support of music in medical contexts such as "benefits of music and its specialized applications in healthcare" (International Association for Music and Medicine 2024, para. 1). Concerts in music and medicine allow people living in healthcare environments to have no restrictions on live performances of music, whether performed as a participant or enjoyed as a spectator (Bayliss 2016).

In this search, 19 research and literature resources ($n = 19$) were screened, resulting in 17 reports ($n = 17$) sought for retrieval and assessed for eligibility. Concerts in music and medicine do not include exposure of music engagements outside of music and medicine settings, such as outdoor music festivals, pop, Rock and Roll concerts, or classical music in venues (Cha et al. 2015; Czepiel et al. 2021; Gjestland and Tronstad 2017; Moreno-Gutiérrez et al. 2023), any logistics related to sound protection and exposure (Alves Araujo et al. 2017; Beach et al. 2020; Kil et al. 2017; Vogel et al. 2014), environmental factors (Chen and Cabrera 2023), lighting effects (Salet et al. 2019), substance use (Ruest et al. 2018), and other general injuries (Schifferle et al. 2023). In this section, two results ($n = 2$) will be discussed with all being experimental designs.

Examples were shared about music's impact on specific situations. This included the "Mozart Effect" (the listening of Mozart's music in the womb or prenatal years) (Verrusio et al. 2015); arts programs in hospitals to promote socialization among adult patients, staff, and artists involved (Preti and Boyce-Tillman 2015); increased cardiovascular health for traditional Djembe drumming (Smith et al. 2014); and singing groups to bring people with dementia together for fun and play (Alzheimer's UK 2015). In addition, MBIs in music and medicine showed promising arts practice with the combination of music and other interdisciplinary arts, such as dance, improvisation, and visual arts. For instance, dance programs have been effective for patients with Parkinson's disease to support physical and psychological benefits with professional dancers (Houston and McGill 2013; Mark Morris Dance Group and Brooklyn Parkinson Group 2010); and enhanced creativity in styles such as hip hop dance (Hip Op-eration Crew 2013). There were also programs in improvisational storytelling in nursing or care facilities (Fritsch et al. 2009); visual arts practice to address recovery and well-being in a sexual assault referral center (Northern Health and Social Care Trust 2013); and art socialization for people with disabilities (Kable 2003).

The impact of music concerts in the experimental articles was focused on dementia care (Shibazaki and Marshall 2017), those diagnosed with Alzheimer's disease (da Rocha et al. 2022), long-term care (Clements-Cortés 2017), and more recently, the implications of music during the COVID-19 pandemic in in-patient care (Ambler et al. 2023). The concerts were facilitated in various ways: music listening for a set number of sessions (da Rocha et al. 2022); ensemble concerts with themes (Clements-Cortés 2017); virtual concerts of visual and sounds performed by professional musicians (Ambler et al. 2023); and music performances of duets by industry musicians that were repetitive (Shibazaki and Marshall 2017). Both in-person (Clements-Cortés 2017; Shibazaki and Marshall 2017) and virtual mediums (Ambler et al. 2023) were sought upon, creating concert programs that impacted experiences of performing musicians, patients, staff, and family members. Patients experienced positive effects from the concert experience with increased levels of cooperation and interaction in conversation (Shibazaki and Marshall 2017); engagement, enjoyment, special moments, and fostering connection (Clements-Cortés 2017); and decreased levels of apathy (da Rocha et al. 2022), patient isolation (Ambler et al. 2023), and agitation and anti-social behavior (Shibazaki and Marshall 2017). For family members and staff, there were also increased levels of care, cooperation, opportunities, and well-being presented by these individuals (Shibazaki and Marshall 2017). Positive benefits were also extended to performing musicians (Clements-Cortés 2017), suggesting the impact of concerts in music and medicine as extending to all participants in the process.

18.4 Discussion

While this chapter aims to report the best practices for MT, MBIs, or a combination of both practices, many articles do not separate the interventions making it difficult to write about them independently. What is an ongoing challenge is the lack of description of the MBIs and MT interventions included in the individual studies, which consist of systematic reviews and other reviews. This vague description is difficult for clinicians to understand how to replicate and implement the MBIs in the care that they provide. Further, a lack of protocols and small sample sizes of studies included in the large reviews are also an issue that was observed in this systematic review. While these concerns are not easy issues to resolve, MT and MBIs require tailoring to some degree (personalization) in order to be effective. Below are specific points of discussion that were found in the resources of this chapter. They are discussed by each healthcare context.

18.4.1 Eating Disorders (EDs)

Testa et al. (2020) noted the inadequate number of randomized control trials within their systematic literature review, thereby challenging the significance of results attributed to group singing and ED. As there was a small number of studies focused on either MT or MBIs for persons with ED, it is difficult to draw large conclusions on this subset. However, given the literature to date, songwriting, improvisation, singing, and combining music with arts-based interventions are demonstrating value and should be further assessed to persons impacted with ED at all ages but also in more inclusive ways to those who identify as non-binary, gender questioning, or those experiencing gender dysphoria.

18.4.2 Work-Related Stress

The quantitative results offered by O'Brien et al. (2021), de Witte et al. (2022), and Beck et al. (2015) emphasized the bio-psychosocial measures of work-related stress in the use of MT and MBIs. While this is important in research, future perspectives on the qualitative nature of music in work-related stress can offer insight into the participant's narratives on the issue. This is seen through works like McFerran et al. (2018), who accounted for self-reported, case study examples on the impact of

MBIs to distress in young people. In addition, through O'Brien's (2021) review, it is discovered that the majority of the studies involve music as medicine and not MT. The main mode of stress reduction in MBIs was listening to music alone with no details on the frequency, duration, or music qualities. In these observations, recommendations by O'Brien et al. (2021) include in-depth examination of the elements in MT protocols to pinpoint the benefits of these music interventions through a certified health professional.

18.4.3 Homelessness

In Gregory et al.'s (2024) study, generalizations cannot be drawn as there are few studies that included children, families, or adults within the last 10 years. The review promoted MT integration into shelter services for empowerment and well-being, but also suggested the need for further methods to address all age groups. As reiterated previously, the development of protocols, specifically in MT, is essential to foster benefits and program development in the field. MT is recommended to be a primary treatment in supporting issues that shelters and other care supports are unable to address, especially for individuals with substance abuse. Music can pose potential risks (e.g., the correlation between music styles and drug consumption) alongside settings where substance use is encouraged and not warranted (Cournoyer Lemaire et al. 2020).

18.4.4 Artists in Residence

For artists in residence, professional training has been a primary intervention to developing their creative arts wisdom in new environments such as healthcare. Scholars such as Beard (2023), Moss and O'Neill (2009), and Sonke et al. (2017) recommend the skills, challenges, and opportunities for artists in residence to work in this environment. In professional training, expressive art therapists (such as art, music, drama, and dance therapy) have been well established in various countries, resulting in the enrollment of post-secondary programs, certification, and work in healthcare settings outside the models of arts therapies (Moss and O'Neill 2009). While there may be overlap of artists in residences and expressive art therapists, artists in residence can have the role of being involved in the decision-making processes of meeting clinical goals of patients with the medical team on site as a creative arts partner. This was seen in Sonke et al. (2017), where artists are valued by nurses as members of an interprofessional care team, as they provided holistic dimensions in patient-centered care and built a culture of collaboration for clinical staff. At the time of Beard's (2023) study, the MT students were not certified as expressive arts therapists; hence, they were classified as artists in residence in this review.

As a result, there is a need for artists in residence to follow organizational policies, practices, and activities within healthcare settings through relevant training courses. Beard (2023) explains that experiences for artists in residences provide the growth of leadership, musical, and clinical skills to MT students, which can be applied to artists that fall outside of expressive arts therapy training like social and interpersonal skills, artistry, and professionalism. Moss and O'Neill (2009) highlight the best practices in training in arts and health through an observation of five organizations. A pilot course structure is recommended for artists with a primary degree in the art form that consists of seminars and shadowing placements that lead to accreditation in a postgraduate certificate or diploma (Moss and O'Neill 2009).

18.4.5 Concerts in Music and Medicine

Music and medicine is practiced internationally but may not be documented in peer-reviewed sources and may not be evidenced in this systematic review. This stands true for Shibazaki and Marshall (2017), whereby researchers attended 22 concerts in England and Japan, interviewing clients with dementia, nursing staff, and families about their experience. The variety of modalities in the music concerts suggests the alternatives to providing care, despite distances between healthcare professionals, and to promote enhanced well-being. The impact of concerts in music medicine was also significantly shown in female older adult patients (da Rocha et al. 2022) and based on the client's musical preferences (da Rocha et al. 2022; Shibazaki and Marshall 2017), implying that recommendations should be developed into concert music programming that is inclusive to all identities.

18.5 Conclusion

Table 18.2 outlines a summary of the key Music Therapy and Music Based Interventions applications effective for each healthcare area or issue.

Table 18.2 Key interventions in each healthcare area/issue

Healthcare area/ issue	Key interventions (MBIs and MT) indicated
Eating disorders (EDs)	Singing, songwriting, guided imagery and music, music listening, improvisation, drumming, creating art, mindfulness, song autobiography, composition, receptive and recreative interventions
Work-related stress	Active and passive MT, music listening, music as medicine, mindfulness breathing and MT, guided imagery and music-modified intervention
Homelessness	Improvisation, songwriting and lyric analysis, instrument playing and composition, progressive muscle relaxation, singing, song sharing, musical game, performance, drumming
Artists in residence	Storytelling and poetry intervention, group singing with highly familiar music
Concerts in music and medicine	Concerts of professional musicians, music listening, virtual concerts

18.6 Future Directions

This chapter offers an extension of a systematic review that has presented an overview of MT and MBIs in several healthcare contexts, including eating disorders, work-related stress, homelessness, artists in residence, and concerts in music and medicine. Similarly to Chap. 17, an overarching theme for further assessment should focus on the efficacy and selection of music, pinpointing on the definitions and descriptions associated with each music intervention. Without this specification, there is difficulty for practitioners who use music in healthcare settings to realize the benefits and its empirical significance. Despite this recommendation, researchers within existing literature have still outlined the benefits and considerations for each healthcare issue or context with a broad perspective in mind. This ranges from passive to active applications, and in combination with other arts-based methods. Also found in Chap. 17, researchers can prioritize the assessment of the preferences for music and note the cultural significance and its responsiveness to users and participants. To do this, necessary protocols are encouraged where applicable, which can enable piloting in global regions and other populations of inclusion, such as equity deserving groups and the voices of marginalized individuals. A key topic that still needs to be addressed is the service user voice, which remains absent in this systematic review. A possible resolution is the ability for researchers to engage in more participatory action studies, stimulating the advancement of the use of MT and MBIs in areas of inclusion and the service user voice.

Acknowledgments Thank you, Elienna Wang, for assisting in the format of the references.

References

Almquist L, Walker SC. Reciprocal associations between housing instability and youth criminal legal involvement: a scoping review. Health Justice. 2022;10:15. https://doi.org/10.1186/s40352-022-00177-7.

Alves Araujo F, Lima Brasil F, Candido Lima Santos A, de Sousa Batista Junior L, Pereira Fonseca Dutra S, Eduardo Coelho Freire Batista C. Auris system: providing vibrotactile feedback for hearing impaired population. Biomed Res Int. 2017;2017:2181380–9. https://doi.org/10.1155/2017/2181380.

Alzheimer's Society. Singing for the brain. 2015. www.alzheimers.org.uk/site/scripts/documents_info.php?documentID=760. Accessed 24 May 2024.

Ambler M, Janss A, Stafford RS, Lin B, Florom-Smith A, Kang AW. Voices of musicians: virtual live bedside music concerts in inpatient care. Healthcare (Basel). 2023;11(22):2929. https://doi.org/10.3390/healthcare11222929.

Bailey BA, Davidson JW. Effects of group singing and performance for marginalized and middle-class singers. Psychol Music. 2005;33(3):269–303.

Bayliss R. Music as medicine. In: Tonkin A, Whitaker J, editors. Play in healthcare for adults. Routledge; 2016. p. 115–23.

Beach EF, Cowan R, Mulder J, O'Brien I. Regulations to reduce risk of hearing damage in concert venues. Bull World Health Organ. 2020;98(5):367–9. https://doi.org/10.2471/BLT.19.242404.

Beard KM. Artists in residence: music therapy students in intergenerational relationships with older adults residing in an assisted living facility. Dissertation, Florida State University. 2023.

Beck BD, Hansen ÅM, Gold C. Coping with work-related stress through guided imagery and music (GIM): randomized controlled trial. J Music Ther. 2015;52(3):323–52. https://doi.org/10.1093/jmt/thv011.

Cha J, Smukler SR, Chung Y, House R, Bogoch II. Increase in use of protective earplugs by rock and roll concert attendees when provided for free at concert venues. Int J Audiol. 2015;54(12):984–6. https://doi.org/10.3109/14992027.2015.1080863.

Chang EX, Brooker J, Hiscock R, O'Callaghan C. Music-based intervention impacts for people with eating disorders: a narrative synthesis systematic review. J Music Ther. 2023;60(2):202–31. https://doi.org/10.1093/jmt/thac018.

Chen Y, Cabrera D. Environmental factors affecting classical music concert experience. Psychol Music. 2023;51(3):782–803. https://doi.org/10.1177/03057356221110631.

Clark DL, Wood L, Sullivan CM. Examining the needs and experiences of domestic violence survivors in transitional housing. J Fam Viol. 2019;34(4):275–86. https://doi.org/10.1007/s10896-018-0010-4.

Clements-Cortés A. Artful wellness: attending chamber music concert reduces pain and increases mood and energy for older adults. Arts Psychother. 2017;52:41–9. https://doi.org/10.1016/j.aip.2016.10.001.

Cournoyer Lemaire EC, Loignon C, Bertrand K. A critical scoping review about the impact of music in the lives of young adults who use drugs. Drug Alcohol Rev. 2020;40(1):135–54. https://doi.org/10.1111/dar.13136.

Czepiel A, Fink LK, Fink LT, Wald-Fuhrmann M, Tröndle M, Merrill J. Synchrony in the periphery: inter-subject correlation of physiological responses during live music concerts. Sci Rep. 2021;11(1):22457. https://doi.org/10.1038/s41598-021-00492-3.

da Rocha LA, Siqueira BF, Grella CE, Gratão ACM. Effects of concert music on cognitive, physiological, and psychological parameters in the elderly with dementia: a quasi-experimental study. Dement Neuropsychol. 2022;16(2):194–201. https://doi.org/10.1590/1980-5764-dn-2021-0088.

Danila MI, Melnick JA, Mudano A, Flood K, Booth K, Kirklin K, Saag KG. A performing arts intervention improves cognitive dysfunction in 50 hospitalized older adults. Innov Aging. 2018;2(2):igy013. https://doi.org/10.1093/geroni/igy013.

de Witte M, Spruit A, van Hooren S, Moonen X, Stams G-J. Effects of music interventions on stress-related outcomes: a systematic review and two meta-analyses. Health Psychol Rev. 2020;14(2):294–324. https://doi.org/10.1080/17437199.2019.1627897.

de Witte M, Knapen A, Stams G-J, Moonen X, van Hooren S. Development of a music therapy micro-intervention for stress reduction. Arts Psychother. 2022;77:101872. https://doi.org/10.1016/j.aip.2021.101872.

Dvorak A. Explanatory sequential descriptive analysis of music therapists' clinical practice for individuals with eating disorders. Arts Psychother. 2023;85:102067. https://doi.org/10.1016/j.aip.2023.102067.

Fritsch T, Kwak J, Grant S, Lang J, Montgomery RR, Basting AD. Impact of timeslips, a creative expression intervention program, on nursing home residents with dementia and their caregivers. Gerontologist. 2009;49(1):117–27. https://doi.org/10.1093/geront/gnp008.

Gjestland T, Tronstad TV. The efficacy of sound regulations on the listening levels of pop concerts. J Occup Environ Hyg. 2017;14(1):17–22. https://doi.org/10.1080/15459624.2016.1207779.

Gregory D, Hernandez F, Beach C. Music therapy in shelters for people who are unhoused: a scoping review. Music Ther Perspect. 2024;42(1):28–35. https://doi.org/10.1093/mtp/miad027.

Gutman S, Precin P, LaForest M. A scoping review examining interventions intended to help LGBTQIA+ youth transition out of homelessness. Int J Homelessness. 2022;2(2):1–28. https://doi.org/10.5206/ijoh.2022.1.14128.

Hepburn P, Rutan DQ, Desmond M. Beyond urban displacement: suburban poverty and eviction. Urban Aff Rev. 2022;59:759–92. https://doi.org/10.1177/10780874221085676.

Hip Op-eration Crew. 2013. https://www.hipop-eration.com/. Accessed 21 May 2024.

Houston S, McGill A. A mixed-methods study into ballet for people living with Parkinson's. Arts Health. 2013;5(2):103–19. https://doi.org/10.1080/17533015.2012.745580.

The International Association for Music and Medicine (IAMM). About us. 2024. https://iammonline.com/about-us/. Accessed 24 May 2024.

Kable L. Caring for caregivers. 2003. Available via Society for the Arts in Healthcare. https://www.americansforthearts.org/sites/default/files/webinar_Caregivers.pdf. Accessed 24 May 2024.

Kil J, Lobarinas E, Spankovich C, Griffiths SK, Antonelli PJ, Lynch ED, Le Prell CG. Safety and efficacy of ebselen for the prevention of noise-induced hearing loss: a randomised, double-blind, placebo-controlled, phase 2 trial. Lancet. 2017;390(10098):969–79. https://doi.org/10.1016/S0140-6736(17)31791-9.

Mark Morris Dance Group and Brooklyn Parkinson Group. Dance for PD. 2010. http://danceforparkinsons.org/about-the-program. Accessed 21 May 2024.

Matoso LML, de Oliveira AMB, de Sousa JC. The effect of organizational musical therapy on reducing the stress level of health care professionals in a public hospital. Psychol Music. 2022;50(4):1225–37. https://doi.org/10.1177/03057356211042090.

McFerran KS, Hense C, Koike A, Rickwood D. Intentional music use to reduce psychological distress in adolescents accessing primary mental health care. Clin Child Psychol Psychiatry. 2018;23(4):567–81. https://doi.org/10.1177/1359104518767231.

Moreno-Gutiérrez JÁ, de Rojas LC, López-González MV, Chao-Écija A, Dawid-Milner MS. Impact of music performance anxiety on cardiovascular blood pressure responses, autonomic tone and baroreceptor sensitivity to a western classical music piano-concert. Front Neurosci. 2023;17:1213117. https://doi.org/10.3389/fnins.2023.1213117.

Moss H, O'Neill D. What training do artists need to work in healthcare settings? Med Humanit. 2009;35(2):101–105. https://doi.org/10.1136/jmh.2009.001792.

Nathan S, Hodgins M, Wirth J, Ramirez J, Walker N, Cullen P. The use of arts-based methodologies and methods with young people with complex psychosocial needs: a systematic narrative review. Health Expect. 2023;26(2):795–805. https://doi.org/10.1111/hex.13705.

Northern Health and Social Care Trust. Northern Ireland's first sexual assault referral centre. 2013. https://www.northerntrust.hscni.net/2013/03/06/northern-irelands-first-sexual-assault-referral-centre/. Accessed 21 May 2024.

O'Brien E, Bedggood J, Ayling A. Evolving and thriving – keeping music therapy alive in a pandemic world: the royal Melbourne hospital music therapy response in 2020. Aust J Music Ther. 2021;32(1):80–96.

Padrao MJ, Coimbra JL. The anorectic dance: towards a new understanding of inner-experience through psychotherapeutic movement. Am J Dance Ther. 2011;33(2):131–47. https://doi.org/10.1007/s10465-011-9113-7.

Page MJ, McKenzie JE, Bossuyt PM, Boutron I, Hoffmann TC, Mulrow CD, Shamseer L, Tetzlaff JM, Akl EA, Brennan SE, Chou R, Glanville J, Gimshaw JM, Hróbjartsson A, Lalu MM, Li T, Loder EW, Mayo-Wilson E, McDonald S, McGuinness LA, Stewart LA, Thomas J, Tricco AC, Welch VA, Whiting P, Moher D. The PRISMA 2020 statement: an updated guideline for reporting systematic reviews. BMJ. 2021;372:n71. https://doi.org/10.1136/bmj.n71.

Pasiali V, Quick D, Hassall J, Park HA. Music therapy programming for persons with eating disorders: a review with clinical examples. Voices. 2020;20(3):15. https://doi.org/10.15845/voices.v20i3.2785.

Preti C, Boyce-Tillman J. Elevate: using the arts to uplift people in hospitals. Salisbury: ArtCare; 2015.

Rio R. Adults in recovery: a year in members of the choirhouse. Nord J Music Ther. 2005;14(2):107–19. https://doi.org/10.1080/08098130509478133.

Ruest SM, Stephan AM, Masiakos PT, Biddinger PD, Camargo CA, Kharasch S. Substance use patterns and in-hospital care of adolescents and young adults attending music concerts. Addict Sci Clin Pract. 2018;13(1):1. https://doi.org/10.1186/s13722-017-0105-x.

Salet N, Visser M, Stam C, Smulders YM. Stroboscopic light effects during electronic dance music festivals and photosensitive epilepsy: a cohort study and case report. BMJ Open. 2019;9(6):e023442. https://doi.org/10.1136/bmjopen-2018-023442.

Savidaki M, Demirtoka S, Rodríguez-Jiménez RM. Re-inhabiting one's body: a pilot study on the effects of dance movement therapy on body image and alexithymia in eating disorders. J Eat Disord. 2020;8(1):1–20. https://doi.org/10.1186/s40337-020-00296-2.

Schifferle A, Eggmann F, Mukaddam K, Kühl S, Filippi A. General and dental injuries sustained at concerts: a questionnaire-based study. Dent Traumatol. 2023;39(1):44–8. https://doi.org/10.1111/edt.12790.

Semborski S, Redline B, Madden D, Granger T, Henwood B. Housing interventions for emerging adults experiencing homelessness: a scoping review. Child Youth Serv Rev. 2021;127:106081. https://doi.org/10.1016/j.childyouth.2021.106081.

Shah P, Mitchell E, Remers S, Van Blydervenn SV, Ahonen H. The impact of group music therapy for individuals with eating disorders. Approaches. 2023;15(1):36–57. https://approaches.gr/shah-a20210718/

Shibazaki K, Marshall NA. Exploring the impact of music concerts in promoting well-being in dementia care. Aging Ment Health. 2017;21(5):468–76. https://doi.org/10.1080/13607863.2015.1114589.

Smith C, Vilijoen JT, McGeachie L. African drumming: A holistic approach to reducing stress and improving health? J Cardiovasc Med (Hagerstown). 2014;15(6):441–446. https://doi.org/10.2459/JCM.0000000000000046.

Son HK, So W-Y, Kim M. Effects of aromatherapy combined with music therapy on anxiety, stress, and fundamental nursing skills in nursing students: a randomized controlled trial. Int J Environ Res Public Health. 2019;16(21):4185. https://doi.org/10.3390/ijerph16214185.

Sonke J. Professionalizing the arts in healthcare field. In: Lambert PD, editor. Managing arts programs in healthcare. 1st ed. London: Routledge; 2015. p. 50–62.

Sonke J, Pesata V, Lee JB, Graham-Pole J. Nurse perceptions of artists as collaborators in interprofessional care teams. Healthcare (Basel). 2017;5(3):50. https://doi.org/10.3390/healthcare5030050.

Testa F, Arunachalam S, Heiderscheit A, Himmerich H. A systematic review of scientific studies on the effects of music in people with or at risk for eating disorders. Psychiatr Danub. 2020;32(3–4):334–45. https://doi.org/10.24869/psyd.2020.334.

Tsai J, Kelton K. Service use and barriers to care among homeless veterans: results from the National Veteran Homeless and Other Poverty Experiences (NV-HOPE) study. J Community Psychol. 2022;51(1):507–15. https://doi.org/10.1002/jcop.22912.

Verrusio W, Ettorre E, Vicenzini E, Vanacore N, Cacciafesta M, Mecarelli, O. The mozart effect: A quantitative EEG study. Conscious. Cogn. 2015;35:150–55.

Vogel I, van de Looij-Jansen PM, Mieloo CL, Burdorf A, de Waart F. Risky music listening, permanent tinnitus and depression, anxiety, thoughts about suicide and adverse general health. PLoS One. 2014;9(6):e98912. https://doi.org/10.1371/journal.pone.0098912.

Wang CC, Lo J, Saunders R, Adama E, Bulsara C, Etherton-Beer C, Yang AWH. Light acupuncture and five-element music therapy for nurses' mental health and well-being during and post-COVID-19: protocol for a randomised cross-over feasibility study. BMJ Open. 2022;12(4):e057106. https://doi.org/10.1136/bmjopen-2021-057106.

Williams E, Dingle GA, Clift S. A systematic review of mental health and wellbeing outcomes of group singing for adults with a mental health condition. Eur J Pub Health. 2018;28(6):1035–42. https://doi.org/10.1093/eurpub/cky115.

Yıldırım D, Çiriş Yıldız C. The effect of mindfulness-based breathing and music therapy practice on nurses' stress, work-related strain, and psychological well-being during the COVID-19 pandemic: a randomized controlled trial. Holist Nurs Pract. 2022;36(3):156–65. https://doi.org/10.1097/HNP.0000000000000511.

Yoshioka-Maxwell A. Predictors of service utilization among homeless former foster youth: implications for intervention. J Soc Work. 2022;22(6):1394–411. https://doi.org/10.1177/14680173221101254.

Part VI

The Research in the Field of Music-Based and Music Therapy Interventions

Music Therapy and Research: Qualitative and Quantitative Points of View

19

Alfredo Raglio and Camilla Figini

Key Points

- This chapter seeks to provide a comprehensive overview of current music therapy research.
- The chapter aims to highlight key considerations for designing research projects, presenting potential methodologies, and distinguishing between quantitative, qualitative, and mixed-methods approaches as a bridge between the two.
- The chapter also addresses pressing critical issues emerging in the field of music therapy research.
- Finally, it underscores the importance of fostering an open-minded approach among music therapy professionals, enabling them to better appreciate the potential of music therapy interventions and develop practical guidelines for clinical practice.

19.1 Introduction

Recently published bibliometric studies report an exponential growth in music therapy research, whether looking at the last decades (Zhi et al. 2024; Li et al. 2021), demonstrating a growing interest, need, and trend toward basing clinical practice on scientifically validated evidence. In support of this assertion, the graphs below,

A. Raglio (✉)
Music Therapy Research Laboratory, Istituti Clinici Scientifici Maugeri IRCCS, Pavia, Italy
e-mail: alfredo.raglio@icsmaugeri.it

C. Figini
University of Pavia, Pavia, Italy

A. Raglio (ed.), *Music and Music Therapy Interventions in Clinical Practice*, Neurocultural Health and Wellbeing,
https://doi.org/10.1007/978-3-031-88578-5_19

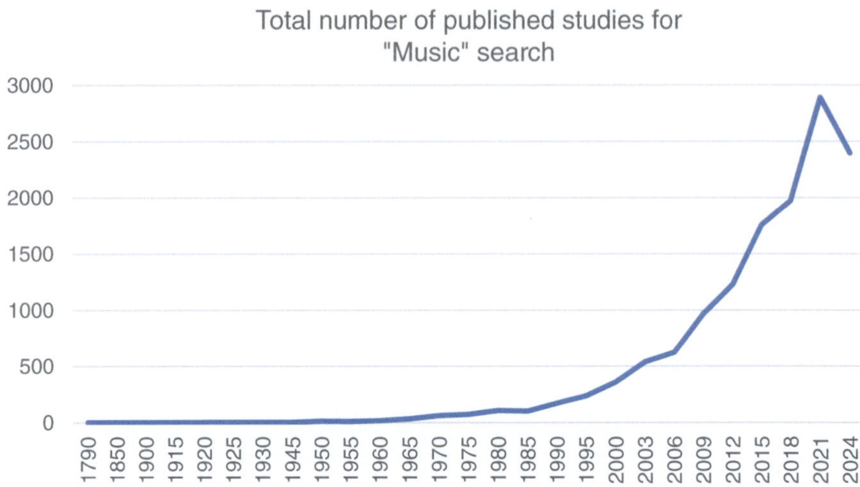

Fig. 19.1 Curve of the number of studies published annually in the PubMed database over the period 1790–2024 for "music" keyword search query

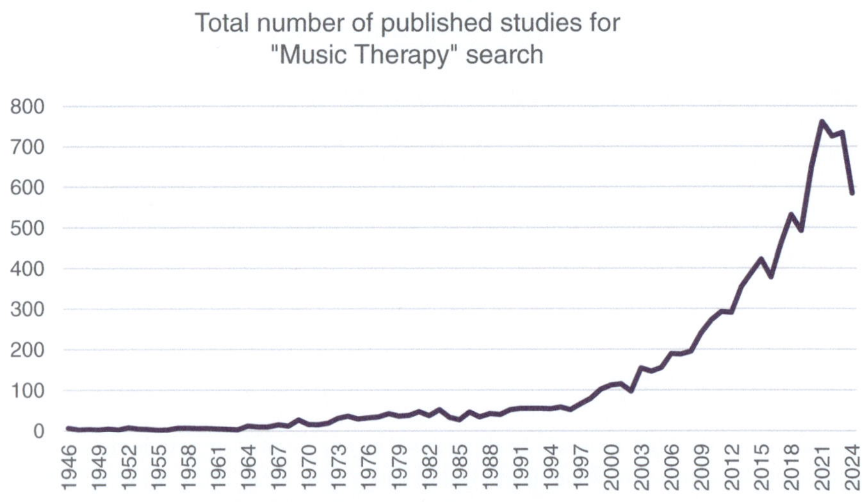

Fig. 19.2 Curve of the number of studies published annually in the PubMed database over the period 1946–2024, for "music therapy" keywords search query

generated by searches of the terms "music" (Fig. 19.1) or "music therapy" (Fig. 19.2) on Pubmed database (one of the largest scientific databases administered by the United States National Library of Medicine-National Institutes of Health), show an absolute increase in the number of studies published since the inception of music therapy as a discipline (Fig. 19.2). The curves in both graphs appear to be reversed in 2024, as many studies still await publication and it is not yet possible to make a precise estimate for this year, as it has not yet been completed. In any case, the increase is exponential for both keywords, but the difference in the number of published studies between the results for the two searches is strikingly significant. Consider, for example, the difference between the studies published in 2023 for the two terms mentioned above: 2797 for the keyword "music" and 734 for the keyword "music therapy." These data show an increase in the use of music in scientific works, but a closer look reveals a nonspecific use of music in most publications, with mainly psycho-educational approaches, adopting pedagogical or humanistic perspectives, leaving out references to the therapeutic use of sound and music or the adoption of models with therapeutic objectives.

Nevertheless, referring to the curve obtained from the search for the string "music therapy," the observable difference is particularly striking when comparing the average annual number of studies published in the decade 1951–1960 ($n = 5.1$) with the number of studies published in the decade 2001–2010 ($n = 175.1$) and in the last decade 2014–2023 ($n = 554.3$).

In summary, these data represent a significant point of evolution, as they show how, despite the critical issues discussed throughout the chapter, the music therapy community is increasingly recognizing the need to integrate the theoretical and practical dimensions of the discipline with research. This shift aims toward a more effective therapeutic application and a clearer definition of the field, ultimately supporting the recognition of music therapy as both a scientific and institutionalized discipline.

From an analysis of the total number of citations of music therapy studies, PLoS One and Cochrane Database of Systematic Reviews appear to be the most influential scientific journals. Moreover, research trends, found through keyword burst and highly cited study analysis, show a specific research focus along the last decade (Zhi et al. 2024), on the effect of music therapy on neurological diseases and the improvement of psychological symptoms such as pain and anxiety, with the top ranked studies being "Music-based interventions in neurological rehabilitation" (Sihvonen et al. 2017) and "Music interventions for improving psychological and physical outcomes in cancer patients" (Bradt et al. 2021).

These data represent a quantum leap if a comparison is made with what is reported in Brooks' work (2003) about the situation in the early 1980s. An analysis of data from various questionnaires submitted to music therapists working in those years reveals a total lack of consideration of the importance of keeping up to date by reading research articles, as well as a belief that scientific literature did not meet one's daily practice needs for further study and, therefore, had little relevance to clinical practice. A push toward the reconsideration of research occurred in the second half of the 1980s. Gregory's (2002) analysis of studies published in the Journal of Music Therapy shows that from the late 1980s onwards, scientific articles dealt with a wider range of clinical pictures, with a main increase in the inclusion of music therapy users not only with intellectual but also with physical disabilities, covering the entire life cycle, from the neonatal population to the later stages of aging.

The issue of research in music therapy is central nowadays, not free of debates and heterogeneous positions. In order for the discipline to progress in its recognition process, it is currently essential to concentrate energies on documenting the effects of music therapy treatment in a rigorous and systematic manner, in terms of efficacy and effectiveness, in line with what has already begun in healthcare systems, for medical and psychological treatments, according to the biomedical model of evidence-based practice (EBP). This work is particularly necessary if we consider the multitude of approaches and theories that currently guide music therapy practice around the world; this, inevitably, leads to a certain complexity and a limited possibility of generalizing the results obtained, especially if the studies do not respect the principles of rigor and systematicity in the modality of collecting and analyzing the data presented to the music therapy community.

The complexity of the musical object, in the variety of its biological, psychological, and sociocultural correlates, makes it difficult to converge the variability of the results found into a single grand explanatory theory, even though we are adopting a forma mentis increasingly oriented toward the documentation of effects, as pointed out by Hillecke et al. (2005). The idea of research as an integral part of the music therapy process was proposed by Gaston (1968), through the image of a tripod formed by the elements of theory, clinical practice and research, all of which are fundamental to ensuring the stability of the discipline, in a process in which research work seeks to provide an answer to the questions arising from clinical practice and addressed through the formulation of theory. Through the research process, it is, therefore, possible to inform clinical practice, with corroborated results useful in providing a foundational structure for all clinical work. We are, therefore, faced with different types of research, structured according to the focus that guides them, distinguishing among a branch that is concerned with analyzing the effectiveness of the treatment, a field that studies the process and all the aspects that make up the treatment itself, and a domain that aims to analyze the consistency of the relationship between the theoretical model and clinical practice. These are interrelated aspects that should guide the daily work of a music therapist. First of all, along this chapter, attention will be drawn to the importance of defining an intervention model that allows the clinician to outline the guidelines of the treatment to be proposed, including all the aspects that concern the definition of typologies of users suitable for treatment, therapeutic objectives, and the appropriate strategies that constitute the intervention techniques. These elements are linked with fundamental importance to the analysis of the process, which would occur through the application of observational tools consistent with the model, allowing to describe the process with precision, and the clinical evaluation of the effects in order to demonstrate the effectiveness of the intervention. On this last point, attention will be paid to the current lack of adequate tools for detecting changes outside the setting, which implies the need to establish collaborations between multidisciplinary teams with professionals from other disciplines in order to develop appropriately standardized and statistically validated tools aimed at adequately evaluating the outcomes of music therapy intervention (Raglio 2013).

Several methods and approaches are used to examine the various facets of this complex object of research, which is music therapy: research methodology uses two main approaches to study the outcome aspects of music therapy intervention and the aspects related to the therapeutic process, relatively defined as quantitative and qualitative methods (Wheeler 1996). While the adoption of quantitative approaches primarily aims at an objective and numerical measurement of effects, the study from a qualitative point of view aims to describe how phenomena are experienced and constructed through description. Moreover, in recent years, a third way of doing research oriented toward integrating these methods is gaining ground, which consists of approaching the study of the phenomenon from a pragmatic point of view, combining the strengths of quantitative and qualitative methods in a mixed-method perspective (Bradt et al. 2013a).

Regardless of the methodology employed or the theoretical framework used to study a phenomenon, a research process—whether in music therapy or other disciplines—should follow a series of preliminary steps. These include the initial identification of a problem, the formulation of a hypothesis to explore it, and the meticulous development of a research design. This design should be as suitable as possible to enable the hypothesis to be either confirmed or refuted. These stages are followed by the actual realization of the therapeutic intervention according to well-defined principles, the subsequent application of observation/evaluation tools, the collection, processing, and subsequent interpretation of the data, which will be, then, presented in the form of results in a clear manner and in compliance with certain standards of scientific rigor.

There are several forms that scientific contributions in the field of music therapy can take for the scientific communication of results: in addition to experimental studies, in which the effects of an intervention are compared with the absence of treatment, relevant information can also be obtained from reviews of studies already presented in previous scientific works on specific population and from studies on a single clinical case or a series of cases or from theoretical and descriptive studies. In the following sections, an in-depth analysis of the different methodologies that can guide the realization of a research project in music therapy is proposed, accompanied by examples and a specific focus on the critical issues that arise in their application.

19.2 Quantitative Approaches

The complexity of the music therapy intervention, which arises from the coexistence of several interacting factors linked to the specificity of the music therapist training, to the reference models and to the characteristics of the users on which to modulate the type of intervention, leads to a series of complications and problems in the evaluation of the effects of the intervention, with outcomes that are often difficult to define. This leads to the need for research projects in which the approaches used are as systematic as possible and the interventions are well-defined by a solid theoretical basis. Quantitative research fits into this framework, with the aim of providing data that are as objective as possible, through numerical quantification and subsequent statistical processing, in order to allow the generalizability of the results found and to reproduce the phenomenon by following a set of guidelines. In the quantitative perspective, which is based on a post-positivist model of reasoning, it will be possible, thanks to a rigorous and systematic research design, to study the object in a cause-effect relationship, i.e., to define that the observed effect is actually due to the treatment and not to other confounding variables (Wheeler 2015). The research designs envisaged by the use of a quantitative approach can be quite varied and differ according to the modulation of parameters such as the reference period (prospective, if it assesses the effects of a study yet to be carried out, or retrospective, if it analyzes variables belonging to the past that may have influenced the present), the type of design (the design can, therefore, be experimental, non-experimental or quasi-experimental), and the number of moments of data collection (e.g., a study may be cross-sectional if there is only one point in time at which the change in a factor is assessed simultaneously in groups of individuals; it may include pre-post analyses, for example, in the case of an intervention, where the same assessments are made before and after a treatment or it may be longitudinal, allowing the change or evolution of the phenomenon to be observed sequentially and repeatedly) (Burns and Meadows 2015).

Table 19.1 shows the main examples of quantitative design that a study can adopt, accompanied by links to guidelines for those study designs implementation and a series of examples of such studies in the music therapy literature.

In music therapy research, it is evident how a quantitative perspective can be adapted to two different macro types of research: descriptive and experimental. A more descriptive way of doing research, using survey and questionnaire techniques, is concerned with collecting numerical data to determine possible ways in which the presence of certain variables and their interaction may influence the processes and outcomes of therapy, without resorting to comparison with a control group. On the other hand, a type of experimental design allows questions focused on the efficacy of music therapy to be answered by actually comparing different treatment conditions, with participants randomly assigned to the different conditions in a balanced manner to maximize control over possible confounding variables.

To be considered experimental, a research design should, therefore, meet a number of requirements and criteria, such as the use of a rigorous experimental design that controls for the influence of possible external variables, the presence of at least two balanced research groups defined by a traceable randomization technique, which should be exposed to different conditions through the direct manipulation of a variable (independent variable that in the case of music therapy is represented by the manipulation of the treatment variable). The comparison of the results obtained in these groups (represented by a dependent or outcome variable), the analysis using inferential statistical techniques and the consequent dissemination of the results of scientific interest are also required (McMillan and Schumacher 2010).

In his publication, Bradt (2012) highlights the different design options that a music therapist may consider in order to test the effectiveness or efficiency of his or her music therapy intervention through experimental research. The most commonly used design options in this field include the pretest-posttest, where the experimental and control groups are given the same assessments before and after the intervention; the posttest-only control group, where no assessment is given before the intervention; the within-subjects design, in which all subjects receive the treatment and the factorial design, a complex research designs that test the effect of more than one independent variable.

The reference literature in the field of music therapy, which can be consulted in the main scientific databases, generally includes different types of experimental research, which can be classified according to the causal strength of the evidence they present: among the evidence with greater external validity, we can find meta-analyses, systematic reviews and randomized clinical trials, followed by exploratory studies and longitudinal (cohort) studies, series of case studies (case series) and single cases (case-control study or case reports) with less scientific impact.

Table 19.1 Main quantitative designs, guidelines, and examples from music therapy literature

Study design	Study characteristics	Guidelines	Music therapy studies examples
Meta-analyses	Quantitative design used to systematically assess the results of previous research on a common question to derive statistically based conclusions.	PRISMA: Preferred Reporting Items for Systematic reviews and Meta-Analyses https://www.prisma-statement.org/	Geretsegger et al. (2022), Bradt et al. (2013c, 2021).
Literature Review (Systematic, Narrative, Scoping…)	Quantitative method used to collect, synthesize, and overview previously published studies on a topic. Systematic review strictly follows a set of guidelines in the process of assessing the quality of each included study. Narrative or scoping reviews use a less formal approach and critically analyze the literature starting from a broad research question.	PRISMA: Preferred Reporting Items for Systematic reviews and Meta-Analyses https://www.prisma-statement.org/ PRISMA guidelines for scoping reviews https://www.prisma-statement.org/scoping	*Systematic* Aalbers et al. (2017) *Narrative* McDermott et al. (2013) *Scoping* Raglio et al. (2024)
Randomized Controlled Trial	An RCT is a study design in which participants are randomly assigned to either an experimental group or a control group. Throughout the study, the only anticipated difference between these groups is the specific outcome variable being examined.	CONSORT: CONsolidated Standards Of Reporting Trials https://www.consort-spirit.org/ SPIRIT: Standard Protocol Items Recommendations for Interventional Trials https://spirit-statement.org/publications-downloads/	Ridder et al. (2013), Raglio et al. (2015), Bieleninik et al. (2017).

(continued)

Table 19.1 (continued)

Study design	Study characteristics	Guidelines	Music therapy studies examples
Nonrandomized Clinical Trials	Nonrandomized trial is a design in which participants are assigned to an experimental or control group using methods other than randomization. This approach may result in baseline differences between the groups that could potentially affect the outcomes being studied.	TREND: Transparent Reporting of Evaluations with Nonrandomized Designs https://www.cdc.gov/hivpartners/php/trend-statement/index.html	Guétin et al. (2009)
Crossover Trials	A crossover study is a trial where participants receive both the experimental and control treatments in sequence, often separated by a washout period to prevent carryover effects, allowing direct within-subject comparisons.		Raglio et al. (2013, 2022).
Cohort Studies	A cohort study involves tracking a group of individuals over time to examine the relationship between certain exposures or risk factors and the development of specific outcomes.	Guidelines for cohort studies STROBE: STrengthening the Reporting of OBservational studies in Epidemiology. https://www.strobe-statement.org/	Baker et al. (2022).
Cases (Single, Case-Control, case series)	A single case study focuses on an in-depth examination of one individual or a unique instance, often to explore rare conditions or generate hypotheses for future research. A case series study analyses multiple cases with a shared characteristic or treatment, providing observational and descriptive insights to identify patterns or trends. A case-control study compares individuals with a specific condition or outcome (cases) to those without it (controls) to retrospectively investigate potential risk factors or exposures.	CARE: CAse REports https://www.care-statement.org/ Guidelines for case-control studies STROBE: STrengthening the Reporting of OBservational studies in Epidemiology. https://www.strobe-statement.org/	Single case: Giovagnoli et al. (2014), Raglio et al. (2018) Case series: Raglio et al. (2014) Case-control: Svansdottir and Snaedal (2006)

Among the experimental studies of modest scientific impact, one of the most common designs can be exploratory studies, which allow the evaluation of an intervention process without the presence of random assignment to groups. Among exploratory studies, one of the most commonly used methods may be the survey, which consists of collecting a large amount of data from a large population of interest that can be used quantitatively and therefore processed by statistical methods to ensure generalizability. In particular, surveys that investigate aspects of clinical practice are generally concerned with the collection of information related to professionals, clients, and the therapeutic process in order to learn more about music therapy practice (Wheeler 2015). Instead, the methodology that involves the collection of data on a single case or a few cases, or to say the single case design, is concerned with the study of a single individual or group behavior over time, examining the real context of practice and the effects of therapeutic change, assessing the impact of particular strategies or therapeutic conditions. In contrast, longitudinal research involves a defined sample being assessed at multiple points over time, and the analysis of the data collected allows comparisons to be made between or among these points.

Among the studies with the greatest scientific impact are definitely randomized controlled trials (RCTs), systematic reviews of the literature, and meta-analyses.

The RCT is a type of design in which the sample of interest is randomly assigned to at least two groups that are compared on a number of outcomes. There are therefore at least two conditions: an experimental condition, in which a clinical intervention is carried out, and a control condition, in which the sample does not receive the treatment and serves as a reference for observing any effects of the treatment itself. The control group, in addition to not receiving the treatment, can be treated in different ways: it can receive the standard treatment, a standard treatment offered in the same way to all members of the sample, known as treatment as usual (TAU), it can be included on a waiting list and receive the experimental treatment at the end of the trial, it can receive a placebo treatment, the experimental treatment in a low dose, or another type of treatment that will be used as a comparison. Of course, there may be more than one experimental group if the object of interest is the comparison of several interventions at the same time. A research design involving the implementation of an RCT thus makes it possible to focus on specific effects of a treatment that are predefined in a set of variables that serve as outcomes. Randomization is used to create balanced groups for a number of potential confounders (controlling for known and unknown characteristics that could influence treatment effectiveness), which would be treated equally except for treatment variable and that would be set up through appropriate inclusion and exclusion criteria so that any differences found in results would be attributable to treatment (Akobeng 2005). An RCT study can be designed in a variety of ways, and feasible designs can be classified into parallel group designs, the most common type of design, in which a group receiving the music therapy intervention is compared with a control group; cross-over designs, in which subjects receive a sequence of different treatments and act as controls for themselves and factorial designs, in which different factors are examined at multiple levels. In addition, RCTs, which are themselves very time- and resource-consuming studies, can often be preceded by a pilot phase, in which small studies are conducted to test the characteristics of the treatments and the trial in general, in order to assess the possible feasibility of a larger trial.

The data obtained from the evaluation of the identified outcomes are statistically processed in the analysis phase in order to examine possible relationships and differences between the variables tested, and the statistical results are interpreted and used to corroborate the hypotheses. This method of conducting scientific research is historically considered to be the only one capable of estimating with a good degree of certainty the causal relationships between variables; it is, therefore, considered to be the gold standard of research, also in the field of music therapy. Its aim is to corroborate the hypothesis of the effectiveness of a music-based intervention with quantitative data capable of attributing the effects on the outcomes of interest to the treatment. Nowadays, there is a growing number of RCTs in the music therapy literature, and it is of paramount importance for a researcher in this field to learn how to report the data from studies in a rigorous and consistent manner, following the best-known guidelines that allow for effective and transparent reporting of information. In this regard, authors of scientific publications are encouraged to follow the CONSORT (Consolidated Standards of Reporting Trials) (Schulz et al. 2010) and TREND (Transparent Reporting of Evaluations with Nonrandomized Designs) guidelines (Des Jarlais et al. 2004) to ensure more specific and shareable reporting; in the specific case of the music-based interventions area researchers could rely on the recommendations proposed in the reporting guidelines by Robb et al. (2011).

The literature provides numerous examples of RCTs that adhere to reporting standards aligned with established guidelines. This approach facilitates scientific exploration of music therapy, both in terms of the intervention's effects on predefined outcomes (Park et al. 2023; Kobus et al. 2022; Yakobson et al. 2021; Raglio et al. 2015; Ridder et al. 2013) and by examining process-related or music-specific aspects to uncover the mechanisms driving the intervention's impact (Raglio et al. 2020).

To give an example, the RCT by Raglio et al. (2015) was concerned with analyzing and comparing the effects of an active music therapy intervention and a therapeutic music listening intervention in a sample of patients with dementia, characterized by the presence of psychological and social symptoms typical of patients in an advanced stage of cognitive impairment. In this case, the participants were randomly divided into three different groups, one of which received standard care (control group) and the other two of which, in addition to standard care, received two different music therapy interventions, in one case an active intervention (based on free musical improvisation) and in the other it was a therapeutic music listening intervention (based on daily listening to a playlist specifically designed to achieve a clinical goal). The effects of the treatments were quantified by administering specific clinical scales to assess the presence of psychological and behavioral symptoms in patients with dementia, such as the Neuropsychiatric Inventory (NPI), which, in the specific case of the study, showed a significant reduction in symptoms scorings in all groups (with some difference between groups in terms of the extent to which symptoms were reduced). On the other hand, the RCT study by Raglio et al. (2020) is a clear example of a study on the internal mechanisms of the music therapy process, in that it aimed to analyze the factors inherent to the musical element capable of producing therapeutic effects, and to identify certain factors predictive of relaxation using machine learning techniques. Listening to different musical pieces on a sample of healthy subjects, with the relative request to quantify the degree of relaxation facilitated by them, made it possible to carry out a parametric analysis of the sound and musical element, which led to the delineation of a series of factors with an important role in predicting the effects of musical listening.

The results of the extensive scientific literature available on a specific research topic in music therapy can be rigorously synthesized using systematic review and meta-analysis methods, which allow all the evidence to be organized and its scientific quality to be assessed. These are systematic processes in which, according to pre-established criteria, a selection is made from the literature present in the databases dedicated to a specific research topic. The selection is, then, processed using statistical procedures with the aim of comparing the effects reported and estimating their magnitude (in the case of meta-analysis), or summarizing them using a series of techniques for risk of bias minimization, in order to provide a complete overview of the state of the art on the phenomenon in question. Knowledge of this type of study plays an essential role in the professional life of music therapists, as it allows them to adopt an evidence-based clinical practice and to find important insights that enable them to make well-founded and informed clinical and research decisions (Hanson-Abromeit and Sena 2014). In this regard, the main database that collects reviews on music therapy practice is the Cochrane Collaboration one (http://www.cochrane.org), an international organization set up with the aim of collecting, evaluating, and disseminating information on the effectiveness of preventive, therapeutic, and rehabilitative interventions. Within this database, there is a whole series of rigorous works that can inform the daily work of the music therapist, dealing with the evaluation of the effects of very different types of intervention on different groups of patients, characterized by the presence of specific features (such as different types of mental or neurological disorders, etc.). A number of relevant examples are listed below (Aalbers et al. 2017; Bradt and Dileo 2014; Bradt et al. 2013b, c, 2021; Geretsegger et al. 2017, 2022; Ghetti et al. 2022; Magee et al. 2017; van Der Steen et al. 2018).

The possibility of adopting a quantitative point of view in music therapy is certainly an option to be considered and privileged, as it promotes a rigorous way of working that allows an adequate elaboration of data that can be used to stimulate reflections that broaden the theoretical and practical awareness of the discipline. Quantifying the aspects of a complex process such as music therapy is a powerful tool for reviewing treatment, as it encourages a deeply analytical attitude toward the many variables at play. A quantitative approach thus makes it possible, in terms of transferability, to highlight important factors concerning the therapeutic mechanisms of music intervention, which, although not fully generalizable, can represent a point of reference and a guide for a rational clinical practice based on a situational assessment of the characteristics of each individual user. The results obtained will, therefore, be a stimulus to question one's own clinical practice, far from being axioms or absolute evidence (Raglio 2013). However, it is clear that an exclusively quantitative approach can be somewhat reductionist in the analysis of a discipline that lacks a certain linearity and includes aspects of discontinuity, such as music therapy, which, basically, consists of the potential of sound and musical elements to embed themselves into a relational context, producing state changes that are difficult to operationalize.

19.3 Qualitative Approaches

A qualitative approach to research means basing the process on the understanding of a phenomenon in its whole complexity and beyond the utopia of objectivity seeking: descriptive strategies are used for speculation and deepening the phenomenon of interest, focusing more on the processes than on treatment outcomes. In music therapy research, a qualitative point of view is currently less applied than a quantitative one although studies investigating the object of music therapy with qualitative perspectives have been increasing in number of publications since the mid-1990s (Brooks 2003; Aigen 2008). This trend shows a relevant evolution of thought in the field of music therapy that is slowly opening up to a comprehensive investigation of the possible mechanisms within therapy.

Bruscia, in his works on the qualitative approach analysis in music therapy research (2005, 1998), has been concerned with defining the possible aims of using qualitative techniques and the research questions that can be addressed. A wide range of possible questions emerges from his reflections, generally concerned with the in-depth study of issues related to the interaction of the therapeutic couple in the actual therapeutic context and to the experiences of the parties involved (therapist, patient(s), third parties such as carers or family members) with a particular focus on exploring the patient's perspective on a problem or object of interest. The material to be micro-analyzed could be, for example, the direct perceptions of an individual on a particular aspect of interest, through the analysis of interviews focusing on personal experiences, through transcripts of verbal exchanges in the therapeutic couple, or through the analysis of the musical product itself resulting from the music therapy sessions. Bruscia (2005, 1998) identifies in the choice of qualitative methods the possibility of achieving a holistic description of the phenomenon, through the discussion of regularities and relationships useful for hypothesizing meaningful explanations, including multiple perspectives, as well as for constructing theories that involve a significant degree of interpretation while leaving space for self-reflection. The centrality of the interpretive aspect is, therefore, the assumption behind the fact that qualitative research adopts an idiographic perspective and is linked to the specific context of investigation, as opposed to quantitative research, in which the context, cultural affiliation, training, and previous experiences of the researcher are used to describe and understand the phenomena under study. In fact, it is often the music therapist himself who takes the role of researcher in order to explore the meaning of his own professional attitudes, to increase his own self-awareness of the mechanisms he puts into action in the therapeutic process and the consequent implications. From this point of view, the researcher plays a key role in the research process, as he/she collects and processes data himself/herself, using multiple resources, through techniques such as observation, the collection perceptions through interviews, the analysis of transcripts of interactions, leaving aside the use of techniques more oriented toward mere quantification, such as the questionnaire.

The methodology used to approach the questions posed varies according to the purpose of the research, in terms of specific data collection techniques, with the aim of constantly monitoring and modifying the techniques used in response to the environmental requirements and the actual context in which the research takes place. However, it is important to start from a solid theoretical base, from a model that guides the research and allows it to take shape, without forgetting the objective of carrying out a holistic analysis in accordance with the principle of trustworthiness, which guarantees a comprehensive vision of the phenomenon (Creswell and Poth 2016).

Table 19.2 shows the main examples of qualitative design that a study can adopt, accompanied by links to guidelines for those study designs implementation and a series of examples of such studies in the music therapy literature.

Among the qualitative methodologies favored in the scientific literature in the field of music therapy, examples include phenomenological research, a technique that consists of the holistic study of human experience through the collection of data that respects a systematic sequence and allows the essence of the experience to be described. Hermeneutic approach is also a commonly used methodology that involves an analytical and circular relationship between the phenomenon of interest and the theories elaborated on the subject. The reference theories are compared with the collected data in a process of continuous modulation and redefinition of the theory applied to the data in order to develop feasible interpretations of the phenomenon (Forinash and Grocke 2005).

Another of the most widely used methodologies in research projects is grounded theory, which is also a methodology that involves a systematic data collection technique that, through comparative analysis and specific data coding procedures, is used to generate, elaborate, and verify inductive theories focused on possible phenomena that emerge in the practice of the music therapy community. Its application in the field of music therapy is privileged in the case of an in-depth study of significant experiences in the real context (naturalistic inquiry), of preexisting scientific material (narrative inquiry), in the case where there is a joint participation of music therapists and patients in the implementation of the research process (participatory action research) or in the case where the researcher decides to conduct research aimed at increasing self-awareness as a music therapy practitioner through introspection (first-person research) (Wheeler 2015).

To give a clearer and more concrete idea of how a data collection process can take place from a qualitative research perspective, consider, as an example of different methodologies, some of the most recent studies that have adopted a qualitative approach to data collection and processing (Schneible et al. 2023; Thompson et al. 2021; Krøier et al. 2021).

Table 19.2 Main qualitative designs, guidelines, and examples from music therapy literature

Study Design	Study characteristics	Tools	Guidelines	Music Therapy Studies Examples
Phenomenological research	Focus on understanding how individuals perceive and interpret a specific phenomenon, capturing the essence of lived experiences from the participants' viewpoints in order to describe and interpret the meanings clients attach to those experiences rather than making generalizations. The goal is to provide a deep understanding of how people make sense of phenomena.	Key tools used for data collection: *Interviews* (in-depth, semi-structured and focus groups) to gather personal experiences. *Observations* to study behaviors and interactions in natural settings. *Text Analysis* (content and thematic analysis) to explore materials for patterns and meanings. *Surveys/ Questionnaires* with open-ended questions for capturing detailed responses. *Visual Methods* (photos and video recording) to gather insights through visual stimuli. *Coding Softwares* (e.g., NVivo, Atlas. ti) to organize and analyze data. *Transcription Tools* (e.g., Otter.ai, Rev) for converting audio or video data into text.	Standards for reporting qualitative research https://journals.lww.com/academicmedicine/fulltext/2014/09000/Standards_for_Reporting_Qualitative_Research__A.21.aspx http://links.lww.com/ACADMED/A218	Krøier et al. (2021), Economos (2018), Pothoulaki et al. (2012)
Hermeneutic approach	Focus on understanding human experiences and social phenomena. It values context and history in shaping meaning, in a dynamic process of interpretation, considering biases and refining understanding through an ongoing dialogue with the data. The aim is to uncover deeper meanings by merging the researcher's and participants' perspectives, leading to a more complete understanding.			Ghetti et al. (2024), Luce (2008),
Grounded theory	Focus on developing theories directly from data, rather than testing existing theories. Researchers collect data, code it to identify patterns, and repeatedly compare new data with existing concepts. This iterative process leads to the creation of theories that are grounded in the real experiences of participants.			Schneible et al. (2023), Daveson and O'Callaghan (2011), O'Callaghan (2012)
Others: Ethnographic design, Narrative Inquiry, Action Research, Content Analysis.	Ethnography: researchers immerse themselves in the culture or community they are studying to observe behaviours, practices, and social interactions. Narrative Inquiry: collection and analyses of personal stories or narratives to understand how individuals make sense of their experiences and construct meaning over time. Action Research: real-world problems solving through collaborative inquiry. Researchers work with participants to identify issues, implement changes, and reflect on the results, Content Analysis: text analysis to identify patterns, themes, and meanings. Researchers examine content systematically to understand underlying messages and cultural patterns.			Baker (2007), Due and Ghetti (2018)

For example, the research project described in Schneible et al. (2023) adopts a grounded theory approach aimed at developing reflections and conceptualizations of the role that music therapy plays within the care that elderly users may receive in long-term care facilities. This work was developed through a collection of perspectives from all stakeholders in care, from residents themselves to staff and their music therapists. Through a rigorous process, including transcription, coding, and appropriate analysis of 17 interviews conducted, the researchers developed a theoretical model describing a process that highlights the role of music therapy intervention in enabling participants to rediscover their best selves. The several beneficial aspects highlighted worked as a stimulus for reflection on the operational phases of clinical assessment and actual intervention, such as accessibility, involvement, personal meaning, facilitation to activate resources, transformation, and integration.

The example of the study by Thompson et al. (2021), on the other hand, also used the interview technique, but with the aim of exploring issues related to the feasibility of including interviews with people with dementia in the evaluation of the music therapy process, based on the experiences of users who had previously contributed to the research by participating in interviews. The data extracted from the transcripts of seven interviews enabled a thematic analysis to be carried out, which was useful in developing reflections and guidelines for researchers and clinicians to refer to when conducting subsequent studies.

The study by Krøier et al. (2021), ultimately, adopted a phenomenological, language-based method of inquiry to delve into challenges of exploring nonverbal and musical interactions through the examinations of six music therapists' lived-experiences about nonverbal interaction with persons with severe dementia, collected with the focus group technique. The transcripts obtained were analyzed and peer validated by the use of musical improvisation as an arts-based analytic approach, with a certain relevance for music therapy practice management. The outcomes resulted from a thematic analysis shed light on what may be some factors influencing music therapists' experiences of nonverbal interaction with their patients, for example, being guided by vitality, awareness of their own reactions, attunement to the person's nonverbal musical parameters, therapeutic presence, and validation. Qualitative approaches to the study of music therapy can indeed be an interesting resource, allowing for the development of useful reflections for professional development. However, these approaches can but complement quantitative ones, which are clearly better suited to understanding whether the effects of therapy are significant in a cause-effect relationship and not limited to speculation.

Mixed methods approaches: a proposal integrating qualitative and quantitative points of view.

Recently, there has been a growing acknowledgement that, in order to provide attentive and quality care to clients, it is important to gather evidence being the result of an integration of different collection methods and different forms of evidence, using an approach that implies the coexistence of qualitative and quantitative methodologies, favoring so-called mixed methodologies (Bradt et al. 2013a). Data collected through the different methodologies complement or explain one another allowing diverse perspectives. An example of a method that is easily adaptable to the combined use of qualitative and quantitative approaches can be represented by case research, which, according to Ridder and Bonde (2019), would be suitable for both descriptive and inferential analyses, thanks to the concrete possibilities it offers for investigating issues related to awareness of clinical practice and how this awareness is translated into practice itself. The feasibility and applicability of this type of design facilitates the collection of different types of data that increase the depth of knowledge about the phenomenon.

However, the combination of methodologies belonging to such distant fields of thought poses a number of challenges that are bound to manifest themselves in new approaches such as mixed methods. First of all, an initial incompatibility becomes evident when we consider issues related to the samples and the respective sampling procedures: whereas quantitative approaches basically require the study of a representative sample large enough to achieve good statistical power, qualitative approaches tend to value the importance of the cases under study according to the extent to which they can facilitate the understanding of the phenomenon. In order to resolve this methodological discontinuity, a mixed methods approach can, simultaneously, consider different samples, which vary according to the needs of the research design, in some cases obtained through sampling guided by predefined strategies, but which can be modified over time, respecting the needs of an emerging approach such as the qualitative one. The result is a prevalent way of structuring these works, in which the different samples are treated sequentially, with a quantitative phase usually followed by a recruitment phase geared toward a qualitative investigation guided by the results of the quantitative phase. Data collected through quantitative and qualitative approaches can be analyzed separately and integrated in a second phase, allowing the uniqueness of each method to be considered and valued but also to be integrated in subsequent comparisons. An example of a sequential design can be found in the recent study by Clements-Cortés (2024), which aimed to evaluate the content, usefulness, and feasibility of a music therapy assessment tool for patients with dementia developed and disseminated in Canada and the United States (Music Therapy Assessment for Older Adults). In this case, a mixed model was used to gather initial feedback and then to study the feasibility of the tool in more detail. A quantitative and exploratory phase of completion of an online questionnaire to investigate the administration experience (on a sample of 18 music therapists) was followed by a second phase consisting of the administration and analysis of follow-up interviews, whose structure was defined after the analysis of the questionnaire compilations. The results of the two study procedures were analyzed and integrated, allowing the assessment instrument to be revised thanks to constructive contributions that helped to better define the language and minimize the risk of bias.

Another interesting example of the application of a mixed-methods design is the study by Stedje et al. (2023), aimed at evaluating possible mechanisms behind the influence of a home-based music therapy intervention on relationship quality in older couples with dementia and caregivers. The study was concerned with integrating the results of an RCT with 68 participating couples with the results of qualitative interviews with four of the couples recruited in the RCT. Relationship quality was, therefore, analyzed using a standardized scale in the quantitative part of the study and by themes emerging from the post-treatment interviews. While the results of the scale did not show any significant differences before and after the intervention, but a certain stability over time, the qualitative analysis made it possible to contribute to important points of reflection that are useful for hypothesizing possible reasons for this lack of significance. A certain ambiguity in the possible mechanisms of influence was highlighted, since although in most cases the music therapy interventions facilitated communication and greater closeness between the couples, situations in which the shared listening led to greater vulnerability and negative emotional reactions were also observed and highlighted. In this case, the integration of the two methods was a very useful resource for further evaluating possible explanations for a result obtained through quantification, with the aim of promoting a whole understanding of the phenomenon.

Finally, a critical point of mixed-methods research concerns the high costs that a two-stage experiment requires with the numerous demands involved, as well as the need for specialized personnel capable of handling both methods. In this sense, receiving training that does not privilege one or the other method and that provides the basis for acquiring a comprehensive expertise is essential today, although it is easy to encounter resistance to change by those professionals who are unwilling to integrate their knowledge or who are rigidly anchored in a traditionalist view (and decidedly against the possibility of collaboration between approaches) that is no longer up-to-date (Bradt et al. 2013a).

19.4 Music Therapy Research: Issues and Future Developments

The points discussed along this chapter highlight an important and emerging trend in music therapy research, which offers clear evidence of the discipline's progress toward recognition and therapeutic legitimacy. This dynamic is particularly evident in advancements in training management, as well as the growing institutionalization and experience of music therapy in clinical and research settings. Although significant efforts have been made to adopt evidence-based approaches and to provide increasing availability of evidence on the effects of music therapy in therapeutic, rehabilitative, and preventive contexts, studies conducted with rigorous scientific criteria remain relatively limited. Additionally, the definition of "music therapy" and its application methods are still not fully established. A key point to consider is that, in many cases, the music therapy community is deeply rooted in pedagogical and humanistic approaches, often overlooking the importance of fostering a scientific culture. As a result, clinicians may struggle to recognize the relevance of research to their practice. One possible explanation for this could be that music therapy students are not sufficiently encouraged to adopt a "research-oriented" mindset throughout their education, which may impact their understanding of the urgency and necessity of research in the field.

In addition to the critical issues mentioned, it is worth noting the limited level of institutionalization that music therapy has achieved to date in treatment and research settings. This is reflected in the insufficient number of facilities available to support and train students in clinical practice and the application of research designs, which affects the continuity of practical experiences and may result in delays in academic training. The partial institutionalization of music therapy also contributes to the limited visibility of the discipline beyond the music therapy community and among other healthcare professionals and experts from different fields. However, involving these professionals in research could provide a valuable multidisciplinary resource, promoting a more integrated approach. This would enable the use of a broader range of research tools, potentially leading to a more refined understanding of how to study the object of music therapy, which exists within a complex, multisystemic framework that benefits from a multidisciplinary approach.

Music therapy indeed intersects with a broad range of scientific fields, including behavioral sciences, social sciences, neuroscience, mathematics, and the arts. As such, training programs should aim to cultivate an open mindset toward scientific approaches, encouraging the development of professionals who engage with the discipline thoughtfully and critically. These professionals should view research not only as a valuable guide for their clinical practice but also as a vital tool for the ongoing growth of the music therapy community. Acquiring foundational skills and terminology in this context is key to professional development and enables music therapists to collaborate effectively with a wide range of other professionals. This promotes shared communication and fosters the integration of diverse perspectives, resulting in a more holistic approach to addressing challenges.

At present, however, there are still relatively few studies that focus on integrated music therapy experiences, clearly defined as therapeutic interventions, rigorously evaluated and incorporating multidisciplinary contributions. Despite the adoption of systematic methods, many studies in the literature fall short of providing detailed descriptions of specific music therapy interventions (Robb et al. 2011). Important elements such as clearly defined therapeutic content, specific frequencies and durations, models guiding the interventions, and the involvement of trained professionals with clear objectives and strategies are often not fully explained. Instead, the literature tends to focus on broader descriptions of musical activities, such as listening exercises or community music-making (e.g., group singing or movement activities with background music), which do not fully meet the criteria for therapeutic interventions. As a result, there is significant variability in the reported experiences, which, instead of focusing on specific methods for assessing the process, tend to evaluate the broad and general effects of music on individuals. This creates a matter of comparability between different experiences. Consequently, the adoption of an evidence-based approach becomes increasingly difficult, further hindering the progress of the discipline's recognition within the wider scientific community.

This issue is likely connected to the limited spread of music therapy knowledge, which may lead to the belief that any use of music in a therapeutic context can automatically be considered a therapeutic intervention. Additionally, this perspective can give rise to the misconception that all aspects of the discipline can be easily quantified and operationalized, sometimes overlooking the need for the adoption of methodologically rigorous approaches. Such approaches should focus on clearly defining the mechanisms behind an intervention, which should be implemented with a well-established and coherent rationale (Raglio and Oasi 2015).

To fully recognize music therapy as a discipline, it is essential to adopt a thoughtful and critical approach to clearly define the object of study. In doing so, researchers should first develop a theoretical model to apply to their clinical practice, identifying potential points of connection or discrepancies. This process will help construct meaningful insights that contribute to a better understanding of the therapeutic process; specifically, on what occurs within a music therapy session and how these experiences translate outside the therapy setting.

The outcome of this approach would be the creation of a set of treatment guidelines that outline all essential components of therapy. It will be necessary to assess which patient groups are most suited for specific treatments, define appropriate therapeutic goals, and apply techniques and strategies based on a clear rationale. This process should be followed by specific assessment procedures that track the progress of treatment over time.

Additionally, adopting a micro-intervention format, as outlined by Hakvoort and Tönjes (2023), which includes a comprehensive framework for all aspects a music therapist should consider when planning treatment, would lead to more detailed descriptions of interventions, including musical mechanisms. A common standard format would enhance comparability across research studies, enabling the music therapy community to observe more accurate and meaningful results, ultimately supporting broader generalizability.

It is clear that in the near future of music therapy, adopting a constructive and proactive approach could foster a mindset open to exploring new research tools that are being developed in contemporary society. This involves a willingness to embrace new methods of investigation, along with a commitment to ongoing learning and continuous research. A key area of importance, in this regard, is the role of new technologies (as discussed in the Introduction of this textbook), including the potential of artificial intelligence (AI), as well as specific assessment methods and the valuable contributions that the field of neuroscience can offer in deepening our understanding of the phenomenon. Integrating these factors would lead to significant progress in understanding the neural and psychophysical aspects involved in clinical and therapeutic work. Therefore, it is crucial to maintain and strengthen the relationship with neuroscience and to invest in the development of new technologies. Over the past few decades, several studies in neuroscience and psychology have explored the relationship between music and the brain (Zatorre and Salimpoor 2013; Koelsch 2009, 2014; Koelsch and Jäncke 2015), unfortunately, the resources needed for neuroimaging techniques or biomarker analysis are often not sustainable.

At this stage, it is vital for music therapy researchers to direct their efforts toward fostering a constructive dialogue between medicine, neuroscience, and music therapy. By integrating various multidisciplinary perspectives, this dialogue can lead to significant advancements in measuring specific outcomes, in line with clinical applications of music therapy. Such collaboration would enable music therapists to develop a more comprehensive view by enhancing their understanding of the biological and neuroscientific aspects that are relevant when analyzing therapeutic effects. This, in turn, would increase the body of scientifically grounded evidence, moving beyond speculative discussions about musical perception and its effects.

The same approach applies to the development of sonification technologies, such as sensors, virtual reality, robots, and noninvasive stimulation devices, which support sensorimotor rehabilitation. These technologies offer additional resources to traditional rehabilitation methods, with previous studies showing promising results, such as accelerated recovery times and more objective assessments (Raglio et al. 2021d, 2023; Colombo et al. 2019). The use of AI and the application of algorithms to study the sound-musical element have also become essential tools for understanding music therapy processes. For example, the algorithmic modulation of musical parameters can help isolate those that influence the psychophysiological effects of music. One such example is the Melomics Health algorithm, designed to explore potential connections between musical parameters and psychophysiological activation or deactivation (Requena et al. 2014; Raglio and Vico 2017; Raglio et al. 2021a, b, c).

While these are early steps in harnessing these technologies, they should serve as a motivation to adopt an open and curious mindset toward studying the field using alternative techniques.

The object of observation in music therapy, as well as the assessment of the process in its full complexity, is another critical aspect to consider, particularly in improvisational approaches that focus on the sound–music interaction within the therapeutic dyad. The goal of research in this area would be to create tools that are as objective, standardized, and validated as possible through appropriate statistical methods. These tools should be capable of recording the changes that occur throughout the therapeutic process and be widely disseminated and promoted within the music therapy community. An example of an effort to develop observational tools for evaluating the process in music therapy, particularly within an intersubjective model framework (Stern 1985, 2004), is the use of grids designed to analyze nonverbal and sound–music communication. These grids aim to capture key aspects, such as the evolving dynamics of the relationship over time. Some of the grids that have been developed for this purpose include the Music Therapy Coding Scheme (Raglio et al. 2006), the Music Therapy Checklist (Raglio et al. 2007), the Music Therapy Rating Scale (Raglio et al. 2011), and the Music Therapy Session Assessment Scale (Raglio et al. 2017).

On the other hand, as far as the evaluation of the results of the music therapy intervention is concerned, the use of the clinical instruments employed has been and will continue to be privileged in order to be able to demonstrate the effectiveness of the intervention. The sensitivity of this issue is underscored by the strong need for collaboration with professionals from various disciplines, which may vary depending on the specific area of intervention and the outcomes to be observed in line with clinical objectives. These effects can span a wide range, from psychological to medical, affecting different systems of the individual, such as emotional, cognitive, motor, and behavioral aspects. In the absence of fully adequate tools to detect changes outside the therapy setting, where such changes may not be immediately observable or measurable, it is crucial to establish a multidisciplinary team focused on developing standardized, validated instruments to assess the outcomes of music therapy. This team should include health professionals such as doctors, clinicians, psychologists, physiotherapists, occupational therapists, and rehabilitation specialists, as well as experts in research methodology and statistical analysis. As such, the music therapist must be prepared to take on multiple roles, whether as a researcher, a therapist implementing the treatment, or a trained observer making detailed observations using the appropriate tools.

19.5 Conclusion

Future progress in music therapy research should focus on several key areas: establishing a clear definition of "music therapy" by outlining specific approaches, objectively assessing intervention effects through collaboration with a network of professionals, staying open to the exploration of new technologies, and promoting a stronger theoretical connection with the field of neuroscience.

Additionally, this effort would lead to the establishment of clear guidelines that contribute to the development of theoretical foundations guiding clinical practice, as well as an enhancement of a more rigorous and reliable scientific approach.

Finally, to achieve these objectives, it will be crucial to explore the use of mixed methods approaches, because of recent methodological advancements, which will enable a more comprehensive study of the phenomenon (Edwards 2015; Erkkilä 2015). This will be encouraged by combining the perspectives of the researcher and the music therapist, but also by favoring the study of the user's "lived experience," which does not have to be underestimated, as music therapy practice is primarily aimed at providing the best possible care to patients.

The human and therapeutic potential of the relationship between humans and the sound-musical element must be recognized and valued (Ghetti and Ray 2023). While music therapy is a relatively new and emerging field, the theoretical study and experimental application of research designs are increasingly guiding practice across various and diverse clinical settings. It is becoming increasingly important for music therapists to feel a strong sense of both the right and responsibility to collaborate with a network of professionals in building the foundations of their profession through a process that integrates theory, practice, and research.

References

Aalbers S, Fusar-Poli L, Freeman RE, Spreen M, Ket JC, Vink AC, Maratos A, Crawford M, Chen XJ, Gold C. Music therapy for depression. Cochrane Database Syst Rev. 2017;11(11):CD004517.

Aigen K. An analysis of qualitative music therapy research reports 1987–2006: articles and book chapters. Arts Psychother. 2008;35:251–61.

Akobeng AK. Principles of evidence based medicine. Arch Dis Child. 2005;90(8):837–40.
Baker F. Enhancing the clinical reasoning skills of music therapy students through problem based learning: an action research project. Nord J Music Ther. 2007;16(1):27–41.
Baker FA, Lee YC, Sousa TV, Stretton-Smith PA, Tamplin J, Sveinsdottir V, Geretsegger M, Wake JD, Assmus J, Gold C. Clinical effectiveness of music interventions for dementia and depression in elderly care (MIDDEL): Australian cohort of an international pragmatic cluster-randomised controlled trial. Lancet Healthy Longev. 2022;3(3):153–65.
Bieleninik L, Geretsegger M, Mössler K, Assmus J, Thompson G, Gattino G, Elefant C, Gottfried T, Igliozzi R, Muratori F, Suvini F, Kim J, Crawford MJ, Odell-Miller H, Oldfield A, Casey Ó, Finnemann J, Carpente J, Park AL, Grossi E, Gold C. Effects of improvisational music therapy vs enhanced standard care on symptom severity among children with autism spectrum disorder: the TIME-A randomized clinical trial. JAMA. 2017;318(6):525–35.
Bradt J. Randomized controlled trials in music therapy: guidelines for design and implementation. J Music Ther. 2012;49:120–49.
Bradt J, Dileo C. Music interventions for mechanically ventilated patients. Cochrane Database Syst Rev. 2014;12:CD006902.
Bradt J, Burns DS, Creswell JW. Mixed methods research in music therapy research. J Music Ther. 2013a;50:123–48.
Bradt J, Dileo C, Potvin N. Music for stress and anxiety reduction in coronary heart disease patients. Cochrane Database Syst Rev. 2013b;12:CD006577.
Bradt J, Dileo C, Shim M. Music interventions for preoperative anxiety. Cochrane Database Syst Rev. 2013c;6:CD006908.
Bradt J, Dileo C, Myers-Coffman K, Biondo J. Music interventions for improving psychological and physical outcomes in people with cancer. Cochrane Database Syst Rev. 2021;10(10):CD006911.
Brooks D. A history of music therapy journal articles published in the English language. J Music Ther. 2003;40:151–68.
Bruscia KE. Standards of integrity for qualitative music therapy research. J Music Ther. 1998;35(3):176–200.
Bruscia KE. First-person research. In: Wheeler BL, editor. Music therapy research. 2nd ed. Gilsum: Barcelona Publishers; 2005. p. 379–91.
Burns DS, Meadows A. Music therapy research. In: Music therapy handbook; 2015. p. 91–102.
Clements-Cortés A. Music therapy assessment for older adults: descriptive mixed-methods study. Behav Sci. 2024;14(5):354.
Colombo R, Raglio A, Panigazzi M, Mazzone A, Bazzini G, Imarisio C, Molteni D, Caltagirone C, Imbriani M. The SonicHand protocol for rehabilitation of hand motor function: a validation and feasibility study. IEEE Trans Neural Syst Rehabil Eng. 2019;27(4):664–72.
Creswell JW, Poth CN. Qualitative inquiry and research design: choosing among five approaches. Sage Publications; 2016.
Daveson B, O'Callaghan C. Investigating the dimension of time: findings from a modified grounded theory study about clients' experiences and descriptions of temporality or time within music therapy. J Music Ther. 2011;48(1):28–54.
Des Jarlais DC, Lyles C, Crepaz N. Improving the reporting quality of nonrandomized evaluations of behavioural and public health interventions: the TREND statement. Am J Public Health. 2004;94(3):361–6.
Due FB, Ghetti CM. Implementation of music therapy at a Norwegian children's hospital: a focused ethnographic study. Voices World Forum Music Ther. 2018;18(2):1–21.
Economos AD. Music therapy when death is imminent: a phenomenological inquiry. J Music Ther. 2018;55(3):309–39.
Edwards J. Music therapy research: context, methodology, and current and future developments. In: Edwards J, editor. The Oxford handbook of music therapy. Oxford library of psychology; 2015. p. 709–19.
Erkkilä J. Mixed methods research in music therapy. In: Edwards J, editor. The Oxford handbook of music therapy. Oxford Library of Psychology; 2015. p. 815–26.

Forinash M, Grocke D. Phenomenological inquiry. In: Wheeler BL, editor. Music therapy research. 2nd ed. Gilsum: Barcelona Publishers; 2005. p. 321–34.
Gaston ET. Music in therapy. New York: Macmillan; 1968.
Geretsegger M, Mössler K, Bieleninik Ł, Chen X, Heldal T, Gold C. Music therapy for people with schizophrenia and schizophrenia-like disorders. Cochrane Database Syst Rev. 2017;5(5):CD004025.
Geretsegger M, Fusar-Poli L, Elefant C, Mössler K, Vitale G, Gold C. Music therapy for autistic people. Cochrane Database Syst Rev. 2022;5(5):CD004381.
Ghetti CM, Ray K. Reflecting on music therapy research on the occasion of the Journal of Music Therapy's 60th anniversary. J Music Ther. 2023;60(3):238–53.
Ghetti CM, Chen XJ, Brenner A, Hakvoort L, Lien L, Fachner J, Gold C. Music therapy for people with substance use disorders. Cochrane Database Syst Rev. 2022;5(5):CD012576.
Ghetti CM, Hjelmbrekke S, Morken K, Dahl T, Stige B. Steering the energy with music: hermeneutic phenomenological study of user perspectives of music and music therapy for co-occurring ADHD and substance use problems. Subst Abuse Treat Prev Policy. 2024;19(1):10.
Giovagnoli AR, Oliveri S, Schifano L, Raglio A. Active music therapy improves cognition and behaviour in chronic vascular encephalopathy: a case report. Complement Ther Med. 2014;22(1):57–62.
Gregory D. Four decades of music therapy behavioral research designs: a content analysis of Journal of Music Therapy articles. J Music Ther. 2002;39:56–71.
Guétin S, Soua B, Voiriot G, Picot MC, Hérisson C. The effect of music therapy on mood and anxiety-depression: an observational study in institutionalised patients with traumatic brain injury. Ann Phys Rehabil Med. 2009;52(1):30–40.
Hakvoort L, Tönjes D. Music-mechanisms at the core of music therapy: towards a format for a description of music therapy micro-interventions. Nord J Music Ther. 2023;32(1):67–91.
Hanson-Abromeit D, Sena MK. The systematic review as a research process in music therapy. J Music Ther. 2014;51(1):4–38.
Hillecke T, Nickel A, Bolay HV. Scientific perspectives on music therapy. Ann N Y Acad Sci. 2005;1060(1):271–82.
Kobus S, Diezel M, Dewan MV, Huening B, Dathe AK, Marschik PB, Felderhoff-Mueser U, Bruns N. Music therapy in preterm infants reduces maternal distress. Int J Environ Res Public Health. 2022;20(1):731.
Koelsch S. A neuroscientific perspective on music therapy. Ann N Y Acad Sci. 2009;1169:374–84.
Koelsch S. Brain correlates of music-evoked emotions. Nat Rev Neurosci. 2014;15(3):170–80.
Koelsch S, Jäncke L. Music and the heart. Eur Heart J. 2015;36(44):3043–9.
Krøier JK, Stige B, Ridder HM. Non-verbal interactions between music therapists and persons with dementia. A qualitative phenomenological and arts-based inquiry. Music Ther Perspect. 2021;39(2):162–71.
Li K, Weng L, Wang X. The state of music therapy studies in the past 20 years: a bibliometric analysis. Front Psychol. 2021;12:697726.
Luce DW. Epistemological development and collaborative learning: a hermeneutic analysis of music therapy students' experience. J Music Ther. 2008;45(1):21–51.
Magee W, Clark I, Tamplin J, Bradt J. Music interventions for acquired brain injury. Cochrane Database Syst Rev. 2017;1(1):CD006787.
McMillan JH, Schumacher S. Research in education: evidence-based inquiry. Pearson; 2010.
McDermott O, Crellin N, Ridder HM, Orrell M. Music therapy in dementia: a narrative synthesis systematic review. Int J Geriatr Psychiatry. 2013;28(8):781–94.
O'Callaghan C. Grounded theory in music therapy research. J Music Ther. 2012;49(3):236–77.
Park JI, Lee IH, Lee SJ, Kwon RW, Choo EA, Nam HW, Lee JB. Effects of music therapy as an alternative treatment on depression in children and adolescents with ADHD by activating serotonin and improving stress coping ability. BMC Complement Med Ther. 2023;23(1):73.
Pothoulaki M, MacDonald R, Flowers P. An interpretative phenomenological analysis of an improvisational music therapy program for cancer patients. J Music Ther. 2012;49(1):45–67.
Raglio A, editor. Musicoterapia: teorie, applicazioni, ricerca, formazione e professione. Aracne Editrice; 2013. p. 79–94.

Raglio A, Oasi O. Music and health: what interventions for what results? Front Psychol. 2015;6:230.
Raglio A, Vico F. Music and technology: the curative algorithm. Front Psychol. 2017;8:2055.
Raglio A, Traficante D, Oasi O. A coding scheme for the evaluation of the relationship in music therapy sessions. Psychol Rep. 2006;99(1):85–90.
Raglio A, Traficante D, Oasi O. Comparison of the music therapy coding scheme with the music therapy checklist. Psychol Rep. 2007;101(3):875–80.
Raglio A, Traficante D, Oasi O. The evaluation of music therapy process in the intersubjective perspective: the music therapy rating scale. A pilot study. Pragmat Obs Res. 2011;2:19–23.
Raglio A, Bellandi D, Baiardi P, Gianotti M, Ubezio MC, Granieri E. Listening to music and active music therapy in behavioral disturbances in dementia: a crossover study. J Am Geriatr Soc. 2013;61(4):645–7.
Raglio A, Guizzetti GB, Bolognesi M, Antonaci D, Granieri E, Baiardi P, Maggioni G, Pistarini C. Active music therapy approach in disorders of consciousness: a controlled observational case series. J Neurol. 2014;261(12):2460–2.
Raglio A, Bellandi D, Baiardi P, Gianotti M, Ubezio MC, Zanacchi E, Granieri E, Imbriani M, Stramba-Badiale M. Effect of active music therapy and individualized listening to music on dementia: a multicenter randomized controlled trial. J Am Geriatr Soc. 2015;63(8):1534–9.
Raglio A, Gnesi M, Monti MC, Oasi O, Gianotti M, Attardo L, Gontero G, Morotti L, Boffelli S, Imbriani C, Montomoli C, Imbriani M. The Music Therapy Session Assessment Scale (MT-SAS): validation of a new tool for music therapy process evaluation. Clin Psychol Psychother. 2017;24(6):1547–61.
Raglio A, Filippi S, Leonardelli L, Trentini E, Bellandi D. The Global Music Approach to Dementia (GMA-D): evidences from a case report. Aging Clin Exp Res. 2018;30(12):1533–6.
Raglio A, Imbriani M, Imbriani C, Baiardi P, Manzoni S, Gianotti M, Castelli M, Vanneschi L, Vico F, Manzoni L. Machine learning techniques to predict the effectiveness of music therapy: a randomized controlled trial. Comput Methods Prog Biomed. 2020;185:105160.
Raglio A, Baiardi P, Vizzari G, Imbriani M, Castelli M, Manzoni S, Vico F, Manzoni L. Algorithmic music for therapy: effectiveness and perspectives. Appl Sci. 2021a;11(19):8833.
Raglio A, De Maria B, Perego F, Galizia G, Gallotta M, Imbriani C, Porta A, Dalla Vecchia LA. Effects of algorithmic music on the cardiovascular neural control. J Pers Med. 2021b;11(11):1084.
Raglio A, Oddone E, Meaglia I, Monti MC, Gnesi M, Gontero G, Imbriani C, Ivaldi GB. Conventional and algorithmic music listening before radiotherapy treatment: a randomized controlled pilot study. Brain Sci. 2021c;11(12):1618.
Raglio A, Panigazzi M, Colombo R, Tramontano M, Iosa M, Mastrogiacomo S, Baiardi P, Molteni D, Baldissarro E, Imbriani C, Imarisio C, Eretti L, Hamedani M, Pistarini C, Imbriani M, Mancardi GL, Caltagirone C. Hand rehabilitation with sonification techniques in the subacute stage of stroke. Sci Rep. 2021d;11(1):7237.
Raglio A, Maestri R, Robbi E, Pierobon A, La Rovere MT, Pinna GD. Effect of algorithmic music listening on cardiac autonomic nervous system activity: an exploratory, randomized crossover study. J Clin Med. 2022;11(19):5738.
Raglio A, De Maria B, Parati M, Giglietti A, Premoli S, Salvaderi S, Molteni D, Ferrante S, Dalla Vecchia LA. Movement Sonification techniques to improve balance in Parkinson's disease: a pilot randomized controlled trial. Brain Sci. 2023;13(11):1586.
Raglio A, Figini C, Bencivenni A, Grossi F, Boschetti F, Manera MR. Cognitive stimulation with music in older adults with cognitive impairment: a scoping review. Brain Sci. 2024;14(8):842.
Requena G, Sánchez C, Corzo-Higueras JL, Reyes-Alvarado S, Rivas-Ruiz F, Vico F, Raglio A. Melomics music medicine (M3) to lessen pain perception during pediatric prick test procedure. Pediatr Allergy Immunol. 2014;25(7):721–4.
Ridder HM, Bonde LO. Music therapy research: an overview. In: Jacobsen SL, Pedersen IN, Bonde LO, editors. A comprehensive guide to music therapy. 2nd ed. Jessica Kingsley Publishers; 2019. p. 391–409.

Ridder HM, Stige B, Qvale LG, Gold C. Individual music therapy for agitation in dementia: an exploratory randomized controlled trial. Aging Ment Health. 2013;17(6):667–78.
Robb SL, Burns DS, Carpenter JS. Guidelines for reporting music-based interventions. J Health Psychol. 2011;16(2):393.
Schneible BK, Beer L, McDermott O, Mulhorn K, Shim M, Bradt J. Development of the music therapy in transition to long-term care model. J Music Ther. 2023;60(4):435–62.
Schulz KF, Altman DG, Moher D. CONSORT 2010 statement: updated guidelines for reporting parallel group randomized trials. Obstet Gynecol. 2010;115(5):1063–70.
Sihvonen AJ, Särkämö T, Leo V, Tervaniemi M, Altenmüller E, Soinila S. Music based interventions in neurological rehabilitation. Lancet Neurol. 2017;16(8):648–60.
Stedje K, Kvamme TS, Johansson K, Sousa TV, Odell-Miller H, Stensæth KA, Bukowska AA, Tamplin J, Wosch T, Baker FA. The influence of home-based music therapy interventions on relationship quality in couples living with dementia—an adapted convergent mixed methods study. Int J Environ Res Public Health. 2023;20(4):2863.
Stern DN. The interpersonal world of the infant. A view from psycho-analysis and developmental psychology. New York: Basic Books; 1985.
Stern DN. The present moment in psychotherapy and everyday life. WW Norton & Company; 2004.
Svansdottir HB, Snaedal J. Music therapy in moderate and severe dementia of Alzheimer's type: a case-control study. Int Psychogeriatr. 2006;18(4):613–21.
Thompson Z, Baker FA, Clark IN, Tamplin J. Making qualitative interviews in music therapy research more accessible for participants living with dementia–reflections on development and implementation of interview guidelines. Int J Qual Methods. 2021;20:16094069211047066.
Van der Steen J, Smaling H, van der Wouden J, Bruinsma M, Scholten R, Vink A. Music-based therapeutic interventions for people with dementia. Cochrane Database Syst Rev. 2018;7(7):CD003477.
Wheeler BL. Music therapy research: quantitative and qualitative perspectives. Arts Psychother. 1996;23(3):277–80.
Wheeler BL. Music therapy research: an overview. In: Edwards J, editor. The Oxford handbook of music therapy. Oxford Library Psychology; 2015. p. 720–47.
Yakobson D, Gold C, Beck BD, Elefant C, Bauer-Rusek S, Arnon S. Effects of live music therapy on autonomic stability in preterm infants: a cluster-randomized controlled trial. Children. 2021;8(11):1077.
Zatorre RJ, Salimpoor VN. From perception to pleasure: music and its neural substrates. Proc Natl Acad Sci USA. 2013;110(Suppl 2):10430–7.
Zhi L, Hou D, Hong Y, Ke M, Zhang Q, Wang Y, Long J. Research on music therapy from 2013 to 2022: a bibliometric and visualized study. Front Psych. 2024;15:1323794.

20 Make the Invisible Visible - Towards Process-Based Outcome Research on Mechanisms of Change in Music Therapy

Jörg Fachner and Sun Sun Yap

Key Points

- Music therapy has been found effective on a range of diseases as reported in case studies, controlled trials, and Cochrane reviews. However, we do not know how music therapy works.
- The social neuroscience of music therapy introduced here offers an adaptive quantitative analysis framework for a highly idiosyncratic therapeutic practice.
- By identifying and contrasting moments of interest, i.e., by identifying crucial sections and nodes of music therapy sessions in which change and therapeutic success develop, we can demonstrate graphically and quantifiably what would otherwise be rendered as "anecdotal evidence" and analyze how change occurs and how music therapy works.
- Apperception, situated cognition, and dialogue are key to analysis of change in creative arts process research.
- This chapter introduces perspectives on adaptive multimodal technologies (e.g., brain imaging and motion capture techniques) that may help to make subtle developments driving change in music therapy processes visible and measurable.

J. Fachner (✉)
Cambridge Institute for Music Therapy Research, Anglia Ruskin University, Cambridge, UK
e-mail: jorg.fachner@aru.ac.uk

S. S. Yap
University Clinic Tulln, Tulln an der Donau, Austria

A. Raglio (ed.), *Music and Music Therapy Interventions in Clinical Practice*, Neurocultural Health and Wellbeing,
https://doi.org/10.1007/978-3-031-88578-5_20

20.1 Introduction

Music has a long tradition of use in recreational, well-being, health, and therapeutic settings. In recent years, forms of music consumption, production, performance, collaboration, and healthcare delivery have changed due to technological progress. However, this process is still in its infancy and is likely to continue with much vigor. Moreover, societal factors such as the aging population and physical distancing during pandemics, add a new dimension to the importance and challenges we will face as we continue to use music in our lives.

Since music therapy has developed, the profession has gone through several waves of interest that have defined its purpose and scope. In essence, it started with musicians experiencing the power of music on themselves and observing distinct responses during performances, educating their pupils, and doing music with other musicians and with patients. When asked to share this information with students, many of the founders pointed to the practical experience that is needed to do music therapy (Bunt and Stige 2014). Music therapists were creating "eclectic" treatment approaches (Taylor 1987) and, consequently, a variety of treatment formats emerged, which reflected the many fields of experience and reference which were based on individual interest, academic backgrounds, and most of all the different clients they were working with. Given the manifold practices, a strong tradition of music therapy is in qualitative research, i.e., methods that allowed to description of the individual interdependencies of health and diseases that were reflected in the therapy domains (Aldridge 1996).

Music therapists look at the interaction between client and therapist and how listening and creating music works in therapy (Fachner 2014). The client is the focus of most case study research into the practice of doing therapy; however, there is a lack of process-related data in the music and health sciences to inform us on what is happening during music therapy (MT) and music-based interventions (MBI), and how responses to music are organized in situ (Fachner 2016b). There is now a well-documented body of evidence comprised of Randomized Controlled Trials (RCT), Cochrane, systematic or scoping reviews on the effect of music therapy on outcome measures of different intervention arms of RCTs, etc. There is also a wealth of case studies reporting about the practice of doing MT and MBI based on subjective process-related experiences of therapists and patients; however, objectivist approaches to case and small-N studies (Ridder and Fachner 2016), especially neuroscience-informed process research into the mechanisms of change in music therapy, are still underdeveloped (de Witte et al. 2021).

20.2 Music Therapy Works—But How?

Music therapy has been established as an allied health profession for more than 50 years, and the last 20 years has seen a surge of outcome studies investigating the efficacy of music therapy. Several Cochrane reviews and RCTs have been published that pointed to the effect of music therapy for specified populations, for example, depression (Aalbers et al. 2017), acquired brain injury (Magee et al. 2017), Autism Spectrum Disorders (ASD) (Geretsegger et al. 2014), Substance Use Disorder (Ghetti et al. 2022), or Schizophrenia (Mössler et al. 2011). Although we know that music therapy can be effective as shown, for example, in Depression RCTs and Cochrane Reviews, we can see that "it seems to work, but how?" (Maratos et al. 2011). To get closer to the action mechanism and describe how, for example, processes of attunement, entrainment, synchronization, inter-subjectivity, and other process-related aspects may contribute to change in depression treatment (see "how the treatment may work" in Aalbers et al. 2017) is of increasing explanatory importance. Multimodal data recordings mixing qualitative and quantitative data streams during music therapy sessions may allow for description and explanation of the changes during the therapy process.

Yet, how music therapy actually works remains an open question (Maratos et al. 2011). While evidence-based research methods rely on quantitative changes in pre–/post-intervention outcome measures (e.g., anxiety or depression levels), the qualitative process-oriented research approaches provide situated and context-rich descriptions of change (Aldridge 2004; Fachner 2014). Both approaches can demonstrate treatment effectiveness, but on different, incommensurable but complimentary levels of evidence. Besides previous anecdotal evidence in narrative case studies and qualitative studies attempting to show the sequence of therapeutic events and their interactions, few studies have allowed for quantitative process and neuromarker-driven analysis of music therapy in action (Ridder and Fachner 2016). The integration of qualitative and quantitative data is a key strength of mixed methods research, enhancing its capacity to interpret complex processes, enhance methodological rigor, creating "opportunities for drawing meta-inferences from conclusions of different methods, such as whether results from one method confirm, expand or diverge from results of another method" (Wollersberger 2022, p. 18). The integration of mixed methods into music therapy research may also reflect a need to demonstrate efficacy to place music therapy in comparison with other evidence-based healthcare interventions (Erkkilä 2016).

In this chapter, we would like to focus on integrating neuroscientific thinking and methods into the field of music therapy. Biomarking of therapeutic outcomes and processes may be of help to understand and measure the nonverbal aspects of therapy more distinct and "make the invisible visible" and to make the idiographic narratives of change count beyond being "anecdotal evidence" (Odell-Miller and Fachner 2021). It is important to note that, for instance, in stroke rehabilitation, we could follow treatment steps according to manuals and guidelines. But apart from following a primarily physiotherapeutic treatment agenda, we are also aware that in developing the therapeutic relationship, the music therapist actually decides at the moment what is of importance for this particular client. And here the emerging esthetic agenda of making music together reveals itself in the audible creative process. To analyze such processes, recent technological developments and esthetic research epistemologies in other fields of the music sciences can be of help to visualize the sometimes-subtle changes that music therapists observe, by using adaptive technology to make the invisible visible.

20.2.1 Moments of Interest

One of the general observations of qualitative data-based evidence is that particular moments of interest (MOI) during therapy can be identified and that these are related to therapeutic progress and establishing a therapeutic relationship (Fachner 2014, 2017; Gavrielidou and Odell-Miller 2017). These moments of interest (MOI) in the therapy can contain different aspects (Fachner 2014, 2017) such as a musical meeting or a shared awareness or perception of a (non)verbal interaction. The content of moments that are of importance and of interest to patients and therapists may vary according to the situation and person. Music therapists refer to "ability in the moment" (Tomaino 2013). For example, if a patient engages in a musical interaction with a music therapist, who closely observes the patient's body language, listens to their musical expressions, and responds and adapts their playing to the qualities of their movements, the patient will be able to move their weak arm better during the musical interaction because the therapist situated their actions in relation to the patient's needs (Tomaino 2013). The patient shares his or her thoughts, imagery, and the feelings evoked by the music, and the therapist interacts with the patient to help solve a problem (Erkkilä et al. 2012). Such a process of shared hearing in a therapeutic process may include the possibility that the therapist's attention is drawn to parts of the music that he or she would neither recognize nor find interesting when listening alone. In therapy, processes of transference and countertransference come into play (Pedersen 2007), and a process of shared hearing may entail sharing a patient's thoughts, images, and emotions, i.e., what he or she perceives and hears.

20.2.2 Music Therapy Intervention Timing, Apperception, and Shared Experience

An important function of music in healing environments is to support the reframing of the patient's focus of attention; to encourage a positive self-perception, and the discovery of new vistas and potentials (Aldridge and Fachner 2006). To induce state change and to alter cognitive frames of reference, intense emotion and imagination processes are evoked during music listening or making (Hove et al. 2016). As extensively discussed elsewhere, how one experiences music depends upon the moment and situation—on where and when you listen to music, how you experience the music, and how you focus your attention on the music (Fachner 2016b, 2017; Schall et al. 2015). Corporeal techniques (dancing, drumming, deep listening, etc.) altering consciousness and the focus of attention offer a way to "empty" the contents of memory, allowing new information to enter (Aigen 1991; Fachner 2011). If the information revealed during the course of a piece of music becomes meaningful to the listener or performer, the brain has various strategies available to enable it to focus on specific parts and process musical elements more distinctly and in a more focused manner.

One of the important issues that arises here is distinguishing between perception (based on sensory data) and apperception. Apperception may be referred to as the "process of constructing mental representations by selecting and integrating mental contents to it" (Helfenstein and Saariluoma 2007, p. 212). Thus, we ascribe meaning to objects based on our existing experience rather than direct sensory input. The "distinction between perception and apperception must be based on explicating the properties of our mental content" (ibid, p. 212). Rather than looking at the chronological order of parts in the music, as successive elements of the entire piece, the focus is on the person's situational relationship to the music; in therapy, this translates into how the perceived musical elements interact with the client's experience of the music in this interactive setting. Whether you would listen closely to the music, be distracted, be lifted, start dancing, or contemplate, is set by the framing (setting) of the listening process, which is dependent on the situation in which you are listening to it. Live music may become boring and recorded music may become alive as long as the music "has got something to say" to you at a particular point in time and space, especially when you share it with someone (Fachner 2014). In music therapy, it is the therapist who is a companion on the patient's imaginary journey into and through the unknown (David Aldridge 2000). In one study, the patient did not know whether her daughter-in-law and her unborn child would survive a cancer treatment. This created a time and therapy situation of shared hearing in which hope and reduction of anxiety were sought by the patient while sharing the imagery evoked by the music (Fachner et al. 2019). The term "therapy," as Plato used it, is "therapeia" (θεραπεία), which means "to accompany patients on their way" into, through, and out of the unknown of their illnesses (Fachner 2014). This original connotation stresses a temporal understanding of the process of doing therapy with a guiding, nurturing, and serving therapist ("therapon"—θεράπων).

20.2.3 Social Neuroscience, Therapeutic Alliance, and Situated Cognition

Bordin (1979) proposed that the working alliance is critical to the change process and defined therapeutic alliance in a psychotherapy context as having three components: agreement on therapy goals, the assignment of tasks, and the development of a bond between patient and therapist (Johnson and Wright 2002). Similarly, in music therapy, the therapeutic relationship is the context within which the therapy process takes place and is seen from the standpoint of common goals, interventions, and the bond within the therapy dyad (Hannibal et al. 2023). Research findings have concluded that the client's expectancy and therapy techniques each account for 15% of the client's improvement. Meanwhile, 40% of the improvement in psychotherapy is attributed to client variables and extra therapeutic influences, and 30% of the client's improvement is accounted for by the therapeutic relationship (Asay and Lambert 1999).

Social neuroscience, researching the functions of the brain in social interaction with others, may give us a good ground to do personalized therapy delivery based on the actual needs and how our embodied but trained reflective music therapy senses are responding in the moment to what is needed and how we can work in an interprofessional multidisciplinary team. How a dialogue between music therapy researchers and neuroscientists will be "driving clinical advances" (O'Kelly et al. 2017) in music therapy research remains to be seen; although a few examples of such dialogue have been discussed showing how different ideas of professional practice and epistemological thinking are driving the discussion (Magee and Stewart 2015), and how research methods employed in the neurosciences with regard to capturing intersubjective, holistic experiences in music therapy can be employed and captured with traditional one-person neuroscience methods (Hunt 2015).

> Whilst music therapy is benefiting from neuroscience collaborations, neuroscience is becoming more enriched by learning about the neural effects of "real world" clinical applications in music therapy. Not only do neuroscientific imaging methods provide biomarking evidence for the efficacy of music therapy interventions, they also offer important tools to describe time-locked interactive therapy processes, feeding into the emerging field of social neuroscience. Music therapy is bound to the process of creating and experiencing music together in improvisation, listening and reflection. Thus, the situated cognition and experience of music developing over time and in differing contexts is of interest in time series data (Fachner 2014, 2016). In (O'Kelly et al. 2017, p. 7)

While neuroscience may help researching and explaining change processes, to know how music is processed in the brain also needs an understanding of how data in neuroscientific research is generated. This may help us to critically distinguish between models explaining the context of human behavior and its ecological validity, i.e., how much it represents transferability into everyday life (Holleman et al. 2020). "Simulated" conditions in music therapy research reflect neither the reality nor the needs of therapists and patients; thus, they hinder the transfer of research outcomes to clinical practice. Although there is a strong trend toward ecological validity, we will not be able to model a real therapy setting. In contrast to experimental research settings in which certain processes are to be measured in a planable manner, it is simply unethically not to follow the needs of the patient asking for help and instead let the experimenter follow a planned schedule that has no therapeutic but scientific goal setting. However, it is possible to accompany actual events in authentic music therapy settings with adaptable and mobile technology and recording it "in situ" (Fachner 2004; Tucek et al. 2022a) according to the limitations and possibilities that the recording technology offers.

The critique from some social scientists and anthropologists of behavioral-measuring procedures in a lab which intends to reduce factors influencing the measures that have an impact on the quality of the data addresses the situation and process of measuring itself (Buytendijk 1967). Humanistic critiques have been based on the uniqueness and contextual nature of human experience, which is dependent on biographical time and place, as well as the uniqueness of the situation in which subjects are involved (Costall and Leudar 1996). Being in a concert or listening to music on the radio adds the contextual dimension of personal experience in an ongoing situation to perceptual processes. This influences intention and selection of what has been heard, focused upon, and perceived consciously during perception. The influence of the experimental setting in a laboratory is an important issue, particularly when we consider how the subject regards his or her control of the situation.

> Not the objective control, as planned by the investigator, determines the changes of physiological measures but the subjectively experienced influence (control) on the process by the subject (Lutzenberger et al. 1985, p. 65).

We have witnessed how for the sake of comparability RCT designs and outcome measures were to some degree superimposed on the arts without reflecting the arts therapy specific performative practice. Results were not always encouraging to the profession (Bieleninik et al. 2017) and yielded corresponding commentaries (Turry 2018). Aldridge pointed toward the importance of the music therapy practice, its art-specific processes and goal setting in medical settings and that outcome measures derived from a different field of practice do not necessarily reflect and measure how music therapy works (Aldridge 2003). One encouraging example of how music therapy practice can be prepared for an RCT while creating treatment fidelity is to bring a group of therapists together to reach a consensus on treatment standards and that a shared practice agenda can contribute to outcomes (Erkkilä et al. 2011; Fachner and Erkkilä 2013). Artists search for uniqueness, while science seeks generalization; we seem to be looking at two contradicting goals, while observing the practice. The key how to this combination lies in the choice of the right tools and the timing. The action mechanism driving change in music therapy needs to be seen through the temporal lens of "situated cognition," in which meaning, knowing and learning are generated in the situation of doing something bound to a (temporal) social, cultural, and physical context (Smith and Semin 2004). *"Change in music therapy is thus dependent on contextual developments and not on a plan made like a scene-play; the music is temporal and emotions signifying meaning are evoked through the interplay of music and the people who do the music"* (Fachner 2014, p. 792/3).

20.3 Research Methods and Technology

Studying the effects of music on the brain has received increasing interest in the past decades. Yet, research is needed into the neural, psychosocial, and clinical aspects and influences of music in real-time and how this amalgamation of science, music, technology, and medicine can be protocolized, implemented, and assessed in clinical populations. Social neuroscience offers methodological access to study social interaction processes in therapeutic domains by blending richness, ecological validity, and contextual factors of real-world designs. To do so, there is a growing demand to forge neuroscience, musicology, digital humanities, medicine, and augmented artificial human intelligence into one de-disciplined cloud. This combination will increasingly utilize big data and AI algorithms to analyze neural and physical data related to biomarkers in therapeutic and clinical settings, striving for excellence not only for the professional field but the heart of all our work: the patient in need of care and/or cure.

20.3.1 Prototypical Use of Music Technology in Therapy Rooms

Using music technology for therapeutic and educational purposes has a long tradition (Magee 2014). The invention of the pianoforte allowed a different way of playing and composing music and is a prototypical example of how technology drives art processes. One of the driving principles of art is the striving for a unique idea with a personal signature that identifies how this unique artist has created a piece of art in a unique way. Artists discuss how they are inspired by unique ideas, and utilizing emerging technologies is one of them. However, the use of technical support has been driven by the wish to revisit what happened in the teaching or in the therapy sessions since musicians have played music with pupils or patients. Early music therapy analysis in the 1960s was based on tape recordings (Nordoff and Robbins 1977, 2007) and writing indices of particular sequences of the musical interactions in the sessions that were then transcribed into scores (Lee and Houde 2011; Wigram 2004). First using analogue audio video technology, but then more widely digital in the 1980 and 1990. The more sophisticated video technology allowed post hoc analysis of movement and embodied action in the music. Inspired by Condon and Sander's (1974) introduction of frame-by-frame analysis of selected moments of interaction microanalysis approaches (Wosch and Wigram 2007) shed more light on how bodies are synchronized in the social domain. Using iPads/iPods/MP3 players and other AV recording tools from the 2000 allowed easy access to samples, rhythmic patterns, and instant recording and playback and also allowed more distinct audio analysis for those interested in these tools. Since wearables have become part of eHealth mainstream culture, emerging ideas of integrating these tools into the educational and therapeutic realm have been discussed. Music therapists are trained to use their intuitive judgment and have started thinking about tools that secure their intuitive judgment in the personalized treatment of patients (J. Erkkilä et al. 2014).

20.3.1.1 The Need for Technological Aid During Situated Decision-Making

In healthcare delivery, there is a strong research tradition that focuses on evidence-based research and practice, i.e., to base judgment on preselected knowledge of evidence-based medicine (EBM) that will then be applied to diagnosed patients and healthcare delivery will be based on manuals that are offering a map of successive steps to change. The manuals are based on the current best evidence and follow a preorganized treatment plan.

However, the daily practice of healthcare delivery is often confounded with many situational variables that impede following a plan. With the 2020 pandemic, we saw how ineffective healthcare delivery can become, when shortages in the supply chain are not allowing best practice and the clinician is asked to rely on improvisation with what is available and intuitive and fast decision-making that is rooted in experience. For decades, researchers on intuitive processes in general medicine (IM) have been asking for tools that allow situated decision-making by adapting to the changing demands of daily practice of healthcare delivery (Fintelmann 2007; Philipp et al. 1999). Both EBM and IM practice share the memory buffer restrictions of relevant information available at the moment of decision-making. In other words, you cannot scroll through a myriad of manuals and medical textbooks to foster your diagnosis when talking to an ill patient in surgery or hospital, but you must rely on your best (but restricted) knowledge. EBM secures decision-making with a long path of selecting the best possible evidence, while IM relies on training awareness on sensual and emotional observation and a gestalt-building process that favors a particular thought that will then be followed as a hypothesis for the treatment (Philipp et al. 1999). What both (EBM and IM) are lacking is access to relevant information that is based on vital parameters of the patient. The physician does a routine diagnosis by measuring pulse, temperature, and other vital signs that may help proving or changing the initial hypothesis but only after analyzing the results. What is needed are tools that instantly support or help revise decision-making.

What has been described for the medical profession is also true for MTs and for music teachers: to decide what the patient or the trainee needs now relies either on a plan or merely on intuition. It is an amalgamated mix of what is at hand in the interactive process of delivering the intervention and the lesson.

What is needed is a radical vision of adapted tools that

1. Help before the intervention to gather the best knowledge about the patient based on an AI-extended anamnesis and music therapy assessment.
2. Help in the therapy with easy and user-friendly access to an array of indices (emotional valence; arousal, alertness; cognitive load; etc.) that allow judgment about the patient's physiological and psychological state.
3. After the therapy by recreating a 3D rewind of the recorded sessions, which allows reconstruction of movement, musical interaction, and synchronous inspection of selectable layers of physiological signals during segments of the interaction process.

20.3.2 Human Body Motion Capture and Analysis

The use of Motion Capture (aka MoCap) in the context of music practice has been explored in a variety of artistic domains in the last 20 years with the advent of reliable active MoCap systems. It has been used to control music and sound, for example, Skogstad et al. (2010), different modes of interaction have been suggested, from direct gestural control (Qian et al. 2004), to a more general analysis of performer movement (Camurri et al. 2004). The recent availability of remote controllers, such as those used for gesture recognition in computer games, as well as RGB-D (red, green, blue—depth) devices and techniques for 3D camera sensing are enabling automated movement analysis for everyday practice of music performance and open up perspectives for music therapy researchers. For example, Hadjakos et al. (2013) presented a method for motion analysis of musical ensembles based on head tracking with a Kinect camera.

Despite such advances, automatic computation and analysis of movement still focus on low-level movement features (e.g., kinematics) mainly. Whereas this is nowadays becoming quite a consolidated area, research is still lagging on the investigation of techniques for computing the expressive qualities of movement. Camurri et al. (2016) conceived a multilayered conceptual framework for the analysis of expressive qualities of movement. They also developed a software platform (EyesWeb XMI) that can capture and process multimodal data, including movement data, in real time. While this framework provides a useful way for conceptualizing and positioning computational methods, more approaches are needed, especially at the higher levels, i.e., those concerning the expressive quality of a movement performance. In the specific domain of music performance, movement was recognized as a major conveyor of expressiveness and emotion to listeners (Leman and Maes 2014). Goebl et al. (2014)summarized quantitative measurement and analysis techniques of three domains of musical expressiveness, including body motion. They outline computational methods to quantitatively assess expressive aspects of the body movements of the performing musicians. Davidson (2012) studied the expressive components of bodily movement in both solo and ensemble musical performances, focusing on flute and clarinet performers and on a pianist.

The mirroring of behaviors comes automatically during interactions, also known as interpersonal synchronization (Feldman 2007). Interpersonal synchronization is integrated into numerous facets of our social lives and helps us in our daily dealings and interactions with others (Hu et al. 2022; Kendon et al. 1976). Infants use this seemingly congenital ability, synchronizing with their parents' voice signals and gestures to interact in proto-conversation (Trevarthen 2008). This ability is practiced and refined while engaging in "motherese," synchronizing movement and nonverbal elements of vocalizing during "baby-talk."

Synchronization of cardiac patterns could also be found among people singing together. Singers in a choir showed higher HRV synchrony during singing (especially in unison) compared to resting, and the conductor's HRV changes when the choir was singing preceded those of the choir members (Lange et al. 2022; Müller and Lindenberger 2011). A significant increase in inter-beat interval from the baseline was also observed in groups drumming together, unaffected by whether they drummed synchronously or asynchronously, which led Gordon et al. (2020) to suggest that the physiological synchrony may depend less on behavioral synchrony but the intention to do so. The authors suggested that this increase in physiological synchrony in both groups could be a result of shared states and joint participation, as previous research has also proposed that physiological synchrony can emerge as a feature of group cooperative tasks or joint activities (Gordon et al. 2020; Palumbo et al. 2017).

20.3.3 Measuring Human Interaction in the Brain

Humans are innately social creatures. Social interaction and social behavior are fundamental components of human life, widely studied in various scientific disciplines, and of growing importance in Information Communication Technologies (ICT), e.g., increased use of digital social networks, online and mobile communities, and enhanced 5G communication technologies. Current artificial intelligence (AI) technologies are capable of exploiting the large amounts of multimodal interaction data ICT provides, allowing quantitative measures of interpersonal communication and conceding the formulation of new interaction models and tools. Cognitive neuroscience, which has traditionally focused on individual brains, has recently begun to investigate social cognition through realistic interpersonal interaction (Redcay and Schilbach 2019). The awareness of the huge impact of social context on neural functions has highlighted the need for experimental paradigms that enable brain functions to be investigated during real social interaction (Acquadro et al. 2016). In this context, music provides an ideal domain for investigating social cognition through realistic interpersonal interaction because it offers a promising approach for balancing the trade-off between ecological validity and experimental control when testing cognitive and brain functions in music therapy (Fachner 2016a).

Musical interaction, including music-based pedagogical and clinical interventions, involves nonverbal communication built on the human predisposition for musicality observable already in infant–caregiver interactions (Malloch and Trevarthen 2009). Such interaction is a multidisciplinary phenomenon based on sensorimotor, cognitive, and social skills, which allows the fulfilment of shared goals to be developed through real-time interpersonal coordination. Furthermore, music is fundamentally interactive, creative, emotional, and social. For social interaction research, music provides ecological validity, avoiding the need to introduce an artificial task; motivation is an inherent part of music and hence it is not necessary to employ extrinsic techniques; musicality is a widespread human capacity, enabling almost everyone to engage in music interaction, and music is a multilevel activity involving sound, movement, and physiological information. Music interaction is one of the most closely synchronized. activities in which human beings engage, and it seems that the ability to entrain to music is unique to humans. Finally, unlike speech, musical interaction is one of the few creative activities allowing simultaneous participation (Cross 2014). All these features of musical interaction, make music a promising avenue for social cognition research.

20.3.3.1 Brain Data Acquisition and Analysis

Hyperscanning, which is the simultaneous measurement of brain activity of two or more persons, is a tool frequently used in social neuroscience research paradigms to study shared neural correlates of social interaction (Pfeiffer et al. 2013; Redcay and Schilbach 2019). Mobile and stationary devices allow hyperscanning of electrophysiological data (EEG) and neurophysiological data (i.e., ECG) from both interactants in a range of scenarios in real-world social interaction in music with high ecological validity and in experimental settings with targeted behavior (Acquadro et al. 2016).

Pioneering music performance research examining two people playing guitar (Lindenberger et al. 2009) or four people playing saxophone (Babiloni et al. 2011, 2012) has shown how physiologic functions synchronize in a coherent manner to produce a social product, i.e., a piece of music performed together. This was, for the guitarists, particularly observed "during the periods of (i) preparatory metronome tempo setting and (ii) coordinated play onset" (Lindenberger et al. 2009, p. 1). Playing a piece together led to synchronous activity in frontal and central brain areas (Sänger et al. 2012), indicating time-locked synching of planning and the creation of a shared activity. Such "hyperscanning" research in the field of social neuroscience tries to trace how brain-to-brain coupling functions in social interaction (F. Babiloni and Astolfi 2014).

A recent investigation into the therapeutic process and interaction during Guided Imagery and Music showed situated Frontal Alpha Asymmetry (FAA) peaks representing valence-related peaks of emotional activity. Strong peaks occurred in the EEG of the patient during important moments of the therapy and a distinct cross-correlation of the therapists and patients FAA during a period of shared emotional intensity (Fachner et al. 2019). Fachner and colleagues ((2019), were interested to know whether shared hearing is mediated via shared emotional networks thus creating a sense of mutuality in knowing about what is shared together. They combined EEG-Hyperscanning with video-rating and in-depth analysis of important moments identified by therapists, patients, and independent raters. This allowed describing the emotional processes, on a second-by-second basis (as indexed by EEG data), that were driving therapeutic change in a particular moment during the music therapy session. The challenge here was to create an ecologically valid research design including the application of brain research tools, while not interfering with the natural course of therapy and its spontaneously developing therapeutic process.

Another study into the dyadic relationship while doing neurological music therapy explored the use of Hyperscanning in children with disabilities describing directionality measures of empathy among the children's brain activity (Kang et al. 2022; Samadani et al. 2021). Analyzing interbrain coupling measures between therapist and a person living with dementia during drum improvisation, we were able to describe increased synchrony values measured from MIDI data of both players and an increased anteriority of therapist's frontal brain-to-brain coupling measures related to the PwD's coupling index during moments of interest compared to moments of no interest (Maidhof et al. 2023). This indicates that the therapist is leading the interaction, here during anamnestic clinical improvisation. Already in the late 1990s, investigations into the socio-physiology of social interaction music therapy were explored from Neugebauer and Aldridge (1998) showing the convergence of HR patterns during important segments in a mock therapy process. As Acquadro et al. (2016) pointed out Hyperscanning is a promising tool for the music sciences in order to understand social interaction in music and studies are evolving that will be taken into account for our endeavors here.

How a mobile EEG Hyperscanning set-up can be feasibly realized in a clinical neurorehabilitation setting was described by Tucek et al. (2022b). In contrast to Samadani et al. (2021) investigating interaction between a child and an observing parent in a music therapy setting, this study tested a dual EEG Hyperscanning (therapist and patient) setup and investigated the synchronization of three AV sources for microanalysis purposes. Samadani et al. recorded the EEG of the parent sitting in another room watching the therapy of the child on a video screen.

20.4 Conclusion: Being Human and Creative Process Research

Being human means to be creative, to relate to others, and to be part of a culture that is developed in places where people produce it as a creative expression of their social identity. Music is one of the cultural assets of regions in which they create a particular expression of their identity that relates to places and ways in which humans interact and create music. At the core of this is the creative process at a certain time and place and the "chemistry" of humans relating to each other in a creative process that can bring about change in practice and outcomes. The "right music at the right time" has an impact on the listener, the expressions of emotions and thoughts in a song can represent and symbolize a common denominator of what many may feel and think at a particular time. Music as the language of emotions allows expressing the momentary multimodal complexity of how things relate to each other and can help to discover ourselves in what we feel and think about the societal challenges and how we join in to bring people and organizations together to support happier and healthier lives.

Music therapy research should be dedicated to study the creative process to bring about change in people's lives, to initiate processes to do things differently, and to overcome the burden experienced when living with disease. Music therapy research may strive for ways in how we can rethink the medical idea of outcomes and treatment processes as we are dealing with interactive creative processes and performances during musical interventions and although performed with a body, the expression of being human is not necessarily identical with the materialistic description of dysfunctions of body parts or physiological processes. To be incorporated in a body is different from its physical functions as we live in our body and being and feeling healthy and creative can also be expressed in an excessive pushing of the body's boundaries for artistic purposes.

In short, music therapy research adds a humanistic, narrative, and temporal perspective of the multimodal human experience to the datasets recorded during creative processes and how change can be described by integrating the creative and physiological processes at a certain time and place. This can be a therapy room in the intimacy of a healing contract between a person seeking help and a professional devoting his/her creative sensitivity to the healing process and not to the artistic outcome, it can be a stage and how the performers are inspired from each other or from the audience, it can be the creation of an audio mix in the studio where shared listening may create a sound that is signified from the people involved, it may be the calibration of audiovisual settings for immersive processes, it may show how a drama therapist mirrors and extends the body language of a person locked in a narrowed regulation of emotion, or how an actor is improvising roles of a play to transform the given narratives.

The methodological repertoire and technical solutions for creative process research should enable us to focus on how the body performs in different settings and how this performance looks like with different lenses of brain and ANS research, how people look at things happening around them during creative processes and track their gaze and objects focused upon, how their bodies move through spaces in which they are involved in creative processes and to utilize the language of current technological measures describing what we can observe, track, and evoke with paradigms that are adequate to represent the creative process of being human.

References

Aalbers S, Fusar-Poli L, Freeman RE, Spreen M, Ket JC, Vink AC, et al. Music therapy for depression. Cochrane Database Syst Rev. 2017;11:CD004517. https://doi.org/10.1002/14651858.CD004517.pub3.

Acquadro MAS, Congedo M, De Riddeer D. Music performance as an experimental approach to hyperscanning studies. Front Hum Neurosci. 2016;10:242. https://doi.org/10.3389/fnhum.2016.00242.

Aigen K. The voice of the forest: a conception of music for music therapy. Music Ther. 1991;10(1):77–98.

Aldridge D. Music therapy and research in medicine – from out of the silence. London: Jessica Kingsley Publishers; 1996.

Aldridge D. Spirituality, healing, and medicine: return to the silence. London/Philadelphia: Jessica Kingsley Publishers; 2000.

Aldridge D. Staying close to practice: which evidence, for whom, by whom? Music Therapy Today. 2003;4(5) Retrieved from http://www.wfmt.info/Musictherapyworld/modules/mmmagazine/issues/20031103132043/20031103132433/DA_Nov03.pdf

Aldridge D, editor. Case studies in music therapy research. London: Jessica Kingsley Publishers; 2004.

Aldridge D, Fachner J, editors. Music and altered states – consciousness, transcendence, therapy and addictions. London: Jessica Kingsley; 2006.

Asay TP, Lambert MJ. The empirical case for the common factors in therapy: quantitative findings. In: Hubble IA, Duncan BL, Miller SD, editors. The heart and soul of change: what works in therapy. American Psychological Association; 1999. p. 23–55.

Babiloni F, Astolfi L. Social neuroscience and hyperscanning techniques: past, present and future. Neurosci Biobehav Rev. 2014;44:76–93. https://doi.org/10.1016/j.neubiorev.2012.07.006.

Babiloni C, Vecchio F, Infarinato F, Buffo P, Marzano N, Spada D, et al. Simultaneous recording of electroencephalographic data in musicians playing in ensemble. Cortex. 2011;47(9):1082–90. https://doi.org/10.1016/j.cortex.2011.05.006.

Babiloni C, Buffo P, Vecchio F, Marzano N, Del Percio C, Spada D, et al. Brains "in concert": frontal oscillatory alpha rhythms and empathy in professional musicians. NeuroImage. 2012;60(1):105–16. https://doi.org/10.1016/j.neuroimage.2011.12.008.

Bieleninik Ł, Monika Geretsegger P, Karin Mössler D, Jörg Assmus P, Grace Thompson P, Gustavo Gattino P, et al. Effects of improvisational music therapy vs enhanced standard care on symptom severity among children with autism Spectrum disorder – the TIME-A randomized clinical trial. JAMA. 2017;318(6):525–35. https://doi.org/10.1001/jama.2017.9478.

Bordin ES. The generalizability of the psychoanalytic concept of the working alliance. Psychother Theory Res Pract. 1979;16(3):252–60. https://doi.org/10.1037/h0085885.

Bunt L, Stige B. Music therapy: an art beyond words. 2nd ed. New York: Routledge; 2014.

Buytendijk FJJ. Prolegomena einer anthropologischen Physiologie. 1st ed. Salzburg: Otto Müller Verlag; 1967.

Camurri A, Mazzarino B, Ricchetti M, Timmers R, Volpe G. Multimodal analysis of expressive gesture in music and dance performances. In: Camurri A, Volpe G, editors. GestureBased communication in human computer interaction. Berlin Heidelberg: Springer; 2004. p. 20–39.

Camurri A, Volpe G, Piana S, Mancini M, Niewiadomski R, Ferrari N, Canepa C. The dancer in the eye: towards a multilayered computational framework of qualities in movement. In: Paper presented at the proceedings 3rd international symposium on movement & computing. Thessaloniki, Greece; 2016.

Condon WS, Sander LW. Synchrony demonstrated between movements of the neonate and adult speech. Child Dev. 1974;45:456. https://doi.org/10.2307/1127968.

Costall A, Leudar I. Situated action I: truth in the situation. Ecol Psychol. 1996;8(1):101–10. https://doi.org/10.1207/s15326969eco0802_1.

Cross I. Music and communication in music psychology. Psychol Music. 2014;42(6):809–19. https://doi.org/10.1177/0305735614543968.

Davidson JW. Bodily movement and facial actions in expressive musical performance by solo and duo instrumentalists: two distinctive case studies. Psychol Music. 2012;40(5):595–633. https://doi.org/10.1177/0305735612449896.

de Witte M, Orkibi H, Zarate R, Karkou V, Sajnani N, Malhotra B, et al. From therapeutic factors to mechanisms of change in the creative arts therapies: a scoping review. Front Psychol. 2021;12(2525) https://doi.org/10.3389/fpsyg.2021.678397.

Erkkilä J. Mixed methods research in music therapy. In: Edwards J, editor. The Oxford handbook of music therapy. Oxford University Press; 2016. p. 815–26.

Erkkilä J, Punkanen M, Fachner J, Ala-Ruona E, Pöntiö I, Tervaniemi M, et al. Individual music therapy for depression – randomised controlled trial. Br J Psychiatry. 2011;199(2):132–9. https://doi.org/10.1192/bjp.bp.110.085431.

Erkkilä J, Ala-Ruona E, Punkanen M, Fachner J. Perspectives on creativity in improvisational, psychodynamic music therapy. In: Hargreaves D, Miell D, MacDonald R, editors. Musical imaginations: multidisciplinary perspectives on creativity, performance and perception. Oxford: Oxford University Press; 2012. p. 414–28.

Erkkilä J, Ala-Ruona E, Lartillot O. Technology and clinical improvisation: from production and playback to analysis and interpretation. In: Stensæth K, editor. Music, health, technology and design, vol. 8. Oslo: The Norwegian Academy of Music; 2014. p. 209–26.

Fachner J. Cannabis, brain physiology, changes in states of consciousness and music perception. In: Aldridge D, editor. Case study designs in music therapy. London: Jessica Kingsley; 2004. p. 211–33.

Fachner J. Time is the key—music and ASC. In: Cardeña E, Winkelmann M, editors. Altering consciousness: a multidisciplinary perspective. Vol. 1. History, culture and the humanities. Santa Barbara: Praeger; 2011. p. 355–76.

Fachner J. Communicating change—meaningful moments, situated cognition and music therapy—a reply to North (2014). Psychol Music. 2014;42(6):791–9. https://doi.org/10.1177/0305735614547665.

Fachner J. The future of music therapy research in neuroscience. In: Dileo C, editor. Envisioning the future of music therapy. Philadelphia: Temple University; 2016a. p. 133–9.

Fachner J. Measuring musical responses. In: Wheeler B, Murphy K, editors. Music therapy research. 3rd ed. Dallas: Barcelona Publishers; 2016b. p. 153–68.

Fachner J. Music, moments and healing processes: music therapy. In: Ashley R, Timmers R, editors. Routledge companion to music cognition. London: Routledge; 2017. p. 89–100.

Fachner J, Erkkilä J. The Finnish research model of a music therapy practice treating depression. Musikther Umsch. 2013;34(1):35–45.
Fachner J, Maidhof C, Grocke D, Nygaard Pedersen I, Trondalen G, Tucek G, Bonde LO. "Telling me not to worry…" Hyperscanning and neural dynamics of emotion processing during guided imagery and music. Front Psychol. 2019;10(1561) https://doi.org/10.3389/fpsyg.2019.01561.
Feldman R. Parent-infant synchrony and the construction of shared timing; physiological precursors, developmental outcomes, and risk conditions. J Child Psychol Psychiatry. 2007;48(3–4):329–54. https://doi.org/10.1111/j.1469-7610.2006.01701.x.
Fintelmann V. Intuitive Medizin – anthroposophische Medizin in der Praxis Grundlagen – Indikationen – Therapiekonzepte. 5., vollst. überarb. Aufl. ed. Stuttgart: Hippokrates; 2007.
Gavrielidou M, Odell-Miller H. An investigation of pivotal moments in music therapy in adult mental health. Arts Psychother. 2017;52:50–62. https://doi.org/10.1016/j.aip.2016.09.006.
Geretsegger M, Elefant C, Mössler KA, Gold C. Music therapy for people with autism spectrum disorder. Cochrane Database Syst Rev. 2014;2014(6):CD004381. https://doi.org/10.1002/14651858.CD004381.pub3.
Ghetti C, Chen X, Brenner A, Hakvoort LG, Lien L, Fachner J, Gold C. Music therapy for people with substance use disorders (review). Cochrane Database Syst Rev. 2022;5:CD012576. https://doi.org/10.1002/14651858.CD012576.pub3.
Goebl W, Dixon S, Schubert E. Quantitative methods: motion analysis, audio analysis, and continuous response techniques. In: Fabian D, Timmers R, Schubert E, editors. Expressiveness in music performance: empirical approaches across styles and cultures. Oxford University Press; 2014. p. 221–39.
Gordon I, Gilboa A, Cohen S, Milstein N, Haimovich N, Pinhasi S, Siegman S. Physiological and behavioral synchrony predict group cohesion and performance. Sci Rep. 2020;10(1):8484. https://doi.org/10.1038/s41598-020-65670-1.
Hadjakos A, Großhauser T, Goebl W. Motion analysis of music ensembles with the Kinect. Paper presented at the international conference on new interfaces for musical expression. Daejeon, Republic of Korea; 2013.
Hannibal N, Pedersen IN, Bertelsen LR, Nielsen RE, Gold C. Process-outcome relations in music therapy versus music listening for people with schizophrenia viewed through a mediational model: the role of the therapeutic alliance. Front Psych. 2023;14 https://doi.org/10.3389/fpsyt.2023.1120003.
Helfenstein S, Saariluoma P. Apperception in primed problem solving. Cogn Process. 2007;8(4):211–32. https://doi.org/10.1007/s10339-007-0189-4.
Holleman GA, Hooge ITC, Kemner C, Hessels RS. The 'real-world approach' and its problems: a critique of the term ecological validity. Front Psychol. 2020;11(721) https://doi.org/10.3389/fpsyg.2020.00721.
Hove MJ, Stelzer J, Nierhaus T, Thiel SD, Gundlach C, Margulies DS, et al. Brain network reconfiguration and perceptual decoupling during an absorptive state of consciousness. Cereb Cortex. 2016;26(7):116–3124. https://doi.org/10.1093/cercor/bhv137.
Hu Y, Cheng X, Pan Y, Hu Y. The intrapersonal and interpersonal consequences of interpersonal synchrony. Acta Psychol. 2022;224:103513. https://doi.org/10.1016/j.actpsy.2022.103513.
Hunt A. Boundaries and potentials of traditional and alternative neuroscience research methods in music therapy research. Front Hum Neurosci. 2015;9(342) https://doi.org/10.3389/fnhum.2015.00342.
Johnson LN, Wright DW. Revisiting Bordin's theory on the therapeutic Alliance: implications for family therapy. Contemp Fam Ther. 2002;24(2):257–69. https://doi.org/10.1023/A:1015395223978.
Kang K, Orlandi S, Lorenzen N, Chau T, Thaut MH. Does music induce interbrain synchronization between a non-speaking youth with cerebral palsy (CP), a parent, and a neurologic music therapist? A brief report. Dev Neurorehabil. 2022;25:426. https://doi.org/10.1080/17518423.2022.2051628.
Kendon A, Harris RM, Key MR. Organization of behavior in face-to-face interaction. Chicago: The Hague; 1976. Mouton; distributed in the USA and Canada by Aldine

Lange EB, Omigie D, Trenado C, Müller V, Wald-Fuhrmann M, Merrill J. In touch: cardiac and respiratory patterns synchronize during ensemble singing with physical contact. Front Hum Neurosci. 2022;16 https://doi.org/10.3389/fnhum.2022.928563.

Lee CA, Houde M. Improvising in styles: a workbook for music therapists, educators, and musicians. Barcelona Publishers LLC; 2011. Workbook edition

Leman M, Maes P-J. Music perception and embodied music cognition. In: Shapiro L, editor. The Routledge handbook of embodied cognition. New York: Routledge; 2014. p. 81–9.

Lindenberger U, Li S-C, Gruber W, Muller V. Brains swinging in concert: cortical phase synchronization while playing guitar. BMC Neurosci. 2009;10(1):22. https://doi.org/10.1186/1471-2202-10-22.

Lutzenberger W, Elbert T, Rockstroh B, Birbaumer N. Das EEG – Psychophysiologie und Methodik von Spontan-EEG und ereigniskorrellierten Potentialen. 1st ed. Berlin: Springer; 1985.

Magee WL. Music technology in therapeutic and health settings. London: Jessica Kingsley Publishers; 2014.

Magee WL, Stewart L. The challenges and benefits of a genuine partnership between music therapy and neuroscience: a dialog between scientist and therapist. Front Hum Neurosci. 2015;9(223) https://doi.org/10.3389/fnhum.2015.00223.

Magee WL, Clark I, Tamplin J, Bradt J. Music interventions for acquired brain injury. Cochrane Database Syst Rev. 2017;1:CD006787. https://doi.org/10.1002/14651858.CD006787.pub3.

Maidhof C, Mueller V, Agres K, Lartillot O, Bloska J, Asano R, et al. Intra- and inter-brain coupling and activity dynamics during improvisational music therapy with a person with dementia: an explorative EEG-hyperscanning single case study. Front Psychol. 2023;14 https://doi.org/10.3389/fpsyg.2023.1155732.

Malloch S, Trevarthen C. Communicative musicality: exploring the basis of human companionship. Oxford/New York: Oxford University Press; 2009.

Maratos A, Crawford MJ, Procter S. Music therapy for depression: it seems to work, but how? Br J Psychiatry. 2011;199(2):92–3. https://doi.org/10.1192/bjp.bp.110.087494.

Mössler K, Chen X, Heldal TO, Gold C. Music therapy for people with schizophrenia and schizophrenia-like disorders. Cochrane Database Syst Rev. 2011;12 https://doi.org/10.1002/14651858.CD004025.pub3.

Müller V, Lindenberger U. Cardiac and respiratory patterns synchronize between persons during choir singing. PLoS One. 2011;6(9):e24893. https://doi.org/10.1371/journal.pone.0024893.

Neugebauer L, Aldridge D. Communication, heart rate and the musical dialogue. Br J Music Ther. 1998;12(2):46–52. https://doi.org/10.1177/135945759801200202.

Nordoff P, Robbins C. Creative music therapy: individualized treatment for the handicapped child. New York: John Day Co; 1977.

Nordoff P, Robbins C. Creative music therapy: a guide to fostering clinical musicianship. 2nd ed. Gilsum: Barcelona Publishers; 2007.

O'Kelly J, Fachner J, Tervaniemi M, editors. Dialogues in music therapy and music neuroscience: collaborative understanding driving clinical advances (eBook ed. Vol. 10). Lausanne: Frontiers Media, SA; 2017. https://www.frontiersin.org/research-topics/3049/pdf.

Odell-Miller H, Fachner J. Changing the lives of people living with dementia (PWD) and their families through music therapy research. REF Impact Case Study; 2021. Retrieved from https://results2021.ref.ac.uk/impact/eb620419-157a-4952-8549-3f7902161d4b?page=1

Palumbo RV, Marraccini ME, Weyandt LL, Wilder-Smith O, McGee HA, Liu S, Goodwin MS. Interpersonal autonomic physiology: a systematic review of the literature. Personal Soc Psychol Rev. 2017;21(2):99–141. https://doi.org/10.1177/1088868316628405.

Pedersen IN. Counter transference in music therapy: a phenomenological study on countertransference used as a clinical concept by music therapists working with musical improvisation in adultpsychiatry. (PhD Doctoral Dissertation). Aalborg: Aalborg University, InDiMedia; 2007.

Pfeiffer U, Timmermans B, Vogeley K, Frith C, Schilbach L. Towards a neuroscience of social interactionFrontiers of neuroscience (eBook ed., pp. 587); 2013. https://doi.org/10.3389/978-2-88919-104-8.

Philipp R, Philipp E, Thorne P. The importance of intuition in the occupational medicine clinical consultation. Occup Med (Lond). 1999;49(1):37–41. https://doi.org/10.1093/occmed/49.1.37.
Qian G, Guo F, Ingalls T, Olson L, James J, Rikakis T. A gesture-driven multimodal interactive dance system. Paper presented at the IEEE International Conference on Multimedia and Expo; 2004, June.
Redcay E, Schilbach L. Using second-person neuroscience to elucidate the mechanisms of social interaction. Nat Rev Neurosci. 2019;20(8):495–505. https://doi.org/10.1038/s41583-019-0179-4.
Ridder HM, Fachner J. Objectivist case study research. Single-subject and small-n research. In: Wheeler B, Murphy K, editors. Music therapy research. 3rd ed. Dallas: Barcelona Publishers; 2016. p. 291–302.
Samadani A, Kim S, Moon J, Kang K, Chau T. Neurophysiological synchrony between children with severe physical disabilities and their parents during music therapy. Front Neurosci. 2021;15 https://doi.org/10.3389/fnins.2021.531915.
Sänger J, Müller V, Lindenberger U. Intra- and interbrain synchronization and network properties when playing guitar in duets. Front Hum Neurosci. 2012;6 https://doi.org/10.3389/fnhum.2012.00312.
Schall A, Haberstroh J, Pantel J. Time series analysis of individual music therapy in dementia: effects on communication behavior and emotional Well-being. GeroPsych: the journal of Gerontopsychology and geriatric. Psychiatry. 2015;28(3):113–22. https://doi.org/10.1024/1662-9647/a000123.
Skogstad S, Jensenius A, Nymoen K. Using IR Optical Marker Based Motion Capture for Exploring Musical Interaction. Paper presented at the Proc. 2010 International conference on new interfaces for musical expression. Sydney, Australia; 2010.
Smith ER, Semin GR. Socially situated cognition: cognition in its social context. Adv Exp Soc Psychol. 2004;36:53–117. https://doi.org/10.1016/S0065-2601(04)36002-8.
Taylor DB. A survey of professional music therapists concerning entry level competencies. J Music Ther. 1987;24(3):114–45.
Tomaino CM. Creativity and improvisation as therapeutic tools within music therapy. Ann N Y Acad Sci. 2013;1303(1):84–6. https://doi.org/10.1111/nyas.12224.
Trevarthen C. The musical art of infant conversation: narrating in the time of sympathetic experience, without rational interpretation, before words. Music Sci. 2008;12(1_suppl):15–46. https://doi.org/10.1177/1029864908012001021.
Tucek G, Maidhof C, Vogl J, Heine A, Zeppelzauer M, Steinhoff N, Fachner J. EEG hyperscanning and qualitative analysis of moments of interest in music therapy for stroke rehabilitation – a feasibility study. Brain Sci. 2022a;12(565) https://doi.org/10.3390/brainsci12050565.
Tucek G, Maidhof C, Vogl J, Heine A, Zeppelzauer M, Steinhoff N, Fachner J. [Preprint] EEG hyperscanning and qualitative analysis of moments of interest in music therapy for stroke rehabilitation – a feasibility study. Preprints. 2022b; https://doi.org/10.20944/preprints202203.0122.v1.
Turry A. Actually, music therapy does work. Music Med. 2018;10(2):113–4. https://doi.org/10.47513/mmd.v10i2.604.
Wigram T. Improvisation: methods and techniques for music therapy clinicians, educators, and students. London/Philadelphia: J. Kingsley Publishers; 2004.
Wollersberger N. Exploring the impact of an indirect music therapy intervention on quality of life for informal caregivers of people living with dementia in the community. (PhD Monograph). Anglia Ruskin University; 2022. https://hdl.handle.net/10779/aru.24835017.v1.
Wosch T, Wigram T, editors. Microanalysis in music therapy: methods, techniques and applications for clinicians, researchers, educators and students. London: Jessica Kingsley Publishers; 2007.

MIX
Papier aus verantwortungsvollen Quellen
Paper from responsible sources
FSC® C105338

If you have any concerns about our products,
you can contact us on
ProductSafety@springernature.com

In case Publisher is established outside the EU,
the EU authorized representative is:
Springer Nature Customer Service Center GmbH
Europaplatz 3, 69115 Heidelberg, Germany

Printed by Libri Plureos GmbH
in Hamburg, Germany